THE
COMBINED VOLUME
COTA Second Edition
and
Practice Issues in
Occupational Therapy

Editor
Sally E. Ryan, COTA, ROH
Faculty Assistant and Instructor
The College of St. Catherine
Department of Occupational Therapy
St. Paul, Minnesota

SLACK Incorporated, 6900 Grove Road, Thorofare NJ 08086-9447

Acquisitions Editor: Amy E. Drummond
Publisher: John H. Bond

ISBN 1-55642-290-3

Published by: SLACK Incorporated
6900 Grove Road
Thorofare, NJ 08086-9447 USA
Telephone 609-848-1000
Fax 609-853-5991
Contact SLACK Incorporated for further information about other books in this field or about the availability of our books from distributors outside the United States.

Last digit is print number: 10 9 8 7 6 5 4 3 2

THE CERTIFIED OCCUPATIONAL THERAPY ASSISTANT

Principles, Concepts and Techniques

2nd Edition

Editor

Sally E. Ryan, COTA, ROH

Faculty Assistant and Instructor
The College of St. Catherine
Department of Occupational Therapy
St. Paul, Minnesota

SLACK Incorporated, 6900 Grove Road, Thorofare, NJ 08086-9447

Dedicated to the Advancement of the Profession of
Occupational Therapy
and to
Colonel Ruth A. Robinson, OTR
who, in an interview before her death in 1989,
stated that she felt her greatest contribution to the
profession of occupational therapy was the
development of the program and curriculum to train
occupational therapy assistants.

Contents

Expanded Contents

About the Editor

A graduate of the first occupational therapy assistant program at Duluth, Minnesota, in 1964, Sally Ryan has just entered her 28th year as a certified occupational therapy assistant and member of the profession. She has taken extensive coursework at the University of Minnesota as a James Wright Hunt Scholar, and at the College of St. Catherine, St. Paul. Her background includes experience in practice, clinical education supervision, and management in long-term care; consultation; and teaching in the professional occupational therapy program at the College of St. Catherine.

In the past, Ms. Ryan has served in a variety of leadership positions at the local, state and national levels. She has served as representative to the American Occupational Therapy Association (AOTA) Representative Assembly from Minnesota; chair of the Representative Assembly Nominating Committee; a member-at-large of the AOTA Executive Board; member and on-site evaluator of the AOTA Accreditation Committee; and member and secretary of the AOTA Standards and Ethics Commission. She has also served the AOTA as a member of the Philosophical Base Task Force and the 1981 Role Delineation Steering Committee, and as a consultant to the COTA Task Force. She is currently the Treasurer and Chair of the Fiscal Advisory Board of the American Occupational Therapy Certification Board.

Ms. Ryan is the recipient of numerous state and national awards. She is the first COTA to receive the AOTA Award of Excellence, has been recognized as an Outstanding Young Woman of America, and was among the first recipients of the AOTA Roster of Honor.

Ms. Ryan has been invited to present numerous keynote addresses, presentations, and workshops, both nationally and internationally. Frequently her topics focus on COTA roles and relationships and intraprofessional team building.

Contributing Authors

Ben Atchison is an Assistant Professor of Occupational Therapy at Eastern Michigan University in Ypsilanti, Michigan. He received his undergraduate degree in occupational therapy at Western Michigan University in Kalamazoo and a Master's Degree in Education from Georgia State University in Atlanta. He is pursuing a doctoral degree in instructional technology at Eastern Michigan University. Professor Atchison is currently serving as Chair of the Physical Disabilities Special Interest Section of the American Occupational Therapy Association. As an Army officer, he holds the position of Assistant Chief, Occupational Therapy Section for the 323rd General Hospital of the United States Army Reserve Medical Department. Professor Atchison has extensive experience in a wide variety of practice areas, including pediatrics, adult outpatient rehabilitation, and home health care. His scholarly contributions have included publications and presentations regarding the elderly, homeless, AIDS, the assessment and management of visual perceptual disorders, and educational design. He has been recognized in *Outstanding Young Men in America* and is the recipient of the Excellence in Teaching Award from Eastern Michigan University and has been designated as a Fellow by the American Occupational Therapy Association.

Harriet Backhaus received her certificate from the occupational therapy assistant program at Westminister College in Fulton, Missouri, and an undergraduate degree in education from Harris College in St. Louis. She is currently employed at the Program in Occupational Therapy at Washington University in St. Louis where she is involved in both clinical practice and undergraduate teaching. Ms. Backhaus is a member of the advisory committee for the occupational therapy assistant program at St. Louis Community College at Meramec, and recently completed a term as a member of the Certification Examination Development Committee of the American Occupational Therapy Certification Board. Her interest in therapeutic media and skills in selecting purposeful activities through activity analysis are widely recognized.

B. Joan Bellman earned a Bachelor of Science degree in occupational therapy from Virginia Commonwealth University in Richmond, Virginia. She held the positions of clinician, clinical education supervisor, and chief of occupational therapy at District of Columbia General Hospital for 29 years, before retiring from government service in 1988. Ms. Bellman has served as a member of the Certification Committee of the American Occupational Therapy Association and as President of the District of Columbia Occupational Therapy Association. Her professional experience has been primarily in the area of adult physical dysfunction, with a special interest and expertise in the fabrication of hand splints and assistive devices. She is currently employed part-time by the Visiting Nurse Association of the District of Columbia and Adventist Home Health Services, Inc. for Northern Prince George's County, Maryland.

Robert K. Bing is Professor Emeritus of Occupational Therapy at the University of Texas School of Allied Health Sciences at Galveston, Texas. He received his undergraduate degree in occupational therapy from the University of Illinois and his Master of Arts and Doctor of Education degrees were conferred by the University of Maryland. His varied clinical experiences include the United States Army, Norwich State Hospital in Connecticut, Nebraska Psychiatric Institute, Illinois Psychiatric Institute, and the University of Texas Medical Branch Hospitals, where he served as the founding dean, School of Allied Health Sciences, and professor of occupational therapy. He has also served as a member of the faculty in occupational therapy departments of six universities. Dr. Bing was elected President of the Maryland and Texas Occupational Therapy Associations and President of the American Occupational Therapy Association. He is the recipient of the Award of Merit and the Eleanor Clarke Slagle Lectureship and was designated as a Fellow of the American Occupational Therapy Association. Dr. Bing was also recently named a Galveston Unsung Hero for his volunteer work and service as a liaison officer for the East Texas AIDS Project. Currently, he is retired and devoting much of his time to professional writing.

Toné F. Blechert received an Associate in Arts degree as an occupational therapy assistant from St. Mary's Junior College and a baccalaureate degree in communications from Metropolitan State University in Minneapolis, Minnesota. She is currently pursuing a master's degree in organizational leadership from the College of St. Catherine in St. Paul. Throughout her career, she has held a number of leadership positions, which have included chair of the American Occupational Therapy Association COTA Task Force and member of the faculty and the steering committee for the Professional and Technical Role Analysis Project (PATRA). Ms. Blechert recently completed a term as a member of the Board of Directors of the American Occupational Therapy Foundation. She has served as a faculty member in the occupational therapy assistant program at the St. Mary's Campus of the College of St. Catherine since 1984. She also serves as the Coordinator of Academic Advising for that campus. In recognition of her numerous professional publications and presentations, she received the Communication Award from the Minnesota Occupational Therapy Association. Ms. Blechert is also a recipient of the Award of Excellence, the Roster of Honor, and the Service Award given by the American Occupational Therapy Association.

Bonnie Brooks earned her undergradute degree in occupational therapy at Indiana University in Indianapolis and also completed a Master of Science Degree in Education at Loyola University in Chicago. Early in her career, she was instrumental in the development of several occupational therapy assistant programs and also served as a faculty member in both technical and professional education. As the Assistant Director of Education at the American Occupational Therapy Association, Ms. Brooks was responsible for assisting in the development of new technical programs and for ongoing activities and initiatives in occupational therapy assistant education. She also served as the liaison to the COTA Task Force and the COTA Advisory Committee, and she was instrumental in providing the COTA perspective for all major AOTA committees and projects. She was also responsible for implementing the first national COTA network. Ms. Brooks has been recognized as a Fellow by the American Occupational Therapy Association, and currently is employed by RehabWorks of Florida in Sarasota where she provides direct service and consultation to long-term care facilities.

Shirley Holland Carr, at the time of her death in 1992, was employed as an occupational therapist at the Pupil Appraisal Service for the East Baton Rouge Parish School in Louisiana, a position she held for more than eight years. Ms. Carr earned her undergraduate degree in education at Tufts University in Boston and received a diploma from the Boston School of Occupational Therapy. Later, she completed her Master of Science degree in psychology at Auburn University. Her many years of practice were community-oriented and included experience in child development, mental health, management, and professional and technical education. In the latter capacity, she was instrumental in planning as well as serving as the director of several occupational therapy assistant programs. Ms. Carr was a recipient of the Award of Excellence for "outstanding performance in professional development" given by the Missouri Occupational Therapy Association, and she was

also been designated as a Fellow by the American Occupational Therapy Association.

Mary K. Cowan is an Associate Professor of Occupational Therapy at Eastern Kentucky University, where she has held a faculty appointment since 1989. Professor Cowan earned her undergraduate degree in occupational therapy at the University of Minnesota and later completed a Master of Arts program in educational psychology at the same institution. She has worked clinically with children with all types of handicapping conditions, particularly in public education settings. Her present study and research focuses on postural stability as it relates to educational performance. She is certified in the Bobath Approach to the treatment of children with cerebral palsy and the administration and interpretation of the Southern California Sensory Integration Tests. Professor Cowan has been recognized as a Fellow of the American Occupational Therapy Association.

Sister Genevieve Cummings was an Associate Professor and Chair of the Occupational Therapy Department at the College of St. Catherine in St. Paul, Minnesota, where she held a faculty appointment since 1960. She received her undergraduate degree in occupational therapy from that institution and later earned a Master of Arts degree in child development from the University of Minnesota. Throughout her career, Professor Cummings was recognized as an outstanding leader, and served in a number of capacities in the American Occupational Therapy Association, including a member of the Executive Board, Chair of the Standards and Ethics Commission, and Representative from the State of Minnesota to the Representative Assembly. She was the recipient of many honors, which include recognition by the Association as one of the first Fellows. She was also the recipient of the Occupational Therapist of the Year and the Communication Awards given by the Minnesota Occupational Therapy Association.

Mary Ellen Lange Dunford is an Assistant Professor and Coordinator for the Occupational Therapy Assistant Program at Kirkwood Community College in Cedar Rapids, Iowa. Professor Dunford received her baccalaureate degree in occupational therapy from the College of St. Catherine in St. Paul, Minnesota, and she is currently pusuing a master's degree in education at the University of Iowa. As a practitioner, she specialized in pediatrics and did pioneering work in the development of methods for adapting and using electronic devices for treatment. An active member of the Iowa Occupational Therapy Association, she held various leadership positions within the organization. Her contributions to the education of certified occupational therapy assistants has had a significant impact on the roles and responsibilities of COTAs practicing in Iowa.

Azela Gohl-Giese is an Associate Professor of Occupational Therapy at the College of St. Catherine in St. Paul, Minnnesota, where she has held a faculty appointment since 1962. Professor Gohl-Giese earned her undergraduate degree in occupational therapy from the College of St. Catherine and later completed a Master of Science degree in management at Cardinal Stritch College. During her tenure at the College her teaching responsibilities have had a primary focus in the areas of psychiatry and group dynamics, where she has placed a strong emphasis on the importance of the therapeutic use of activity in collaboration with team members, especially the certified occupational therapy assistant. Currently she serves as the fieldwork coordinator, working closely with clinical educators in designing learning experiences for students, many of whom are practicing COTAs working toward a baccalaureate degree. A number of these students are enrolled in the Weekend College Occupational Therapy Program, where Ms. Gohl-Giese served as the first coordinator.

Nancy Kari is an Associate Professor of Occupational Therapy at the College of St. Catherine in St. Paul, Minnesota, where she has been a faculty member since 1978. She received her baccalaureate degree in occupational therapy from the University of Wisconsin at Madison and a Master's Degree in public health from the University of Minnesota. Pursuing her interests in organizational governance and institutional change, she also serves as adjunct faculty with Project Public Life, a national initiative to reengage citizens in public life, at the Humphrey Institute of Public Affairs at the University of Minnesota. Associated with this work, she co-directs the Lazarus Project, an action-research pilot program that investigates issues of empowerment within nursing homes. The goal of her pioneering work is to create a community model, which is an alternative to the traditional medical and therapeutic models of governance. Professor Kari has published papers on team building and on the politics of empowerment and is a recent recipient of the Communication Award given by the Minnesota Occupational Therapy Association. She is also a recipient of the Cordelia Meyers Writer's Award, given by the American Occupational Therapy Association.

M. Jeanne Madigan has been Professor and Chair of the Department of Occupational Therapy at Virginia Commonwealth University in Richmond, Virginia, since 1984. She received her undergraduate degree in occupational therapy from the College of St. Catherine in St. Paul, Minnesota; her Master of Arts degree in occupational therapy from the University of Southern California; and her Doctorate in Education, with an emphasis in curriculum and instruction, from Loyola University in Chicago. Dr. Madigan has served on numerous education and evaluation-related committees and task forces of the American Occupational Therapy

Association, including Chair of the Certification and Program Advisory Committees, Essentials Review Committee, and the Role Delineation Committee; and she has been designated as a Fellow by the Association. She has served as a consultant and a member of advisory committees of several occupational therapy assistant educational programs, and she is currently serving as a member of the advisory committee of the first occupational therapy assistant program in Virginia at J. Sargent Reynolds College.

LaDonn People is an instructor in the Department of Occupational Therapy at Eastern Michigan University in Ypsilanti where she has held a faculty appointment since 1990. Formerly, she was employed for 18 years as an instructor in the occupational therapy assistant program at Wayne County Community College in Detroit and as the fieldwork coordinator in that institution for ten years. Ms. People earned her undergraduate degree in occupational therapy from Eastern Michigan University and later completed a Master of Arts degree in occupational education at the University of Michigan in Ann Arbor. She is presently pursuing a doctoral degree in instructional technology at Wayne State University in Detroit. Her professional interest and expertise are in the areas of physical dysfunction and gerontology.

Brian J. Ryan received his Bachelor of Science degree in electrical engineering from the University of Minnesota in Minneapolis. His interest in computers grew out of a need to collect and analyze large data sets in relation to his work in failure analysis, parts control and quality control. As a private pilot, he also found numerous computer applications for navigation and communication. Mr. Ryan currently serves as a Principle Engineer at Alliant Tech Systems in Hopkins, Minnesota, in the Reliability, Maintainability and Safety Departments. He also serves as a consultant to the Pavek Wireless Museum in Minneapolis and the Experimental Aircraft Association Museum in Oshkosh, Wisconsin, where he has been instrumental in research and development of new electronic communications exhibits. His interest in occupational therapy was brought about through marriage to a COTA.

Patrice Schober-Branigan is an occupational therapist at the Minnesota Center for Health and Rehabilitation in Minneapolis, Minnesota. Ms. Schober-Branigan earned her Bachelor of Arts degree in occupational therapy from the College of St. Catherine in St. Paul, Minnesota. She has completed considerable advanced study and training in hand rehabilitation and was previously an active member of the American Society of Hand Therapists. Ms. Schober-Branigan has lectured on the topic of hand rehabilitation and splinting to occupational therapists, occupational therapy assistants, physicians, nurses and students. She has also published, and has designed and presented programs to industry on prevention of cumulative trauma. In her clinical work in a hand surgery practice, she has trained and supervised a COTA in static splinting techniques. Her specialization has broadened to the larger field of industrial rehabilitation and ergonomics, and she especially enjoys her work in a holistic, multidisciplinary rehabilitation center.

Phillip D. Shannon is the Coordinator of the Community Health Education and Medicaid Access Enhancement Project, co-sponsored by the Cameron County Health Department in San Benito, Texas, and by Project HOPE in Millwood, Virginia. His undergraduate degree in occupational therapy from California State University at San Jose was followed by two graduate degrees from the University of Southern California, a Master of Arts degree in occupational therapy and a Master of Public Administration degree. He has served as a program director in both technical and professional occupational therapy educational programs and is a retired officer of the United States Army. Mr. Shannon has published extensively in professional journals, primarily on the philosophy and theory of occupational therapy, and he has published chapters in three books as well. In addition to developing and presenting numerous workshops in the United States, he developed and conducted workshops for the United States Army Seventh Medical Command in Germany from 1985-1990. He was also the principal speaker for the Sixth National Congress of the Occupational Therapy Association, Bogata, Columbia. He has been the recipient of several awards, including the Chair's Service Award from the State University of New York at Buffalo, the Service Award of the American Occupational Therapy Association, and the Retired Educator's Award from the Association's Commission on Education. He has also been recognized as a Fellow by the American Occupational Therapy Association. Mr. Shannon served as Chair of the Certification Examination Development Committee and member of the Board of Directors of the American Occupational Therapy Certification Board.

Rhonda Stewart holds an Associate of Arts degree from Wayne County Community College in Detroit, Michigan, and a Bachelor of Science degree in occupational therapy from Eastern Michigan University at Kalamazoo. She is currently pursuing a Master of Science degree in Health Administration from Central Michigan University. Ms. Stewart has practiced as both a COTA and an OTR in physical medicine and rehabilitation, mental health, and home health settings where all age groups and a variety of diagnostic problems are treated. She has taught occupational therapy assistant courses and presented workshops at Wayne County Community College and is currently employed as a staff therapist and clinical supervisor at William Beaumont Hospital in Royal Oak, Michigan, and a part-time consultant

for community rehabilitation programs. Ms. Stewart is a governor-appointed member of the Michigan Licensing and Regulation Board for Occupational Therapists and also serves as the current President of the Michigan Occupational Therapy Association. In addition, she is Chair of the Board of Directors of the Michigan Black Occupational Therapy Caucus. She has presented papers at national and state conferences on issues related to practice, management and students.

Javan E. Walker, Jr. is Director of the Division of Occupational Therapy and Associate Professor of Occupational Therapy at Florida Agricultural and Mechanical University in Tallahassee, Florida, where he developed the program. Before assuming this position he was the Director of the Occupational Therapy Assistant Program at Illinois Central College in Peoria. Professor Walker began his occupational therapy career as a COTA in the United States Army. He earned his undergraduate degree in occupational therapy from Wayne State University in Detroit and a Master of Arts degree in education from Bradley University. He is currently a doctoral candidate at Illinois State University. After 15 years of active duty as an occupational therapist, Mr. Walker currently holds the rank of Lieutenant Colonel in the United States Army Reserves. In addition to his work as an educator and a clinician, he was recently elected as the Alternate Representative to the American Occupational Therapy Association Representative Assembly for the state of Florida. Professor Walker has provided consultation to long-term care facilities and mental health programs for the past 15 years, and he is actively involved with computer technology professionally and as a leisure time pursuit.

Doris Y. Witherspoon is the Director of Industrial Technology at Henry Ford Community College in Dearborn, Michigan. Formerly she was employed at Wayne County Community College for 20 years where she held the positions of Director of the Occupational Therapy Assistant Program, Director of Allied Health, and Dean of Vocational Technology. Ms. Witherspoon developed the occupational therapy assistant program at the college and taught classes in the program for 18 years. She earned her undergraduate degree in occupational therapy from Eastern Michigan University in Ypsilanti, and later completed a Master of Science degree in occupational education from the University of Michigan. She is currently a doctoral student at Wayne State University in Detroit. As an occupational therapy assistant educator, Ms. Witherspoon served on numerous state and national committees, including the American Occupational Therapy Association Certification Committee, Chairperson of Occupational Therapy Assistant Educators for the Association's Commission on Education; she was also President of the Black Occupational Therapy Caucus.

Acknowledgments

I am indeed indebted to a number of individuals who assisted in the preparation of this book. In the early stages of planning, many occupational therapy assistant program directors, faculty members, clinicians and practitioners responded to a lengthy survey. These OTRs and COTAs provided thoughtful critiques and comments, which were of great help in determining the focus of this second edition. Special thanks is offered to Dr. Louise Fawcett who assisted with the interpretation of survey data, and to Phillip Shannon, who served as a primary reviewer and consultant during the early planning stages of this edition.

The contributions of the highly skilled contributing authors are gratefully acknowledged. Their work, individually and collectively, is the great strength of this text. Twenty-one occupational therapists and assistants have provided their extensive knowledge and expertise to this text. They come from diverse practice, education and research backgrounds; eight OTR contributors are or were occupational therapy assistant program directors. Many of the 21 authors, representing 12 states and the District of Columbia, have been actively involved in leadership roles in their state associations as well as in the American Occupational Therapy Association, the American Occupational Therapy Foundation and The American Occupational Therapy Certification Board. Nine of the authors have been recognized by AOTA as Fellows or members of the Roster of Honor. The contributions of an electrical engineer have enhanced the chapter on computers. It has been a great privilege to work with these outstanding writers, and I convey my most sincere thanks to each of them.

I would also like to offer my thanks to the reviewers who provided critiques of all of the manuscripts. Their objectivity and critical analysis of the content was most helpful in this developmental process.

Appreciation is also offered to M. Jeanne Madigan who assisted in writing a number of the related learning activities, which appear at the conclusion of each chapter.

Cheryl Willoughby, Editorial Director, and Elaine Schultz, Associate Editor, at Slack Inc., provided me with numerous resources, advice, critiques, and overall editorial assistance. Their patience, coupled with expert problem-solving skills, helped me immeasurably in this enormous task. Publication of this text would not have been possible without their expertise and assistance.

I would like to acknowledge and express my personal gratitude to Sister Genevieve Cummings, chairperson, and all of the members of the faculty of the Department of Occupational Therapy at the College of St. Catherine for their support and encouragement during the many phases of this task. Their willingness to share resources and offer critiques and support was of great help.

To the many therapists, assistants, friends and family members who provided ideas, listened to my concerns, and responded to my endless questions, I offer my most sincere appreciation. I regret that space does not allow me to list each of them individually.

My daughter Mary deserves very special thanks for assuming many tasks, which ranged from proofreading, editing, duplicating, and mailing to house cleaning, cooking, shopping and walking the dogs. Deep appreciation is offered to this versatile young woman, whose generosity of time and talent allowed me to complete a most arduous project.

Thanking my husband Brian is most difficult. He filled many supportive roles, including active listener, thoughtful reactor, consultant, reviewer, typist, illustrator, errand runner, FAX sender, telephone monitor, and household manager. Suffice it to say that this project would never have been accomplished without his sense of humor, inspiration, insight, patience, and remarkable ability to adapt. I am ever grateful.

—Sally E. Ryan

Foreword

Without a doubt, Sally Ryan is a pioneer in the professional development of the certified occupational therapy assistant, and this book is a concrete example of her many contributions. This publication is the most complete and comprehensive textbook ever compiled for the OTA, and it has become the standard for others to emulate.

Before the first edition was published, educators would have to collect information from numerous sources and create their own materials in order to instruct OTA students in their vocational responsibilities. Frequently, these materials had to be adapted to accommodate the specific needs of the occupational therapy assistant. This approach gave students the impression that there was no body of knowledge designed specifically for them. This informational deficit sent the implicit message to OTA students that they needed to know what the occupational therapist knows, only at a lower level.

The Certified Occupational Therapy Assistant: Principles, Concepts and Techniques establishes the knowledge base for the occupational therapy assistant. A more clear identification of this knowledge base will enable health care administrators to recognize the value of the COTA in helping to meet many of the staffing problems occurring in our health care settings today. Once their responsibilities have been defined, occupational therapy assistants will be able to assume the roles for which they were trained and which sometimes have been assigned to other specialists. In the national climate of managed health care costs, this appropriate use of the COTA will be an important strategy in providing cost-effective health care.

Over the past few years, Sally Ryan has focused on the concept of team building, believing that many of the current problems in our profession and health care in general are due to difficulties in team building. This lack of team work has been an impetus to incorporate team building concepts in her professional activities, and this textbook itself represents a major team-building effort. The variety and quality of the authors are outstanding, each contributor providing an essential component to the total body of knowledge, and each chapter complementing and building on the others.

The central theme of this book is occupation, the major construct of our profession. Proper emphasis is placed on purposeful activity, rather than exercises and "talk therapies," illustrating the importance of activity to the health of human beings. The use of activity as a major tool of the COTA is nicely integrated into the descriptions of functional treatment programs.

The book also emphasizes the human element of health care and the role the occupational therapy assistant performs in providing this component. Because the OTA becomes the close partner of the patient, working with the patient to facilitate an improvement in lifestyle, it is the assistant who really provides the caring and touching component that is known to be a major contributor to the healing process. This element is crucial because the human touch is too often forgotten in health care, for professionals have a tendency to do things to people without really interacting with them as human beings. This book illustrates how the quality of time the OTA spends with the patient dealing with daily life skills facilitates the provision of this necessary component.

New areas of practice are evolving for the occupational therapy assistant and they will continue to evolve. In the future, I envision areas of practice in which the OTA practices independently, with an occupational therapist available for consultation. Certainly the area of tool adaptation in industry could be such an area, as the knowledge and skills used in analyzing activities and adapting tools and equipment are basic to the practice of the OTA.

Finally, the Army is extremely proud that Sally Ryan has dedicated her book to COL Ruth Robinson, OTR (Retired). COL Robinson recognized early the critical role the assistant would play in the profession. She knew that the certified occupational therapy assistant would become a "prime mover" of the profession by allowing occupational therapists to provide health care to many more patients while increasing the quality of care. I know she would have been very proud of this textbook, its authors and its editor.

—COL Roy Swift, PhD, OTR, FAOTA
Chief, Army Medical Specialists Corps

Preface

TO THE SECOND EDITION

Work on the second edition of this text began in earnest in January of 1989. That year was particularly significant because it marked the 30th anniversary of certified occupational therapy assistants (COTAs) working in the profession.

Discussions with technical level faculty, occupational therapists and assistants serving as clinical supervisors and practitioners, as well as results of a survey directed at this audience, emphasized the need to readopt the fundamental objectives of the first edition: 1) focus on the basic principles, concepts and techniques of the profession; 2) provide both an extensive and a realistic view of the roles and functions of certified occupational therapy assistants in entry-level practice and beyond; 3) provide examples of how to successfully build intraprofessional relationships; and 4) be useful in the clinic as well as the classroom. These objectives were again used as a foundation for developing, organizing and sequencing content areas.

The content in the first edition has been greatly expanded and updated. Therefore, it was decided to publish this edition in a two-book format. This volume is an introductory text; the second volume, *Practice Issues in Occupational Therapy*, is a more advanced text, focusing on specific practice applications, as well as related knowledge and skills.

Several documents published by the American Occupational Therapy Association (AOTA) were used as primary guides for content development: The *Entry-Level Role Delineation for Registered Occupational Therapists (OTRs) and Certified Occupational Therapy Assistants (COTAs)*, the *Essentials and Guidelines for an Accredited Educational Program for the Occupational Therapy Assistant, Uniform Terminology for Reporting Occupational Therapy Services*, 2nd Edition, and the *1990 Member Data Survey*. Preliminary data from the *Job Analysis Study*, conducted by the American Occupational Therapy Certification Board, was also considered.

Eight new chapters have been added to this edition, as well as a glossary and related learning activities. Other chapters have been expanded and updated. The reader will also find more photographs, illustrations, charts and forms to enhance and emphasize important points. In addition, all chapters now open with a set of key concepts and a list of essential vocabulary terms. The key concepts are designed to assist the students in focusing their study on the fundamental subjects in each chapter. The essential vocabulary words are terms important to chapter content and occupational therapy practice, and appear in bold type at first mention. Every effort has been made to define each term clearly, both in context and in the glossary.

The book is divided into five major sections. The first section focuses on historical, philosophical and theoretical perspectives, providing the reader with a basic understanding of some of the important principles that have guided the profession. The heritage of the COTA is emphasized, with prominent developmental milestones interwoven in the story.

Section II focuses on the core concepts of occupational therapy, which include principles of human development and the components of occupation that influence role performance. Another important emphasis is the occupational performance areas of activities of daily living, work and play/leisure. Following chapters point to some of the skills necessary for effective therapeutic intervention with emphasis placed on the teaching/learning process, interpersonal communication and applied group dynamics. The section concludes with a discussion of important aspects of the individualization of occupational therapy, with factors such as environment, sociocultural considerations, change and prevention stressed. Throughout this section, short case studies are included to provide the reader with examples of occupational therapy personnel working with patients of varying ages in a variety of traditional and nontraditional treatment settings.

Technology is emphasized in Section III. The use of video, small electronic toys and devices, and computers in occupational therapy evaluation and treatment are presented. The reader is provided with basic terminology and information as well as numerous applications and resources for these technologies.

Section IV is devoted to the discussion of selected contemporary media techniques. Thermoplastic splinting and adaptive equipment construction provide the reader with a variety of examples, practical applications and methods for developing skills in these important areas.

In Section V, the final segment, the focus is on purposeful activity, emphasizing the application of arts and crafts and the analysis of activities. Fundamental principles are discussed as a means for integrating many of the core concepts presented in preceding chapters. Strategies for building skill in these important aspects of practice are stressed.

When using this book, it is important for the reader to note the following:

1. In addition to the main chapter designations, all important chapter subheadings also appear in the Expanded Contents. They are titled to reflect the major objectives of the writers and the editor.

2. Every effort has been made to use gender-inclusive language throughout the book. In some instances, it was necessary to use "him or her," recognizing that this may be awkward for the reader. Exceptions to the use of gender inclusive pronouns occur in the discussion of historical material, philosophical principles and in some quotations.

3. The term *patient* has been used frequently to describe the recipient of occupational therapy services. The authors and the editor recognize that this term is not always the most appropriate; however, it is believed to be preferable to other options currently being used. Exceptions have been made in some instances where such terms as the *individual*, the *student*, the *child*, etc. have been used.

4. Related learning activities have been included at the conclusion of each chapter. Some of these were published previously in *The Certified Occupational Therapy Assistant: Roles and Responsibilites Workbook.*

5. Whenever a writing project of this magnitude is undertaken, inadvertent omissions and errors may occur. Although every attempt has been made to prevent such occurrences, it is the hope of the editor and the authors that these will be called to their attention, so that they may be corrected in the next printing.

In conclusion, it is my belief that this book and its companion volume will serve as a model and a guidepost for occupational therapy teamwork in the delivery of patient services. It will serve as an incentive for the technically and professionally educated practitioners to discover the many ways in which their skills and roles complement each other. It will also serve as a catalyst for developing new skills and roles in response to the ever-changing needs of our society.

The former President of the American Occupational Therapy Association, Carolyn Manville Baum, summed it up best in her 1980 Eleanor Clarke Slagle Address when she stated

As a profession and as professionals, let us put our resources, intelligence, and emotional commitment together and work diligently toward the ascent of our profession. The health care system, the clients (patients) we serve, and each of us individually will benefit from our commitment.

—Sally E. Ryan
1991

Preface
TO THE FIRST EDITION

Work on this text began in the spring of 1984. That year was particularly significant because it marked the 25th anniversary of certified occupational therapy assistants (COTAs) working in the profession.

The project was given impetus from the fact that there was no comprehensive book written expressly for occupational therapy assistants. Discussions with technical level faculty, occupational therapists (OTRs) serving as clinical supervisors, and assistants emphasized the need for a text that would focus on the basic principles of the profession; a book that would provide both an extensive and a realistic view of the roles and functions of certified occupational therapy assistants in entry-level practice and beyond; a book that would provide examples of how to successfully build intraprofessional relationships; and, finally, a book that could be used in the clinic as well as the classroom. These objectives were adopted as a foundation for developing, organizing and sequencing content areas.

Four documents published by the American Occupational Therapy Association (AOTA) also served as primary guides for content development: the *Entry-Level OTR and COTA Role Delineation,* the *Essentials of an Approved Educational Program for the Occupational Therapy Assistant, Uniform Terminology for Reporting Occupational Therapy Services,* and the *1982 Member Data Survey.* All but the latter are included as appendices.

The book is divided into six major sections. The first section (Historical Perspectives) introduces the themes and perspectives of the book. Section II focuses on the core knowledge of occupational therapy, which includes philosophical and theoretical material as well as principles of human development and basic influences contributing to health. The daily living skills of self-care, work, and play/leisure are also addressed as the primary foundations of the profession, along with descriptions of some of the skills necessary for effective therapeutic intervention. Emphasis is placed on the teaching/learning process, interpersonal communication, group dynamics and the occupational therapy process.

In Section III (Intervention Strategies), case studies demonstrate the roles of occupational therapy assistants and occupational therapists working with selected patients to illustrate specific ways in which the profession's role delineation can be used to provide efficient and effective health care delivery.

Section IV (Models of Practice) provides numerous examples of the team approach in working with patients of varying ages in a variety of traditional and non-traditional treatment settings. The roles of the OTR/COTA team in a hospice setting are delineated, and the roles of the COTA in work and productive occupation programs and as an activities director are addressed.

Concepts of Practice are reviewed in Section V, which includes discussions of contemporary media techniques as well as management and supervision principles and issues.

The final section (Contemporary Issues) discusses ways of enhancing intraprofessional relationships through the effective use of supervision, mentoring, and conflict management fundamentals, and reviews the maturation process of the assistant and related professional socialization elements. Principles of occupational therapy ethics are presented, and future trends for the profession are outlined.

In addition to the main chapter designations, all important chapter subheadings appear in the Table of Contents. Their titles reflect the major objectives of the writer and editor. *The Certified Occupational Therapy Assistant: Roles and Responsibilities Workbook,* also published by SLACK, Inc., provides the student with study and discussion questions and exercises, as well as additional learning resources.

Every effort has been made to use gender-inclusive language throughout the book. In some instances, it was necessary to use "him or her," recognizing that this may be awkward for the reader.

In conclusion, it is my belief that this book will serve as a model and a guidepost for occupational therapy teamwork in the delivery of patient services. It will serve as an incentive for technically and professionally educated practitioners to discover the many ways in which their skills and roles complement each other. It will also serve as a catalyst for developing new skills and roles in response to the ever-changing needs of our society.

The former President of the American Occupational Therapy Association, Carolyn Manville Baum, summed it up best in her 1980 Eleanor Clarke Slagle Address when she stated

As a profession and as professionals, let us put our resources, intelligence, and emotional commitment together and work diligently toward the ascent of our profession. The health care system, the clients (patients) we serve, and each of us individually will benefit from our commitment.

—Sally E. Ryan
1986

Introduction

OCCUPATIONAL THERAPY—A PROFILE*

Occupational therapy is the art and science of directing participation in selected tasks to restore, reinforce and enhance performance; to facilitate learning of skills and functions essential for adaptation and productivity; to diminish or correct pathology; and to promote and maintain health. Its fundamental purpose is the development and maintenance of the capacity to perform those tasks and roles essential to productive living and to the mastery of self and the environment.

Because the primary focus of occupational therapy is the development of adaptive skills and performance capacity, its concern is with factors that serve as barriers or impediments to the individual's ability to function, as well as those factors that promote, influence or enhance performance.

Occupational therapy provides service to those individuals whose abilities to cope with tasks of living are threatened or impaired by developmental deficits, aging, poverty and cultural differences, physical injury or illness, or psychosocial and social disability.

The term *occupation* refers to a person's goal-directed use of time, energy, interest and attention. The practice of occupational therapy is based on concepts that acknowledge the following principles:

1. Activities are primary agents for learning and development, and they are an essential source of satisfaction.

2. In engaging in activities, the individual explores the nature of his or her interests, needs, capacities, and limitations; develops motor, perceptual and cognitive skills; and learns a range of interpersonal and social attitudes and behaviors sufficient for coping with life tasks and mastering elements of the environment.

3. Task occupation is an integral part of human development; it represents or reflects life-work situations, and is a vehicle for acquiring or redeveloping those skills essential to the fulfillment of life roles.

4. Activities matching or relating to the developmental needs and interests of the individual not only afford the necessary learning for development or restoration, but provide an intrinsic gratification that promotes and sustains health and evokes a strong investment in the restorative process.

5. The end product inherent in a task or an activity provides concrete evidence of the ability to be productive and to have an influence on one's environment.

6. Activities are "doing," and such a focus on productivity and participation teaches a sense of self as a contributing participant rather than as a recipient.

These principles are applied in practice through programs reflecting the profession's commitment to comprehensive health care.

*Adapted with permission from "Occupational Therapy: Its Definition and Function," Reference Manual of Official Documents of the American Occupational Therapy Association, 1980 (revised 1983), American Occupational Therapy Association, Inc.

Section I
HISTORICAL, PHILOSOPHICAL AND THEORETICAL PRINCIPLES

Living Forward, Understanding Backward:
   A History of Occupational Therapy Principles

The COTA Heritage: Proud, Practical, Stable, Dynamic

History may be defined as a recorded narrative of events that have occurred in the past. It is a collection of information drawn from many sources that include speeches, letters, minutes of meetings, photographs, diaries, articles and interviews. In learning about history, the student is provided with an appreciation for, and understanding of, the important roots of the profession. It gives insight to the rich legacy of events, experiences and people that have shaped our past.

This first section details significant aspects of the history of occupational therapy from the perspective of the profession's priniciples. Lessons from our past, reflecting basic concepts, values and beliefs, continue to influence contemporary practice and will have a marked impact on our future. The developmental milestones of the certified occupational therapy assistant (COTA) are also chronicled, and the heritage of the COTA is characterized by Carr as "proud, practical, stable and dynamic."

As Bing has stated, "Fundamentally, history is experience, rather than the mere telling of quaint stories or reminiscing about past feats or failures. It is knowing enough about what has come before to know what to consider or rule out in evaluating the present, on our way to the future."

Living Forward, Understanding Backward

A HISTORY OF OCCUPATIONAL THERAPY PRINCIPLES

Robert K. Bing, EdD, OTR, FAOTA

INTRODUCTION

The renowned 19th century American philosopher, physician and psychologist, William James, is reputed to have observed that "We live forward; we understand backwards." We exist in the present, yet are future oriented. To make sense of the present or future, we must have knowledge about and an appreciation of the past.

Today, occupational therapy personnel face numerous predicaments. Educational preparation for practice is based predominantly on knowledge and skills that are marketable in a very competitive health care environment. The *what* of our art, science and technology is emphasized, often at the expense of the *why*. What is missing is the sense of what has come before, of those recurring patterns that offer legitimacy and uniqueness in the health care profession.

History is an invaluable tool to assess the present and determine future courses of action. The recording of an occupational life or medical history is a testament to the past's influence on current conditions and its ability to offer approaches to alleviate problems. Fundamentally, history is experience, rather than the mere telling of quaint stories or reminiscing about past feats or failures. It is knowing enough about what has come before to know what to consider or what to rule out in evaluating the present, on our way to the future. As Neustadt and May point out, we must learn "...how to use experience, whether remote or recent, in the process of deciding what to do today about the prospect for tomorrow."[1]

KEY CONCEPTS

Age of Enlightenment

Moral treatment

The York Retreat

Hull House and Consolation House

Invalid Occupations

National Society for the Promotion of Occupational Therapy

Habit training

Purposeful work and leisure

Interaction of mind and body

Time-honored principles

AGE OF ENLIGHTENMENT—THE 1700S

To place the history of occupational therapy in proper perspective, we could go as far back as the Garden of Eden. Dr. William Rush Dunton, Jr., one of the founders of the 20th century's occupational therapy movement, insisted that those fig leaves had to have been crocheted by Eve. She was trying to get over her troubles, which had something to do with her being "beholden" to Adam and his rib. But let us pass over all of that and begin this story in Europe over 200 years ago. This era became known as the Age of Enlightenment or, in some quarters, the Age of Reason. Those engaged in science and philosophy were known as *natural philosophers*. Nearly a century later (the late 1800s), the two disciplines separated and the term *scientist* came into the language.

In the late 1700s, Western Europe was astir with a new view of life. Social, political, economic, and religious theories promoted a general sense of human progress and perfectibility. Notions about intolerance, censorship and economic and social restraints were being abandoned and replaced by a strong faith in rational behavior. Universally valid principles governing humanity, nature and society directed people's lives and interpersonal relationships.

The changing ethic of work added a rich ingredient to this new, heady brew. Fundamental was Martin Luther's viewpoint, which declared that everyone who could work should do so. Illness and begging were unnatural. Charity should be extended only to those who could not work because of mental or physical infirmities or old age.

John Calvin added to these ideas. Although he was a theologian, he expressed a number of ideas from which contemporary capitalism sprang. Production, trade and profit were encouraged. Work was to be disciplined, rigorous, methodical and rational. There was no room for luxuries or any activities that softened the soul. deGrazia summed up this period: "Once man worked for a livelihood, to be able to live. Now he worked for something beyond his daily bread. He worked because somehow it was the right or moral thing to do."[2] By the late 1800s much of work had become a calling.

MORAL TREATMENT

Near the center of all of this invigorating change was the treatment of sick people, particularly the **mentally ill** (those with diseases and conditions causing mental impairment). Whereas long-term survivors of physical disease with physical disabilities were still rare because treatment was so inadequate, the mentally ill were a significant portion of the population.

Up to this time the insane had been housed and handled no differently than criminals and paupers and were often chained in dungeons. Moral treatment of the insane was one product of the Age of Enlightenment. It sprang from the fundamental attitudes of the day: a set of principles that govern humanity and society; faith in the ability of the human to reason; purposeful work as a moral obligation; and the supreme belief in the individual. Fast disappearing were the centuries old notions that the insane were possessed of demons; that they were no better than paupers or criminals; that crime, sin, vice and inactivity were the core of insanity.

Two men of the 18th century working in different countries, and unknown to each other, initiated the moral treatment movement. These two could not have been more dissimilar. Phillippe Pinel was a child of the French Revolution, a physician, a scholar, and a natural philosopher. William Tuke was an English merchant, wealthy, a deeply religious Quaker and a philanthropist.

Father of Moral Treatment—Phillippe Pinel

According to Pinel, moral treatment meant treating the emotions. He believed the emotionally disturbed individual was out of balance and the patient's own emotions could be used to restore equilibrium. The compassionate Pinel believed the loss of reason was the most calamatous of all human afflictions. The ability to reason, he claimed, principally separates the human from other living forms. As Pinel wrote in his famous treatise in 1806, because of mental illness, the human's "...character is always perverted, sometimes annihilated. His thoughts and actions are diverted...His personal liberty is at length taken from him...to this melancholy train of symptoms, if not early and judiciously treated...a state of most abject degradation sooner or later succeeds."[3]

Some medical historians believe Pinel was stating that moral treatment was synonymous with humane care. His writings do not bear out this assumption. He strongly believed that each patient must be critically observed and analyzed before treatment is begun. The moral method is well reasoned and carefully planned for the individual patient. Pinel's biographer, Mackler, describes moral treatment as

...combined gentleness with firmness. It meant giving each patient as much liberty as he could manage, but it also taught him respect for authority. Firmness was necessary at times, but no harm must come to the patient. Moral treatment meant an unvarying routine which was necessary to maintain the patient's feeling of security and respect for authority. These would help him gain control over his emotions.[4]

Occupation figured prominently in Pinel's scheme, primarily to take patients' minds away from emotional distress and to develop their abilities. Music and various forms of literature were used. Physical exercise and work were a part of institutional living. Pinel advocated patient farms on the hospital grounds. This period was largely an agricultural era, where one's life revolved around producing products necessary for survival and one's emotional content was elaborately interwoven. The care of animals and the necessary routines of growing crops provided patients with a respect for the authority of nature and yet with as much liberty as could be tolerated. The unvarying routine to maintain farming as part of the institution made a strong appeal to moral concepts, such as respect, self-esteem and dignity for the patient.

The York Retreat—William Tuke

During this same time, English society was in ferment. Gossip about King George III, who was giving the American colonies "fits," suggested that he was in similar trouble; he was said to be possessed by mania. While some questioned his right to rule, including close relatives, the general public sympathized with the king.

Part of this new humane concern was influenced by the beliefs and work of the **Society of Friends,** derisively known as the Quakers. They emerged in 17th century England and became one of the most distinctive movements of Puritanism. In the last decades of the 18th century, William Tuke and various members of his family established The York Retreat, primarily because of their religious-based concerns about the deplorable conditions in public insane **asylums.** Until this time, the term *retreat* had never been applied to an asylum. Tuke's daughter-in-law suggested the term to convey the Quaker belief that such an institution may be ". . .a place in which the unhappy might obtain refuge, a quiet haven in which (one). . .might find a means of reparation or of safety."[5]

Several fundamental principles became evident within a short time. The approach was primarily one of kindness and consideration. The patients were not thought to be devoid of reason or feelings or honor. The social environment was to be as nearly like that of a family with an atmosphere of religious sentiment and moral feeling. Tuke and Thomas Fowler, the visiting physician, believed that most insane people retain a considerable amount of self-command. The staff endeavored to gain the patient's confidence, to reinforce self-esteem, and to arrest the attention and fix it on objects that are opposite to the illusions the patient might possess.

Employment in various occupations was expected as a way for the patient to maintain control over his or her disorder. As Tuke reported

. . .regular employment is perhaps the most efficacious; and those kinds of employment. . .to be preferred. . .are accompanied by considerable bodily actions; that are most agreeable to the patient; and

which are most opposite to the illusions of his disease.[5]

The Retreat staff came to realize that inactivity

. . .has a natural tendency to weaken the mind, and to induce (boredom) and discontent. . .(therefore) every kind of rational and innocent employment is encouraged. Those who are not engaged in any useful occupation, are allowed to read, write, draw, play at ball, chess, etc.[5]

Because of Quaker beliefs, patients were specifically not allowed to play for money or participate in gaming of any kind.

Occupations and amusements were prescribed to elicit emotions opposite to those of the disorder. For instance, the melancholy patient was introduced to the more active and exciting kinds of activities, and the patient with mania was encouraged to engage in sedentary tasks. The writing of poetry and essays was occasionally used; however, this activity was closely monitored so that such writings did not reinforce or continue undesirable behavior. When writing was used it was found ". . .to give the patients temporary satisfaction and make them more easily led into suitable engagements."[5]

Other activities included mathematics and natural science. These disciplines were thought to be most useful, since they had a kinship to everyday work and could be applied to other pursuits within The Retreat or after patients were released. It was believed that they helped bring back more normal patterns of thinking and attention. The **habit of attention** (Tuke's phrase) was a key element in the use of occupations. Tuke realized the various kinds of concentration required to perform a variety of tasks helped limit undesirable stimuli. Thus, work was broken into components, which were used to limit undesirable thoughts and to expand positive feelings.

The pioneer work of the Tuke family opened a new chapter in the history of the care of the insane in England and, eventually, in the United States. Mild management methods, infused with kindness and the building of self-esteem through the judicious use of occupations and amusements, brought forth more desirable behavior. Patients recovered and rarely needed to return for further care.

Pinel's major work on moral treatment was published in 1801 and Tuke's description of The Retreat appeared in 1813. These brought on a rush of reforms in institutions in Europe and, ultimately, the United States.

Sir William and Lady Ellis

Sir William Charles Ellis and his wife were in charge of newly founded county asylums in England during the first half of the 19th century. They regarded the hospital as a community—"a family," as Sir Ellis called it. He paid little attention to medical remedies and concentrated on moral treatment principles, which he believed to be difficult but most likely to result in the "gradual return to reason and happiness." Lady Ellis carried the title of *workwoman,* and she organized female patients in classes to make useful and fancy articles, which were sold at fairs and bazaars. Men were encouraged to follow their own trades or to learn new ones from tradesmen employed by the institution. As Hunter and Macalpine report:

> *Ellis and his wife. . .proved there was less danger of injury from putting the spade and hoe into the hands of a large proportion of insane persons, than from shutting them up together in idleness, under the guards of straps, strait-waistcoats, or chains.*[6]

A remarkable innovation of Sir and Lady Ellis was the establishment of **after-care houses** and night hospitals. Keenly aware of environmental and social influences on insanity, they envisioned these halfway houses ". . .as stepping-stones from the asylum to the world by which the length of patients' stay would be reduced and in many cases completed. . .to go out and mix with the world before their discharge."[6]

Moral Treatment in the United States

The roots of moral care and occupations as treatment were brought to the United States by the Quakers. They established asylums and immediately implemented the Tuke's programs. The programs were popular because they helped maintain relatively low costs by having patients perform most of the necessary work of the asylum: growing crops and vegetables, maintaining herds, and manufacturing clothing and other goods. The typical institution was a beehive of activity largely designed to help it remain as self-sufficient as possible.

Reformers were in abundance. Borrowing heavily from the York Retreat, Thomas Eddy, a member of the board of governors of the Society of the New York Hospital, proposed in 1815 the construction of a building for exclusive use by mental patients.[7] He envisioned a balanced program of exercise, entertainment and occupations. Patients

> *. . .should freely partake of bodily exercises, walking, riding, conversations, innocent sports, and a variety of other amusements. . . .Those kinds of employments are to be preferred, both on a moral and physical account which are accompanied by considerable action most aggreeable to the patient and most opposite to the illusion of his disease.*[7]

In the mid 1800s, just when it seemed that the moral movement was expected to be fully realized, unanticipated trouble came from all directions. A reform-minded humanitarian, Dorthea Lynde Dix, had been campaigning vigorously for better care of the mentally ill, including moral principles. State legislatures were responding positively by establishing public mental hospitals. By 1848 Dix decided to approach the Federal government. Her vision was the establishment of a federal system of hospitals. After six years of wearying work, Dix was rewarded when Congress passed her bill. President Franklin Pierce, however, vetoed it, claiming states' rights would be endangered if the federal government took on the care of mentally ill patients. How differently our institutional system would be today if the Dix bill had been signed.

State hospitals were experiencing great difficulties with new types of patients: immigrants from Europe who were unable to adjust to the new conditions. They became public wards, often unable to use the language, and were considered unemployable. Several hospitals attempted to introduce moral principles, even establishing English instruction. The Bloomingdale, New York, Asylum made such an attempt in 1845. Classes were also held in chemistry, geometry and the physical sciences. These classes were coupled with manual labor suitable for men and women. This approach eventually failed for many reasons. Patients often were unaccustomed to the American forms of labor. Bilingual instructors could not be found. Foreign-born mechanics and artisans could not find familiar labor. Finally, large numbers of patients were too ill to participate in the available occupations.[7]

By the mid 1800s, the American agenda largely consisted of expansionism and slavery issues. These did not bode well for improving or increasing public care of the insane. Moral treatment, including occupations, rapidly began to disappear. By the onset of the Civil War, virtually none existed in state or public-supported institutions. Custodial care continued well into the 20th century. According to Bockhoven,[8] moral treatment disappeared because 1) the founders of the US movement retired and died, leaving no disciples or successors; 2) the rapid increase in foreign-born and poor patients greatly overtaxed existing facilities and required the construction of more institutions with diminished tax support; 3) racial and religious prejudices on the part of alienists (soon to be named psychiatrists) reduced interest in humane treatment and care; 4) state legislatures became increasingly more interested in less costly custodial care; 5) trained personnel were in short supply; and 6) the incurability of insanity became a dominant belief. Deutsch quotes one eminent psychiatrist in the latter decades of the 19th century: "I have come to the conclusion that when a man becomes insane, he is about used up for this world."[9]

20TH CENTURY PROGRESSIVISM

The 20th century brought with it unparalleled exuberance. The United States had largely recovered from the Civil War and acquired considerable overseas possessions as a result of the Spanish-American War. For a few years before 1900 and for some years after, nearly all Americans had become ardent believers in progress, although they did not always agree about what the word meant. Historians generally agree that *progressivism* resulted from the realization in America of the Age of Enlightenment. Prosperity was fueled by science and technology and with a flurry of industrial inventions. Cities grew rapidly, particularly in the East and Middle West. Railroads punched their way through all kinds of barriers, and in all directions, linking the country's population. The newly invented automobile served important economic purposes and became useful in leisure pursuits, with opportunities to escape the inherent stress of change. Bates describes the era of progressivism:

Conditions of prosperity deeply affected the tone of American life. The hope and buoyancy were extraordinary. Indeed, the attitude of Americans on many subjects can hardly be appreciated apart from the facts of prosperity and promise of more to come. . . .Seldom in history had a country experienced so much activity, so many diversions and (apparent) opportunities.[10]

There was more than a modest amount of zaniness during this era. Many physicians regarded increased female education as the primary cause of decreased women's health. These men felt the woman's brain simply could not assimilate a great deal of academic instruction beyond high school. Some physicians went further and claimed that women who worked were in danger of acquiring predominantly male afflictions—alcoholism, paralysis, and insanity. Women were thought to have an inborn immunity to such ills.

Drug therapy was also unusual by today's standards. The pharmaceutical firm that helped to usher in the aspirin craze introduced a new medication for bad coughs—heroin. Other across-the-counter products included cocaine tablets for the throat and general nervousness. Baby syrups were spiked with morphine, and miscarriage-producing pills, according to the ads, were a sure and great remedy for married ladies.

The Progressive Era was not always progressive. Poverty, racial injustice, ethnic unrest, sterilization of *mental defectives* (as they were known) and possible sterilization of social misfits, repression of women's rights because of leftover Victorian ideals, a marked increase in industrial accidents resulting in chronic disabilities, and a continued lack of concern about the institutionalized insane were all part of the times.

One significant feature was the emergence of an aristocracy, which came from successes in trade, industry and land acquistion. Many of the offspring of the new aristocracy, particularly women who did not marry and bear children, dedicated themselves to public service. Few of these women pursued nursing, since it was unseemly to deal with bodily fluids and excrement and the unsavory conditions surrounding illness and disease. Rather, they chose social work and, ultimately, occupational therapy because of the inherent status gained from accomplishing good work.

As one might expect from all the contradictory activity, several movements arose in this period of relative prosperity: individualism versus nationalism, racial justice versus nativism, women's rights versus men's rights, labor versus management, social justice, conservation. Bates concluded: "Much of life seemed to be changing. Somehow the old and new struggled to reach a new synthesis."[10] Two major emphases finally emerged from progressivism: a belief in freedom or the restoration of individual freedom, and the creation of a positive state wherein the government was expected to provide a variety of services to its citizens.

Chicago's Hull House

Social experiments abounded during this period, particularly in urban areas. One such experiment was Hull House, opened by Jane Addams in 1889. Hull House was intended to serve the immigrants and the poor through a variety of educational, social, and investigative programs. Along with Julia Lathrop and Florence Kelley, Addams created an environment that helped bring occupational therapy to the forefront, as a part of the restorative process of individual freedom. Eleanor Clarke Slagle, a pioneer in occupational therapy, spent two periods as a staff member at Hull House and established the first training program for occupation workers (the forerunner of occupational therapy personnel).

Invalid Occupations—Susan Tracy

The first individual in the 20th century to use occupations with acutely ill patients was Susan Tracy, a nurse. She initiated instruction in activities to student nurses as early as 1902. She coined the term **occupational nurse** to signify a specialization. By 1912 she was working full-time to apply moral treatment principles to acute medical conditions. She was convinced that remedial activities ". . .are classified according to their physiological effects as stimulants, sedatives, anesthetics. . . .Certain occupations possess like properties."[11] Tracy was also interested in experimentation and observation to enhance her practice. In 1918 she published a research paper on 25 mental tests derived from occupations. For example, by instructing the patient in using a piece of leather and a pencil, ". . .require him to make a line of dots at equal distances around the margin and at uniform distances from the edge. This constitutes a test of judgment in estimating distances."[12] Continuing with the same piece of leather, the patient is instructed to punch a hole at each dot. To do this, the patient must consider the two sides of leather and the two parts of the tool and must bring these together, thus making a *simple construction* test.[12]

Tracy determined that high-quality work was therapeutic. "It is now believed that what is worth doing at all is worth doing well and that practical, well-made articles have a greater therapeutic value than useless, poorly made articles."[13] Tracy's major work, *Studies in Invalid Occupations,* published in 1918, is a revealing compendium of her observations and experiences with different kinds of patients.[14] Among her many lasting principles, one stands out: "The patient is the product, not the article he makes."[15]

Reeducation of Convalescents— George Barton

The Progressive Era spawned a number of reformers who, although dissimilar in background, character and temperament, strove to work together on common goals. Two individuals significant to occupational therapy were George Edward Barton and William Rush Dunton, Jr. Barton, by profession an architect, contracted tuberculosis during adulthood. His constant struggle led him into a life of service to physically disabled persons.

Barton founded Consolation House in Clifton Springs, New York, in 1914, an early prototype of a rehabilitation center. Today he would be considered an entrepreneur. He was an effective speaker and writer, although often given to exaggeration. Barton's main themes were hospitals and their responsibilites to the discharged patient, the conditions the discharged patient faces, the need to return to employment after an illness, and occupations and **reeducation** of convalescents.

Barton's first published article in 1914 was based on a speech given to a group of nurses, in which he described a weakness in hospitals: "We discharge them not efficients, but inefficients. An individual leaves almost any of our institutions only to become a burden upon his family, his friends, the associated charities, or upon another institution."[16] Later in the article he warms to his subject: "I say to discharge a patient from the hospital, with his fracture healed, to be sure, but to a devestated home, to an empty desk, and to no obvious sustaining employment, is to send him out to a world cold and bleak. . ." His solution: ". . .occupation would shorten convalescence and improve the condition of many patients." He ended his oration with a rallying cry: ". . .It is time for humanity to cease regarding the hospital as a door closing upon a life which is past and to regard it henceforth as a door opening upon a life which is to come."[17]

At Consolation House, physically impaired individuals underwent a thorough review, including a social and medical history, and a consideration of their education, training, experience, successes, and failures. Barton believed that ". . .by considering these in relation to the condition (the patient) must presumably or inevitably be in for the remainder of his life, we can find some form of occupation for which he will be fitted."[18]

The word reeducation was firmly a part of Barton's terminology after World War I. He believed that hospitals should become reeducation institutions for the war-wounded to return the veteran to his rightful place in society. He declared: ". . .By a catalystic concatenation of contiguous circumstances we were forced to realize that when all is said and done, what the sick man really needed and wanted most was the restoration of his ability to work, to live independently, and to make money."[17]

Barton's major contribution to the reemergence of moral treatment principles was an awakening of physical reconstruction and reeducation through employment. Convalescence, to him was a critical time for the inclusion of something to do. Activity

. . .clarifies and strengthens the mind by increasing and maintaining interest in wholesome thought to the exclusion of morbid thought. . .and a proper occupation during convalescence may be made the basis. . .of a new life upon recovery. . .I mean [a job, a better job, or a job done better] than it was before.[18]

Judicious Regimen of Activity— William Dunton

A medical school graduate of the University of Pennsylvania and a psychiatrist, William Rush Dunton, Jr., devoted his entire life to occupational therapy. A prolific writer, he published in excess of 120 books and articles related to occupational therapy and rehabilitation. He also served as treasurer and president of The National Society for the Promotion of Occupational Therapy (the forerunner of The American Occupational Therapy Association), and for 21 years he was editor of the official journal. As a physician, he spent his professional career treating psychiatric patients in an institutional setting. Key to his treatment methods was what he called a *judicious regimen of activity*. He read the works of Tuke and Pinel, as well as the efforts of significant alienists (an early term for psychiatrists) of the 19th century.

In 1895, Dunton joined the medical staff at Sheppard and Enoch Pratt Asylum in Towson, Maryland. From his readings and observations of patients there he concluded that acutely ill patients generally were not amenable to occupations because their weakened attention span would make involvement in activity fatiguing and harmful. Later, activities might be prescribed that use energies not needed for physical restoration. Stimulating attention and directing the thoughts of the patient in regular and healthful paths would ensure an early discharge from the hospital. Dunton developed a wide variety of activities from knitting and crocheting to printing, the repair of dynamos, and farm work to gain the attention and interest, as well as to meet needs, of all patients. He stated it this way: "It has been found that a patient makes more rapid progress if his attention is concentrated upon what he is making and he derives stimulating pleasure in its performance."[19] **Interest** in the activity was paramount in Dunton's thinking. He wrote:

> By "interest" is meant the state of consiousness in which the attention is attracted to a task, accompanied by a more or less pleasurable emotional state. It is believed that attention, as distinguished from interest, lacks the emotional content or accompaniment. That is, an emotion is produced by the performance of a task, motor action, or by sensory stimulus. . . .As yet there are no studies which tell us why or how certain desires or emotions are created by auditory, visual, or other stimuli.[20]

At the second annual meeting of the National Society for the Promotion of Occupational Therapy in 1918, Dunton unveiled his nine cardinal principles to guide the emerging practice of occupational therapy and to ensure that the new discipline would gain acceptance as a medical entity. These principles were the following:[21]

1. Any activity should have as its objective a cure.
2. The activity should be interesting.
3. There should be a useful purpose other than to merely gain the patient's attention and interest.
4. The activity should preferably lead to an increase in knowledge on the patient's part.
5. Activity should be carried on with others, such as a group.
6. The occupational therapist should make a careful study of the patient and attempt to meet as many needs as possible through activity.
7. Activity should cease before the onset of fatigue.
8. Genuine encouragement should be given whenever indicated.
9. Work is much to be preferred over idleness, even when the end product of the patient's labor is of poor quality or is useless.

The major purposes of occupation in the case of the mentally ill were outlined in Dunton's first book, *Occupation Therapy: A Manual for Nurses*, published in 1915.[22] The primary objective is to divert attention either from unpleasant subjects, as is true with the depressed patient, or from daydreaming or mental ruminations, as in the case of dementia praecox (schizophrenia)—that is, to divert the attention to one main subject.

Another purpose of occupation is to reeducate—to train the patient in developing mental processes through ". . .educating the hands, eyes, muscles, just as is done in the developing child."[22] Fostering an interest in hobbies is a third purpose. Hobbies serve as present and future safety valves and render a recurrence of mental illness less likely. A final purpose may be to instruct the patient in a craft until he or she has enough proficiency to take pride in the work. However, Dunton noted: "While this is proper, I fear. . .specialism is apt to cause a narrowing of one's mental outlook. . . .The individual with a knowledge of many things has more interest in the world in general."[22]

The Origin of the Term *Occupational Therapy*

There is a continuing controversy about who was initially responsible for the term *occupational therapy*—Dunton or Barton. At Sheppard and Enoch Pratt Asylum, Dunton directed the therapeutic occupations program. A special building was completed in 1902 and named The Casino. It was dedicated space for a wide variety of occupations and amusements. In 1911, Dunton initiated a training program for nurses in patient occupations, and here he first used the term *occupation therapy*. This term appeared in his handwritten lecture notes, dated October 10, 1911. This is the earliest known record of the use of this term. In later years Dunton indicated that Adolph Meyer, a renowned psychiatrist and personal and professional friend, was the first to use the term *therapy* and *therapeutic* in connection with occupations; but that he was the first person to put *occupation* and *therapy* together as one phrase.

Barton's claim to the first use of the term appeared initially in March, 1915, in *The Trained Nurse and Hospital Review*.[23] The article was based on a speech given in Massachusetts on December 28, 1914. Before then, Barton had preferred the term *occupation reeducation*, which accurately described his efforts at Consolation House. During preliminary discussions between Barton and Dunton about a national organization, during 1915 to 1916, a series of squabbles took place, mostly through correspondence. Terminology figured heavily in these differences of opinion. Barton preferred his *occupational reeducation* and Dunton held tenaciously to *occupation therapy*. Barton finally countered with *occupational therapy*, preferring the adjectival form. They did agree on the term *occupational workers*, since the word *therapist* was considered the sole property of the psychiatrist. Dunton did not change his mind until well into the 1920s.[23,24]

Habit Training—Eleanor Clarke Slagle

Eleanor Clarke Slagle is considered the most distinguished 20th century occupational therapist. One of five founders of the national professional organization, she served in every major elective office. She was also Executive Secretary for 14 years. In the first decade of this century, she was partially trained as a social worker and completed one of the early special courses in curative occupations and recreation at the Chicago School of Civics and Philanthropy, which was associated with Hull House. She worked subsequently in a number of institutions, most notably the new Henry Phipps Clinic, Johns Hopkins Hospital, in Baltimore, Maryland. There she served under the direction of the renowned psychiatrist, Adolf Meyer. At this same time, she became a devoted friend of William Dunton's family. Later, she moved to New York where she pioneered in developing occupational therapy in the State Department of Mental Hygiene.

Slagle was knowledgeable about moral treatment principles and embraced them as the core of her thinking and practice. She emphasized that occupational therapy must be a "...consciously planned, progressive program of rest, play, occupation, and exercise..."[25] She often spoke of the need for the mentally ill person to spend a fairly well-balanced day. In addition, she placed considerable emphasis on the personality of the therapist:

> ...the proper balance of qualities, proper physical expression, a kindly voice, gentleness, patience, ability and seeming vision, adaptability...to meet the particular needs of the individual patient in all things....Personality plus character also covers an ability to be honest and firm, with infinite kindness.[26]

Her most long-lasting contribution to the care of the mentally ill was what she entitled *habit training*. This plan was first attempted at the Rochester, New York State Hospital in 1901, but it was Slagle who developed and refined the basic principles for those patients who had been hospitalized for five to 20 years and whose behavior had steadily regressed. Habit training was 24 hours long and involved the entire ward staff. It was a reeducation program designed to overcome disorganized habits, to modify other habits, and to construct new ones, with the goal of restoring and maintaining of health. She declared: "In habit training, we show...the necessity of requiring attention, of building on the habit of attention—attention thus becomes application, voluntary and, in time, agreeable."[26]

A typical habit training schedule called for patients to arise at 6:00 A.M., wash, toilet, brush teeth, and air beds. After breakfast, they returned to the ward and made beds, and swept. Classwork followed and lasted for two hours. It consisted of a variety of simple crafts and marching exercises. After lunch, there was a rest period; continued classwork; and outdoor exercises, folk dancing, and lawn games. After supper, there was music and dancing on the ward, followed by toileting, washing, teeth brushing, and preparing for bed.[27]

After maximum benefit was achieved from habit training, the patient progressed through three phases of occupational therapy. The first was what Slagle called the *kindergarten group*. "We must show the ways of stimulating their special senses. The employment of color, music, simple exercises, games, and storytelling along with occupations, the gentle ways and means...(used) in educating the child are equally important in reeducating the adult."[26] Occupations were graded from simple to complex. The next phase was *ward classes in occupational therapy*: "...graded to the limit of accomplishment of individual patients."[28] When able to tolerate it, the patient joined in group activities. The third phase was *the occupational center*. "This promotes opportunities for more advanced projects...a complete change in environment; ...comparative freedom; ...actual responsibilities placed upon patients; the stimulation of seeing work produced; ...all these carry forward the readjustment of patients."[28]

In 1922 Slagle summarized her philosophy as follows:

> Of the highest value to patients is the psychological fact that the patient is working for himself....Occupational therapy recognizes the significance of the mental attitude which the sick person takes toward illness and attempts to make that attitude more wholesome by providing activities adapted to the capacity of the individual and calculated to divert his attention from his own problems.[26]

Further, she declared: "It is directed activity, and differs from all other forms of treatment in that it is given in increasing doses as the patient improves."[29]

Figure 1-1 shows Eleanor Clarke Slagle (standing) when she was the Director of Occupational Therapy at the New York Department of Mental Hygiene. She is inspecting the weaving of a woolen rug by Mrs. Margaret Kransee, instructor at the Manhattan State Hospital, Wards Island, in 1933.

THE PHILOSOPHY OF OCCUPATION THERAPY— ADOLPH MEYER

A history of this type would not be complete without at least a brief mention of Adolph Meyer, a Swiss physician who immigrated to this country in 1892. By the end of 1910 he became professor of psychiatry at Johns Hopkins University and the first director of the Henry Phipps Clinic. Meyer "borrowed" Eleanor Clarke Slagle from Hull House for two years, during which time she founded the therapeutic occupations program in the clinic. Meyer's lasting contribution to psychiatry is the psychobiologic approach to mental illness and health. He coined this term to indicate that the human is an indivisible unit of study, rather than a composite of symptoms: "Psychobiology starts not from the mind *and* body or from elements, but from the fact that we deal with biologically organized units and groups and their functioning. . .the 'hes' and 'shes' of our experience—the bodies we find in action"[30] (see Chapter 6).

Meyer's commonsense approach to the problems of living was his keynote:

> *The main thing is that your point of reference should always be life itself. . . .As long as there is life there are positive assets—action, choice, hope, not in the imagination but in the clear understanding of the situation, goals, and possibilities. . . .To see life as it is, is one of the fundamentals of my philosophy. . .[31]*

Because of his friendship with Slagle and Dunton, Meyer agreed to deliver a major address at the Fifth Annual Meeting of the National Society for the Promotion of Occupational Therapy in Baltimore, October, 1921. This address has become a classic in occupational therapy literature. Meyer emphasized occupation, time, and the productive use of energy. He stated:

> *The whole of human organization has its shape in a kind of rhythm. . . .There are many. . .rhythms which we must be attuned to: the larger rhythms of night and day, of sleep and waking hours. . .and finally the big four—work and play and rest and sleep, which our organisim must be able to balance even under difficulty. The only way to attain balance in all this is actual doing, actual practice, a program of wholesome living is the basis of wholesome feeling and thinking and fancy and interests.[32]*

In this address, Meyer successfully brought the fundamental moral treatment principles of more than a century before into contemporary occupational therapy practice, and established the foundation of what now is known as **occupational behavior,** the *Model of Human Occupation* and *occupational performance* (see Chapters 3 and 4).

FOUNDING OF THE AMERICAN OCCUPATIONAL THERAPY ASSOCIATION

The American Occupational Therapy Association (AOTA) archives hold all of the correspondence between George Barton and William Dunton and, later, Eleanor Clarke Slagle, during the era when discussions were held about creating a national organization[33] to be a mechanism for exchanging views and extending information about the fledgling "new line of medicine." The first letter in the series was from Dunton to Barton on October 15, 1915, wherein he suggested that Barton take the lead in organizing

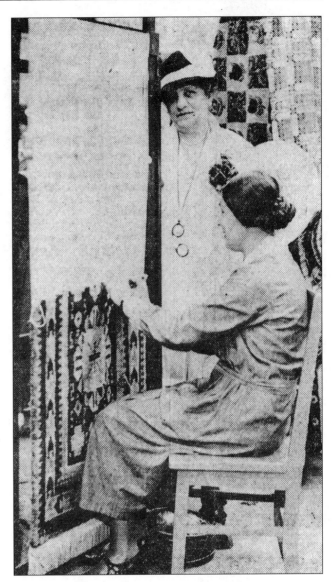

Figure 1-1. Eleanor Clarke Slagle (standing) and Margaret Kransee, 1933. (From personal archives. Robert K. Bing.)

"a central bureau for occupation workers." Barton wrote back, agreed, and suggested a title, Society for the Promotion of Occupation for Reeducation. A series of false starts ensued and Dunton became exasperated with the lack of progress. Local groups of occupation workers were forming to exchange views, and he felt they needed support and guidance from a national group. On December 7, 1916, Dunton wrote Barton again, proposing a five-member national executive committee. Disagreements between the two arose about who should be invited. They were settled on December 20, 1916, when Barton wrote Dunton with a new title, National Society for the Promotion of Occupational Therapy.

After some juggling of dates, March 15-17 were set for the organizational meeting and incorporation of the Society. Barton invited the "big five," as he called the executive committee, to use his Consolation House for the event, as he wished to be host. The invitees, other than Dunton, included Eleanor Clarke Slagle, then the General Superintendent of Occupational Therapy at Hull House; Susan Cox Johnson, the Director of Occupations, New York State Department of Public Charities; and Thomas B. Kidner, the Vocational Secretary, Canadian Military Hospital Commission. Susan E. Tracy, Instructor in Invalid Occupations, Presbyterian Hospital, Chicago, was also invited but declined because of her work schedule. Isabelle Newton, Barton's secretary at Consolation House, was invited to attend in that capacity (Figure 1-2). Barton was elected President, a position he nominated himself for a few weeks before the meeting.

The next six months proved critical. Barton became increasingly annoyed at Dunton and Slagle, who was Vice President. He suspected they were trying to overshadow his presidency. He also became involved in a heated debate about finances with Dunton, the Treasurer. Subsequently, Barton refused to attend the first annual meeting on Labor Day weekend, September, 1917, in New York City. He cited poor health. Dunton was elected the new President. There is no record that Barton attended any meetings of the national organization for the remainder of his life; however, he did remain a member.[34]

OCCUPATIONAL THERAPY'S CREED

To solidify and publicize the fundamental principles of occupational therapy a Pledge and Creed was developed in 1925 and adopted by the AOTA the next year.[35] The efforts toward developing a creed began in late 1924 when Marjorie B. Greene, Dean, Boston School of Occupational Therapy

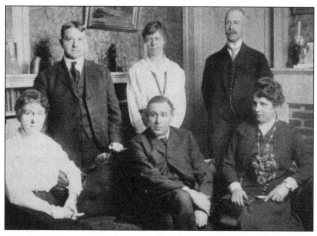

Figure 1-2. The founders of the National Society for the Promotion of Occupational Therapy. Front Row L-R: Susan Cox Johnson, George E. Barton, Eleanor Clarke Slagle. Back Row L-R: William R. Dunton, Isabel Newton, Thomas Kidner.

wrote the Association's President, Thomas B. Kidner, seeking his counsel in modifying the Pledge and Creed originally created by *Modern Hospital* and adopted by the American Hospital Association in early 1924. She indicated: "This sums up so splendidly the spirit of service and the outstanding factors of our work that we too (presumably the Boston School) are most anxious to adopt it." In due time, Dean Greene, with suggestions from Eleanor Clarke Slagle, William Dunton, and Thomas Kidner developed the desired modifications. It was adopted by AOTA at the tenth annual meeting in Atlantic City in 1926. It remains today, just as it was approved more than 60 years ago, although there have been some discussions about revising it.[36]

Pledge and Creed for Occupational Therapists

REVERENTLY AND EARNESTLY do I pledge my whole-hearted service in aiding those crippled in mind and body;

TO THIS END that my work for the sick may be successful, I will ever strive for greater knowledge, skill, and understanding in the discharge of my duties in whatsoever position I may find myself;

I SOLEMNLY DECLARE that I will hold and keep inviolate whatever I may learn of the lives of the sick;

I ACKNOWLEDGE the dignity of the cure of disease and the safeguarding of health in which no act is menial or inglorious;

I WILL WALK in upright faithfulness and obedience to those under whose guidance I am to work in the holy ministry to broken minds and bodies.

The 1925 Principles

A committee of AOTA, made up of physicians and chaired by William Rush Dunton, Jr., compiled an outline of lectures on occupational therapy for medical students and physicians.[37] The members developed a definition, objectives, statements of the use of a variety of activities with different kinds of patients, therapeutic approaches, and the qualities and qualifications of practitioners. This was the first such effort since Dunton had created his principles in 1918.[21]

The first principle states: "Occupational therapy is a method of training the sick or injured by means of instruction and employment in productive occupation."[37] One is struck by the importance of the connection between learning by doing and purposeful activity. This was the dominant theme in several of the principles. The act of doing should be seen from the patient's point of view. For example, the treatment objectives stated: ". . .sought are to arouse interest, courage, and confidence; to exercise mind and body on healthy activity; to overcome disability; and to re-establish capacity for industrial and social usefulness."[37]

Rules were established about the extent of activities, and attention was given to their qualities and effect on the patient. The use of crafts and work-related occupations was emphasized. Games, music and physical exercise were not to be overlooked. "Novelty, variety, individuality, and utility of the products enhance the value of an occupation as a treatment measure."[37] A warning was offered: whereas quality, quantity and salability may serve some objectives, these must not override the main purpose of the activity. Belief in the various properties of occupation is evident in the statement: "As the patient's strength and capability increase, the type and extent of occupation should be regulated and graded accordingly."[37]

The committee made a statement about the quality of work to be expected as a therapeutic approach: ". . .inferior workmanship or employment in an occupation which would be trivial for the healthy, may be (used) with the greatest benefit to the sick or injured, but standards worthy of entirely normal persons must be maintained for proper mental stimulation."[37]

The relationship between purposeful activity and the connections between the mind and body is found in this principle: "The production of a well-made. . .article, or the accomplishment of a useful task, requires healthy exercise of mind and body, gives the greatest satisfaction, and thus produces the most beneficial effects."[37] Involvement in group activity is advised ". . .because it provides exercise in social adaptation. . ."[37] The importance of occupational therapy is evident in the statement: ". . .the treatment should be prescribed and administered under constant medical advice and supervision, and correlated with the other treatment of the patient."[37] In regard to application it was stated: ". . .system and precision are as important as in other forms of treatment."[37] Evaluation rests with measuring the effect of the occupation on the patient, the extent to which objectives are being realized.

One final principle addresses the qualifications of the practitioner: "Good craftsmanship. . .ability to instruct. . .understanding, sincere interest in the patient, and an optimistic, cheerful outlook and manner. . .are essential."[37] Elsewhere in the lecture outline, the committee recommended that therapists and aides should have ". . .a therapeutic sense, the teaching instinct, and good mental balance. Personality constitutes 50 percent of the value of these workers."[37]

During this period, a number of issues were combined, including the following:

1. Purposeful work and leisure
2. The intricate involvement of the mind and body (interdependence of mental and physical aspects, also known as holism)
3. Occupational therapy as a learning process
4. The therapeutic use of one's personal qualities

The literature of the next several decades, which was a period of remarkable development in the profession, gives evidence of how these principles became operational.

Purposeful Work and Leisure. In her early endeavors as a practitioner, Clare Spackman explored the perplexing problem of engaging the patient's interests.[38] "One of the therapist's problems is in approaching the patient who refuses occupational therapy; yet, he is often the one who needs it the most. Many patients scorn occupational therapy as being child's play or beneath their dignity, or are frankly uninterested and apathetic. . ."[38] Her recommendation was to approach the patient through his or her interests. "There are few people who have not some interest and to make the right suggestion at the right time takes both experience and imagination."[38] Spackman advised: "The therapist's greatest danger in her approach is failure to make first contacts. . .sufficiently vital. Being in a hurry, and a tendency to consider only the physical motion necessary is her greatest pitfall. The need of psychological treatment. . .is as necessary as any other."[38]

Martha Gilbert, an occupational therapist at the Choctaw-Chickasaw Sanitorium in Oklahoma built her entire treatment program around purposeful work and leisure for children.[39] The sanitarium was a federal institution with 75 beds for Indian children with tuberculosis and related diseases. In 1929, times were difficult, not only because of the Great Depression, but also because Indian children were not highly valued, except by those who cared for them on a daily basis.

Gilbert developed her comprehensive program of appealing activities that activated the interest and attention of her patients. She reported:

> Supplies for craftwork were very meager but the children were eager to learn, loved to draw and march to music and do calesthenics to. . .records. There was no playground apparatus but long walks were permitted and. . .after supper (there) was often a hunt for wild flowers or for nuts and wild berries.[39]

For handwork, she used native materials to ". . .fashion objects of interest. . . .In summer, clay from the hillsides; in fall leaves from the trees; and in winter, anything from paper dolls to hooked mats and rugs were fashioned. . ."[39] Gilbert and her patients also cultivated a garden out of the barren, wind-driven soil. The more able patients transported creek bottom soil in small cans and jars. They formed a "bucket brigade" and kept the plants alive during harsh weather. "We harvested our peanuts with much gusto, used them in candy-making and picked our flowers to adorn the shops and schoolroom."[39]

The children's cultural background was an important part of her treatment program. "We try to make much of the (various) holidays; we invent a game to use with our Indian puppets or try a health or ceremonial play or pageant to give us an excuse for 'dressing up.' "[39]

Gilbert's approach may be seen today, as therapists and assistants carry out innovative and imaginative programs in impoverished areas of the United States, and indeed, throughout the world.

Involvement of the Mind and Body. In 1927, Ida Sands, the chief occupational therapist at Philadelphia General Hospital addressed the AOTA annual conference.[40] She stated that occupations are curative through three spheres:

Occupational therapy, through carefully selected and graded work, develops resistance: 1) spiritually, by keeping up self-respect and developing ambition and initiative; 2) mentally, by developing coordination and mental poise; and 3) physically, by developing weak muscles through adapted occupation.[40]

She defended the importance of spirituality in occupations in this way:

I have put spiritual rehabilitation first because it is often a delicate process. This form of rehabilitation is approached by the occupational therapist through understanding;. . .that subtle quality which enables a person to estimate the needs and. . .possibilities of another.[40]

The interaction of mind and body has remained a basic principle throughout our historical evolution. Beatrice Wade, a renowned clinician, educator and administrator, spoke of the treatment of the total patient in an address in 1967.[41] She stated: "This approach is unique to occupational therapy among the. . .health disciplines. . . .There has always existed a strong component concerned with the behavior of the physically ill or disabled, as well as the mentally sick; with the entirety of man and his functioning as a patient."[41] This occupational therapy concept, she continued, ". . .prevented (as has occurred in medical practice) an undesired separation of the psychiatric therapist from those who develop knowledge and skills centered in the treatment of the physically disabled."[41] Stated another way:

The major emphasis in occupational therapy is not the body as such but the individual as such. The therapist's background is strongly weighed in an understanding of personality adjustment and reactions to social situations. . .and in the patient's attitudes toward an adjustment to acute and chronic disabilities.[42]

Occupational Therapy as a Learning Process. Throughout the formative years, occupational therapy and education

held much in common, not so much in how patients were instructed, but, in the outcomes of that instruction through changes in behavior and performance of a more complex nature. Harriet Robeson, a distinguished therapist, addressed a group of social workers in 1926 and affirmed some longstanding principles:

Many think of occupational therapy as only handwork. It is far more than that. (It) is a program of work, play, and medicine to meet the mental, physical, and social needs of each patient. It is reeducation.[43]

The reeducation process follows the same pathway as as normal education: ". . .a gradual growth through progressive development. . . .We must teach (the patient) to creep and to creep in the right direction."[43]

Robeson also faced the challenge of crafts being central to practice: "Handicrafts are only some of the tools with which we work, not primarily with the idea that patients will earn a future livelihood. . .but because since Adam people have found expression through work with their hands; a primitive outlet, creative, educative, constructive."[43] She went on to speak about physical and emotional functions and adaptation:

Crafts may also be adapted to meet nearly all needs in mental and physical adjustments. Movements required in physical restoration of function can be found in. . .various crafts. These same techniques can produce definite results in mental cases in substituting purposeful occupation for scattered and destructive activity. . .and ideational deterioration. Furthermore, crafts can meet all degrees of scholastic background and intelligence.[43]

(See Chapter 16 for more information on the historical and contemporary use of crafts.)

Irene O'Brock, director of occupational therapy at the University of Oklahoma Hospitals in 1932, indicated that her program for children had an ". . .additional value, a deeper more intangible significance: the natural tendencies of life, play, and companionship."[44] She based her treatment program on five **lines of readiness:** 1) to construct things, 2) to communicate things, 3) to find out things, 4) to compete in things, and 5) to excel in things. The first line of readiness included a workshop with tools and materials, such as wood, metal, textiles, clay, yarn, and the like. Books and magazines were also available. The second line of readiness, to communicate things, involved ". . .stories, music, dramatizations, songs, and pictures, . . .even making musical instruments. . ."[44] The third line, to find out things, involved ". . .occupations and natural phenomena of community life, such as the building of a dog house for a pet or digging a cave for the gang to meet in. Too, gardening is of great importance in the developing of a community spirit."[44] To compete in things, the fourth line of readiness, O'Brock had a playground and gym: "Competition does much to teach good sportsmanship. We occasionally have afternoons of play. The children always help to plan these days. . .prizes are given for (those) excelling in games."[44]

Learning played an important role in what was known as *fieldwork*, treating patients who were homebound. In 1926, a therapist named Martha Emig related an experience she had with a 31-year-old homebound man, born with cerebral palsy, and living in Duluth, Minnesota.[45] He was confined to a small alcove between the kitchen and the dining room. His mother showed a great deal of concern and love, but she felt the therapist would be wasting her time, ". . .as the (mother thought the) young man was helpless and had no mind."[45] According to Emig:

During my visit I found he was mentally alert and he became interested in a few (handmade) articles I had with me, pointing to the baskets and saying "I like that." He complained that his hands were stiff, that he could hold nothing, that his mother always fed him. I had him flex and extend his fingers, which he did slowly and with difficulty, so I told him how, by using his hands, they would become stronger.[45]

In time, his skill and speed in basketry increased to such a point that the therapist was delivering additional materials almost on a daily basis. He found an outlet for his finished products and made enough money to purchase his own materials. "I helped him keep his accounts. He seldom made a mistake in calculating."[45] The patient went on to read and indulge in other studies with the family's help. Emig reported: "The home atmosphere changed; the family all are interested and they help him."[45]

Figure 1-3 shows two men engaged in activites that were typical of the times. These patients were receiving occupational therapy treatment at the Jewish Sanitorium and Hospital for Chronic Disease in Brooklyn, New York. They were painting colorful designs on wooden plates, which were sold at a bazaar, with the proceeds used to augment the hospital fund, which provided care for more than 500 disabled men, women, and children.

The Practitioner's Personal Qualities. As noted earlier, one of the 1925 principles stated that the essential qualities of the therapist and aide were at least of equal value to any instruction or procedures used in applied occupations. One of the first student papers published in *Occupational Therapy and Rehabilitation*, the official journal of the AOTA, appeared in 1930. Nelda McKee of the University of Minnesota wrote on "Ethics for the Occupational Therapist." She discussed ". . .the ideals, customs, and habits which members of the profession are. . .accumulating around the name and character

of the trained therapist."[46] Essential attributes in dealing with patients include honesty, frankness, and wisdom. She showed her insight when she stated:

A therapist should endeavor to develop a symmetrical life. We all have a physical, mental, spiritual, and social side to our make-up which needs care and cultivation. The (therapist) is under personal obligation to keep herself from growing narrow. . . .Above all, (she) must keep the quality of being "teachable." Then she will never stop developing the possibilities which she possesses.[46]

McKee ends her ethical statements with: ". . .the ideal therapist never forgets that our ambitions are all directed towards one common end. We are working for the advancement of understanding and the enlargement of human life."[46] (More information on ethics may be found in the companion volume to this text, *Practice Issues in Occupational Therapy: Intraprofessional Team Building*).

Joseph C. Doane, MD, who later became president of AOTA, gave an impromtu address to conferees at the 1928 AOTA annual meeting.[47] He distinguished between two kinds of workers, the *occupationalist* and the *therapist*:

I regret to say that the occupationalists include not a few physicians and many laymen. (They believe) that occupational therapy is a very interesting and very useful plaything which begins and stops there; they see the product, rather than the patient; they comment on the beautiful colors and difficult weaves. . . .They see nothing beyond the mere physical thing which has resulted from the activity.

Then there is the other party—the therapist. The therapist looks at yarn and raffia, not as materials to be used. . .but as the implements or tools to be employed in the handling of much more difficult material, the disposition of the persons who are ill, a most varying and a most uncertain commodity.[47]

For Doane, the critical importance is for the therapist ". . .to know what sick people do and think and why dispositions, when mixed with sickness, behave as they do—much more important than to know how to make something."[47]

WE LIVE FORWARD

Contemporary occupational theorists and visionaries, such as Mary Reilly, Phillip Shannon, Gary Kielhofner, Janice Burke, and Elizabeth Yerxa, find ample support for

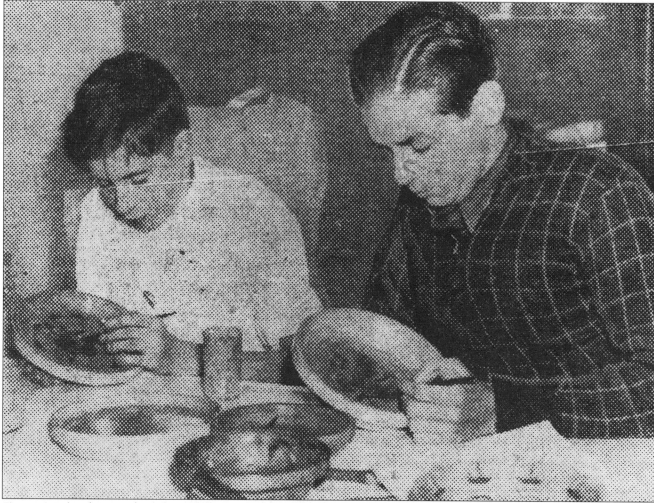

Figure 1-3. Patients in Occupational Therapy Department Jewish Sanitorium and Hospital for Chronic Diseases, Brooklyn, New York, 1937. (From personal archives. Robert K. Bing.)

their concepts in the founding, time-honored principles. In 1961, Reilly observed:

> My reexamination of our early history revealed that our profession emerged from a common belief held by a small group of people. This common belief is the hypotheses upon which our profession was founded. It was, and indeed still is, one of the truly great and even magnificent hypotheses of medicine today: That man, through the use of his hands as they are energized by mind and will, can influence the state of his own health. The splendor of its vision goes far beyond rating it as an idea conceived once in a lifetime or even once in a century. Rather, it falls in the class of one of those great beliefs which has advanced civilization.[48]

For nearly two decades, between 1958 and 1977, Reilly wrote extensively about occupational therapy principles and the profession's changing role in medicine and health care. As Madigan and Parent point out:

> She stated that the medical model is designed to prevent and reduce illness and does not address the reduction of incapacity that results from illness. It is the occupational therapist's (and assistant's) responsibility to activate residual adaptation of patients and to help deficit humans achieve life satisfaction through work and social involvement.[49]

Reilly repeatedly called for a renewed conceptualization of occupational therapy as reflected in the ideals of Dunton, Slagle and Tracy. In addition, Reilly argued that occupational therapy needed to be concerned about the difficulties people have with their occupations all along the developmental continuum, including play and work. This she called **occupational behavior**, ". . .and proposed it as the unifying concept about which occupational therapists could develop a body of theory to support practice."[49]

By 1977, much of occupational therapy practice had markedly shifted away from its foundation in the original principles. Phillip Shannon viewed with alarm what was taking place. He called it a derailment:

> . . .*a new hypothesis has emerged that views man not as a creative being capable of making choices and directing his own future, but as a mechanistic creature susceptible to manipulation and control via the application of techniques. . .is a derailment from those. . .values and beliefs that legitimized the practice of occupational therapy. If occupational therapy persists in this direction, what was once and still is one of the great ideas of 20th century medicine will be swept away by the tide of technique philosophy. Should this happen the ligitimacy of occupational therapy may be revoked and. . .its services absorbed by other health care professions.*[50]

Shannon was one of many graduate students under Reilly who advanced occupational behavior theory.

Six years later, in 1983, Kielhofner and Burke completed an exhaustive review of the early literature and were left "with a deep respect for the ideas and accomplishments of the. . .first generation of therapists. Both a science of occupation and the art of using occupation as a medical therapy were conceived, clearly articulated, and applied."[51] Yet, something was missing, something had been dropped out in the intervening years between the development of the principles and the time of their review:

> *A sense of confidence and enthusiasm for occupational therapy seems to have waned, and today we seem bewildered in the face of clinical problems which early occupational therapists readily embraced. Furthermore, our confusion over the identity of occupational therapy seems inexplicable compared with the unified view of early occupational therapists concerning the nature of their service.*[51]

Kielhofner and his associates proceeded with the development of what they term *a model of human occupation,* using the concepts of occupational behavior theory[52] (see Chapter 4).

The latest addition to this evolution, starting with the original principles, is called *occupational science* and is viewed by many as a foundation for occupational therapy well into the next century. Occupational science is believed to be an emerging basic science that supports occupational practice. Supporters state:

> *By identifying and articulating a scientific foundation for practice, occupational science could provide practitioners with support for what they do, justify the significance of occupational therapy to health, and differentiate occupational therapy from other disci-*

> *plines. It could provide new understanding of what it means to be chronically disabled in American society, thereby enabling occupational therapists (and assistants) to be more effective advocates for, and allies with, people who are disabled. The science of occupation could help the profession contribute new knowledge and skills to the eradication of complex problems affecting everyone in society.*[53]

OCCUPATIONAL THERAPY: POETRY OF THE COMMONPLACE

What might we carry away from this story of our profession's principles? History tells us that in turbulent times we tend to turn to structure for stability. Contrary to what many of us believe, we will not find any safety in our technology; it changes too rapidly; it is but shifting sand. Where we will find comfort and security is in the centuries-old fundamentals and principles still quite evident in today's occupational therapy practice. We will find assurance in our belief system that has emerged and will continue to develop as time moves on. Our principles and our belief that human beings can survive castastrophes of illness, disease and disabling situations and learn, perhaps for the first time, how to live life well—that is fundamental to our unique efforts.

Occupational therapy's realm consists of a carefully compounded, great vision, transforming the poetry of the commonplace into a vital sustainer and prolonger of precious life. Through the judicious use of a unique technology—human occupation—that has been grounded in research confirming the art and science, and cautiously blended with timeless values, beliefs, and principles, we will inevitably succeed where others have failed. The grand tasks of occupational therapy remain: to attend to the multiple, complex, interrelated, and critical human activities of not just living, but living well. Through the habits of attention and interest we engage the human in regaining the harmony of functions that ensure survival, in retaining those characteristics that facilitate and push balanced growth and development; and in attaining those interrelated meanings of a purposeful, fulfilled life within the context of a personal and social order.

SUMMARY

Occupational therapy's beginnings reach back more than 200 years, to the Age of Enlightenment when human beings were emerging with a new, expanded view of "why on earth they were on earth." There was a sense of economic, political, social, and religious progress. Ideas were forming about the importance of each human being, about the human ability to think and learn, about labor as the central focus of life, and about human existence being governed by a prevailing set of principles directed toward everyday living. These same ideals became significant in caring about and for the mentally ill.

In Europe, the birthplace of this new age, men and women, such as Phillippe Pinel, William Tuke, and Sir William and Lady Ellis, engaged their mental patients in a variety of occupations and amusements for a number of purposes: to restore reason; to provide feelings of security and self-worth; to allow as much freedom of choice and movement as possible, regardless of mental conditions; and to arrest delusional attention and fix it on objects that would help restore reason. From their experience, the caregivers established certain principles that were handed down to the present day. For more than 50 years, during the latter decades of the 19th century and the early 20th century, these principles all but disappeared because of social, economic, and political upheavals. They reemerged in the second decade of this century as occupational therapy.

In the United States, during the Progressive Era, a diverse collection of men and women restated and added to the inherited principles. Among these people were William Rush Dunton, Jr., a psychiatrist; Eleanor Clarke Slagle, a partially-trained social worker; Susan Tracy, a nurse; George Edward Barton, a disabled architect; and Adolph Meyer, a psychiatrist. Their contributions remain today as the cornerstone of occupational therapy principles:

1. Activity contains ingredients by which an ill or disabled individual may gain understanding of and control over one's own feelings, thoughts, and actions; habits of attention and interest; usefulness of occupation; creative expression; the process of learning by doing; skill; and concrete evidence of personal accomplishment.

2. Variations of activity provide opportunities to balance the larger rhythms of life: work, play, rest, and sleep, which must remain balanced if health is to be regained, maintained or attained.

3. Purposeful occupation involves the intricate interplay of the mind and body, which cannot be separated if the human being is to engage in activity.

4. Involvement in remedial activity has as a major purpose the acquiring or restoring of usefulness to oneself and others as a happy, productive human being.

5. The patient is the product of his or her own efforts, not the article made nor the activity accomplished.

6. One's approach to the patient is as significant to treatment and rehabilitation as is the selection and use of an activity.

7. A knowledge of the patient's needs, an appreciation of the pain that accompanies an illness or disability, a strong desire to reduce or remove it, and a gentle firmness are among the major characteristics of the provider of therapeutic occupations.

These principles remain intact, although often restated and reworded. There is considerable evidence they will remain a part of our practice through the efforts of such individuals as Mary Reilly, Phillip Shannon, Gary Kielhofner, Janice Burke, and Elizabeth Yerxa and her associates. Occupational behavior, the model of human occupation, and occupational science offer assurances that these principles will still be with us well into the next century.

Acknowledgments

The author wishes to express his profound gratitude to those people who so generously assisted in the search for materials and in the preparation of the manuscript: Lillian Hoyle Parent, OTR, FAOTA; James L. Cantwell, OTR; Gary A. Wade, OTR; Florence S. Cromwell, OTR, FAOTA; and Inci Bowman, PhD, Director, Truman Blocker History of Medicine Collection (AOTA Archives), Moody Medical Library, The University of Texas Medical Branch at Galveston.

Thanks also to the staff of the *American Journal of Occupational Therapy* for permission to use excerpts from previously published articles: "Occupational Therapy Revisited: A Paraphratic Journey," volume 35, no 6, 1981 and "Living Forward, Understanding Backwards, Part 1 and 2," volume 38, nos 6 and 7, 1984.

Related Learning Activities

1. Construct a historical timeline identifying the important events and people that shaped the profession's history.

2. Much of the impetus for the development of the profession grew out of the principles of moral treatment, yet adherence to moral treatment "died out." What implications does this have for occupational therapy today?

3. Review the summary of principles and compare and contrast them with those you see in occupational therapy literature and practice environments today. Discuss the similarities and differences.

4. If you could have spent time talking with Barton and Dunton, what would you have discussed?

5. Identify ways in which the early beliefs about habit training are reflected in occupational therapy practice today.

References

1. Neustadt RE, May ER: *Thinking in Time: The Uses of History for Decision-Makers.* New York: The Free Press, 1986, p. xxii.

2. deGrazia S: *Of Time, Work, and Leisure.* New York: Twentieth Century Fund, 1962, p. 45.

3. Pinel P: *A Treatise on Insanity in Which Are Contained The Principles of a New and More Practical Nosology of Manical Disorders.* Translated by DD Davis. London: Cadell and Davis, 1806, pp. xv-xvii.

4. Mackler B: *Phillippe Pinel: Unchainer of the Insane.* New York: Franklin Watts, 1968, p. 76.

5. Tuke W: *Description of The Retreat: An Institution Near York for Insane Persons of The Society of Friends.* London: Dawson of Pall Mall, 1813, pp. 20, 156, 180-182.

6. Hunter R, Macalpine I: *Three Hundred Years of Psychiatry: 1535-1860.* London: Oxford University Press, 1963, pp. 871-872.

7. Hass LJ: One hundred years of occupational therapy. *Arch Occup Ther* 3(2):83-100, 1924.

8. Bockhoven JS: *Moral Treatment in Community Mental Health.* New York: Springer Publishing, 1972, pp. 20-31.

9. Deutsch A: *The Mentally Ill in America: A History of Their Care and Treatment from Colonial Times,* 2nd ed. New York: Columbia University Press, 1949.

10. Bates JL: *The United States, 1898-1928: Progressivism and a Society in Transition.* New York: McGraw-Hill, 1976, pp. 18-19, 40.

11. Tracy SE: The place of invalid occupations in the general hospital. *Mod Hosp* 2 (5):386, 1914.

12. Tracy SE: Twenty-five suggested mental tests derived from invalid occupations. *Maryland Psychiatric Q* 8:15-16, 1918.

13. Tracy SE: Treatment of disease by employment at St. Elizabeth's Hospital. *Mod Hosp* 20 (2):198, 1923.

14. Tracy SE: *Studies in Invalid Occupations.* Boston: Witcomb and Barrows, 1918.

15. Barrows M: Susan B. Tracy, RN. *Maryland Psychiatric Q* 6:59, 1917.

16. Barton GE: A view of invalid occupation. *Trained Nurse and Hospital Review* 52 (6):328-330, 1914.

17. Barton GE: Occupational nursing. *Trained Nurse and Hospital Review* 54 (6):328-336, 1915.

18. Barton GE: The existing hospital system and reconstruction. *Trained Nurse and Hospital Review* 69 (4):309,320, 1922.

19. Dunton WR: The relationship of occupational therapy and physical therapy. *Arch Phys Ther* 16 (1):19, 1935.

20. Dunton WR: *Prescribing Occupational Therapy.* Springfield, Illinois, Charles C. Thomas, 1945, pp.5-6.

21. Dunton WR: The principles of occupational therapy. In *Proceedings of the National Society for the Promotion of Occupational Therapy, Second Annual Meeting.* Catonsville, Maryland, Spring Grove State Hospital Press, 1918, pp. 25-27.

22. Dunton WR: *Occupation Therapy: A Manual for Nurses.* Philadelphia, WB Saunders, 1915, pp. 25-26.

23. Barton GE: Occupational therapy. *Trained Nurse and Hospital Review* 54 (3):135-140, 1915.

24. Bing RK: Who orginated the term "occupational therapy?" Letter to the editor. *Am J Occup Ther* 41:3, 1987.

25. Slagle EC: Occupational therapy: Recent methods and advances in the United States. *Occup Ther Rehabil* 13:289, 1934.

26. Slagle EC: Training aides for mental patients. *Arch Occup Ther* 1:13-14, 1922.

27. Slagle EC, Robeson HA: *Syllabus for Training Nurses in Occupational Therapy.* Utica, New York, State Hospital Press, 1933, p. 29.

28. Slagle EC: A year's development of occupational therapy in New York state hospitals. *Ment Hosp* 22:100, 102, 1924.

29. Kidner TJ: Occupational therapy: Its development, scope, and possibilities. *Occup Ther Rehabil* 10:3, 1931.

30. Meyer A: The psychobiological point of view. In Brady JB (Ed): *Classics in American Psychiatry.* St Louis, Warren H. Green, 1975, p. 263.

31. Leif A: *The Commonsense Psychiatry of Dr. Adolph Meyer: Fifty-Two Selected Papers.* New York, McGraw-Hill, 1948, pp. vi-xi.

32. Meyer A: The philosophy of occupation therapy. *Arch Occup Ther* 1:6 1922. (Reprinted *Am J Occup Ther* 31:10, 1977).

33. Unpublished correspondence. AOTA Archives 1914-1917, Series 1. Truman Blocker History of Medicine Collection, Moody Medical Library, The University of Texas Medical Branch at Galveston.

34. Licht S: The founding and founders of the American Occupational Therapy Association. *Am J Occup Ther* 21:269-271, 1967.

35. Historical documents. AOTA Archives 1924-1970, Series 5. Truman Blocker History of Medicine Collection, Moody Medical Library, The University of Texas Medical Branch at Galveston.

36. McDaniel M: Letter to the editor. *Am J Occup Ther* 24:517, 1970.

37. Adams JD et al: An outline of lectures on occupational therapy to medical students and physicians. *Occup Ther Rehabil* 4:277-292, 1925.

38. Spackman CS: The approach to the patient in a general hospital. Unpublished paper delivered at Tri-State Institute on Occupational Therapy, Farnhurst, NJ, March 9, 1936, pp. 3-5.

39. Gilbert ME: Occupational therapy program at Chocktaw-Chickasaw Sanitorium. *Occup Ther Rehabil* 15:110-113, 1936.

40. Sands IF: When is occupation curative? *Occup Ther Rehabil* 7:117-119, 1938.

41. Wade BD: Occupational therapy: A history of its practice in the psychiatric field. Unpublished paper delivered at the AOTA 51st annual conference, October, 1967.

42. Illinois Advisory Committee on Occupational Therapy. The basic philosophy of occupational therapy. In *The University of Illinois Faculty-Alumni Newsletter of the Chicago Professional Colleges,* 6 (4):9, 1951.

43. Robeson HA: How can occupational therapists help the social service worker? *Occup Ther Rehabil* 5 (4):279-381, 1926.

44. O'Brock I: Occupational treatment for crippled children. *Occup Ther Rehabil* 11 (3):204-205, 1932.

45. Emig MR: Fieldwork: Some experiences and observations. *Occup Ther Rehabil* 5 (2):129-130, 1926.

46. McKee N: Ethics for the occupational therapist. *Occup Ther Rehabil* 9 (6):357-360, 1930.

47. Doane JC: Occupational therapy. *Occup Ther Rehabil* 8 (1):13-14, 1929.

48. Reilly M: Occupational therapy can be one of the great ideas of 20th century medicine. *Am J Occup Ther* 26:1-2, 1962.

49. Madigan MJ, Parent LH: Preface. In Kielhofner G (Ed): *A Model of Human Occupation: Theory and Practice*. Baltimore, Williams & Wilkins, 1985, pp. 25-26.

50. Shannon PD: The derailment of occupational therapy. *Am J Occup Ther* 31:233, 1977.

51. Kielhofner G, Burke JP: The evolution of knowledge and practice in occupational therapy: Past, present, and future. In Kielhofner G (Ed): *Health Through Occupation: Theory and Practice in Occupational Therapy*. Philadelphia, FA Davis, 1983.

52. Kielhofner G (Ed): *A Model of Human Occupation: Theory and Application*. Baltimore, Williams & Wilkins, 1985.

53. Yerxa EJ et al: An introduction to occupational science, a foundation for occupational therapy in the 21st century. *Occup Ther Health Care* 6(4):3, 1989.

The COTA Heritage
PROUD, PRACTICAL, STABLE, DYNAMIC

Shirley Holland Carr, MS, LOTR, FAOTA

INTRODUCTION

This chapter is a story about the birth of the certified occupational therapy assistant (COTA). The story begins in the post-World War II era with Ruth Robinson and Marion Crampton, and later Ruth Brunyate Wiemer and Mildred Schwagmeyer. With one exception, these early participants are active retirees. Colonel Robinson's thoughts were taken from the *American Occupational Therapy Association's Visual Taped History Series*.[1] Described here are 1) the circumstances that led to the creation of the COTA, 2) the roles of some individuals who were instrumental in the development of the concept, educational training, and practice of the occupational therapy assistant, and 3) COTA accomplishments.

You are carried from the "beginnings" to your own entry into our profession, with emphasis on the early years. If you discern more anecdotes than usual, consider that while you are reading contemporary history the writer was reminiscing.

USE OF PERSONNEL BEFORE 1960

Before World War II, many registered occupational therapists (OTRs) worked in psychiatric institutions. Psychiatric hospitals often had large patient populations of between 1,000 and 6,000.[2] With a shortage of therapists, occupational therapy services often were provided by a number of aides, assistants, or technicians who were supervised by one or two occupational therapists. After 1945 and influenced by military experience, increasing numbers of therapists practiced in medical and rehabilitation settings.[3,4] This added to the already severe shortage of OTRs in psychiatric settings during and after World War II.[3,4]

Supportive personnel (OT aides and technicians) working in psychiatric facilities were valuable and valued employees, having learned the "tricks of the trade" by modeling therapist behaviors or by trial and error. In contrast to the mobility of OTRs, the employment stability of aides and technicians often made them the most knowledgeable personnel about individual patient behavior and the

ESSENTIAL VOCABULARY

Supportive personnel

Inservice training

Committee on OTAs

Grandfather clause

Guide for supervision

Career mobility

Practice settings

COTA Task Force

COTA Advisory Committee

Award of Excellence

KEY CONCEPTS

Early use of personnel and training

Role of AOTA

Educational patterns

Rights and privileges

Developmental milestones

Roster of Honor

availability of activities and equipment in a given setting. Supportive personnel knew how to do things, but lacked goal-oriented intervention methods necessary to work without immediate supervision. This deficit motivated supervisory personnel to organize courses for occupational therapy assistants.[3,5]

EARLY TRAINING NEEDS AND SHORT COURSES

Several states and the military recognized the need for **inservice training** (on-the-job educational oppurtunities) for occupational therapy personnel and developed courses of varying lengths. As early as 1944, the US Army developed a one-month course. Crampton, employed by the state of Massachusetts, developed and conducted four- and six-week courses before approval by the American Occupational Therapy Association (AOTA). Other states with early short courses were New York, Wisconsin and Pennsylvania (for activity aides).[6]

AOTA'S ROLE IN THE DEVELOPMENT OF THE COTA

The overlapping employment and Association roles of Marion Crampton, Colonel Ruth Robinson, Mildred Schwagmeyer and Ruth Brunyate Wiemer were fortuitous to the development of the COTA. Each of these women had a long-standing interest in the use of supportive occupational therapy personnel, and all but Wiemer were members of the **Committee on Occupational Therapy Assistants.**[7] This committee was delegated responsibility for all developmental aspects of the occupational therapy assistant, including needs assessment, educational program standards, new program proposal and on-site review, and program approval.[8]

In addition, members of the Committee on Occupational Therapy Assistants reviewed applications for certification under the **grandfather clause.**[9] Of 460 applications, 336 individuals became COTAs.[10] The committee also undertook the continuing education of OTRs by preparing documents and acquiring grant funds to sponsor national workshops.[8] The focus was twofold: appropriate supervision and use of COTAs.

Schwagmeyer joined the AOTA office staff,[8] and later Wiemer became president of the AOTA from 1964 to 1967, six years after Robinson's term.[11] Those four—Robinson, Crampton, Schwagmeyer, and Wiemer—"tell it best," as they were the key players in the creation and nurturing of occupational therapy assistants.

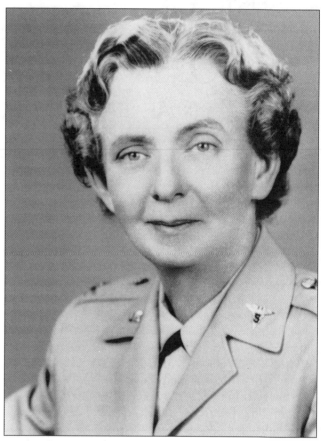

Figure 2-1. Ruth A. Robinson.

Ruth A. Robinson

Colonel Ruth A. Robinson was president of the AOTA from 1955 to 1958 (Figure 2-1). About the same time, she became Chief of the Occupational Therapy Section of the Women's (later Army) Medical Specialist Corps, and then the first Chief of the Women's (later Army) Medical Specialist Corps. Both her military and Association roles involved advocacy for the training of supportive occupational therapy personnel. She served on the Committee on Occupational Therapy Assistants from its inception, as a member, chair, and consultant.[11,12]

In an interview[1] a few years before her death in 1989, Colonel Robinson stated that she thought her greatest contribution to the occupational therapy profession was the development of the program and curriculum to train occupational therapy assistants. She also stated:

We may not realize how far advanced the occupational therapy profession was. We set a standard for other professions to follow. At first our program concentrated on the care of the psychiatric patient, just as in the early days of occupational therapy. It was frightening to some of us who felt we were not far enough advanced ourselves or secure in our own identities to be able to accept the responsibility of supervising others. We still have a long way to go. I thought the COTA ultimately would be what we thought of then as the occupational therapist, and that the COTA would be the best job in occupational therapy, leaving the OTR to do the intake work and program planning for individual patients. Recognition of the COTA through certification made me the proudest.[1]

Marion W. Crampton

Marion W. Crampton was a member of the House of Delegates, a delegate member of AOTA's Board of Management, and finally a member of the board itself (Figure 2-2). She was employed by the Massachusetts Department of Mental Health to work with the state psychiatric facilities as well as the state schools under the Division of Mental Retardation. Crampton's employment involved meeting the need for occupational therapy services in her state's institutions at a time of OTR shortages. She understood the problems and the needs of personnel with less than optimal preparation because that was her daily work. She already was involved in Massachusetts when the Committee on Occupational Therapy Assistants was formed and she was appointed chair. Crampton included "members of the loyal

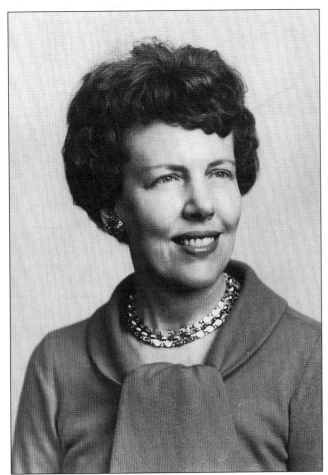

Figure 2-2. Marion W. Crampton, OTR.

opposition" as she made appointments to the committee, so all sides were heard.[6]

As noted earlier, implementation of the occupational therapy assistant program brought a deluge of applications from occupational therapy personnel seeking credentialing under the grandfather clause. She recalled, "During the two year period, applications were reviewed in a 'round robin' composed of all committee members, who worked evenings, weekends, holidays, and even vacations to process these forms."[6]

The occupational therapy assistant education program in Massachusetts was an inservice program for employed individuals with experience in occupational therapy. Crampton noted:

The first group of students thought long and hard before applying to the course, which required leaving families for a month and returning to school after many years. Exams were especially threatening, since some students had only tenth grade educations, and had school-aged children who questioned their grades.[6]

Mildred Schwagmeyer

Mildred Schwagmeyer worked in tuberculosis hospitals until recruited as assistant director of education at the AOTA national office in 1958 (Figure 2-3). Nine years later she became director of technical education, remaining in this position until 1974.[13] She became the most knowledgeable person on the subject of occupational therapy assistants at the national office and in the United States. She continued to work in occupational therapy assistant educational services through several title changes until her retirement.

In recalling those years Schwagmeyer commented:

I knew in a general way about what was going on, but not that the COTA would have a real impact on my working life. After only four months as assistant director of the education, the division became responsible for occupational therapy assistant education. I became liaison to the Committee on Occupational Therapy Assistants, which reported directly to the Board of Management. At first, occupational therapy assistants were only part of my job, but the work became increasingly time consuming, demanding, and absorbing. By the 1960's, being technical education director and working with the Committee on Occupational Therapy Assistants was a full time position.[8]

She went on to recount:

As educational programs moved from hospital-base to academic-base training, concern and discussion in-

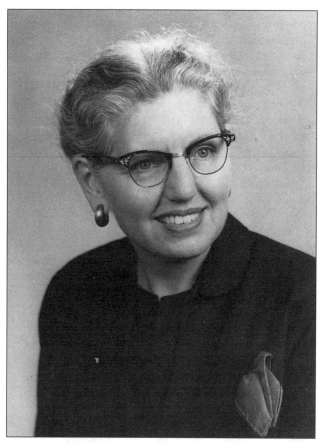

Figure 2-3. Mildred Schwagmeyer, OTR.

creased on topics such as career mobility, entry level skills, laddering, behavioral objectives, lack of appropriate textbooks and teaching aids, shortage of faculty, and over education by some programs leading to dissappointment in graduates' work experience.[8]

Five federally funded invitational workshops were held at yearly intervals between 1963 and 1968.[14] Four were attended primarily by academic and clinical faculty, and the last included an equal mix of OTRs and COTAs. Topics included role and function, COTA/OTR relationships, and supervision.[8] Excellent teaching materials came from these workshops, including a **Guide for Supervision,**[15] concepts from which are included in the 1990 document, *Supervision Guidelines for Certified Occupational Therapy Assistants.*[16] State associations were encouraged to hold meetings to disseminate information developed at the last workshop.

Schwagmeyer brought a precise use of language to her work. Among other things, she taught us that the term *certified occupational therapy assistant program* was a non sequitur. Programs are approved, but students cannot seek certification until they graduate. Even today you may sometimes hear the incorrect terminology.

After the 1964 restructuring of AOTA,[17,18] the func-

tions of the Committee on Occupational Therapy Assistants slowly were integrated into the council structure,[8] and the committee was dissolved. Seldom have so few accomplished so much.

Ruth Brunyate Wiemer

Ruth Brunyate Wiemer was employed as an occupational therapy consultant for the Maryland Department of Health and in 1964 became president of the AOTA (Figure 2-4).[11] Wiemer guided the Association through the difficult period of reorganization.[19] Of that period she said:

Communication was slow and labored, with few secretaries in the national office, or in occupational therapy departments. Flying was not common; one usually traveled by car or train. Expense accounts were unheard of, either at AOTA or on the job. Little money was available for phone, retreats, or any type of face-to-face confrontation.[20]

She continued:

Our world changed rapidly in 1965 after Medicare, with an explosion in the number of proprietary nursing homes and home health agencies. Occupa-

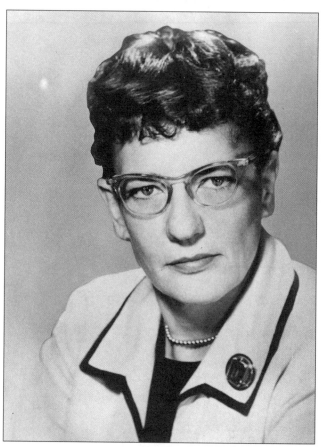

Figure 2-4. Ruth Brunyate Wiemer, OTR.

tional therapy was a small unrecognized profession without precedent for adopting such a concept (as the COTA). Nursing had supportive personnel, but were protected by licensure; we were not.[20] *For professional occupational therapists, COTAs became an added issue because of the following:*

1. *OTRs feared the unknown, especially those with no experience working with or supervising supportive personnel.*
2. *OTRs feared the AOTA was imposing the COTA on the profession.*
3. *OTRs feared giving representation to the COTA, and the consequences of COTAs voting.*
4. *Abilities of the COTA highlighted weaknesses in OTR skills such as deficits in supervisory techniques and current clinical practice, contentment in their own comfortable niche, naivety, and insufficient business acumen.*
5. *There was a lack of country-wide consensus on the appropriate role of occupational therapy, itself.*[20]

In such an environment, how then were COTAs nurtured? My belief is that the leadership came from those therapists used to hierarchical order, chain of command, and discipline, such as in the military, veterans administration, or health departments. Therapists from psychiatric settings also were familiar with working with supportive personnel.[20]

While others argued, Wiemer often seemed to be collecting her thoughts. Her responses were graceful, direct, organized, and reasoned; and they did not hide her advocacy for COTAs. She used a convincing metaphor in referring to the OTR/COTA problem: "Able seamen far outnumber captains and commodores, yet ships do not sink, and new ship forms, from sail to nuclear power, have evolved to meet man's need. So too the varied levels of our profession can be coordinated to achieve efficiency and growth."[21]

Therapists who had not stayed abreast of current clinical practice had reason to be concerned about the role of the COTA.[22] According to a 1967 "Nationally Speaking" column in the *American Journal of Occupational Therapy,* "Therapists away from current practice should be aware that what was taught fifteen years ago as functional treatment is taught to COTAs today as maintenance and supportive therapy."[23] This writer's attempt to motivate other therapists may sound harsh, but the basic premise about current practice was true.

According to Wiemer:

Change eventually came about in the profession, brought about by the advent of the COTA; these included the sharpening of the roles and functions which opened up part-time positions, increased legis-

lative efforts, and increased state licensure. A physician once asked how the occupational therapy profession had the vision to establish a subprofessional group. The profession did not; a few within it did and urged that we follow, and we did.[20]

FEELINGS OF DISTRUST

Feelings of distrust among some OTRs perodically ran high for a number of years, reigniting each time new COTA rights and privileges were initiated. The following anecdote is an example of such an emotional response in the early 1970s, when the AOTA Delegate Assembly considered **career mobility** to allow COTAs to become OTRs by fulfilling certain fieldwork requirements and passing the national certification examination for occupational therapists.[22] One evening two AOTA national office staff members spoke on the subject at a district occupational therapy meeting. Heated discussion followed the presentations as a few vocal therapists expressed concern that such legislation would directly threaten their jobs. Others disagreed, and still others sat quietly, because the hour was late and the response had become familiar. A stenotypist took notes throughout the meeting so the proceedings could be distributed to therapists statewide. Apparently to prevent such dissemination, the stenotypists tapes were "lost," but later were retrieved from a lavatory trash can. The proceedings were published,[24] the Delegate Assembly voted COTAs career mobility rights terminated in 1982,[25] and OTRs' employment was unaffected as a consequence of this or any other action pertaining to COTA rights.

"As the first COTAs practiced and practiced well at the technical level,"[20] OTRs and COTAs began building on each other's strengths, learning to identify and complement each other's skills to the betterment of the profession. As you read furthur in this and in subsequent chapters, you will see how the COTA/OTR relationship continues to mature.

OCCUPATIONAL THERAPY ASSISTANT EDUCATION

The initial short-term courses, such as those conducted under the auspices of the state hospital systems in Massachusetts, Wisconsin and New York, were inservice programs.[6] In 1961, a program in Montgomery County, Maryland, was approved in general practice to train students to practice in nursing homes.[26] The first approved program combining psychiatric and general practice was at the Duluth Vocational-Technical School in Minnesota; it also targeted student training for nursing homes.[27] Another Minnesota program at St. Mary's Junior College became the first approved two-year college program.[28] By 1966,[29] the original single-concept programs were being eliminated, and soon all students were enrolled in programs that prepared them to work in general areas of occupational therapy practice, rather than in a specialized setting.

Within the parameters set by AOTA guidelines for the number of program hours, program length remained variable depending on the academic setting, length of school day, length of fieldwork and student backgrounds. One interesting program consolidated all of the academic work into a summer. The program used the college campus and employed faculty members when the campus would otherwise be closed. All students had prior experience in occupational therapy or associated departments, or at least two years of college and experience working in a health facility. Such students had fewer professional socialization needs than typical junior college students, but received the same occupational therapy education in an eight-hour classroom day. Fieldwork was arranged when the other college students returned to campus.[30]

PRACTICE SETTINGS

As we have seen, COTAs were trained initially to work in psychiatric hospital **practice settings** and then in nursing homes and other general medical settings. Many still work in those facilities. The dispersion of COTAs into nontraditional settings came about, not because of training, but because of federal legislation.[23] Initially, Titles XVIII and XIX of P.L.89-97 (1965),[31] more commonly known as Medicare and Medicaid, opened employment in nursing homes, related facilities, and home health agencies. Other funding opened opportunities in community health and mental health centers, day care centers, and centers for the well aging. Numbers of COTAs increased at the same time some OTRs began moving from hospitals to less traditional community practice settings.[32] COTAs joined the move to community settings, sometimes in larger numbers than OTRs. Carr commented, "It may be either COTA or OTR who meanders away from traditional to new settings, but whichever goes first the other will accompany or soon follow."[24] Current employment settings for COTAs are the following:[33]

Nursing Homes and Related Facilities 20.1%
General Hospitals 18.6%
Public School Systems 14.4%
Psychiatric Facilities/Programs 8.4%
Rehabilitation Centers/Programs 8.4%

Residential Care Facilities 7.5%
Day Care Centers 4.3%
Community Mental Health Centers 3.8%
Others under 2% each 14.5%

With the passage of P.L. 94-142, The Education for All Handicapped Children Act of 1975,[34] occupational therapy personnel were recruited as a related service by public schools to assist children three through 21 years to learn skills necessary to participate in their individualized special education programs. P.L. 99-457, the Handicapped Amendments of 1986,[35] gave a direct occupational therapy role in early intervention with children from birth through two years, and COTAs and OTRs again modified their roles as they moved into schools.

As you read later in this chapter about some individual COTAs who have been singled out for honors, be aware how many have moved to nontraditional roles, some requiring OTR supervision and some not. Even in roles requiring no OTR supervision, it is observed that COTAs continue their relationships informally with their counterparts.

PRIDE IN RIGHTS AND PRIVILEGES HARD WON

The Chronology of COTA Developmental Milestones shown in Figure 2-5 chronicles hard-won rights and privileges, as well as a few not yet won. In 1980, the AOTA Executive Board formed the **COTA Task Force** to identify COTA concerns and formulate suggestions.[36,37] A year later the Task Force reported the following recommendations:[37,38]

1. Submit a resolution to the Representative Assembly to establish COTA representation. This was to include a proposal for a nationwide communication network.
2. Increase COTAs' participation on key committees and commissions and national office advisory committees.
3. Maintain a roster of COTAs qualified and interested in serving on committees at state, regional and national levels.
4. Establish "COTA Share" column in *OT Newspaper*.
5. Design COTA workshops to improve technical skills.
6. Encourage utilization of COTAs as educators in professional and technical education programs.
7. Appoint a COTA liaison in the national office.

The COTA Task Force was funded for several years[39] and then replaced by a **COTA Advisory Committee** in 1986.[40] All of the original objectives were accomplished, along with many others identified by the networking of the COTA Advisory Committee. Although a proposal to elect a COTA member-at-large in the Representative Assembly was defeated in 1982,[41] a similar measure in 1983[42] created a COTA representative with voice and vote elected by the membership. It is anticipated that when COTAs are routinely elected to the Representative Assembly from their states, such a special at-large position will be unnecessary. Two COTAs have been elected to the Representative assembly from their states, but none are currently serving.

COTAs describe the 1980s as having had two phases. In the early part, they expended their energy claiming a fair share of responsibility in the Association. Their effort paid off, and in the latter part of the decade increasing numbers of COTAs were involved in local, state and national professional activities. The maturity of the COTA group was especially obvious when the COTA Advisory Committee voluntarily withdrew the proposal to change the title of COTAs and discouraged any further action on that long-held dream because the legal and economic implications outweighed the benefits.[36]

In 1989, 21 full-time and 20 part-time COTAs were employed as faculty in technical education programs, and six full-time and 20 part-time COTAs were on faculties of professional curricula. Nine COTAs were members of state regulatory (licensure or registration) boards. Can the day be far off when COTAs are directors of educational programs?[43] Ten years ago only the visionaries among us would even have dreamed that in 1987 the American Occupational Therapy Association would change its by-laws,[44] allowing no distinction between COTAs and OTRs running for elected national office, including the office of president. Jones commented that with the labor shortage (where this chapter began), COTAs are becoming administrators, hiring OTRs as consultants and clinicians.[43]

MULTIPLYING SLOWLY

The fears of some OTRs, as outlined by Wiemer, that COTAs would become more numerous than OTRs,[20] has not yet happened. The number of COTAs has increased,[45,46] but their impact on the profession is far greater than numbers indicate. As you read the information on outstanding COTAs, compare it with the membership statistics shown in Figure 2-6 and see if you agree.

The decrease in membership from 1986 to 1988 was expected, due to a change in the method of counting after the separation of certification and membership in 1986.[45,46]

ROSTER OF HONOR

The Roster of Honor recognizes COTAs with at least five years of experience "who, with their knowledge and expertise, have made a significant contribution to the continuing education and professional development of members of the Association, and provide an incentive to contribute to the advancement of the profession."[47] Become familiar with their names so you will recognize them when you meet them (and you will). Many of the recipients also received the **Award of Excellence,**[47] which recognizes the contributions of COTAs to the advancement of occupational therapy and provides an incentive to contribute to the development and growth of the profession.

The following recipients of these honors, which the American Occupational Therapy Association bestows on COTAs, are presented here with our pride in their accomplishments:

Sally E. Ryan of Mounds View, Minnesota, received the Roster of Honor (1979) and the Award of Excellence (1976) for "outstanding achievements and contributions in education, committee work in professional organizations at affiliate and national levels, and for identifying the needs of the COTA as a membership group."[48,49] She is a member of a professional occupational therapy curriculum faculty and is both an editor and author of textbooks for occupational therapy assistant students.

Betty Cox of Baltimore, Maryland, received the Roster of Honor (1979) and the Award of Excellence (1977) for "leadership in increasing the involvement of COTAs both in the practice arena and in the Association."[48,49] Her own business offers professional seminars in health-related subjects, both nationally and internationally. She is also president of a publishing company that produces books on occupational therapy.

Terry Brittell of New Hartford, New York, received the Roster of Honor and the Award of Excellence (1979) for "outstanding contributions to occupational therapy in the areas of practice and clinical education and for service to the profession and for services to the community."[48,49] At the same psychiatric facility where he was a traditional COTA, he was the coordinator of a stress management program for employees, and of the Mental Health Players, a community prevention program based on role playing.

Charlotte Gale Seltser of Chevy Chase, Maryland, received the Roster of Honor (1981) "in recognition of her program development for the visually handicapped."[48,49] Seltser, now retired, is employed as a volunteer at the National Eye Institute of the National Institutes of Health teaching patients appropriate independence and coping skills, and referring them to community agencies.

Toné Frank Blechert of Excelsior, Minnesota, received the Roster of Honor and the Award of Excellence (1981) "in recognition of her outstanding contributions to occupational therapy in the area of occupational therapy technical education."[48,49] As a faculty member of a junior college, she teaches mental health concepts and group dynamics to occupational therapy assistant students and coordinates

1949	AOTA Board of Management discussed a proposal to the AMA for a one-year training program for "assistants" by Guy Morrow, OTR of Ohio.[50]	1974	First COTAs take certification examination as part of career mobility plan to become OTRs.[64]
1956	AOTA Board of Management approved a task force to investigate occupational therapy aides and supportive personnel.[51]	1974	COTAs get *American Journal of Occupational Therapy* as a membership benefit.[64]
1956	AOTA Board of Management changed name of Committee on Recognition of Non-professional Personnel to Committee on Recognition of OT Aides to avoid use of term "non-professional" in all correspondence. In October of the same year, the name was changed to Committee on Recognition of Occupational Therapy Assistants.[52]	1975	Award of Excellence created for COTAs.[65]
		1975	COTAs became eligible to receive the Eleanor Clarke Slagle Lectureship Award and the Award of Merit.[66]
		1976	First COTA elected member-at-large of the Executive Board.[67]
		1977	First national certification examination administered to occupational therapy assistants.[68]
		1978	Roster of Honor award established.[69]
1957	AOTA Board of Management accepted the committee's plan and agreed to implement plan in October, 1958.[53]	1979	Policy adopted that the acronym "COTA" can be used only by assistants currently certified by AOTA.[70]
1958	First *Essentials and Guidelines of an Approved Educational Program for Occupational Therapy Assistants* adopted.[53]	1980	Funding for two year (later refunded) COTA advocacy position for AOTA office.[71]
1958	Plan implemented.[53,54]	1981	COTA Task Force established.[37]
1958	Grandfather clause established.[53,54]	1981	Eight COTAs are faculty members of professional occupational therapy curricula.[65]
1959	First OT assistant education program approved at Westborough State Hospital in Massachusetts.[14]	1981	Entry-level OTR and COTA role delineations adopted.[25]
1960	336 COTAs certified through grandfather clause.[10]	1982	Career mobility plan terminated.[24]
1961	First general practice program approved at Montgomery County, Maryland.[25]	1982	"COTA Share Column" introduced in *Occupational Therapy Newspaper.*[73]
1962	First COTA directory published.[14]	1983	Representative Assembly agreed a COTA member-at-large elected to the assembly would have voice and vote.[42]
1963	Board of Management established COTA membership category.[55]		
1965	First paper authored by a COTA published in the *American Journal of Occupational Therapy.*[56]	1985	First COTA representative and alternate to serve in the Representative Assembly elected.[74]
1966	All future educational programs must prepare occupational therapy assistant students as generalists, including both psychosocial and general practice input.[28,57]	1987	AOTA Bylaws Revision allowed no distinction between COTA and OTR in running for or holding office, including president of the Association.[44]
1967	First COTA meeting held at AOTA Annual Conference.[58]	1989	Twenty-one full-time and 20 part-time COTAs employed in occupational therapy assistant education programs.[43]
1968	Eight COTAs served on various AOTA committees.[59]	1989	Six full-time and twenty part-time COTAs employed in professional occupational therapy curricula.[43]
1969	Tenth anniversary of COTAs noted in Schwagmeyer paper.[60]	1989	Nine COTAs are members of state regulatory boards.[43]
1970	Effort to change name of COTA to "associate" or "technician" failed in Delegate Assembly.[61]	1990	New guidelines for supervision of COTAs adopted by the Representative Assembly.[16]
1971	Military occupational therapy technicians eligible for certification as COTAs.[61]	1991	Treatment in Groups: A COTA Workshop was sponsored by the AOTA as the association's first continuing education program specifically for COTAs.[75]
1972	Fifth Annual COTA Workshop held in Baltimore on subject of COTA/OTR relationships.[14,62]		
1972	First book review written by COTA published in the *American Journal of Occupational Therapy.*[63]	1991	First AOTA COTA/OTR Partnership Award received by Illena Brown and Cynthia Epstein.[76]
1973	Career mobility plan endorsed by Executive Board.[3]	1992	17,000 COTAs certified by AOTCB.[77]

Figure 2-5. Chronology of COTA Developmental Milestones.

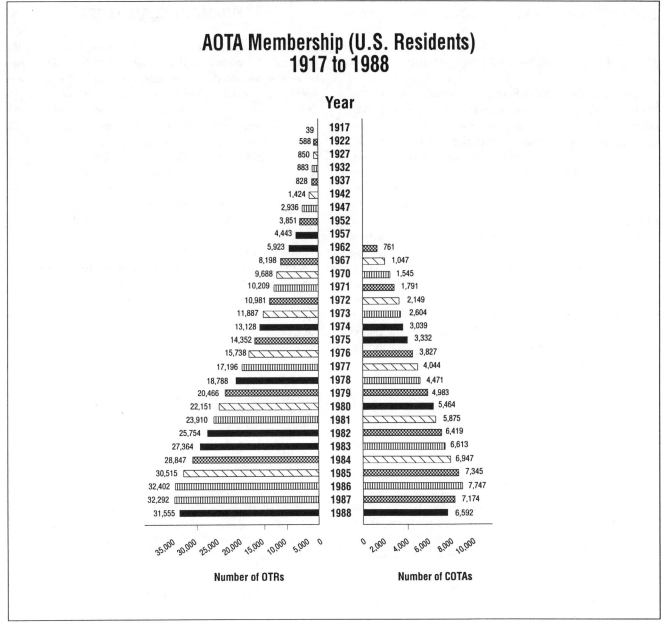

AOTA Membership (U.S. Residents) 1917 to 1988

Year

	Number of OTRs	Year	Number of COTAs
	39	1917	
	588	1922	
	850	1927	
	883	1932	
	828	1937	
	1,424	1942	
	2,936	1947	
	3,851	1952	
	4,443	1957	
	5,923	1962	761
	8,198	1967	1,047
	9,688	1970	1,545
	10,209	1971	1,791
	10,981	1972	2,149
	11,887	1973	2,604
	13,128	1974	3,039
	14,352	1975	3,332
	15,738	1976	3,827
	17,196	1977	4,044
	18,788	1978	4,471
	20,466	1979	4,983
	22,151	1980	5,464
	23,910	1981	5,875
	25,754	1982	6,419
	27,364	1983	6,613
	28,847	1984	6,947
	30,515	1985	7,345
	32,402	1986	7,747
	32,292	1987	7,174
	31,555	1988	6,592

Figure 2-6. AOTA membership statistics for OTRs and COTAs.

academic advisement for all students. She is currently pursuing a master's degree in organizational leadership.

Ilenna Brown of Plainfield, New Jersey, received the Roster of Honor (1984) for "fostering pride and pursuit of excellence for COTA practitioners."[48,49] In a 550-bed nursing facility, Brown is supervising COTA and rehabilitation coordinator for programs carried on cooperatively by occupational therapy, physical therapy and rehabilitation nursing.

Barbara Larsen of Mahtomedi, Minnesota, received the Roster of Honor (1985) for "exemplary leadership and promotion of the profession."[48,49] Larson returned to school

and is now an OTR. She is the coordinator of an industrial rehabilitation clinic and is the past president of her state association.

Patty Lynn Barnett of Birmingham, Alabama, received the Roster of Honor (1986) for "dynamic leadership in the promotion of COTAs."[48,49] Barnett is a faculty member of a university occupational therapy curriculum where she teaches activity classes and coordinates clinical education for assistant students.

Margaret S. Coffey of Russiaville, Indiana, received the Roster of Honor and Award of Excellence (1986) for "excellence in role expansion, and commitment to

COTAs."[48,49] Before becoming a COTA, she completed a master's degree. She currently cares for two toddlers, coordinates a weaver's group, and recently co-authored *Activity Analysis Handbook* with two occupational therapists.[78]

Barbara Forté of Palm Springs, California, received the Roster of Honor and the Award of Excellence (1986) because "through exemplary qualities of dedication and commitment, (she) provides outstanding leadership in local, state, and national organizations. She articulates the emerging role of COTAs and serves as a role model."[48,49] Forté has broad experience in delivering community-based clinical services and is currently employed in a private mental health facility.

Robin Jones of Chicago, Illinois, received the Roster of Honor and the Award of Excellence (1987) because she "exemplifies excellence and professionalism and is recognized as a strong COTA role model by her peers. [She is] recognized as an outstanding practitioner, teacher and advocate for occupational therapy."[48,49] Jones is the director of an independent living center, and is currently enrolled in a master's degree program in public services administration. She is vice chair of her state's licensure board.

Teri Black of Madison, Wisconsin, received the Roster of Honor and Award of Excellence (1989) for "leadership modeling for COTA-OTR professional development."[48,49] She teaches in an area technical college and practices in a nursing home. Black served two terms as chair of her state's licensure board.

Sue Byers of Gresham, Oregon, received the Roster of Honor (1989) for "exemplary role modeling for COTAs and students."[48,49] As a member of the faculty of an occupational therapy assistant education program, Byers teaches in the occupational therapy assistant education program and keeps her clinical skills sharp by working in home health.

Diane S. Hawkins of Baltimore, Maryland, received the Roster of Honor (1991) in recognition of her "significant contributions in staff development and communications." Currently, Diane is a faculty consultant for the AOTA workshop "Treatment in Groups: A Workshop for COTAs" and an associate faculty member for the Sheppard and Enoch Pratt National Center for Human Development.

ELEANOR CLARKE SLAGLE AWARD

As yet, no COTA has received the Eleanor Clarke Slagle Award, the highest honor given by the American Occupational Therapy Association to any COTA or OTR. This honor may be waiting for you or one of your peers.

SUMMARY IN ALLEGORY

Picture a young fruit tree growing well, but having the potential of producing a limited amount of fruit. On advice of well-experienced practitioners, a graft of another tree is applied to increase productivity and quality of fruit. Although tramatic to the tree and to the graft bud at first, the surgery is successful. The graft takes well, and the whole tree develops and becomes stronger than before, even stronger than it could have been if left alone to grow naturally. Now after more than 30 years, the subtle difference in a part of the tree is indistinguishable, unless you are up close or know fruit trees very well.

Editor's Note

At the request of the author, the writing style has not been modified to third person, to conform with other chapters. Rather, the terms *you* and *your* have been retained where appropriate to assist in engaging the reader in the story as it unfolds.

Acknowledgments

Marion Crampton, Mildred Schwagmeyer, and Ruth Wiemer shared their early COTA stories and allowed me to use their materials; I avow my appreciation. I also thank those who helped me document memories and flesh out the intervening years. These individuals include the thirteen "ROHers," especially Patty Barnett and Sally Ryan, Robert Bing, Bonnie Brooks, Marie Moore, Dottie Renoe, Lauren Rivet, and Ira Silvergleit. Lisa Dickey has been a patient co-proofreader, and Joel G. Swetnam has generously shared his computer graphic skills in the development of the AOTA membership figure.

Related Learning Activities

1. Identify some of the barriers to acceptance of the COTA in the profession, both historically and currently.

2. Interview at least three COTAs and three OTRs and determine what the current issues are relative to supervision. What efforts are being made to resolve the issues?

3. Write a short paper discussing how COTAs will be viewed by the profession in the next decade. What challenges will assistants face? What new roles will be assumed?

4. List some of the characteristics that contribute to a positive OTR and COTA team relationship.

5. If you had the opportunity to talk to Wiemer, Schwagmeyer or Crampton, what questions would you ask? What advice would you seek?

References

1. Cox B: *American Occupational Therapy Association's Visual Taped History: Ruth A, Robinson.* Galveston, Texas, AOTA Archives, Moody Medical Library, University of Texas Medical Branch, 1977.
2. East Louisiana State Hospital: *Historical Outline.* Jackson, Louisiana, undated.
3. Hopkins H, Smith H: *Willard and Spackman's Occupational Therapy,* 5th edition. Philadelphia, JB Lippincott, 1978.
4. Willard HS, Spackman C: *Occupational Therapy.* Philadelphia, JB Lippincott, 1947.
5. Crampton M: Educational upheaval for occupational therapy assistants. *Am J Occup Ther* 21:317-320, 1967.
6. Crampton M: Presentation at 30th anniversary COTA forum. Baltimore, 1989.
7. AOTA: Annual report, committee on occupational therapy assistants. *Am J Occup Ther* 18:45-46, 1964.
8. Schwagmeyer M: Presentation at 30th anniversary COTA forum. Baltimore, 1989.
9. AOTA: Executive director's report. *Am J Occup Ther* 13:36, 1959.
10. AOTA: Board of management, midyear meeting report. *Am J Occup Ther* 14:232, 1960.
11. AOTA: Presidents of the American Occupational Therapy Association (1917-1967). *Am J Occup Ther* 21:290-298, 1967.
12. West W: In memoriam. *Am J Occup Ther* 43:481-482, 1989.
13. M. Schwagmeyer personal correspondence to S. Carr, January 4, 1990.
14. AOTA: *Development of the Certified Occupational Therapy Assistant* undated.
15. AOTA: *Guide for Supervision,* 1967.
16. AOTA: *Supervision Guidelines for the Certified Occupational Therapy Assistant.* Representative assembly minutes, 1990.
17. AOTA: Annual business meeting report. *Am J Occup Ther* 19:33, 1965.
18. AOTA: Bylaws, October 27, 1964. *Am J Occup Ther* 19:37-41, 1965.
19. Wiemer R: AOTA conference keynote address. *Am J Occup Ther* 20:9-11, 1966.
20. Wiemer R: Presentation at 30th anniversary COTA forum. Baltimore, 1989.
21. Wiemer R: Workshop Summary. Workshop on the Training of the Occupational Therapy Assistant, Detroit, Michigan, August 2, 1964.
22. AOTA: 52nd annual conference, annual business meeting. *Am J Occup Ther* 36:808-826, 1982.
23. Carr SH: A modification of role for nursing home service. *Am J Occup Ther* 21:259-262, 1971.
24. Texas Occupational Therapy Association, Southeast District: Proceedings of meeting. October 15, 1973.
25. AOTA: 1982 representative assembly report. *Am J Occup Ther* 36:808-826, 1982.
26. Caskey V: A training program for occupational therapy assistants. *Am J Occup Ther* 15:157-159, 1961.
27. Occupational Therapy Assistant Education Program brochure. Duluth Area Vocational Technical School, Duluth, Minnesota, 1964.
28. AOTA: Board of management report. *Am J Occup Ther* 19:100, 1965.
29. AOTA: Delegate assembly minutes. *Am J Occup Ther* 20:49-53, 1966.
30. Occupational Therapy Assistant Education Program Brochure. Westminister College-William Woods College, Fulton, Missouri, 1976.
31. U.S. Senate, Committe on Finance. The Social Security Act and Related Laws. December 1978 edition. Washington DC, US Government Printing Office, 1978.
32. Carr SH: Models of manpower utilization. *Am J Occup Ther* 25:259-262, 1971.
33. AOTA: 1986 Member Data Survey. *Occup Ther News* September, 1987.
34. Education for All Handicapped Children Act (Public Law 94-142), 1975, 20 U.S.C. 1401.
35. Education of the Handicapped Act Amendments of 1986 (Public Law 99-457), 20 U.S.C. 1400.
36. AOTA: 1980 Representative assembly minutes. *Am J Occup Ther* 43:844-870, 1980.
37. AOTA: COTA task force chart of concerns. *Occup Ther News* 35:8, 1981.
38. Barnett P: COTA task force report. *Occup Ther News* 35:(August) 1981.
39. AOTA: 1983 Representative assembly minutes. *Am J Occup Ther* 37:592,1983.
40. Brittell T: AOTA COTA advisory committee final report, 1986.
41. AOTA: 1982 Representative assembly minutes. *Am J Occup Ther* 36:808-926, 1982.
42. AOTA: Representative assembly minutes. *Am J Occup Ther* 37:831-840, 1983.
43. Jones R: Presentation at 30th anniversary COTA forum, Baltimore, Maryland, 1989.
44. AOTA. Bylaws revision, 1987.
45. AOTA: Member Data Survey, 1986. (Data combined with #46).
46. AOTA: Membership Data Base, 1989. (Data combined with #45).
47. AOTA: Award Nomination Form, Roster of Honor.
48. AOTA: Annual Conference Awards Ceremony Programs, 1979 to 1989.
49. Brayley CR: AOTA awardees 1977-1988. *Occup Ther News* 2(July) 1988.
50. AOTA: Education committee report. *Am J Occup Ther* 4:221, 1949.
51. AOTA: Annual reports *Am J Occup Ther* 11:41, 1957.
52. AOTA: Committee for recognition of occupational therapy assistants. *Am J Occup Ther* 12:669-675, 1958.
53. AOTA: Annual reports. *Am J Occup Ther* 12:38, 1958.
54. West W: From the treasurer. *Am J Occup Ther* 12:31, 1958.
55. AOTA: Board of management meeting. *Am J Ocup Ther* 18:34-35,45, 1964.
56. Johnson AA: Tool holder. *Am J Occup Ther* 19:214, 1965.
57. AOTA: Annual business meeting. *Am J Occup Ther* 21:95, 1967.
58. AOTA: Annual business meeting. *Am J Occup Ther* 22:99-118, 1968.
59. AOTA: Annual business meeting. *Am J Occup Ther* 23:168-169, 1969.

60. Schwagmeyer M: The COTA today. *Am J Occup Ther* 23:69-74, 1969.

61. AOTA: Delegate assembly minutes. *Am J Occup Ther* 24:438-443, 1970.

62. AOTA: 51st conference, minutes of meeting. *Am J Occup Ther* 26:95-113, 1972.

63. Knapp RL: Activity programs for senior citizens. *Am J Occup Ther* 26:224, 1972.

64. AOTA: Delegate assembly. *Am J Occup Ther* 28:549-566, 1974.

65. AOTA: Delegate assembly, *Am J Occup Ther* 29:552-564, 1975.

66. AOTA: Guidelines for AOTA recognitions. *Am J Occup Ther* 29:632-633, 1975.

67. AOTA: Annual business meeting. *Am J Occup Ther* 31:196-203, 1977.

68. AOTA: Delegate assembly. *Am J Occup Ther* 30:576-590, 1976.

69. AOTA Annual business meeting. *Am J Occup Ther* 32:671-677, 1978.

70. AOTA: Representative assembly. *Am J Occup Ther* 33:780-813, 1979.

71. AOTA 1980 representative assembly. *Am J Occup Ther* 34:844-870, 1980.

72. AOTA: Research information division, Dataline. *Occup Ther News* 36(March) 3, 1982.

73. AOTA: 1981 representative assembly. *Am J Occup Ther* 35:792-808, 1981.

74. AOTA: Newly elected officers for 1985-1986. *Occup Ther News* 39(May) 1, 1985.

75. Robertson S: COTA workshop first of its kind. *OT Week,* March 28, 1991.

76. The Association: 1991 Awards and Recognitions Recipients *Am J Occup Ther* 45:1148, 1991.

77. Gray M: Personal communication, May 1992.

78. Lamport N, Coffey M, Hersch G: *Activity Analysis Handbook* Thorofare, New Jersey, SLACK, Inc., 1989.

Section II
CORE KNOWLEDGE

Philosophical Considerations for the Practice of Occupational Therapy

Theoretical Frameworks and Approaches

Basic Concepts of Human Development

Components of Occupation and Their Relationship to Role Performance

Occupational Performance Areas

The Teaching/Learning Process

Interpersonal Communication Skills and Applied Group Dynamics

Individualization of Occupational Therapy

Building on the historical principles outlined in the beginning of the book, Section II focuses on the core concepts of the profession. These concepts are introduced through a discussion of philosophical considerations—the values and beliefs about the nature of human existence and the nature of the profession—which serve as a guide for action. These actions are further discussed in the context of theoretical frameworks and approaches frequently used as a basis for the delivery of occupational therapy services. The core elements of human development and the components of occupation that influence role performance are also presented. Another important emphasis is the occupational performance areas of activities of daily living, work and play/leisure. Following chapters address some of the people-to-people skills necessary for effective therapeutic intervention, with emphasis placed on the teaching/learning process, interpersonal communication and applied group dynamics.

The section concludes with a discussion of the important aspects of the individualization of occupational therapy, stressing such factors as environment, sociocultural considerations, change and prevention.

Consideration of the unique needs of the whole person is a prevailing theme throughout this segment. As Witherspoon stresses in regard to the profession: "[we] assist individuals in adapting to society, in assuming their occupational roles, in receiving gratification, and in reaching their full potential."

Philosophical Considerations

FOR THE PRACTICE OF OCCUPATIONAL THERAPY

Phillip D. Shannon, MA, MPA

INTRODUCTION

A vital aspect of the educational preparation of the occupational therapy assistant is an appreciation of the philosophy on which the practice of occupational therapy is based. Why is this so vital? There are at least four reasons that provide a rationale.

First, the philosophy of any profession represents the profession's views on the nature of existence. These views reflect the reasons for its own existence in responding to the needs of the population served. For example, a somewhat complex question addressed in philosophy is: "What is man?" Is man a physical being, a psychological being, a social being, or all of these? If man is perceived by a profession as a physical being only, then in responding to the needs of "man the patient" the action is quite clear: the practitioner deals only with the body, not with the mind. As incon-

ceivable as this particular belief might appear, the practices of some professions reflect a narrow perspective of man. Sometimes, as it will be discussed later, a profession does not practice what it believes.

Guided by its philosophical beliefs, a grand design evolves to specify the purposes or goals of the profession. Lacking an understanding of the philosophical basis for this grand design, the practitioner cannot be sure that the goals he or she is pursuing are worth pursuing or that the services provided are worth providing.

A second reason for understanding the philosophy of the profession is that philosophy guides action. Indeed, it is only within the context of a profession's philosophy that actions have meaning. Attending to the leisure needs of the patient, for instance, is one of the major concerns of occupational therapy, because its practitioners believe that man seeks a sense of quality to life. One aspect of a **quality**

KEY CONCEPTS

Rationale for philosophy

Metaphysical principles

Epistemological principles

Axiological principles

Philosophy of Adolph Meyer

Therapist/patient versus therapist/client relationship

life, like a satisfying work life, is a satisfying leisure life. Consequently, using arts and crafts to promote the leisure interests and skills of the patient and, therefore, the quality of life of the patient, is an action that makes sense because the action has philosophical meaning.

One of the primary reasons for studying philosophy, according to Thomas, is to clarify beliefs so that the action "which stems from those beliefs is sound and consistent."[1] Clarifying the beliefs of the profession should be regarded as a critical component of the occupational therapy assistant's education to ensure that his or her actions are sound and consistent; that is, that the occupational therapy assistant's entry-level behaviors are based on and consistent with a set of guiding philosophical beliefs.

A third rationale for understanding the philosophy of occupational therapy is the direct relationship between the growth of the profession and the ability of its practitioners to explain their "reasons for existence." In the present era of accountability, where the justification for programs and the competition for resources to support these programs is greater than in previous years, one cannot assume that those external to the profession, such as physicians, will perceive occupational therapy as an intrinsically good or essential service. Claims of goodness must be substantiated with evidence. That evidence must be supported philosophically, otherwise it will lack a context for its interpretation. For example, documented evidence that a patient's range of motion in the left elbow was increased by five degrees as a result of occupational therapy's intervention is important. What strengthens this evidence, however, are the reasons for intervening in the first place. These reasons are linked to the philosophical beliefs of the profession.

Finally, it is not sufficient for the occupational therapy assistant to be skilled in applying the techniques of the profession. On the contrary, he or she must have some appreciation, philosophical and theoretical, of the reasons why these techniques are applied. Lacking this appreciation, the occupational therapy assistant will apply these techniques without being able to communicate their value to the patient, thereby failing to motivate the patient's active involvement in treatment.

Certainly from the initial stage of patient referral to the last stage of discontinuing the patient's treatment, the philosophical beliefs of the profession must remain in the foreground. For the occupational therapy assistant, who has major responsibilities along the entire continuum of health care, these beliefs and the actions that stem from them must be understood and practiced. Indeed, this is the first duty of the occupational therapy assistant.

WHAT IS PHILOSOPHY?

To appreciate fully the philosophy of occupational therapy, one must appreciate and understand philosophy in general. Basically, philosophy is concerned with the "meaning of human life, and the significance of the world in which man finds himself."[2] Man is, by nature, a philosophical creature. Questions such as who am I?, what is my destiny?, and what do I want from life? are questions of meaning and purpose that concern all human beings. Each individual, in responding to questions such as these, develops a personalized view of oneself and the world, commonly referred to as a **"philosophy of life."** This philosophy represents a fundamental set of values, beliefs, truths and principles that guide the person's behavior from day to day and from year to year.

The philosophy of a profession also represents a set of values, beliefs, truths and principles that guides the actions of the profession's practitioners. Typically, as with individuals, the philosophy evolves over time and sometimes changes as a profession matures. Each profession, in shaping and reshaping its philosophy, has choices to make in three philosophical dimensions. These include metaphysics, epistemology and axiology.

Metaphysics

Metaphysics is concerned with questions about the ultimate nature of things, including the nature of man. With regard to the nature of man in particular, the **mind/body relationship** is of special interest to the philosopher. Are mind and body two separate entities, one superior to the other, or are mind and body a single entity representative of the "whole"—the whole person? The first position, that of mind/body separation, is the **dualistic** position. The second position, that of mind/body as one entity, is the position of **holism.**

While most (if not all) professions claim to be holistic, the truth in this claim is seen to the extent to which the actions of the profession are consistent with its beliefs. Assume, for example, that the actions of "profession X" are directed toward exercise as the means for promoting a healthy body, (ie, a healthy "physical" body). Assume also that profession X claims to be holistic, asserting a concern for the whole person. In actuality it is dualistic because the body is viewed as superior to the mind; the goal of exercise, in this case, is a healthy body, not a healthy body and a healthy mind. There is a contradiction, therefore, in what profession X believes and what it does. Its actions do not follow from its beliefs, and the claim of holism is illegitimate. When exercise is seen as promoting the health of the "whole," a more holistic approach is demonstrated.

Epistemology

The second dimension pertinent to shaping and reshaping the philosophy of a profession is the dimension of epistemology, which is concerned with questions of truth. What is truth? How do we come to know things? How do we know that we know? One way of knowing is by experience. One knows, for example, that the flame of a fire brings pleasure in terms of the warmth it provides, but also that it produces pain if it is touched by the bare hand. Usually, one only needs to experience this pain once to "know that he or she knows." Is experience the only route to truth or knowing? From a holistic perspective, there are many routes to truth and knowing. Intuition, for instance, is considered to be as truthful as experiential learning or the logic reasoned by the powers of the intellect. For the dualist, on the other hand, the subjective realities of intuition and experience cannot be accepted as truths. On the contrary, only the objective reality of rational thought can be admitted as truth; truth is logic.

Axiology

The third dimension of philosophy is axiology, which is concerned with the study of values. Two types of questions are addressed by axiology: questions of value with regard to what is desirable or beautiful in the world (aesthetics), and questions of value with regard to the standards or rules for right conduct, or **ethics.** Most people would agree that a long life is a desirable thing—something that is valued. Some people might argue that a long life without a sense of quality to one's life is a life that is not worth living. Almost everyone would maintain that it is wrong to take a life, yet, there are those who believe that "a life for a life," might be justified in some instances.

Conflicting values and standards often produce dilemmas that are difficult to resolve. If life is valued, for example, is it right or moral to disconnect the support systems maintaining the life of the person who has been certified as "brain dead?" Is it right or moral to prolong a life that may not be a life worth living? These are difficult questions of value about what is desirable or beautiful in the world and about the standards that will be applied in pursuing that which is valued.

Each profession has choices to make about what it considers beautiful and desirable in the world and the ethical principles that it will follow in achieving its goals. For medicine, the preservation of life is the first priority, and perhaps this is as it should be, for medicine. But, is this the highest priority of the other health care professions? Should it be the highest priority? A profession that claims to be holistic cannot be satisfied with saving lives. Instead, a holistic profession would maintain that a life worth saving must be a life worth living.

Given this brief glimpse of metaphysics, epistemology and axiology, each dimension can be discussed as it relates to the philosophy of occupational therapy. Specifically, four questions will be addressed:

1. The metaphysical question of "what is man?"
2. The epistemologic question of "how does man know what he knows?"
3. The aesthetic question of "what is beautiful or desirable in the world?"
4. The ethical question of "what are the rules of right conduct?"

Two approaches will be taken in responding to these questions. First, the philosophy of Adolph Meyer, who was primarily responsible for providing occupational therapy with a philosophical foundation for practice, will be examined. Second, the extent to which this philosophical base has survived the test of time will be explored.

THE EVOLUTION OF OCCUPATIONAL THERAPY

Occupational therapy evolved from the moral treatment movement that began in the early 19th century.[3] If there was a single purpose to which the champions of this movement were committed, it was to humanize and to provide more humane forms of treatment for the mentally ill incarcerated in the large asylums in this country and abroad. Marching under the banner of humanism, the leaders of this movement sought to defend and preserve the dignity of all human beings, particularly the sick and the disabled.

Among these humanists who carried the movement into the 20th century was the psychiatrist Adolph Meyer (Figure 3-1), whose paper on "The Philosophy of Occupation Therapy"[4] laid the foundation for the practice and promotion of occupational therapy. Meyer's philosophy was based on his observations of everyday living. From his beliefs about the nature of man, about life, and about a life worth living, the pioneers of the profession emerged to chart its course. Although Meyer has been quoted frequently in the literature of recent years, a more extensive discussion of his philosophy is provided here because, to date, his thoughts have not been examined within the context of metaphysics, epistemology, and axiology.

A Retrospective Glance at the Philosophy of Adolph Meyer

What is Man? Meyer's perspective of man was holistic:

Our body is not merely so many pounds of flesh and bone figuring as a machine, with an abstract mind or

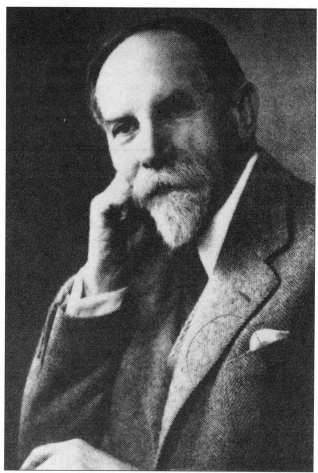

Figure 3-1. Dr. Adolph Meyer, psychiatrist and early occupational therapy proponent and philosopher (Fabian Bachrach Photo). Courtesy of the Archives of the American Psychiatric Association.

soul added to it. (Rather it is a live organism acting) in harmony with its own nature and the nature about it.[4]

For Meyer, three characteristics distinguished man from all other organisms: sense of time, capacity for imagination, and need for occupation.

A sense of time—past, present and future—was the central theme of Meyer's philosophy. He believed that a sense of time, and particularly time past, (experience) provides man with an advantage over other living organisms in terms of adapting in the present and manipulating the future. This capacity to learn from experience, when blended with the capacity for imagination or creativity, allows man to alter his environment. The squirrel, for example, is totally dependent on its environment for food and shelter during the winter months. Man, on the other hand, through experience and imagination, has been able to alter his environment to ensure survival from hunger through food preservation techniques and protection from the cold via heat-producing systems.

The need for occupation was regarded by Meyer as a distinctly human characteristic. He defined occupation as

"any form of helpful enjoyment,"[4] which clearly transcends the notion of occupation as being limited to work. On the contrary, the meaning of occupation was extended by Meyer to include all of those activities that comprise a normal day, particularly work and play. He considered occupation important to all, the sick as well as the healthy. Each individual must achieve a balance among his occupations, a balanced life of not only work and play, but also of rest and sleep.[4]

How Does Man Know That He Knows? Man learns not only by experience, but also by **"doing"**: engaging mind and body in occupation. By doing, man is able to achieve. Fidler and Fidler, in reiterating this theme in the 1970s, maintained that doing is linked to becoming, to realizing one's potential.[5] Fundamental to achieving and becoming is doing. In doing, man comes to know about himself and the world. In doing, man knows that he knows.

What is Desirable or Beautiful in the World? For Meyer, man is not content simply existing in the world. Instead, man seeks a sense of quality to life that comes from the pleasure in achievement.[4] It is in engaging the total self that man comes to experience the pleasure in achievement, which Reilly, in her Eleanor Clarke Slagle lectureship, articulated so beautifully: "That man, through the use of his hands as they are energized by mind and will, can influence the state of his own health."[6] Again, it is in doing that man achieves and is able to acquire a sense of quality in his life.

What are the Rules of Right Conduct? Meyer, in outlining the guiding principles for the practice of occupational therapy, maintained that the occupation worker should provide **opportunities**, not **prescriptions**.[4] Prescriptions tend to constrain the development of one's potential, whereas opportunities nourish it. To apply prescriptions is to treat the patient as an object; to offer opportunities is to regard the patient as a person. Inherent in this principle of right conduct is a belief in the type of relationship that the occupation worker should maintain with the patient—a helping relationship, a caring relationship, a relationship where patients are indeed treated as persons and not as objects.

To summarize, Meyer's perspective of man was holistic. He emphasized doing as the primary route to truth and to achieving a sense of quality in one's life. Prerequisite to doing, however, is opportunity. Lacking the opportunity to do, man, like the squirrel, cannot control his own destiny. On the contrary, man becomes the squirrel, controlled and manipulated by his environment.

The Test of Time

Has the philosophy of Adolph Meyer, which provided the direction for the practice and promotion of occupational therapy, survived the test of time; or has the profession, as it matured, changed its direction, based on a different set of values, beliefs, truths, and principles? The answer is reflected in the report to the American Occupational Therapy Association on the Project to Identify the Philosophical Base of Occupational Therapy, which was submitted to the Executive Board of the AOTA in 1983.[7] This report does not represent "an official position" of the AOTA with regard to the philosophy of occupational therapy, but it is the documentation of a six and one-half-year project designed to trace the philosophical beliefs of the profession historically and to interpret those beliefs within the context of more modern times. In reviewing the degree to which the beliefs of Adolph Meyer have withstood the test of time, the four philosophical questions addressed earlier are once again discussed in the following sections.

What is Man? The belief in holism has persisted in the profession.[7] Indeed, one of the unique aspects of occupational therapy is its integrating function, where mind and body are activated to promote the patient's total involvement in the treatment process. To lose sight of this function is to lose sight of one of the major contributions of occupational therapy—attending to the "whole person."

One might speculate that it is the profession's commitment to holism that has attracted people to occupational therapy rather than to some of the other health professions that appear less holistic. Even in occupational therapy, however, the concept of holism, although universally professed, is not uniformly applied in practice. Action is not always consistent with belief. When practice takes the form of dealing only with the mind, only with the body, or worse yet, with only parts of the body, the commitment to holism has been compromised; and there is a contradiction between what one believes and what one does.

For example, hand rehabilitation has become a highly specialized area of practice. Unquestionably, there is a significant contribution to be made to health care in this area. However, when some of the practitioners in rehabilitation begin to refer to themselves as "hand therapists" versus "occupational therapists," there is an implicit shift away from holism. The belief in holism may remain, but the explicit actions that follow are sometimes not holistic. Only when hand rehabilitation focuses on the whole person does it retain its holistic function.

Another contradiction between belief and action is in mental health practice. Probably one of the first signs indicating the shift away from holism in mental health is when the practitioner uses the title "psychiatric occupational therapist" or "psychiatric occupational therapy assistant." "Psychiatric occupational therapy" personnel tend to focus only on the mind of the patient to the exclusion of the patient's body. Furthermore, when the practitioner's actions are directed primarily toward the unconscious mind, as in providing activities for the sublimation of innate drives,

attention is not even focused on the whole mind, much less the mind and body. Again the belief in holism may be contradicted by the practitioner's actions.

Surely these examples are not characteristic of most practitioners in mental health; nor is "hand therapy" necessarily limited to the treatment of the hand. However, when the broad concerns of occupational therapy are narrowed, the patient is somehow cheated in the process.

Also surviving the test of time is the belief in Meyer's distinguishing characteristics of man. Indeed, in responding to the needs of "man the patient," occupational therapy has placed a high priority on time as a continuum in the life of a patient, designing programs of treatment within the context of the patient's past, present and future. In implementing these programs, the patient's capacity for imagination or creativity is challenged in the interest of serving the need for occupation.

Occupation, as defined in the report from the AOTA Project to Identify the Philosophical Base of Occupational Therapy, is "goal-directed behavior aimed at the development of play, work and life skills for optimal time management."[7] If, as Reilly proposed, man's need for occupation is "that vital need of man served by occupational therapy,"[6] then to reduce the concept of occupation to the level of exercising bodily parts with weights and pulleys, or to the level of occupying the patient's mind with activities that bear little or no relationship to the nature of his or her occupation, is to deny this vital need. In addition, another unique aspect of the profession is somehow lost in the transformation of belief into action.

In contrast, by drawing on the patient's past experiences in work and play and in exploring the patient's values, capacities, and interests, the therapist should provide experiences that will serve the patient's need for occupation. In addition, in tapping the creative potential of the patient in areas such as problem solving and decision making, the therapist can expand the patient's capacities for altering the environment, thereby, expanding the potential for adapting in the present and for controlling his or her own destiny into the future.

How Does Man Know That He Knows? From the beginning, occupational therapy has believed in the active versus the passive involvement of the patient in treatment, that is, in doing. As Meyer believed, however, doing is but one way of knowing. There are multiple routes to truth— experience, thinking, feeling and doing—which the modern-day practitioner also accepts as reality.[7] One knows, for example, what happiness means because it has been experienced and because it can be felt. Happiness cannot be measured, but this does not make it any less real.

Among the many ways of knowing, doing is emphasized in the profession as the means for acquiring the skills for daily living and knowing one's capabilities in the present and one's potential for the future. Here again, the opportunities for doing must be framed within the context of the whole person. Consider, for example, the active engagement of the patient in sensory-integration activities. One of the major reasons for involving a patient in this type of activity is that the ability to receive and process sensory information is one way of knowing. For example, one knows that it is cold, and, therefore, that the body should be protected with warm clothing because one is able to feel cold, process this input, and take the appropriate steps to protect oneself.

Lacking the ability to process sensory information, the person is denied an important, if not critical, source of information. In this case, doing, in the form of involving the individual in sensory-integration activities, is an important step in the process of knowing. On the other hand, if the patient benefits from involvement in occupational therapy are limited to those derived by applying the techniques of sensory-integration, then occupational therapy has not served its holistic function; nor has it served the patient's need for occupation.

The practitioner takes a step away from this belief in doing when the action of "having the patient do" is replaced with the action of "doing to the patient." Another unique aspect of occupational therapy is obscured when the patient is denied the opportunity for doing.

What is Desirable or Beautiful in the World? To subsist, according to Meyer, is not enough for man. Man seeks something beyond subsistence or survival: the "good life," a life of quality. In maintaining this position over the years, occupational therapy has focused its attention in two directions, minimizing the deficits and maximizing the strengths of the patient.[7] Attending to one without attending to the other is incomplete and insufficient if the goals go beyond mere survival.

Traditionally, occupational therapy has minimized its contribution to the survival aspects of care and maximized its role in promoting a life of quality for its patients. Perhaps this is as it should be, perhaps not. Perhaps it is a matter of interpretation, that is, how one defines survival in terms of whether or not this position is legitimate. Consider, for example, the patient who has not learned the techniques of wheelchair mobility. This individual will not survive, at least not as a self-sufficient being. Consider also the patient who cannot dress him- or herself and is unable to organize time to meet the demands of daily living. This patient will not survive with any degree of autonomy or self-respect. Furthermore, as Shannon stated, "bodies and minds that are not active will atrophy from disuse, they will die. Also, people who lack quality in their lives sometimes engage in self-destructive behaviors, such as alcoholism, that lead to deterioration and death."[8] Does occupational therapy contribute to the preservation of life? Surely, as these examples suggest, occupational therapy contributes to the survival of the patient directly, if survival is interpreted to mean the ability to care for self, and indirectly, by adding a sense of quality to the lives of those served by the profession.

Reilly stated that "the first duty of an organism is to be alive; the second duty is to grow and be productive."[6] If survival is the first priority of the organism, then perhaps the position of the profession can be strengthened by developing an argument for the practice and promotion of occupational therapy that includes a commitment to the survival of the patient, as well as to the quality of his or her life.[8] In developing this argument, it must be made clear that the first priority of the profession is to teach the patient skills that will ensure survival. The second priority is to guide the patient toward the realization of his or her potential and social worth as a member of society, as evidenced, according to Heard, by the ability to perform an **occupational role**.[9] Indeed, it is for these reasons that man engages in occupation; it is also for these reasons that occupational therapy exists.

Occupational therapy has expressed its commitment to the second priority, but its actions are often directed to the first.[7,8] As Heard maintained, it is in addressing the second priority, and particularly the social worth of the patient, that occupational therapy has been most negligent.[9] Yet, in attending to the social worth of the patient, the profession is making a major contribution to a more healthy society. Certainly, in making this contribution, as Yerxa argued that it must,[10] the profession's value is increased and its survival guaranteed.

What are the Rules of Right Conduct? Meyer's principle of providing opportunities, not prescriptions, for patients has been one of the distinguishing characteristics of the profession. In applying the rule of non-prescription, the patient becomes an active partner in treatment. Why is this important?

First, the skills and habits necessary for the performance of occupational roles cannot be administered to the patient, but must be acquired by the patient. Second, prescriptions tend to foster pawnlike behaviors (externally controlled), whereas opportunities encourage origin-like behaviors (internally controlled), as defined by Burke.[11] In applying prescriptions, the patient is treated as a pawn, externally controlled by those responsible for his or her care; in offering opportunities, the patient is treated as origin, drawing upon the strengths within him- or herself to assume control for his or her own life. If taking charge of one's own life is important and assuming control for one's own destiny is valued, providing opportunities and not prescriptions is a necessary first step.

In offering opportunities for patients to take charge of their own lives, two major ethical principles guide the actions of the practitioner. The first of these is the principle *nonmaleficence*, which states that not only should one do no

Table 3-1
Summary of Philosophical Beliefs, Principles and Contradictory Practices

Philosophical Beliefs	Principles for Practice	Beliefs/Principles Compromised
Metaphysical Position		
The belief in holism, in mind and body as one entity	Attending to the whole person	Attending only to the mind or only to the body or parts of the body
The belief in the uniqueness of or in man's distinctly human qualities, which include an appreciation of time, past, present and future	Designing intervention programs within the context of the patient's past, present and future	Attending to the present needs of the patient without considering the patient's past experiences and goals for the future
The capacity for imagination	Challenging the patient's capacity for imagination or creativity	Providing prescriptions versus opportunities
The need for occupation	Promoting a balanced life of work, play, rest and sleep	Placing an emphasis on the treatment of pathology to the extent that the acquisition of skills that will support occupational role is minimized or ignored
Epistemologic Position		
The belief that there is not just one, but many routes to knowing or learning	Valuing experience, thinking and feeling in the process of doing en route to knowing or learning	Treating the patient as a passive versus active participant during the process of intervention
Axiologic Position— **The Aesthetic Component**		
The belief that man seeks a life beyond subsistence, a life of quality	The first principle: teaching survival skills by minimizing deficits and maximizing strengths	Teaching survival skills without attending to the patient's potential beyond survival and to the patient's social worth
	The second principle: providing opportunities for achievement, for the realization of one's potential and one's social worth	
Axiologic Position— **The Ethical Component**		
The humanistic belief that patients should be treated as persons, not objects	Protecting the patient from harm; promoting good	Neglecting the patient's safety or security needs and/or failing to protect the patient's rights as a patient and as a human being
	Demonstrating kindness and caring	Promoting a therapist-client versus therapist-patient relationship
	Providing opportunities versus prescriptions	Applying remedies that discourage individual initiative

harm, but also that one should promote the good. The second is the principle of *beneficence,* or the rule that one should show kindness and caring.[12] Perhaps no profession can lay greater claim to applying these principles than occupational therapy. The principle of showing kindness and caring, however, raises the issue of patient versus client.

Which is more legitimate: a therapist-client relationship or a therapist-patient relationship?

In a therapist-client relationship, the client is perceived as an object, an "it," because only one aspect of the client becomes the focus of attention. The therapist-client relationship is similar to that of a used car salesperson who has only one goal: to sell the client a used car regardless of whether the client can afford gasoline to operate the car, or whether the client has the financial resources to insure and maintain it.

In a therapist-patient relationship the patient is perceived not as an object, but as a person. Patients expect that their total well-being will be improved when seeking health care. Reilly argues that there is a special bond in the therapist-patient relationship, similar to the bonding relationship of teacher-student, that is not present in a therapist-client relationship. Like teacher-student, the therapist-patient relationship is reciprocal, one involving mutual loyalties, obligations and caring.[13]

Over the years occupational therapy has prided itself on the fact that it cares. In caring about its patients, the profession has demonstrated that it is holistic and humanistic. If a different type of caring evolves, as implied by the use of the term "client," then any future claim of being a holistic, humanistic enterprise will have to be denied.

SUMMARY

The philosophical beliefs guiding the contemporary practice of occupational therapy can be traced to Adolph Meyer, whose philosophy of *occupation therapy* was framed within the context of metaphysics, epistemology and axiology. Meyer's philosophy was both holistic and humanistic. As it persists in the present to guide the actions of the occupational therapy practitioner, so will it persist in the future to provide direction for the profession as it continues to mature.

The philosophical beliefs identified in this chapter and the principles for practice that evolved from these philosophical beliefs are summarized in Table 3-1, which also contains descriptions of situations when these beliefs and principles are compromised. The COTA owes allegiance to these beliefs and principles when responding to the needs of those served by the profession.

Editor's Note

In the context of this chapter, the term "man," in the philosophical sense, refers to the generic term "mankind," which is considered standard and gender inclusive.

Related Learning Activities

1. The author cited several ways in which occupational therapy practitioners fail to retain a holistic approach to rehabilitation. Outline how occupational therapy personnel in a physical dysfunction setting and in a psychosocial dysfunction setting would proceed with evaluation and treatment applying a holistic approach.

2. Reilly, Heard and Yerxa were cited regarding whether the profession of occupational therapy should be concerned with survival or with quality of life. What are the pros and cons of each position? What are the implications of each course of action?

3. Make a list of your basic beliefs about occupational therapy. Compare and discuss your list with a classmate or peer.

4. List at least four reasons why it is important for COTAs to be able to communicate the philosophy on which the profession of occupational therapy is based.

5. Discuss the following questions with a peer: According to Meyer, what three characteristics distinguish man from all other organisms? What are the implications for occupational therapy practice?

References

1. Thomas CE: *Sport in a Philosophic Context.* Philadelphia, Lea and Febiger, 1983, p. 19.
2. Randall JH, Buchler J: *Philosophy: An Introduction.* New York, Barnes and Noble, Inc., 1960, p. 5.
3. Bockhoven JS: Legacy of moral treatment 1800's to 1910. *Am J Occup Ther* 25:223-225, 1971.
4. Meyer A: The philosophy of occupation therapy. *Am J Occup Ther* 31:639-642, 1977.
5. Fidler GS, Fidler JW: Doing and becoming: Purposeful action and self-actualization. *Am J Occup Ther* 32:305-310, 1978.
6. Reilly M: Occupational therapy can be one of the great ideas of 20th century medicine. *Am J Occup Ther* 16:1-9, 1962.
7. Shannon PD: Report on the AOTA Project to Identify the Philosophical Base of Occupational Therapy. January, 1983. Condensed under the title: *Toward a Philosophy of Occupational Therapy.* August, 1983.
8. Shannon PD: From another perspective: An overview of the issue on the roles of occupational therapists in continuity of care. *Occup Ther Health Care* 2:3-11, 1985.
9. Heard C: Occupational role acquisition: A perspective on the chronically disabled. *Am J Occup Ther* 31:243-247, 1977.
10. Yerxa E: The philosophical base of occupational therapy. In *Occupational Therapy: 2001 AD.* Rockville, Maryland, American Occupational Therapy Association, 1979, pp. 26-30.
11. Burke JP: A clinical perspective on motivation: Pawn versus origin. *Am J Occup Ther* 31:254-258, 1977.
12. Beauchamp TL, Childress JF: *Principles of Biomedical Ethics.* New York, Oxford University Press, 1983, pp. 106-107, 148.
13. Reilly M: The importance of the patient versus client issue for occupational therapy. *Am J Occup Ther* 6:404-406, 1984.

Theoretical Frameworks and Approaches

M. Jeanne Madigan, EdD, OTR, FAOTA
Sally E. Ryan, COTA, ROH

INTRODUCTION

Confusion about the terminology related to theory has been reflected in the occupational therapy literature. Terms that have been used by occupational therapy personnel include *theory, paradigm, model of practice, frame of reference, and conceptual framework.* These terms have been used very specifically by some to differentiate levels of theory development, whereas others have used the terms loosely and interchangeably.

This chapter emphasizes the term *theoretical frameworks,* which is defined as the interrelated set of ideas that provide a way to conceptualize the fundamental principles and applications inherent in the practice of occupational therapy. The reader should note that some theoretical frameworks are more fully developed than others.

In addition, some are much more general, allowing application in many areas of practice with a variety of patients, whereas others are more appropriate to specific populations and conditions. The chapter is organized based on this fact with the more general theoretical frameworks presented in the beginning. With this understanding, the purposes of this chapter are twofold: to indicate why the consideration of theoretical frameworks is important and to introduce the occupational therapy assistant student and practitioner to a variety of theoretical frameworks proposed and used by members of the profession.

Parham[1] has pointed out that theory is critically important for occupational therapy to be recognized as a profession and valued as a unique and necessary service to patients. She indicated that theory provides reasons

KEY CONCEPTS

Occupational behavior

Model of human occupation

Adaptive responses

Facilitating growth and development

Doing and becoming: purposeful action

Mosey's four frameworks

Sensory integration

Spatiotemporal adaptation

Neuromotor approaches

Cognitive disabilities model

for making decisions and taking actions in regard to patients. Theory is also the key to systematic research and increased development of a knowledge base.

When one engages in theory-based practice, one selects certain things to consider when evaluating patients and determining goals and the methods to accomplish those goals.

Parham[1] has stated that theory helps us "set the problem" (by identifying the appropriate problem to solve) and "solve the problem" (by applying the appropriate procedures for intervention). Sands[2] indicated that *setting the problem* is the responsibility of the occupational therapist, but that the COTA collaborates with the OTR in *solving the problem*. This approach indicates that both must have some knowledge of the theoretical foundations for practice, although at different levels of understanding.

This chapter focuses on some of the more well-known and used theoretical frameworks proposed by occupational therapists. Basic information is provided to acquaint the reader with primary principles, concepts and applications. The reference and bibliographic listings should be used for more in-depth study.

OCCUPATIONAL BEHAVIOR

In her Eleanor Clarke Slagle address, Mary Reilly concluded "that man, through the use of his hands, as they are energized by mind and will, can influence the state of his own health."[3] This hypothesis was formulated from her examination of the heritage of our founders. She returned to the principles of moral treatment and the concepts of health-restoring properties of occupation; habit training; and a balance of work, play, rest, and sleep, proposed by Adolph Meyer, Eleanor Clarke Slagle, Louis Haas, Susan B. Tracy, George Barton, and other founders of the profession (see Chapter 1).

Using these basic ideas and borrowing related concepts from many other disciplines, she built her framework, which emphasizes the critical importance of occupation to the well-being of the individual—that each person has a need to master his or her environment, to alter and improve it. She stated that the goal of occupational therapy is "to encourage active, open encounter with the tasks which would reasonably belong to (one's) role in life"[3] and the occupational therapy clinic is a "laboratory setting for human productivity."[3] According to this framework, occupational therapy practice is based on the assumption that "the mind and will of man are occupied through central nervous system action and that man can and should be involved consciously in problem solving and creative activity."[3] Reilly defined the developmental continuum of play and work as occupational behavior. She proposed that this definition should be the

unifying concept around which occupational therapists could build a body of knowledge to support practice in all areas of the profession and to guide education and research.

Using a psychiatric occupational therapy clinic as a proving ground for her ideas, Reilly examined life roles relative to community adaptation and to identify various skills that would support these roles. She then built a milieu to encourage competency, arouse curiosity, and develop appropriate skills and habits. Patients' daily living was to be balanced among work, play and rest at appropriate times and with opportunities for decision making. Occupation, therefore, would become the integrating factor for improving patient behavior.[4]

During the 1960s and the 1970s, Reilly and her students at the University of Southern California researched, discussed and refined the various concepts that became the occupational behavior body of knowledge. Since reduction of disease does not necessarily lead to improved function and increased engagement in activity, the purpose of occupational therapy was "to prevent and reduce the incapacities resulting from illness" and to "activate the residual adaptation forces within the patient."[5] Occupational therapy's focus was the patients' achievement and the ability to carry on the daily activities required by their social roles. It was proposed that the achievement drive generates interests, abilities, skills and habits of competition and cooperation. The environment for this was engagement in play and work (occupational behavior). Play was seen as both preparatory and facility to work, oftentimes offering support to a work pattern through the application of adaptive skills learned through play activities.

Temporal adaptation was also considered to be an important element. How one occupies time and the appropriate balance of activities within specific and general time frames was considered a sign of one's ability to adapt.[6] According to Reilly, organization of time and behavior to carry out one's roles was necessary and involved a complex process that follows a ranked system (in ascending order), which moves from *rules* to *skills* to *roles*.[7]

Evaluation was viewed as identifying role-function problems. Treatment planning and implementation were aimed at role reconstitution so that individuals could go about their activities of daily life having achieved the necessary competence and deriving a level of satisfaction as they fulfilled their occupational roles.[5]

MODEL OF HUMAN OCCUPATION

As students of Reilly, Gary Kielhofner and Janice Burke were involved in identifying concepts and adding to the theoretical foundation of the occupational behavior framework. They developed a theoretical framework based in part on occupational behavior framework. Since then, Kielhofner has enlisted the aid of many students and associates in developing the model of human occupation and in further defining and refining the basic concepts.

Kielhofner and Burke organized the concepts of occupation into a **general systems** theoretical framework. They conceptualized humans as an open system composed of input, throughput, output and feedback.[8] Thus there is a dynamic interaction between the parts of the system and with the environment. The parts are defined as follows:[8]

- *Input* describes information received from the environment.
- *Throughput* refers to one's internal organizational processes.
- *Output* is defined as the mental, physical and social aspects of occupation.
- *Feedback* means information received regarding consequences of actions taken, which guides future behavior.

This system is self-transforming; that is, output and feedback provide input and, in turn, throughput modifies output. Society makes demands of the system in the form of norms and role requirements. The internal part of the system (throughput) is composed of the three following subsystems:[8]

- **Volition** guides individual choices and is influenced by values, goals and interests. It refers to motivation and the resulting actions. If the will to act is not present, action will not occur.
- **Habituation** refers to the individual's habits and internalized roles. It helps to maintain activity and action and is characterized by activities that tend to be routine.
- **Performance** means actions produced through skill acquisition. It is seen through the individual's performance and operates on rules and procedures for using skills.

The interaction of these three subsystems is critical for determining the composition of the systems output; higher subsystems control the lower ones and the lower subsystems constrain the higher ones.[8]

Three levels of motivation in the volitional subsystem govern change in other subsystems:[8]

- *Exploration* promotes generation of skills.
- *Competency* helps organize habits.
- *Achievement* influences the acquisition of competent role behavior.

"Occupation is the purposeful use of time by humans to fulfill their own internal urges toward exploring and mastering their environment that at the same time fulfills the requirements of a social group to which they belong and personal needs for self-maintenance."[9] It is a lifelong series of experiences and a changing balance of play and work. The occupational therapy clinic should provide a hierarchical set of challenges that corresponds to the exploration,

competency and achievement hierarchy of motivation.[9]

The goal of therapy is to achieve a balance among the subsystems, which is necessary for fulfilling both internal satisfaction and external demands. Changes in the system must begin with the lowest level of the subsystem (exploration) and the lowest level of behavior (skills). Occupational therapy creates an environment that presents demands for performance and elicits enactment of responses that can result in positive feedback. Challenges should then be increased to elicit a sense of competency.[10] Therapy is a process in which the system experiences the organizing involvement in planned occupations.[11]

Kielhofner views the occupation of human beings as a dominant activity, which is the result of evolutionary development. It is reflected in the individual's need for both productive and enjoyable behavior.[12] Roann Barris has also contributed to the development of this model, particularly in relation to the environmental aspects. Figure 4-1 illustrates the model of human occupation.

ADAPTIVE RESPONSES

Lorna Jean King believes that occupational therapy needs a unifying theory that ensures cohesiveness between the different areas in which occupational therapy personnel practice, especially in this time of specialization. The theory should also distinguish occupational therapy from other disciplines. In her Eleanor Clarke Slagle lecture in 1978, King said that she was struck by A. Jean Ayre's phrase "eliciting an adaptive response." After reviewing the literature, she concluded that adaptation was the common thread which ran throughout the history of occupational therapy.

She outlined the following four characteristics of the adaptive response:[13]

1. It requires active participation (the person must act rather than being acted on by another).
2. It must be evoked by the demands of the environment.
3. It is usually most efficiently organized subcortically (conscious attention directed to objects or tasks rather than specific movements).
4. It is self-reinforcing (each success acts as a motivation for greater effort or a more complex challenge).

Occupational therapy personnel must know principles and milestones of **human development** and which adaptive response is needed so that they can provide the proper environment and stimuli for a given action. The stimuli must also be given at an opportune time when a successful response is most likely to occur. King[13] states that occupational therapy consists of structuring the surroundings, materials, and especially the demands of the environment in

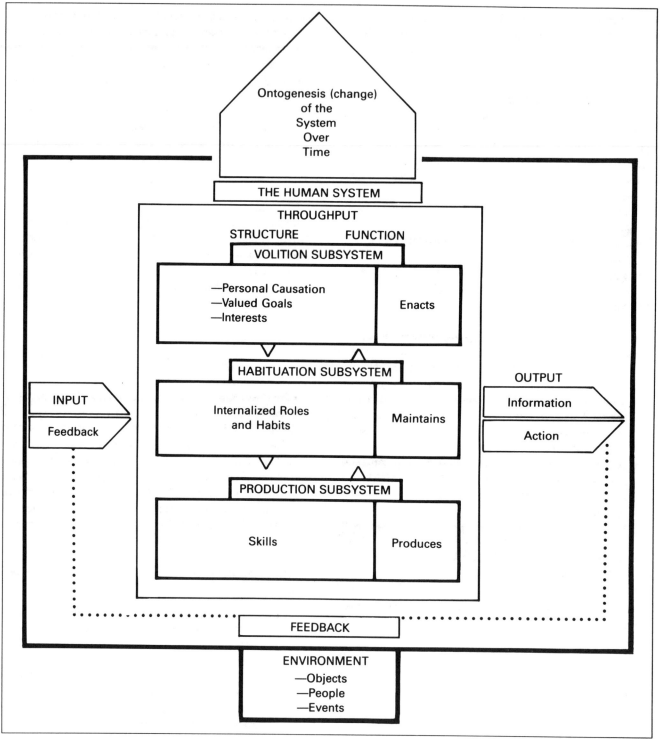

Figure 4-1. Model of human occupation. From Kielhofner G and Burke JP: A model of human occupation. Part I: Conceptual framework and content. *Am J Occup Ther* 34:572-581, 1980. Used with permission.

such a way as to call forth a specific adaptive response.

Kleinman and Bulkley,[14] in attempting to apply King's theoretical framework in 1982, presented an adaptation continuum, consisting of the following basic categories:

1. Homeostatic reactions
2. Adaptive responses
3. Adaptive skills
4. Adaptive patterns

They pointed out that the first relates to the capacity to perform, the second and third relate to performance, and the fourth relates to the constellations of performance over time. They also stated that the major function of all health disciplines is to foster adaptation. However, the second and third levels of the continuum are more appropriately the responsibility of occupational therapy because the focus is an integrated response to the whole person.[14]

FACILITATING GROWTH AND DEVELOPMENT

The facilitating growth and development framework was presented by Lela Llorens in her 1969 Eleanor Clarke Slagle address. The following premises were cited as a basis for her theory:[15]

1. Human development occurs horizontally in the areas of neurophysiologic, physical, psychological, and psychodynamic growth and in the development of social language, daily living, and sociocultural skills.
2. Humans develop longitudinally in the preceding areas in a continuous process as they age.
3. Mastery of skills, abilities, and relationships in each of these areas is necessary for satisfactory coping behavior and satisfactory relationships.
4. This mastery usually occurs naturally through the experience with the environments of home, school and community.
5. When physical or psychological trauma interrupts this growth and development process, a gap in development occurs, resulting in a disparity between expected behaviors and skills necessary to the adaptation process.
6. Through the skilled application of activities and relationships, occupational therapy can provide growth and development links to assist in closing this gap by increasing skills, abilities and relationships.

Using the work of many other theorists, Llorens constructed a matrix detailing selected development expectations, facilitating activities and adaptive skills. She pointed out that the occupational therapist is the enculturation agent who must understand the needs of the individual (determining function and dysfunction). The therapist then chooses activities and relationships to attain the following goals:[15]

1. Ameliorate (improve) or modify dysfunction.
2. Enhance remaining function.
3. Facilitate growth consistent with the individual's developmental stage.

She stressed that, while emphasis may be put on facilitating growth in a specific area of dysfunction, simultaneous attention should be given to all other areas of development so that an integrating experience will take place. The occupational therapist must determine the level at which the individual is functioning in the various aspects along the developmental continuum and program activities accordingly. It is necessary to meet the individual's needs at the present level of development and to monitor progress so that treatment can move to a higher level. If all areas of development are not considered, it is unlikely that there will be much success in restoring *integrated* function.[15]

In 1984, Llorens indicated that functional adaptation is the goal of occupational therapy. This adaptation depends on the dynamic interaction between the individual and the environment. She differentiated between three levels of environment as follows:[16]

1. First level—the individual (interior environmental factors are biologic, psychophysiologic, and sociologic
2. Second level—family, spouse, and partner interactions
3. Third level—community relationships

Through research that she and her students have carried out, Llorens concluded that occupational therapy objectives are concerned first with the patient as an environment that needs to gain or regain integrity to function adaptively within the sociocultural and person-made environments.[16]

DOING AND BECOMING— PURPOSEFUL ACTION

Gail Fidler and her husband Jay, a psychiatrist, first introduced a framework for occupational therapy as a communication process. This framework was concerned with action and its use in communicating feelings and thoughts as well as nonverbal communication. The occupational therapy experience was structured according to the following factors:[17]

1. The action itself
2. Objects used in the **action process** and ones that result from the action process
3. Interpersonal relationships that influence the action and, in turn, are influenced by it

They concluded that activity and objects function as catalytic agents or stimuli eliciting intrapsychic and interpersonal responses.[17]

Fourteen years later the Fidlers introduced a framework that modified these ideas somewhat and became known as "doing and becoming—purposeful action." They concluded that we realize our being in doing; what is potential becomes actual.[18] Their work was based on the belief that doing is a sense of performing, producing or causing; it is purposeful in contrast to random and is directed toward the following:[18]

1. Intrapersonal—testing a skill
2. Interpersonal—relationships
3. Nonhuman—creating an end product.

Through action and feedback, individuals know their potentials and limitations of self and the environment and achieve a sense of competence and worth. Becoming occurs when actions are transformed into behavior that satisfies individual needs and contributes to society. Activity must match maturation, developmental needs, and skill readiness and be recognized by the group as relevent to values and needs.[18] This framework has been used primarily in mental health.

MOSEY—FOUR FRAMEWORKS

Anne Cronin Mosey has long been a contributor to enunciating the parameters of occupational therapy and its theoretical frameworks. Four of her contributions, spanning more than 20 years, are presented here. It is interesting to identify various concepts and to note their evolution and relative emphasis over time.

Recapitulation of Ontogenesis

In 1968, Mosey developed a theoretical framework for the practice of occupational therapy called *recapitulation of ontogenesis*. This model was influenced by Mosey's clinical work with Gail Fidler.[19] The term reflects the biologic concept that there is a "repetition of evolutionary stages of a species during embryonic development of an individual organism."[19] She stated that an individual is able to move from a state of dysfunction to a state of function through participation in activities similar to those object interactions believed to be responsible for the development of an adapting human organism. She outlined the following seven adaptive skills:[20]

1. Perceptual-motor   *hand eye roordination*
2. Cognitive   *- thinking*
3. Drive-object   *motivation*
4. Dyadic interaction   *with one or more people*
5. Primary group interaction   *family, peers etc*
6. Self-identity   *self esteem.*
7. Sexual identity

Each of these adaptive skills was further divided into hierarchical components, so that one must learn a lower-level component before learning a higher-level one. She also said that these components are interdependent; one must learn some components in one skill before being able to learn certain components in another skill. She concluded that a state of function was the intergrated learning of those adaptive skills components needed for

successful participation in the social roles expected of the individual in the usual environmental setting.[20] Learning occurs through involvement in activities that allow the individual to progress sequentially through those stages of development that previously were never completely mastered. She stressed the importance for occupational therapy personnel to analyze activities, first according to **skill components** and then according to their environmental elements. Initial, immediate goals are related to learning the most elementary skill components, whereas long-term goals are the patient's successful participation in expected social roles.[20]

Activities Therapy

The **activities therapy** framework, developed by Anne Mosey and introduced in 1973, is based on the assumption that many individuals who are unable to learn to function in the community have mental health problems.[21] These problems occur due to basic skill deficits, such as failure in planning and carrying out activities of daily living, and inability to express feelings in a socially acceptable way, among others.[22]

Activities therapy takes place in the present in a therapeutic community; both one to one and groups are used in treatment. It is immediate and action-oriented, with the treatment focusing on the patient's future needs and the knowledge and skills necessary to meet these needs.[19] Individual values are also considered in planning the treatment activities, which emphasize learning by doing.[22] Examples include how to plan meals, shop and prepare nutritious food, or read a bus schedule and take a bus to and from a specified location. This model is used primarily in adult mental health.

Biopsychosocial Model

In 1974, Mosey proposed the biopsychosocial model for the profession of occupational therapy as an alternative to the medical model and the health model. She stated that it directs attention to body, mind and environment of the individual.[23] The major assumption of this model is that humans have a right to a meaningful and productive existence—not only to be free from disease, but to participate in the life of the community. It is oriented toward the delineation of the learning needs of the person and the teaching/learning process (see Chapter 8). Initial evaluation is the assessment and delineation of the individual's learning needs. Next is the specification of what knowledge, skills and attitudes should be the focus of the treatment program (learning sequence and priorities). The selection and organization of learning experiences are a statement of the teaching plan. Occupational therapy personnel should follow the principles of teaching and learning, which include the following:[23]

1. Beginning where the learner is and proceeding at a rate that is comfortable for the learner

2. Involving the learner as an active participant
3. Facilitating learning through frequent repetition and practice
4. Moving from simple to complex

This model is oriented to the client-in-the-community and views occupational therapists, assistants, and the individual receiving services working together to solve problems of living. It focuses on humans as a biologic entity, a thinking and feeling person, and a member of the community[23] (see Chapter 6 for related information).

Domains of Concern and Tools

In 1981, Mosey outlined what she considered to be a model for the practice of occupational therapy. She identified the following domains of concern: performance components (sensory integration, neuromuscular function, cognitive function, psychological function, and social interaction) within the context of age, occupational performance, and an individual's environment.[24] She also stated that the legitimate tools of occupational therapy are the nonhuman environment, conscious use of self, the teaching-learning process, purposeful activities, activity groups, and activity analysis and synthesis.[24]

SENSORY INTEGRATION

The sensory integration approach to occupational therapy intervention was introduced by A. Jean Ayres in the 1960s and resulted from her various and extensive research projects, which were an integral part of her clinical practice. It was based on her earlier work with perceptual motor deficits.[21,25] Sensory integration may be defined as the ability to develop and coordinate sensory information, motor response, and sensory feedback.[26]

Deficits were originally found through the administration of the *Southern California Sensory Integration Tests,* which included visual, kinesthetic, tactile and motor areas. The tests were revised and extended in the 1980s and renamed the *Sensory Integration and Praxis Tests.* As with the original battery, it measures sensory integration processes that provide a foundation for learning and behavior. Test scores are viewed as a "total picture" rather then individually.[27] They provide information about how the human brain receives and processes sensory messages and organizes a response to the sensory information.[21]

Sensory integration treatment procedures focus on "control of sensory input that proceeds according to a developmental sequence and requires an adaptive response."[19] Activities and appropriate therapeutic equipment are selected to obtain the desired sensory input and response. For example, treatment might include rubbing the skin with terry cloth to provide tactile stimulation or having a child lie prone on a scooterboard and move about in a specific way to provide vestibular stimulation.[21] This approach has been widely used with children. Other applications have been proposed, eg, King, with adult schizophrenics, and Lewis,[28] with elderly patients.

SPATIOTEMPORAL ADAPTATION

Spatiotemporal adaptation is a model developed by Elnora Gilfoyle and Ann Grady based on the human development milestones and learning sequence of Gesell and Piaget, respectively, as well as biopsychosocial elements and the Bobath approach.[21] The model focuses on adaptation to space and timing of movements to build postural and movement strategies, which are adapted to achieve purposeful behaviors such as creeping, crawling and walking. The behaviors are a foundation for development of skills and the performance of purposeful activities.[21] Gilfoyle and Grady view the behaviors in a spiraling continuum in which adaptation begins before birth. When considering the present status of a child, past behaviors are called up to improve the present situation and enhance future skill acquisition and adaptation. Figure 4-2 illustrates the sequence of the model and the relationship of sensory input, motor output and sensory feedback. The following are brief definitions of the terms used in the continuum to achieve spatiotemporal adaptation:[29]

1. **Assimilation**—the ability to absorb, to make information a part of one's thinking
2. **Accommodation**—the ability to modify or adjust in response to the environment
3. **Association**—the ability to relate factors from the past to experiences in the present
4. **Differentiation**—the ability to determine what differences exist between objects and events

To provide further illustration, the following scenario describes a little boy who is just beginning to crawl. The child learns that reciprocal movement of the arms and legs will move him forward a given distance. He also learns that he can crawl that distance at a fast or slow rate. This information is assimilated and recalled the next time the child has an opportunity to crawl. The child is crawling on another occasion and becomes distracted. He crawls too close to the wall and hits his head. The child then crawls away from the wall thus accommodating to this environmental barrier. He continues crawling about the room and touches a lamp cord. The mother responds by lightly tapping the child's hand and saying "no." He touches the cord again and the mother responds in the same way (association). Eventually the child learns to differentiate what he can touch and what should not be touched.

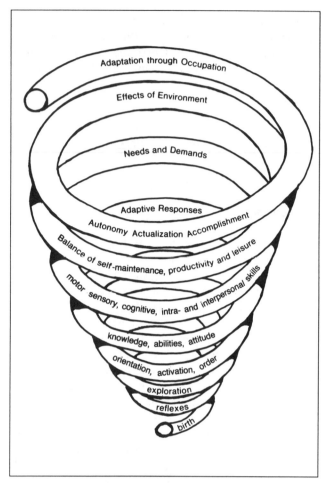

Figure 4-2. Spatiotemporal adaptation model. From Gilfoyle, Grady, and Moore: *Children Adapt.* Thorofare, New Jersey, Slack Inc., 1981.

NEUROMOTOR APPROACH

Neuromotor approaches are a group of treatment strategies based on a reflex (peripheral) model and/or a hierarchical (central) model of motor control. In the reflex model, sensory input controls motor output. Another way of stating this is that sensation is essential for movement to occur. Various sensory stimuli, such as vibration, tapping and quick stretch, are used to elicit more normal motor output. In the hierarchical model of motor control, motor programs in the brain control movement. To enhance motor performance, normal movement patterns are practiced repeatedly to develop motor programs that are thought to underlie all movement patterns. All of the neuromotor approaches emphasize that the nervous system controls movement, and view other systems within the body and the environment as subservient. These approaches also emphasize the importance of the normal developmental sequence in treatment. Proponents believe that the changes seen during development are a result of the maturation of the nervous system.

The Rood Approach

Margaret Rood was a physical and occupational therapist who developed her neurophysiologic approach to treatment while working with patients having cerebral palsy and hemiplegia.[21,30] Her treatment centered on the principles that sensory stimulation can assist in developing normal muscle tone and motor response, and that stimulation of reflex responses is the first step in motor control development.[31]

Sensory stimulation is a central focus to effect the desired motor response. Treatment includes relaxation techniques, such as slow stroking of the spinal column, slow side-to-side rolling, and neutral warmth, which entails wrapping the patient or a part of the patient in a blanket. Sensory stimulation may be provided by using a vibrator or brush or through rubbing the belly of a muscle to facilitate or make the desired response easier.[32]

Rood was a strong advocate of purposeful activity and promoted the use of her techniques in conjunction with such woodworking tasks as sanding a bread board. Through engagement in an activity, the patient's attention is focused on the task at hand and achievement of that task rather than the correct motor response.[32]

Proprioceptive Neuromuscular Facilitation

The proprioceptive neuromuscular approach (PNF) was developed by the physiatrist Herman Kabat. It was later expanded by Margaret Knott and Dorothy Voss, both physical therapists. PNF is used with patients with cerebral palsy as well as those with spinal cord injuries, orthopedic problems and other disabilities affecting the neuromuscular system. The basic thrust of this approach is stimulation of the proprioceptors. **Proprioceptors** are located in the muscles, tendons, and joints, which, through movement, make the patient aware of position, balance and equilibrium changes. Mass movement patterns are developed first through activities such as washing a floor in a creeping position or finger painting on the floor on "all fours." Making a macramé project is an example of how fine motor coordination might be used. Diagonal patterns of motion are stressed to facilitate the appropriate motor responses. The patient's active participation in the process is emphasized.[33]

Neurodevelopmental Approach

The late Karel Bobath, a neuropsychiatrist, and Berta Bobath, a physical therapist, developed the neurodevelopmental approach to treatment (NDT) while they were practicing in London. This approach, used with cerebral palsy and hemiplegia patients primarily, is based on the following concepts:[31]

1. Patterns of movement are learned and refined to enable the individual to develop skills.
2. Abnormal patterns of posture, balance and movement occur when the brain has been damaged.

3. Abnormal patterns interfere with the individual's ability to carry out normal activities of daily living.

Basic treatment centers on the inhibition or restraint of abnormal reflex patterns through handling and sensory stimulation. The goal is to help the patient produce the desired normal movement pattern. For example, the therapist might place a child on top of a large, inflated ball and roll the ball from side to side. The desired response is that the child will extend his or her hands and arms to maintain balance and as a protection against falling off the ball.[31] As this activity is repeated, changes will occur in muscle tone that promote normal movement.[32]

Movement Therapy

The movement therapy approach to treatment was developed in the 1950s by a physical therapist, Signe Brunnstrom, as a method for treating patients with hemiplegia. Based on the principles of neurodevelopment, she defined specific states of recovery of the hand, arm and leg. She also developed related techniques to establish patterns of motion or **synergies**.[31] Some of these techniques include tapping the belly of a muscle, applying pressure on a tendon, and quickly stroking a muscle.

Primitive reflexes, present in the early stages of normal development, often reappear in a patient who has had a cerebral vascular accident. These reflexes are facilitated in occupational therapy through activities that offer resistance (eg, weaving and woodworking) to promote the functional return of movement patterns. Such activities allow a neurologic impulse to spread to other muscles in a group. Visual and verbal clues are also a very important part of the total treatment process.[31,34] Brunnstrom noted that the movement therapy patterns that deal primarily with the lower extremities should be dealt with by a physical therapist.[31]

COGNITIVE DISABILITIES MODEL

In the early 1980s, Claudia Allen proposed a theory to guide occupational therapy practice. She indicated that identification of functional units of the brain would help specify elements that could assist in uniting our profession.[35] She constructed a matrix of six levels of cognitive function, which indicates the complexity of sensorimotor association formed during the process of performing a task:[36]

1. Automatic actions
2. Postural actions
3. Manual actions
4. Goal-oriented actions
5. Exploratory actions
6. Planned actions

She defined a *cognitive disability* as a series of functional units of behavior that cut across diagnostic categories and interfere with task behavior. According to her findings, cognitive disability is a restriction in sensorimotor actions originating in the physical or chemical structures of the brain. These changes produce observable and measurable limitations in routine task behavior. These dysfunctions restrict performance of social roles, limit ability to function in carrying out activities of daily living, and signal that disease exists.[36]

Allen devised a method of measuring the degree of social dysfunction and constructed another matrix, identifying levels of cognitive disability that corresponded to the the the six levels of cognitive ability and disability. These range, in ascending order, from level 1, severe impairment, to level 6, no impairment. At each cognitive level, specific motor actions and associated sensory cues are provided. For example, the following characteristics would be exhibited by a level 4 patient:[37]

1. Spontaneous motor actions are goal-directed
2. Can copy or reproduce a task from an example, such as chopping vegetables or sanding wood
3. Responds to visual sensory cues, ignoring what is not in immediate view

A third matrix, task analysis for cognitive disability, indicates the type and amount of assistance required to complete the task and specifies the kinds of directions a care giver needs to provide for each of the six cognitive levels.[35]

Allen pointed out that other disciplines frequently focus on verbal behavior and that occupational therapists who emulated them did little to help patients or the profession. Now, more neuroscientists are recognizing the importance of voluntary motor actions as a way to clarify the brain-behavior association. Occupational therapy personnel are unique in their approach, however, because of what we can do with motor action by applying task analysis.

According to Allen *task analysis* refers to the examination of each step that is followed in a typical procedure to achieve a goal. Occupational therapists and assistants use task analysis to modify the task procedure so that patients can achieve greater independence. The task analysis is a guideline for selecting and designing activities that correspond to the patient's level of ability (see Chapter 17). The structure of an activity is modified by using elements of the physical environment as substitutes for deficient patterns of thought.[35]

Allen also points out that occupational therapy treatment objectives differ according to the medical condition of the patient (unstable, acute versus stable, chronic). These objectives can be directed toward treatment (changing the condition) or compensation (modifying the task to offset deficits). In the case of cognitive deficit, the therapist or assistant can do little to improve the deficit. By reporting changes in the patient's behavior, however, occupational therapy personnel as well as other team members can identify what kinds of therapy would be most appropriate and report on the effectiveness of drugs and other forms of treatment. Another extremely important use of this framework is the ability to identify when a patient should be discharged and to plan the appropriate community support and placement.[35,36]

Originally used with psychiatric patients, this framework is also effective across other diagnostic categories and can be used whenever cognitive limitations are involved, such as stroke, head injury, dementia and mental retardation. This model focuses on measurement and management rather than improvement as goals of occupational therapy treatment. Allen emphasizes, however, the importance of providing activities that require increasingly complex abilities as the patient's cognitive functioning changes. Occupational therapy personnel can also provide tasks that a person can do successfully during acute illness or recovery by changing a task to place it within the patient's range of ability. In addition, Allen points out that the cognitive disabilities model can provide a mechanism to objectively assess occupational therapy services. She believes that we must achieve greater specificity about objectives and methods to increase the ability to facilitate independence through activity.[35]

FUTURE CONSIDERATIONS

The profession has not yet identified or adopted a singular theoretical framework or group of frameworks.[38,39] The debate continues as to the relative advantages and disadvantages of taking such a position. Some advocates of endorsing one comprehensive framework point to the need to achieve a greater degree of professional unity and to guide important research. Others feel that this is a narrow approach, emphasizing that multiple theoretical perspectives are more appropriate for the multifaceted practice of occupational therapy.[39] Although some practitioners indeed believe that it is advantageous to use more than one theory, Parham[1] cautions therapists to be sure that the theories they combine are compatible (based on similar assumptions and values).

It is unlikely that this issue will be resolved in the near future. As both the profession and society continue to grow and change, some frameworks and approaches will be discarded, others will be combined, and new ones will emerge. Certain common denominators, however, will survive the test of time: historically significant guiding principles, philosophical values and beliefs, ethics, and core concepts of *occupation*. These elements will continue to be in the forefront and provide a strong influence in further defining the theoretical foundations and guiding the profession in its research and continued development of its knowledge base.

SUMMARY

Definitions and basic concepts relative to some of the theoretical frameworks and approaches proposed by occupational therapists and others have been presented. The importance of using theoretical frameworks is stressed as a means of helping practitioners "set the problem" and "solve the problem," as well as being a key to systematic research and the continued building of a knowledge base specific for occupational therapy. Examples are provided that are general and have application to all areas of practice, such as occupational behavior and the model of human occupation, whereas others deal with specific clinical settings, such as psychiatry and pediatrics. Theoretical approaches related to the application of definitive techniques, such as sensory integration, proprioceptive neuromuscular facilitation, and cognitive disabilities, are also addressed. Reference is often made to human development and occupation as a base for many of these theories. Nevertheless, the profession has yet not adopted a singular theoretical framework or group of frameworks. This is currently evidenced by the pioneering work being done by the faculty and students at the University of Southern California in developing an emerging science of occupation (see Chapter Six).

Acknowledgment

Appreciation is extended to Virgil Mathiowetz, PhD, OTR, for his provision of content related to neuromotor approaches.

Related Learning Activities

1. Select any two of the more general theoretical frameworks and compare and contrast them in terms of basic values and beliefs, variety and age of patients, specific treatment techniques, and any additional pertinent factors. Use references and bibliographic material as needed. Organizing the material into a chart may be helpful.

2. Write a list of the theoretical frameworks and approaches you have personally observed being carried out in practice. Compare the list with at least two peers and determine which frameworks and approaches seem to be used most often in your area.

3. Develop a list of at least 20 different treatment activities for a variety of different patients with varying diagnoses. Adapt these activities to at least two different theoretical frameworks and approaches. Demonstrate some of these modifications to peers.

4. Stage a debate with your peers focusing on whether the profession should adopt a single theoretical framework as a foundation for practice. Provide a rationale for the stand taken.

5. Which of the many theoretical frameworks and approaches discussed in this chapter could be combined? What would be gained? What would be lost?

References

1. Parham D: Toward professionalism: The reflective therapist. *Am J Occup Ther* 41:555-561, 1987.
2. Sands M: Applying theory to practice: A response from technical education. In: *Occupational Therapy Education: Target 2000.* Rockville, Maryland, American Occupational Therapy Association, 1986, pp. 125-126.
3. Reilly M: Occupational therapy can be one of the great ideas of 20th century medicine. *Am J Occup Ther* 16:1-9, 1962.
4. Reilly M: A psychiatric occupational therapy program as a teaching model. *Am J Occup Ther* 20:61-67,1966.
5. Reilly M: The educational process. *Am J Occup Ther* 23:299-307, 1969.
6. Shannon P: Occupational behavior frame of reference. In Hopkins HL, Smith HD (Eds): *Willard and Spackman's Occupational Therapy* 7th edition. Philadelphia, JB Lippincott, 1988.
7. Reilly M: Defining a cobweb, an explanation of play. In Reilly M (Ed): *Play as Exploratory Learning.* Beverly Hills, California, Sage Publications, 1974.
8. Kielhofner G, Burke JP: A model of human occupation. Part 1: Conceptual framework and content. *Am J Occup Ther* 34:572-581, 1980.
9. Kielhofner G: A model of human occupation, Part 2: Ontogenesis from the perspective of temporal adaptation. *Am J Occup Ther* 34:657-663, 1980.
10. Kielhofner G: A model of human occupation, Part 3: Benign and vicious cycles. *Am J Occup Ther* 34:731-737, 1980.
11. Kielhofner G, Burke JP, Igi CH: A model of human occupation, Part 4: Assessment and intervention. *Am J Occup Ther* 34:777-788, 1980.
12. Kielhofner G: Occupation. In Hopkins HL, Smith HS (Eds): *Willard and Spackman's Occupational Therapy* 6th edition. Philadelphia, JB Lippincott, 1983, p. 31.
13. King LJ: Toward a science of adaptive responses. *Am J Occup Ther* 32:429-437, 1978.
14. Kleinman BL, Bulkley BL: Some implications of a science of adaptive responses. *Am J Occup Ther* 36:15-19, 1982.
15. Llorens LA: Facilitating growth and development: The promise of occupational therapy. *Am J Occup Ther* 24:93-101, 1970.
16. Llorens LA: Changing balance: Environment and individual. *Am J Occup Ther* 38:29-34, 1984.
17. Fidler GS, Fidler JW: *Occupational Therapy: A Communication Process in Psychiatry.* New York, McMillan, 1964.
18. Fidler GS, Fidler JW: Doing and becoming: Purposeful action and self-actualization. *Am J Occup Ther* 32:305-310, 1978.
19. Miller BRJ et al: *Six Perspectives on Theory for the Practice of Occupational Therapy.* Rockville, Maryland, Aspen, 1988.
20. Mosey AC: Recapitulation of ontogenesis: A theory for practice of occupational therapy. *Am J Occup Ther* 22:426-438, 1968.
21. Reed KL: *Models of Practice in Occupational Therapy.* Baltimore, Williams & Wilkins, 1984.
22. Mosey AC: *Activities Therapy.* New York, Raven Press, 1973.
23. Mosey AC: An alternative: The biopsychosocial model. *Am J Occup Ther* 28:137-140, 1974.
24. Mosey AC: *Occupational Therapy: Configuration of a Profession.* New York, Raven Press, 1981.
25. Ayers AJ: The development of perceptual motor abilities: A theoretical basis for treatment of dysfunction. *Am J Occup Ther* 17:221-225, 1963.
26. *Uniform Terminology for Reporting Occupational Therapy Services.* Rockville, Maryland, American Occupational Therapy Association, 1979.
27. Vezie MB: Sensory integration: A foundation for learning. *Acad Ther* 10:348, 1975.
28. Lewis SC: *The Mature Years.* Thorofare, New Jersey, Slack Inc., 1979, p. 93.
29. Gilfoyle EM, Grady AP, Moore, JC: *Children Adapt.* Thorofare, New Jersey, Slack Inc., 1981.
30. Cromwell FS: In memoriam. *Am J Occup Ther* 39:54, 1985.
31. Trombly CA, Scott AD: *Occupational Therapy for Physical Dysfunction.* Baltimore, Williams & Wilkins, 1977, pp. 70, 78, 87, 91, 98.
32. Huss AJ: Overview of sensorimotor approaches. In Hopkins HL, Smith HD (Eds): *Willard and Spackman's Occupational Therapy,* 6th edition. Philadelphia, JB Lippincott, 1983, pp. 116-117.
33. Voss DE: Proprioceptive neuromuscular facilitation: Application of patterns and techniques in occupational therapy. *Am J Occup Ther* 13:193, 1959.
34. Huss AJ: Sensory motor treatment approaches. In Willard H, Spackman C (Eds): *Occupational Therapy* 4th edition. Philadelphia, JB Lippincott, 1971, pp. 379-380.
35. Allen CK: Independence through activity: The practice of occuptional therapy (psychiatry). *Am J Occup Ther* 36:731-739, 1982.
36. Allen CK, Allen RE: Cognitive disabilities: Measuring the social consequences of mental disorders. *J Clin Psychiatry* 48:185-190, 1987.
37. Early MB: *Mental Health Concepts and Techniques for the Occupational Therapy Assistant.* New York, Raven Press, 1987, pp. 47-53.
38. Hopkins HL: Current basis for theory and philosophy of occupational therapy. In Hopkins HL, Smith HD (Eds): *Willard and Spackman's Occupational Therapy,* 6th edition. Philadelphia, JB Lippincott, 1983, p. 28.
39. Punwar AJ: *Occupational Therapy Principles and Practice.* Baltimore, Williams & Wilkins, 1988, p. 221.

Basic Concepts of Human Development

Sister Genevieve Cummings, CSJ, MA, OTR, FAOTA

INTRODUCTION

Human development is the essential basis for all occupational therapy practice. Although the subject of human development is vast and cannot be covered completely in this discussion, the elements most applicable to the practice of occupational therapy are addressed here: motor, cognitive and psychosocial development. Language development, although important, is not considered.

Basic theorists who will be discussed are Arnold Gesell, Jean Piaget, Erik Erikson, Robert Havighurst, and Abraham Maslow. There are, of course, many others who could be included and have contributed greatly to the field of human development. This chapter should be regarded as a summary and as a review of material studied in detail in courses in human growth and development.

MOTOR DEVELOPMENT

Many investigators have contributed to the body of knowledge about motor development. Among the most important is Arnold Gesell. Gesell studied and developed his theories first at Yale University and eventually at the Gesell Institute of Child Development. His important work is in the area of infant and child development.

Motor development occurs in a relatively unvaried sequence; however, the timing of each step in the sequence may be highly varied. Some of the principles that guide motor development are the **cephalocaudal development** and **proximal-distal development** (ie, development proceeds from the head to the lower extremities [tail] and from the parts close to the midline to the extremities, respectively). Control of the head occurs before

---

KEY CONCEPTS

Gesell's principles of motor development

Piaget's principles of cognitive development

Erikson's stages of psychosocial development

Havighurst's developmental life tasks

Maslow's hierarchy of needs

Relationship to disability

ESSENTIAL VOCABULARY

Cephalocaudal development

Proximal-distal development

Reciprocal interweaving

Reflex

Perception

Manipulation

Organization

Equilibration

Ego strength

Self-actualization

control of the limbs; control of the trunk and shoulder occurs before the hand.[1] The principle of **reciprocal interweaving** has been defined as well. This term refers to the fact that immature behavior and more mature behavior alternate in a constantly spiraling manner until, eventually, the mature behavior is firmly established. Therefore, development does not occur in a straight-line manner, but by this interweaving or circling pattern. Through careful studies, Gesell determined milestones of development that the infant should accomplish at particular times. The major milestones are shown in Table 5-1.[1-3]

Most children follow this sequence, although sometimes the sequence is altered or a stage is omitted. The actual time spent becoming stable in these tasks varies greatly. Reciprocal interveaving may be of short or long duration, or it may not be apparent to observers of the development. There is also a distinction between the time when the child is capable of performing these tasks, given optimal conditions, and when the tasks appear spontaneously. How strongly the parents desire to have a child perform the particular task seems to influence the development; children who are encouraged and given many opportunities to practice or perform may master a task sooner than those not having that encouragement. Motor development depends highly on both reflex and sensory development.

Reflex Development

A **reflex** is a constant response to a given stimulus. Reflexes generally precede voluntary movement control and later are integrated with motor function. Reflex action is observed as early as the seventh week in utero. By the 14th week in utero, the fetus reacts to stimulation with multiple motor responses.[4] Primitive reflexes, present at birth, involve the entire body and limbs. Rooting, sucking, incurvatum, crossed extension, withdrawal, Moro's reflex, primary righting, primary walking, and grasp are the major reflexes present at birth[4-5] (see Appendix A). A discussion of these reflexes and their development is beyond the scope of this chapter.

Sensory Development

At birth, the sensation of touch is highly developed and serves as the main source of sensory information for the neonate. All of the somatosensory **perceptions,** such as pain, temperature and touch, are present.

Visual perception is also present at birth, but is probably limited to light/dark perception and vague visual images. Fixing on an object for a brief time occurs at approximately one month, with more stable fixation occurring at three to four months. The visual system continues to develop for about ten years. Hearing appears to become acute a few days after birth. Smell and taste are present at birth and well developed by the second and third months[4] (see Appendix A).

Table 5-1 Milestones in Gross Motor Development and Postural Control	
Accomplishment	**Age in Months**
Lift head to 45° when prone	2
Lift chest off floor when prone	3
Sit up when supported	4
Sit by self	7
Crawl	8
Pull self up on furniture	9
Creep	10
Walk when led	11
Stand alone	14
Walk alone, straddle-toddle (feet far apart, full sole step)	15
Toddle (longer steps, narrower width, lower step height)	18
Run	21

Reach and Early Manipulation

Reaching in the supine position using small incipient movements occurs between eight and 12 weeks of age. Spontaneous regard of objects occurs at about 16 weeks, accompanied by greatly increased arm activity. Bilateral approach movements begin around 20 weeks, and at 24 weeks bilateral grasp of the object occurs. Beyond 28 weeks, the activity becomes more and more unilateral.

In the sitting position only passive and brief regard for reaching occurs from 12 to 16 weeks. At 20 weeks, the child makes movements that are likely to cause contact with the object. At 24 weeks, the child grasps the object and can **manipulate** it somewhat. A 28-week-old child can move an object such as a rattle from hand to hand and manipulate it in a variety of ways. By 18 months, the toddler reaches for near objects easily and automatically, but reaches for distant ones more awkwardly. This reaching for distant objects gradually becomes smoother and more coordinated by five years of age.

Grasp and Release

Grasp occurs as a reflex prenatally. There are two aspects to this reflex action: finger closure and gripping. Light pressure or stroking on the palm elicits closure; stretching the finger tendons elicits gripping. The closure aspect of the reflex disappears from 16 to 24 weeks after birth; the gripping aspect weakens and then disappears from 12 to 24 weeks.

Voluntary grasping, in contrast to reflex grasping, follows a relatively precise pattern. Initially, the ulnar side of the hand is used in a raking manner. Objects are palmed rather then handled precisely by the fingers. At 18 months the hand is open until it contacts the object; the thumb is in opposition.[2,3]

At 24 weeks, squeeze grasp is normally achieved. By 28 weeks, hand grasp is accomplished, and a palm grasp usually is performed by 32 weeks. At 52 weeks, the baby shows improved ability to use a four-finger grasp. Other milestones, which may be termed predrawing, include the ability to hold a crayon or object of similar size at 12 months, to "scribble" at 18 months, and to follow a horizontal line with a crayon at 30 months.

When the infant is eight weeks, a swiping movement is used to reach an object, but contact is not made; at three months, swiping results in some contact. By four months, the child is using a palmar grasp (ie, all fingers and the palm are in contact with the object). At six months, a mitten pattern of grasp appears whereby all of the fingers are together and the thumb is in opposition. At the baby reaches the age of seven months, the fingers, particularly the middle finger, are used as a rake to get an object into the palm with the thumb in opposition. At eight months, there is a beginning palmar prehension-thumb, index and middle fingers in opposition to each other. By one year, the child can use a more advanced palmar or fingertip prehension.[6]

Releasing is a more difficult motor activity than grasping. At nine months, the child begins to release objects voluntarily. At this age, the child will drop things spontaneously or will release an object when an adult takes it. At approximately 11 to 12 months, the child will release things on request.[7] Table 5-2 presents a list of grasp, release and manipulation milestones.[1]

COGNITIVE DEVELOPMENT

Jean Piaget is primarily responsible for the theory of cognitive development. Born in Switzerland in 1896, he did his early work in biology, but he eventually became interested in normal child development, particularly in the cognitive area. He used a clinical method of careful observation of children, beginning with his own, to study and analyze behavior and thinking. He did not use control groups, random sampling, or other research techniques of that type; but instead studied children in their natural environment doing their normal activities. He later developed a series of tasks to be presented to children as a basis of observation and analysis. Piaget died in 1983.[6,8-10]

Piaget's theory of intellectual development includes the concepts of organization and adaptation. **Organization** refers to a person's tendency to develop a coherent system, ie, to systematize. Adaptation is the tendency to adjust to the environment. As new knowledge is attained, it must be brought into balance with previous experience. This balance is called **equilibration**.[6,8]

Organization and adaptation are two tendencies within each person. Experiences are changed into knowledge through two complementary processes: assimilation and accommodation. Assimilation is a process by which an experience is incorporated into existing knowledge; in accommodation what is known is adjusted to the environment.

Knowledge is gained when experiences are organized, systemized, and related to previous experiences. This knowledge is adjusted according to the outside environment, the reality of things around the individual. A dynamic balance is being sought between what is known and what is objectively present. "Accommodation and assimilation, which are two complementary aspects of adaptation, are

Table 5-2
Milestones on Grasp, Release and Manipulation

Accomplishment	Age
Hands fisted	4 weeks
Hands open; scratches and clutches	16 weeks
Grasps cube in palm; rakes at pellet	28 weeks
Crude release	40 weeks
Prehends pellet with neat pincer grasp	52 weeks
Builds tower of 3 cubes; turns 2-3 pages at once	18 months
Builds tower of 6 cubes; turns pages singly	24 months
Builds tower of 10 cubes; holds crayon adult-fashion	36 months
Traces with lines	48 months

perpetually in action, are trying to maintain an equilibrium which is perpetually disrupted."[11]

Piaget described four stages of cognitive development: *sensory-motor* period, *preoperational* period, the *concrete-operational* period, and the *formal-operations* period (Table 5-3). The order of acquiring the skills in each period is constant, but the timing is not. Piaget emphasized the integrative aspect of stages, ie, structures of each stage become an integral part of the next stage. Each stage includes a period of preparation and a level of completion.[12]

Table 5-3
Piaget's Four Major Stages
of Cognitive Development

Stage	Name	Age
I	Sensorimotor	Birth to 2 years
II	Preoperational	2 to 7 years
III	Concrete Operations	7 to 11 years
IV	Formal Operations	12 to 15 years

Sensory-Motor Period

The sensory-motor period extends from birth until the appearance of language, or about two years of age. It is a period that begins with reflex activity, particularly sucking, eye movements and the palmar reflex. Through the use of reflexes, the baby brings information in and begins the process of assimilation. The child reacts to objects through reflex activity and gradually develops habits of response. These habits become organized as the baby learns to perceive and identify objects. The child learns to relate actions to objects and to see objects as something outside self. As children move through this stage, they learn the names of objects but do not name them because this is a preverbal stage. A child will search for objects that are not visible, try out different means of securing objects, and experiment with different properties of objects. At this point, the child begins to relate the means (actions) to the end (achieving what he or she wants).

Preoperational Period

The preoperational period is the time from approximately two to seven years of age. An operation is defined as a mental action that can be reversed; Preoperational refers to the period in which the child is unable to reverse mental actions. The child's reasoning is from the particular to the particular.[11] Generalization is not possible, and neither inductive nor deductive reasoning is present. The child is not

able to distinguish between reality and fantasy. One strong characteristic of this period is animistic thinking. The child regards inanimate objects as living and gives feelings and thoughts to them. The child is able to be aware of past and future, as well as present, but of short durations in each direction. Concepts of time are limited but present.

Concrete-Operational Period

The concrete-operational period occurs between about seven and 11 years. In this stage the child is able to use logic in thinking and is able to reverse mental actions. The child can analyze, understand part and whole relationships, combine or separate things mentally, put things in order, and multiply and divide. This stage is concrete because the mental processes are limited to those that are present and deal with the concrete. The child is not able to generalize. Abstract thinking begins to occur at the end of this period.

Formal-Operational Period

Toward the end of elementary school age and into the high school age, the young person develops the ability to reason hypothetically. The person in the formal-operational period is able to think about thinking. He or she is able to think abstractly; objects need not be present. Logical thinking and the ability to reason with syllogisms (a form of reasoning involving three propositions) are present. Theories can be developed and understood.

The development of the abilities in this stage lead to adult thinking patterns. Experience has shown that many adults do not think with adult thinking patterns, but may use concrete-operational patterns. It is also apparent, that the development of cognition is closely related to sensorimotor development. Lack of normal sensorimotor development will limit the child's ability to experiment with and explore cognitive skills. When a disability or condition interferes with the active exploration of the environment, it is necessary to make such exploration central in treatment.

PSYCHOSOCIAL DEVELOPMENT

Erik Erikson contributed greatly to the development of theories of psychosocial development and provided a framework for looking at development throughout the life span. He is usually classified as a neo-Freudian. He defined "eight ages of man," first described in his book *Childhood and Society* (Table 5-4). For each of the eight ages he identified a pair of alternative attitudes toward life, the self and other people. The person must resolve each of the issues identified as the alternatives. **Ego strength** develops from this process at each age, and these strengths continue throughout life; this development is cumulative.[13,14]

Table 5-4
Erikson's Eight Stages of Psychosocial Development

Stage	Name	Age
I	Basic Trust versus Mistrust	Birth to 18 months
II	Autonomy versus Shame and Doubt	18 months to 3 years
III	Initiative versus Guilt	3 to 5 years
IV	Industry versus Inferiority	6 to 11 years
V	Identity versus Role Confusion	12 to 17 years
VI	Intimacy versus Isolation	Young Adulthood
VII	Generativity versus Stagnation	Maturity
VIII	Ego Integrity versus Despair	Old Age

First Stage: Trust Versus Mistrust

Erikson's first stage centers on the polarity between trust and mistrust. This stage occurs during infancy when there is complete dependence on others who provide care. How this care is given determines the basic outlook of the infant. If the quality of the care is good and loving, then the infant develops a sense of expecting the good. If the child's needs are not fulfilled in a caring manner, a sense of expecting the worst develops. Trust, then, is the result of the relationship between feeling comfort and having that feeling relate to the world. This does not mean that mistrust does not occur or is not appropriate in some situations. Part of the balance is the recognition of when to trust and when not to trust.

The appropriate resolution of trust-mistrust leads to hope. Hope refers to an expectancy that needs will be met. As growth and development proceed, a basic attitude of hope means that the person expects the good and will have an optimistic approach to all aspects of life. If mistrust is emphasized, the person lacks this expectancy, is pessimistic, and usually looks at the dark side of any situation. This stage corresponds to Freud's oral stage of development.

Erikson points out that it is not the quality of food and basic care that influences this feeling of trust, but the quality of the relationship between the provider, usually the mother, and the infant. The mother-child relationship is crucial.[13]

Second Stage: Autonomy Versus Shame and Doubt

The second stage, autonomy versus shame and doubt, is the beginning of independent action by the child. As the child begins to move independently by standing and walking, develops control over bodily functions, and clearly distinguishes self from others, he or she begins to establish control over self and the environment. How the parents react to these efforts at independence and how much control they feel they must exert determines the balance between auton-

omy and shame. Again, this is a dynamic balance, not a matter of all or none.

Resolution of this stage results in will or free choice, the ability to choose to behave in a certain way because it is the best way to behave under the circumstances. A person who successfully resolves this conflict will be able to accept law and act independently within it as an adult.[13,14]

Third Stage: Initiative Versus Guilt

The third stage focuses on the balance between initiative and guilt. At this stage, the child is highly active, is able to use language effectively, and is learning to control the environment. The balance needed is between having confidence to try new activities and fearing the consequences of behavior. Questions of what others will think, how they will react to behavior, and what will happen as the result of the behavior are factors. This balance may result in a person who is confident to strike out on new things, to explore possibilities, and to work for goals; or a person who is fearful, feels guilty about doing or not doing, and is overly concerned about what will happen as a result of behavior. The resolution of this stage is purpose, the ability to establish goals and act to reach them.

Play, particularly the use of toys, is of great importance in the development and the resolution of this stage. The child uses this method to try new behaviors to learn of the reactions of others. Toys and play can help to develop initiative and confidence at this stage.

Fourth Stage: Industry Versus Inferiority

As the child reaches school age, which in most societies is approximately five years of age, the world becomes a wider arena. Play becomes the child's work. Tasks take on a greater degree of importance; how the child relates to these tasks determines the balance within this stage. Industry versus inferiority is the focus of this fourth stage. If the child succeeds and gains confidence from the tasks attempted, the ability to take on new tasks and the feeling of being able to achieve whatever is desired is fostered. If the child feels a failure in comparison with other children, a sense of inferiority results. This feeling can interfere with the ability to experiment and enjoy new activities. The use of tools, generally the same tools used by adults, is an important task at this stage.

The resulting quality of the dynamic balance in this stage is competence, described by Erikson as the ability to use dexterity and intelligence in the completion of tasks, which implies a sense of satisfaction in the completion. This developmental stage spans the elementary school ages of approximately five to 13 years of age.

Fifth Stage: Identity Versus Role Confusion

The fifth stage is that of identity versus role confusion and is the stage of adolescence. Erikson describes this stage as that in which youths are concerned with how they appear in the eyes of others in comparison to how they appear to themselves.[13] It is a time of great physiologic change. It is also a time of solidifying the skills developed in earlier stages and focusing these on the adult world of work. Knowing who they are and how they will relate to the world is an essential task. Peer relationships are highly important. Casual observation of adolescents confirms that being a part of a group, experimenting with all aspects of behavior, being different from those of any other age, and at the same time seeking acceptance are characteristics of this time.

Role confusion is the other end of this dynamic balance. It is characterized by an individual's inability to identify with the adult world of work and define his or her role in the environment. Much of the behavior of adolescence is an attempt to avoid this role confusion and to seek out and establish the appropriate boundaries.

The quality that develops in the successful fulfillment of this stage is fidelity. This is the ability to maintain loyalties in spite of differences. This loyalty is the result of strong peer identification.

Sixth Stage: Intimacy Versus Isolation

Young adulthood, the early twenties, focuses on the development of the capacity for intimacy. Erikson defines intimacy as "the capacity to commit oneself to concrete affiliations and partnerships and to develop the ethical strength to abide by such commitments, even though they may call for significant sacrifices and compromises."[14] Sexual relations are an important part of achieving this intimacy. The achievement of unity with another person and the development of a new identity that includes that person within it is the purpose and the result of a sexual relationship. Previous sexual relationships may have had the different purpose of establishing and solidifying self-identity.[14] The opposite pole is isolation: avoiding contacts that might lead to intimacy.[13]

Love is the result of the successful resolution of this stage. Although marriage is often the societal expression of this stage, marriage itself does not necessitate true intimacy.

Seventh Stage: Generativity Versus Stagnation

Generativity refers to the concern for the establishment and the guidance of the next generation. It does not necessarily include the bearing and rearing of children, although this is a common way for this stage to be expressed, but centers on a concern that what is important to human beings and society be passed on to the next generation. Erikson indicates that productivity and creativity are facets of this stage, but cannot replace generativity itself.[13] Older, more mature persons need to be able to share and to give. Generativity implies giving without expecting return. Care (concern for what has been generated) is the quality that emerges from the resolution of this stage.

The opposite pole of generativity is stagnation. Without sharing or giving, the person becomes preoccupied with self, without concern for growth or change. Erikson likens stagnation to having self as a child or pet. People may turn in on themselves and lavish the love and care they would give their children or pets on themselves.

Eighth Stage: Ego Integrity Versus Despair

Ego integrity includes an acceptance of self, of nature, and of one's life. It means that the person recognizes the value of the particular life led and does not grieve over what might have been. Such a person has inner satisfaction and is not compelled to try desperately to "live life to the fullest" or to make up for lost time. No time is regarded as "lost."

The opposite pole is despair, in which the person fears death with a feeling of unfulfillment: "There's so much left to do and no time to do it." This is characterized by an agonizing concern and penetrating dissatisfaction.

The quality of the resolution of this stage is wisdom. A person who is wise has knowledge of what is true and has the necessary judgment to act on what is right. This is a culmination of all the qualities described. As indicated, these qualities are cumulative, each being incorporated into the next, and surviving in the subsequent stage. Thus, a fully developed person has a sense of hope, determines options by free choice, establishes purpose, is competent, is faithful to self and to others, is capable of loving and caring, and is able to know and act on the truth.

Erikson made a major contribution to the field of development by the exploration of psychosocial development throughout the life span. He has pointed out that each of these stages presents a crisis or critical choice. This does not mean that it is catastrophic, but rather what emerges is particular to the stage. The way in which each polarity is resolved serves as the basis for the development in the next stage.

DEVELOPMENTAL LIFE TASKS

Robert Havighurst is credited with the concept of developmental life tasks. His book, *Developmental Tasks and Education,* is the primary source of information on this concept.[15] This approach is based on the idea that living and growing involve learning. Both inner and outer forces influence the development of life tasks. For instance, a child does not have the life task of walking until the physical condition and nervous system development allow for it. These are inner forces. The fact that the child is expected, encouraged, and helped to walk at a certain age is an outer force. In addition, some forces come from personal motives and values. These three types of forces combine to create the need to accomplish tasks.

Developmental life tasks must be accomplished by each person for successful living. It is also necessary to learn tasks at the most appropriate time. It is useless to try to teach a developmental task before the time when the combined physical, psychological, and personal forces are present to make the task appropriate.

Havighurst divides development into six age periods and discusses six to ten developmental tasks for each period (Table 5-5). He emphasizes that this is an arbitrary presentation of the tasks and that additional tasks may occur within each period. Each set of developmental tasks needs to be accomplished for adequate development and to form the basis for development in the next period.

Infancy and Early Childhood

Havighurst lists nine developmental life tasks of this period, in which the age range is from birth to about six years of age. He indicates that many of these tasks could be broken down into a number of separate tasks. However, the principal tasks are as follows:
1. Learning to walk
2. Learning to take solid foods
3. Learning to talk
4. Learning to control the elimination of bodily wastes
5. Learning sex differences and sexual modesty
6. Achieving physiologic stability (the only one of these tasks that appears to be purely biologic)
7. Forming simple concepts of social and physical reality
8. Learning to relate oneself emotionally to parents, siblings and others
9. Learning to distinguish right from wrong and developing a conscience

Middle Childhood

Middle childhood extends from about six to 12 years of age and is equivalent to Erikson's school age (industry versus inferiority). Havighurst points out that there are three "great outward pushes" on the child during this period: into

Table 5-5 Havighurst's Developmental Stages		
Stage	**Name**	**Age**
I	Infancy and Early Childhood	Birth to 6-7 years
II	Middle Childhood	6 to 12 years
III	Adolescence	12 to 18 years
IV	Early Adulthood	19 to 30 years
V	Middle Age	30 to 60 years
VI	Later Maturity	Over 60 years

the peer group, into games and work requiring neuromuscular skills, and into adult concepts and communication. Nine developmental life tasks relate to these three outward thrusts:
1. Learning physical skills necessary for ordinary games (throwing, catching, handling simple tools)
2. Building wholesome attitudes toward oneself a growing organism (habits of self-care, cleanliness, ability to enjoy using the body, wholesome attitudes toward sex, etc.)
3. Learning to get along with peers
4. Learning an appropriate masculine or feminine social role (the cultural basis of this is the most important, since there appears to be no basis for sexual differences in motor skills, and since role expectations are changing)
5. Developing fundamental skills in reading, writing and calculating
6. Developing concepts necessary for everyday living ("The task is to acquire a store of concepts sufficient for thinking effectively about ordinary occupational, civic, and social matters"[15])
7. Developing conscience, morality and a scale of values (the latter develops slowly during this period)
8. Achieving personal independence (developing the authority to make choices for oneself)
9. Developing attitudes toward social groups and institutions (religious and economic groups)

Adolescence

Adolescence extends from 12 to 18 years of age. The principal developmental life tasks during this period, according to Havighurst, are as follows:
1. Achieving new and more mature relationships with peers of both sexes (The goal is to "become an adult among adults"; working with others and leading without dominating are the most crucial part of the adolescent's life.)

2. Achieving a masculine or feminine social role (a changing phenomenon in our society—It is now more difficult to define the appropriate and acceptable sex role, or to be certain that there is one, then it was when Havighurst considered these tasks.)

3. Accepting one's physique and using the body effectively (Physiologic maturity affects the chronologic age at which this becomes an important task.)

4. Achieving emotional independence of parents and other adults (The important task is the development of affection and respect for parents and older adults without dependence on them.)

5. Achieving assurance of economic independence (feeling able to make a living—Today most adolescents begin some type of work early in this period, but are not financially independent until later.)

6. Selecting and preparing for an occupation

7. Preparing for marriage and family life (There is a great deal of variation in how adolescents view marriage and their own desire for it.)

8. Developing intellectual skills and concepts necessary for civic competence (Direct or vicarious experiences in government, economics, politics and psychology are the bases for the development of concepts necessary for civic competence.)

9. Desiring and achieving socially responsible behavior (Older adolescents often develop altruism and want to be able to "make a difference" in society.)

10. Acquiring a set of values and an ethical system to guide behavior (Solidifying present values, developing new ones, and becoming aware of values held are aspects of this task.)

Early Adulthood

This period extends from 18 to 30 years of age. For most individuals, a great many things happen during this time. It is usually the period in which marriage takes place, children are born, full-time career-oriented employment is begun, and independent living arrangement is achieved. Havighurst feels that this is a time when the person is most able to learn, but that it also is a time when there is little effort to teach.[15] The eight developmental tasks are as follows:

1. Selecting a mate (the most interesting and disturbing of the tasks, it is usually considered almost totally the responsibility of the persons involved.)

2. Learning to live with a marriage partner (success is built on successful fulfillment of the previous life tasks.)

3. Starting a family (both mother and father assume new roles and adapt psychologically to the changes that this brings.)

4. Rearing children (meeting the physical and emotional needs of the child, adapting to new circumstances, and taking on responsibilities for another person.)

5. Managing a home physically (furnishing, repairing, decorating, cleaning, and providing an atmosphere conducive to living), psychologically (providing an environment that allows those living in the place to feel comfortable and to be themselves), and socially (providing for relationships between the persons who reside there). Havighurst indicated that much of this was the responsibility of women, although men also contributed.[15]

6. Getting started in an occupation (Havighurst first related this task to men, and noted that this is so important that a young person may delay fulfilling other tasks, such as choosing a partner, until this task has been accomplished.)

7. Taking on civic responsibility (This task is less important early in the period; young adults begin to see the advantages of belonging to and influencing organizations of all kinds once the other tasks have become more solidified.)

8. Finding a congenial social group (The group of friends from adolescence is often psychologically and geographically distanced, so new friendships must be established.)

Middle Age

From about 30 to 55 years of age the individual is exceedingly active in fulfilling what are perceived as life goals. It is a time of great productivity. The life tasks of those who are married and have a family have a different focus from tasks of those who have not married. For family members, the tasks will be reciprocal as individuals react to each other.[15] Havighurst lists seven developmental tasks for this period:

1. Achieving civic and social responsibility by taking part in organizations and taking on responsibilities in effecting change (Middle age is the period in which most people are able to make their best contributions in this area—they have the greatest interest, the most energy to give, and the most available time.)

2. Establishing and maintaining an economic standard of living (This is the most important task of the period for many people, with social and even psychological needs sacrificed for econmic necessity.)

3. Assisting teen-aged children to become responsible and happy adults (being a good role model—The middle-aged parent has the task of facilitating the adolescent in maturing and becoming independent.)

4. Developing adult leisure-time activities (This task results from the increase in leisure time and changes in the kinds of leisure activities that appeal to the person.)

5. Relating oneself to one's spouse as a person (Husbands and wives relate to each other in different ways as parenting becomes less demanding and securing economic stability is of less concern.)

6. Accepting and adjusting to the physiologic changes of middle-age (The gradual aging that went unnoticed earlier is replaced by more dramatic changes that can no longer be ignored, particularly the stress of female menopause.)
7. Adjusting to aging parents (Taking on the care of parents and working out new psychological relationships, which reflect the way developmental tasks were handled early in life, the socioeconomic realities, the ages and physical and mental conditions of both parents and adult children, and a host of other factors.)

Later Maturity

This later time of life is still a period of learning. Many new circumstances require adaptation by the older person. Usually retirement from the occupation that has sustained the person for decades will occur. Marked economic changes often occur during this period, as well as major changes in interpersonal relationships. The life tasks are many. Havighurst lists the following six:

1. Adjusting to decreasing physical strength and health (The rate of decrease is different for each person, but all must adjust to a loss of vigor and independence in action, and many older persons have health problems affecting the cardiovascular system, the nervous system, and the joints.)
2. Adjusting to retirement and reduced income (Work is often intimately related to self-worth, although some people look forward immensely to retirement.)
3. Adjusting to death of a spouse (This task is probably the most difficult life task faced by individuals, often including a change of living arrangements, learning to do things that the spouse always did, dealing with loneliness, and handling changes in financial stability.)
4. Establishing an explicit affiliation with one's age group (This task includes receiving social security payments, moving to a retirement village, requesting a senior citizen discount, joining a senior citizen group, etc.)
5. Meeting social and civic responsibilities (as the population ages, it becomes increasingly important for older people to maintain their interest and concern with the political and social climate.)
6. Establishing satisfactory living arrangements (This task includes preferably making housing decisions themselves, keeping the physical condition of one's home in satisfactory repair and cleanliness, moving into smaller quarters while remaining independent, living with relatives, becoming acclimated to some form of congregate living, or accepting skilled nursing care.)

Havighurst's life tasks were originally published in 1948. Society has changed in many ways since then, but most of the life tasks remain valid for most people. One of the areas to which he did not refer is adjustment to divorce by both the couples and children.

Havighurst's work has formed an important basis for occupational therapy. When completion of the life tasks is disrupted by illness or disability, an essential role of therapy is to provide the opportunities for those life tasks to be accomplished.

PSYCHOSOCIAL NEEDS

Another approach to the consideration of human development was formulated by Abraham Maslow. Maslow described a hierarchy of needs, which must be fulfilled to achieve full development as a human being. Maslow feared the misapplication of his theories and emphasized the flexibility of this hierarchy and the importance of other motivating factors.[16]

Maslow's theory centers on the idea that the individual has basic needs, which are never completely satisfied, but which approach satisfaction to varying degrees. These needs are in a hierarchy: Usually the most basic must be partially met before the next set emerges. This progression is in many ways cyclical: One always moves back to more basic needs and then further up the hierarchy before coming back to the basics. There are five sets of needs: physiologic, safety, belongingness and love, esteem, and self-actualization; and two sets of needs that are integrated throughout the hierarchy, cognitive and aesthetic (Figure 5-1).[16]

Physiologic Needs

The physiologic needs are the basic drives to attain what is necessary to maintain homeostasis in the body. The needs related to homeostasis usually are food and water to supply nutrients to the body. There are other basic physiologic needs, however, that do not appear to relate closely to homeostasis, such as the need for sexual activity, sleep and activity.[16] These needs must be met to some extent before other needs emerge. Maslow points out that if these needs are seriously unmet, no other needs exist; a person who is starving is unable to appreciate any other needs. Gratification of the basic physiologic needs will lead to the emergence of the next level of needs (safety), whereas deprivation of these needs will lead to an all-encompassing concern for their fulfillment.

Safety Needs

Safety needs include the need for security, protection, structure, law and similar components that create a feeling of safety. Maslow indicates that this need can be seen more clearly in infants and young children, but that the needs are also important in the adult. All people appear to have a need

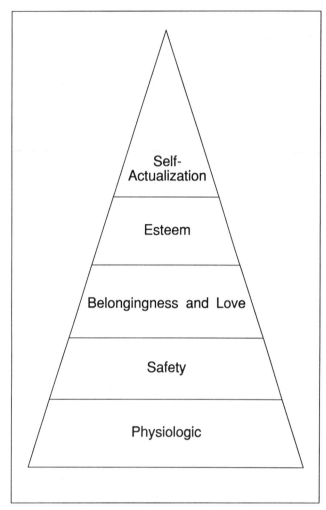

Figure 5-1. Maslow's hierarchy of needs.

for routine, predictability, and protection from danger. The infant reacts strongly to any threat to security; adults have learned to be more controlling of reactions.

The need for adequate housing is a prominent safety need that is often lacking in society. Many elderly people feel that they are in danger whenever they leave their own homes. People also seek to give themselves structure and routine, both of which meet safety needs.

Belongingness and Love Needs

The needs to experience love and affection, to have deep relationships with people, to have friends, and to feel a secure place in one's family or group are some of the aspects of this level of Maslow's hierarchy. When physiologic and safety needs are met, these needs for belongingness become prominent.

Maslow points out that mobility in our society creates problems in relation to these needs. Adjusting to new neighborhoods, making new friends, leaving old friends, establishing new roots, and relating to a totally new set of

persons cause upheaval in the fulfillment of these needs. Developing loyalties to country, city, neighborhood, employer, and family are ways in which this need is demonstrated. Persons who are alienated do not feel a sense of belonging; their needs on this level are thwarted. The great interest in tracing family history may well be a response to the difficulties people in our mobile society are experiencing and a strong expression of the need to belong.

The more severe psychological disorders may be traced to the person's lack of fulfillment of these needs.[16] One of the major problems of aging is the gradual loss of relationships with spouse and friends, and consequent isolation.

Esteem Needs

These needs are divided by Maslow into those related to the concept of self (feelings of adequacy, sense of competency, self-esteem and self-respect) and those related to other people's estimation of the person. Reputation, status, attention and recognition are some of the elements of these needs that come from outside the person and may or may not be correlated with the person's own perceptions. A person with an excellent reputation and high status and recognition may still feel inadequate and incompetent. Maslow also includes the need for independence and freedom in this category.

Cognitive Needs

Maslow discussed the needs to know and understand as cognitive needs that were integrated with the basic hierarchy of needs. He saw these as related to both the need for safety and the need for self-actualization. Curiosity, the desire to seek out answers, and the need to give meaning to events, circumstances and life itself are some of the aspects of cognitive needs. Active searching for explanations for what is observed or perceived is an on-going expression of this need. Cognitive needs are present in infancy and early childhood, and persist throughout life.

Aesthetic Needs

The need for beauty, for what is aesthetically pleasing, is a motivating factor for at least some persons. Maslow believed that healthy children universally demonstrate this need. As with the cognitive needs, he proposed that these needs are integrated into the basic hierarchy of needs, rather than being a step in the hierarchy.

Need for Self-Actualization

Self-actualization is the highest level of need. It is the desire to be fulfilled and to be all that one is capable of being. This need includes the ability to carry out most capably what one is most fitted for. Many people search for a number of years yet never find their real place in the world. For these needs to emerge, it is usually necessary for the physiologic, safety, belongingness and love, and esteem needs to be at least partially filled.

Although these five levels of needs are described as a hierarchy, there is a great deal of flexibility. For some people, the need for self-actualization is so strong that it overrides hunger or the need for status. Maslow also points out that one's values may change the relative importance of the levels of need. The framework of the hierarchy, however, is valid for most people.

CONCLUSION

It is essential that all occupational therapy personnel be knowledgeable in the areas of human development. Development occurs over the entire life span. There are a number of areas of development (motor, social, speech and language, psychological, cognitive, and sensory) but a person should be thought of as a whole person. It is necessary to think of the patient as *person* and to consider all of the areas of development at the particular stage of that individual. To facilitate the correlation of some of the developmental data from birth to adolescence, Mary K. Cowan, MA, OTR, FAOTA has developed a useful chart, which is shown in Appendix A.

Disability, whether physical, psychological, or both, affects development at all ages. Understanding the appropriate aspects of development will help to direct the formation of occupational therapy treatment goals and assist in the selection of suitable treatment approaches and media.

SUMMARY

Basic concepts of human development have been presented. These include motor development from birth through five years of age, primarily as described by Gesell and associates; cognitive development as studied by Piaget; psychosocial development throughout the life span according to Erikson; the developmental tasks first discussed by Havighurst; and the basic needs hierarchy of Maslow.

Related Learning Activities

1. Start a collection of children's drawings that represent the acquisition of fine motor skills at various stages of development.

2. Observe a group of children six to 12 years of age who are playing in a school yard during a recess period. Describe the play activities taking place and identify specific physical and social skills observed.

3. Chaperone an adolescent party at which both young men and women are guests. Compare and contrast behaviors seen with the work of two developmental theorists.

4. Develop a short, ten-item questionnaire that focuses on the life tasks defined by Havighurst. Use the questionnaire as a guide for interviewing a young adult, a middle aged person, and an elderly person, each of whom has a physical or mental disability.

5. Discuss the results of the questionnaire information from item four with peers. Were any additional life tasks identified? Did sociocultural background, economic status, educational level, or disability have an influence on the achievement of any life tasks?

References

1. Knoblock H, Pasamanick B (Eds): *Gesell and Amatruda's Developmental Diagnosis.* Hagerstown, Maryland, Harper & Row, 1974.
2. Gesell A: *The First Five Years of Life.* New York, Harper and Row, 1940.
3. Ames L et al: *The Gesell Institute's Child from One to Six.* New York, Harper & Row, 1979.
4. Noback CR, Demarest RJ: *The Human Nervous System,* 3rd edition. Lisbon, McGraw-Hill, 1981.
5. Fiorentino MR: *Normal and Abnormal Development.* Springfield, Illinois, Charles C. Thomas, 1972.
6. Biehler RF: *Child Development.* Boston, Houghton Mifflin, 1976.
7. Barclay LK: *Infant Development.* New York, Holt, Rhinehart & Winston, 1985.
8. Ginsberg H, Opper S: *Piaget's Theory of Intellectual Development.* Englewood Cliffs, New Jersey, Prentice Hall, 1969.
9. Flavell JH: *The Developmental Psychology of Jean Piaget.* Princeton, New Jersey, D. Von Nostrand, 1963.
10. Rosen H: *Pathway to Piaget.* Cherry Hill, New Jersey, Postgraduate International, 1977.
11. Wursten H: *Jean Piaget and His Work.* Unpublished paper presented at the American Occupational Therapy Conference, Los Angeles, 1972.
12. Gruber H, Coneche JJ: *The Essential Piaget.* New York, Basic Books, 1977.
13. Erikson EH: *Childhood and Society.* New York, WW Norton, 1963.
14. Stevens R: *Erik Erikson.* New York, St. Martin's Press, 1983.
15. Havighurst RJ: *Developmental Life Tasks and Education.* New York, David McKay Company, 1952.
16. Maslow AH: *Motivation and Personality.* New York, Harper & Row, 1970.

Components of Occupation

AND THEIR RELATIONSHIP TO ROLE PERFORMANCE

Ben Atchison, MEd, OTR, FAOTA

The same stream of life that runs through my veins night and day, runs through the world and dances in rhythmic measure.

—Rabindranath Tagore

INTRODUCTION

One concept that drives the practice of occupational therapy is the idea of occupation. Both the student and practitioner must understand the importance of occupation and its impact on biological, psychological, and sociocultural mechanisms. Putting that understanding into action to enhance role performance is the essence of the profession and appropriate intervention.

This chapter reviews the concept of *occupation* and describes three components that are vital to successful occupation. A review of the literature related to the impact of occupation on these three mechanisms is presented. Illustrations of the connection among these components, or their integration, are presented through brief case studies, which provide examples of how role performance is influenced. Elements of the teaching/learning process are also addressed.

THE MEANING OF OCCUPATION

In the development of a profession like occupational therapy, it is vital to define and articulate the unique aspects of the field. As occupational therapy personnel examine the basic philosophical beliefs of practice as described in Chapter 3, a return to the profession's early roots is evident. In this vein, as early as 1917, the founders of the National Society for the Promotion of Occupational Therapy established these objectives (see Chapter 1):[1]

1. The advancement of occupations as a therapeutic measure
2. The study of the **effects of occupation** (outcome of purposeful, meaningful activity) on the human being
3. The dissemination of scientific knowledge on this subject

KEY CONCEPTS

Meaning of occupation

Biologic components

Psychologic components

Sociocultural components

Relationship of components to role performance

ESSENTIAL VOCABULARY

Effects of occupation

Occupational science

Human activity

Choice of occupation

Biopsychosocial

Integrative school

Immunity

Culturally sensitive

Teaching/learning process

Disruption

Based on these founding ideas, a movement is currently underway to establish an academic discipline called **occupational science,** which is clearly rooted in these early principles set forth by the founders of the occupational therapy profession.[2] To understand the rationale for developing such a discipline, one needs to look at the concept of occupation and, in doing so, appreciate the complexity of its components as well as its relevance as a field of study that will ultimately increase the knowledge base of the profession.

Occupation refers to **human activity** and includes those basic needs for survival, as well as those activities we choose to pursue to live a productive, full life. The term *to occupy* does not connote passivity; rather, it conveys action, employment and anticipation.[3] Occupation includes the full repertoire of our daily activities, which are self-directed, purposeful, and socially acceptable.[4] Our **choice of occupation** comes from our cultural exposure, individual values and interests, and special abilities. It is a choice that is individualized and complex. Occupation is of symbolic importance to humans.[5] What a person does to occupy time has significance in social, cultural and spiritual contexts.[6] According to Reed,[7] occupation is dynamic and occurs through the influence of biologic, psychologic and sociocultural environments.

The occupational therapy assistant will have the opportunity to affect the occupational well-being of patients through intervention in the areas of self-maintenance (activities of daily living), work, play and leisure, and rest. Each recipient of occupational therapy treatment must be given the opportunity to teach the assistant what those areas mean in his or her life before effective therapeutic intervention can take place.

COMPONENTS OF OCCUPATION

Occupation can be seen as an end product of the human systems that interact to enable one to function. The interaction of these systems is of interest to many health practitioners, including occupational therapy personnel. These systems, including biologic, psychologic and sociocultural, are concepts on which rehabilitation is founded.[8] The impact of these systems, individually and in an integrated form, has been put forth as one model of intervention in occupational therapy practice. According to Reed, "The **biopsychosocial** model is designed to weigh the relative contributions of social and psychologic, as well as biologic factors, in determining the degree of health and illness and dysfunction."[7] The occupational therapy process of analyzing individuals through a systems approach provides understanding that a change in any subsystem may affect the whole human system.[7] The person is not to be viewed in

terms of a diseased organ or traumatized limb, but as a total organism with psychologic, social and biologic factors all being equal. If one considers the impact of amputation, it is not difficult to think beyond the obvious biologic changes. One must also appreciate the impact on the individual's psychologic and social functioning. Consideration is critical in therapeutic assessment and appropriate intervention. However, it is not easy to quantify the degree of impairment in all three areas, which is a limitation of this model.[7] For example, observation of biologic and physiologic changes after amputation of a limb are quantifiable, whereas psychological recovery, which may involve a change in values, interests, self-esteem, and emotions, is not as easily measured (Figure 6-1).

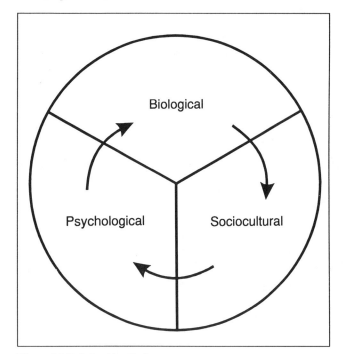

Figure 6-1. Relationship of subsystems.

Among several schools of thought in psychiatry is the **integrative school,** also known as the biopsychosocial school. Tiffany[8] points out that this approach is based on the idea that psychologic behaviors are determined by the complexity of physical, emotional, social and cultural processes that are interrelated. The theoretical frameworks that address the broad areas of knowledge that compose this school of thought include occupational behavior and those based on human development[9] (see Chapter 5).

Mosey[10] described the advantages of viewing the biopsychosocial model as a frame of reference for occupational therapy. She stresses that the first advantage is that our information about an individual is composed of information about the body, mind and environment. An appreciation of the relevance of this information strongly parallels the holistic approach to intervention, which is generic to occupational therapy philosophy. The second advantage is that this model addresses teaching/learning theory, which is a practical aspect of occupational therapy. The following sections detail information on these points, beginning with the first advantage.

Biologic Component

Biologic components include those internal systems that the individual must have to function, ie, the anatomic and physiologic components of the body. Disease and illness have an impact on these functions, as in the case of a cerebral vascular accident. The therapeutic intervention strategy for such a condition, which requires increasing musculoskeletal function (among others), includes engagement in activities to gain greater range of motion, muscle strength, and coordination. This approach has its basis in knowledge of the biologic component.

There are numerous reports in the scientific literature about the relationship of engagement in activity and biologic health. Bortz[11] presents a review of biologic changes that take place with aging. These changes are similar to those that take place as a result of enforced physical inactivity. The physiologic changes that take place at the cellular level and across total organs suggest that changes take place by disuse and not just from the aging process.[11] Specific studies related to the impact of exercise and activity on **immunity** are more prevalent. Simon[12] summarizes ten studies indicating that athletes, because of their habitual engagement in activity, have special defenses against illness. His studies focus on the effects of exercise on various "host-defense" factors, indicating that an active body has decreased potential for infection.

The study by Valliant[13] on the effect of exercise on older adults concluded that those who were actively involved experienced a significant reduction in depression and body fat concentration, leading to improved biologic health. Siscovick et al.[14] present information that outlines the benefits of physical activity on specific diseases. Many other studies clearly support the notion that humans who are actively engaged in physical activity have a healthier biologic profile. A number of these studies, including those specifically noted, present evidence of actual cellular changes as a result of physical activity. It is important for the occupational therapy assistant to be aware of these research findings because they provide needed justification for the inclusion of activity in a patient's overall health care management program.

Psychologic Component

The psychologic component is based on developmental, learning and behavioral theories. The occupational therapist's and assistant's knowledge of activity design and implementation is based on these theories as well. The certified occupational therapy assistant should review the literature for a basic understanding of these theories to appreciate their relevance in the intervention process. When planning activity, occupational therapy personnel consider the psychologic components of occupational performance, which include role acquisition, development and clarification of values and interests, initiating and terminating activity, and development of self-concept.

There is support for the relationship between engagement in activity and enhanced psychologic behavior. Soenstrom and Morgan[15] present a detailed analysis of self-esteem theory and provide an empirically based (experiential) rationale for self-esteem enhancement through engagement in activity. Valliant[13] also reports increased cognitive performance among older adults as a result of participation in an exercise program on a regular basis. Cook[16] describes the "alternatives approach" to drug abuse prevention based on the concept that individuals provided with healthful, nonchemical ways of gaining rewards and pleasures will be less likely to engage in drug or alcohol abuse. He presents a series of guidelines for the selection and development of activities from a "biopsychological" model of alternatives.

Sociocultural Component

The sociocultural component of this model addresses issues of individual values, roles and social patterns that must be a focus in effective intervention. The social skills related to occupational performance include social conduct, conversational skills, and self-expression. Although patients are expected to function within general social norms, it is critical that each of these skills be addressed in the context of the individual's cultural background. For intervention to be truly effective, the variation among patients with respect to ethnic values, interests, requirements, needs and roles must be considered. The social dynamics of one group will be unique from others and intervention must be sensitive to this fact.

Boyle[17] addresses these points in an excellent article on the multiple issues related to rehabilitation of individuals with physical performance deficits. She recommends that the profession of occupational therapy become more **culturally sensitive** (ie, aware of others' traditions, customs and beliefs) to meet the needs of the varied groups of patients who receive services. Recruitment of a more heterogenous group of therapists and assistants is one important way to address this issue. Further, she suggests that occupational therapy educational programs require certain courses that lead to a better understanding of and interaction with various cultural groups, including requirement of foreign language courses (see Chapter 10).

The Teaching/Learning Process

The second advantage of the model is that it focuses on the **teaching/learning process.**[10] This process emphasizes team effort in rehabilitation—the team being the therapist or the assistant and the patient. One guiding principle of occupational therapy intervention emphasizes "doing with" rather than "doing to." This model presents less emphasis on "treating" and more on "teaching." The therapist or assistant begins where the patient is and proceeds at a rate appropriate to the individual's ability. The teaching/learning process takes into account the learner's biologic, psychologic and sociocultural capacities and requirements (see Chapter 8).

ILLUSTRATIONS OF THE BIOPSYCHOSOCIAL CONNECTION

The occupational therapy assistant who views intervention from a biopsychosocial point of view will have an appreciation of the impact of dysfunction on role performance. It is important to remember that each system, if dysfunctional, can precipitate breakdown of function in the others. Illustrations of this point follow in brief case examples.

Case Study 6-1

Joe. Joe has a serious respiratory disease. He needs to be supported by a mobile oxygen unit, which causes a great deal of emotional discomfort. Because of this disease, he has great difficulty breathing during any activity, is often nauseated, and has a poor appetite. Since he is unable to perform many activities, he is deconditioned, which leads to fatigue and further discomfort. He is afraid that he is going to continue to get worse. His previously active social life is no longer as full. Joe spends a great deal of time alone, worrying about his health. When he worries, he feels his need to take in more oxygen as his respiration and demands for oxygen increase.

Joe's case illustrates the impact of biologic dysfunction on social and psychologic components and the disruptive cycle that can occur among the components. His biologic disease leads to disruption of his mental health, which creates a breakdown in socialization. This in turn continues to contribute to his biologic dysfunction. The cycle continues.

Case Study 6-2

Katherine. Katherine has been diagnosed with rheumatoid arthritis. The course of her condition has been stable for about five years. She has been able to maintain a high level of function, in spite of the disabling hand condition typified by this disease. Recently, she learned that her father was diagnosed as having pancreatic cancer and would not likely survive beyond one year. She has

suffered considerable grief over this news and has noted increased swelling and pain, and decreased motion in all her joints. She also is experiencing increased inflammation. Her appetite is decreasing, she feels very fatigued, and she is not sure she can continue to work every day, as she has done in past years. Her anxiety grows over the impending loss of her father, as well as her potential loss of function.

Katherine's case presents an example of someone who is suffering exacerbations of a dormant condition due to psychosocial stressors. The biologic manifestations are real, but precipitated by emotional stress.

Case Study 6-3

Tom. Tom sustained a head injury as a result of a swimming accident two years ago. He had rather intensive rehabilitation, including residency for six months at a community reentry program for head-injured individuals. His discharge from the program and subsequent return to his home has been difficult. The rehabilitation team at the community reentry program has made great efforts to assist Tom in developing functional skills to allow a transition to independent living. Yet, after a short time at home, Tom is lonely, depressed, and unable to cope independently. He also drinks heavily, a behavior that led to the accident causing his injury. Tom's premorbid lifestyle, a critical factor in the overall success of his rehabilitation program, was not addressed. He is again at risk.

RELATIONSHIP TO ROLE PERFORMANCE

The ability of an individual to achieve success in role performance is a result of biopsychosocial competence. **Disruption** of any of these three components will result in dysfunctional patterns of role performance. The term "disruption" refers to a forced interruption in a person's life. It is the degree of disruption that the occupational therapy assistant should question. That is, some individuals will be unaffected by biopsychosocial stressors that cause total breakdown in others. This difference is due to adaptation and, as demonstrated by the case studies, occurs within the limits of the individual. Thus, it is important to provide opportunities that allow for adaptation and manipulation of the environment. This goal might be accomplished in a clinical setting initially and then gradually approached in "real world" situations. The process of adaptation must be approached through engagement in occupation. Through occupational therapy intervention, the patient can learn problem-solving methods that will assist in occupational performance and effective adaptation.[18] To illustrate this idea, application of the process will be applied to the cases described earlier.

Joe

Because of the severity of his respiratory disease, Joe will have considerable difficulty in performing all of his previous occupations. He requires mechanical adaptations and adaptive devices to allow for energy conservation, so that he may be able to achieve independently self-care tasks. Allowing him to dress himself, through work simplification techniques, will result in his feeling more capable and less regressive. Feeling less exhausted due to simple environmental adaptations will allow Joe to resume some aspects of his role as a husband. Although alteration of the biologic deficit is not possible, adaptation of his environmemt will lead to enhanced competence in some activities leading to improved psychologic health and resulting in less stress on an already taxed biologic system.

Katherine

Katherine is clearly suffering biologic symptoms as a result of psychologic stressors. Allowing her to work through her grief by expressing her feelings of loss, fear and anxiety will provide the "nourishment" needed to replenish her physical strength. Symptoms as noted will decrease along with her opportunity to express her grief.

Tom

Tom's case represents a critical problem in rehabilitation. To provide proper treatment for Tom, the rehabilitation team must better understand his background, particularly his social history. An understanding of his lifestyle and experiences that place him at high risk for disability is needed if rehabilitation is to be effective. Boyle[17] speaks to this issue when she points out that a single impulsive act, such as drinking and driving, "may cause a person to cross the threshold for disability, that point at which a physiologic or psychologic effect begins to be produced."[17] Boyle recounts the story of John Callahan, a successful cartoonist with quadraplegia. His disability was the result of an automobile accident, caused by driving while intoxicated. It wasn't until six years after his injury that he realized that the true source of his disability was not his physical limitations, but the fact that he was an alcoholic.[17]

IMPLICATIONS FOR OCCUPATIONAL THERAPY

Taking a holistic view of the individual, with consideration as to how the biologic, psychologic and sociocultural components impact on occupation and role perfomance, is critically important for all members of the profession if we are to be successful in our intervention efforts. When specializing in areas such as neurodevelopmental therapy or hand therapy, it is important to continue to view the whole person, not just the immediate problem.

SUMMARY

The concept of occupation was reviewed, together with the three important components: biologic, psychologic and sociocultural. All must be considered to have a holistic approach to therapeutic intervention. Case studies were presented to illustrate the interrelationship of the components and their impact on role performance and the health of the individual. Scientific evidence was introduced that clearly demonstrates that changes at the cellular level, as well as changes in psychological behavior, occur as a result of engagement in occupation. Biologic conditions are often exacerbated by sociocultural conditions, which must be addressed as a part of a therapeutic intervention program. The importance of the teaching/learning process was also emphasized.

Editor's Note

This chapter builds on the content found in the preceding chapters. To gain maximal appreciation for the information presented here, the reader should have a good understanding of historical, philosophical, theoretical and developmental principles of the profession. The author's discussion of the components of occupation in relation to role performance provides the necessary background for the student to proceed to the study of the remaining chapters, particularly those on occupational performance areas.

Acknowledgment

The author and the editor wish to thank Sr. Genevieve Cummings, CSJ, MA, OTR, FAOTA for her content and editorial suggestions.

Related Learning Activities

1. Define the term *occupation* in your own words.

2. Discuss your primary occupations and roles with a peer. Identify similarities and differences.

3. Interview a child, a teenager, an adult and an elderly person, all of whom have a physical or psychosocial disability. Determine in what ways, if any, their disability changed their primary roles and occupations.

4. What were some of the specific biologic, psychological, and social factors that had an influence on the patients interviewed in item 3?

5. Review the case study about Katherine. List potential treatment activities that could be used as a part of an occupational therapy program.

References

1. Dunton WR: The principles of occupational therapy. *Proceedings of the National Society for the Promotion of Occupational Therapy: Second Annual Meeting.* Catonsville, Maryland, Spring Grove State Hospital, 1918.

2. Yerxa E et al: An introduction to occupational science, a foundation for the occupational therapy in the 21st century. *Occup Ther Health Care* 6:1-17, 1989.

3. Englehardt HT: Defining occupational therapy: The meaning of therapy and the virtues of occupation. *Am J Occup Ther* 31:666-672, 1977.

4. University of Southern California, Department of Occupational Therapy: A proposal for a new doctor of philosophy degree in occupational science. Unpublished manuscript, 1987.

5. Campbell J: *The Power of Myth.* New York, Doubleday, 1988.

6. Fraser JT: *Time, the Familiar Stranger.* Amherst, Massachusetts, University of Massachusetts Press, 1987.

7. Reed KL, Sanderson S: *Concepts of Occupational Therapy.* Baltimore, Williams & Wilkins, 1983.

8. Tiffany E: Psychiatry and mental health. In Hopkins HD, Smith HL (Eds): *Willard and Spackman's Occupational Therapy,* 5th edition. Philadelphia, JB Lippincott, 1978.

9. Adams JE, Lindemann E: Coping with long-term disability. In Coelho GV, Hamburg DA, Adams JE (Eds): *Coping and Adaptation.* New York, Basic Books, 1974.

10. Mosey AC: An alternative: The biopsychosocial model. *Am J Occup Ther* 28:137-140, 1974.

11. Bortz WM: Disuse and aging. *J Am Med Assoc* 248:1203-1208, 1980.

12. Simon HB: The immunology of exercise. A brief review. *J Am Med Assoc* 252:2735-2738, 1894.

13. Valliant PM: Exercise and its effects on cognition and physiology in older adults. *Percept Mot Skills* 61:1031-1038, 1985.

14. Siscovick DS, LaPorte RE, Newman JM: The disease specific benefits and risks of physical activity and exercise. *Public Health Rep* 100:180-188, 1985.

15. Soenstrom RJ, Morgan WP: Exercise and self-esteem: Rationale and model. *Medicine and Science in Sports and Exercise* 21:329-337, 1989.

16. Cook R: The alternatives approach revisited: A biopsychological model and guidelines for application. *Int J Addict* 20:1399-1419, 1985.

17. Boyle M: The changing face of the rehabilitation population: A challenge for therapists. *Am J Occup Ther* 44:941-945, 1990.

18. Ryan SE: Theoretical frameworks and approaches. In Ryan SE (Ed): *The Certified Occupational Therapy Assistant: Roles and Responsibilities.* Thorofare, New Jersey, Slack Inc., 1986.

Occupational Performance Areas

Doris Y. Witherspoon, MS, OTR

INTRODUCTION

Occupational performance areas are those things accomplished each day that sustain and enhance life. Everyday life presents few problems to individuals who have "good" physical and emotional health. Occupational therapy personnel work with patients with health problems brought about by causes such as birth defects, injury or illness. These impairments can affect a person's ability to meet needs and fulfill desired roles and life goals.[1] Early occupational therapy practice was founded on the idea that activity promotes mental and physical well-being and that, conversely, absence of activity leads to deterioration or loss of mental and physical function.[2]

Occupational therapy assumes that daily activities play a central part in everyone's life. This assumption grew out of knowledge and concern that people must be able to perform certain tasks at prescribed levels of competence.[3] These activities have been identified as occupation.

The three major **categories of occupation** are referred to collectively as occupational performance areas and include activities of daily living (ADLs), work activities, and play or leisure activities. Healthful living and self-esteem depend on the balance established among these three types of occupational performance. Individuals who fail to develop balanced living routines or whose routines have been disrupted may learn to regain their occupations through participation in occupational therapy.[3]

The individual's view of an activity varies considerably. In one situation a task may be considered work, but in another setting it may be a leisurely activity. For example, a woman does house cleaning in clients' homes and considers her tasks gainful employment. When she cleans her own home in preparation for guests, however, the same activity could be described as leisurely.

KEY CONCEPTS

Occupational therapy process

Activities of daily living: physical and psychological components

Play classifications

Contributions of play to development

Purposes, functions, and goals of leisure

Recreation

Significance of work

Relationship of work to physical and psychosocial elements

Where does work fit into the daily living routine? Because of cultural dictates, ADLs, also referred to as self-care, are a precursor to work; and work, a precursor to leisure. American culture, for the most part, dictates that one's grooming and hygiene be completed before going to the work place. It is also generally accepted that leisure is a reward activity for one's hard work. In addition, many of the functional abilities acquired through work activities and training are used in everyday leisure activities. The interrelationship of the primary components of occupational performance areas is shown in Figure 7-1.

The relationship among ADLs, work and leisure changes markedly as individuals progress from infancy to adulthood. Consequently, the daily living routines of infants and adults are very dissimilar.[4] One's **cultural environment** (ie, human and non-human elements that relate to traditions,

customs and beliefs) and related social status help in defining the balance among activities. Routine activity for blue collar workers will differ substantially from the regular activity of executives and homemakers.

A lack of balance in healthful activity can cause withdrawal, depression, or deterioration in the individual's capacity to meet daily needs. Occupational therapy assists in developing, redeveloping, or maintaining necessary activity skills for occupational performance, which lead to productive and satisfying lifestyles. **Skill acquisition** allows the impaired individual to return to independent, wholesome living in the community.[3]

Everyone needs balanced activity to adapt to societal living. An important goal of occupational therapy is to correct deficiencies that interfere with the exercise of independence by teaching ADLs, work, and play and leisure activity skills.

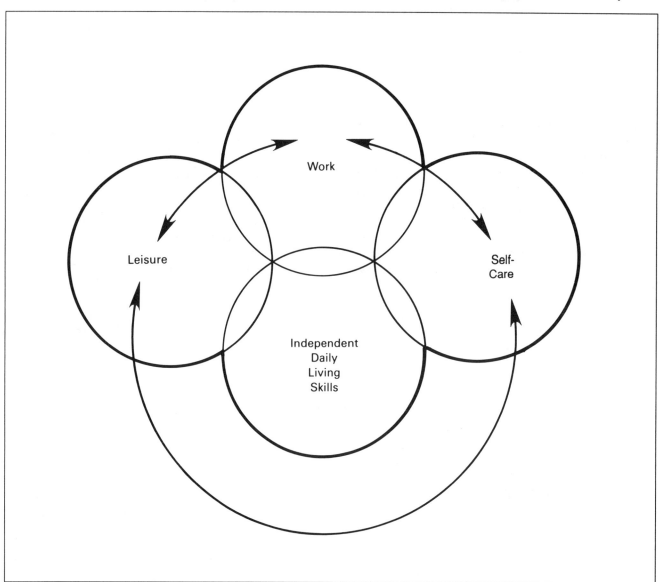

Figure 7-1. The interrelationship of primary components of occupational performance areas.

THE OCCUPATIONAL THERAPY PROCESS

The essential focus of the occupational therapy evaluation is on the occupational skills and roles of the patient in relation to occupational performance responsibilities. Occupational therapy personnel study these skill levels, roles, and responsibilities and determine how the patient's normal patterns of dealing with them have changed. Both the family and the patient are involved in determining the specific discrepancies between past and present activities and the level of performance, and discovering what level of function is necessary and acceptable to the patient in the personal environment and social/cultural setting. An objective assessment of the patient's needs and potential is essential for the registered occupational therapist and the certified occupational therapy assistant to plan and implement a treatment program that will allow the patient to gain or regain as many functional abilities as possible. ADLs are a primary focus of the occupational therapy process.

Occupational therapy assistants must understand and appreciate the importance of occupational performance activities to provide the most effective therapeutic intervention strategies in meeting the patient's needs. They can assist patients in determining their present status and the additional skills and attitudes they may need to acquire to achieve their goals.[5]

ACTIVITIES OF DAILY LIVING

While play/leisure and work activities are equally important skills, ADLs (self-care) are presented first because they are prerequisite to work and play/leisure, and are paramount to independent survival.[6]

An individual is expected to perform routine tasks such as dressing, feeding, and grooming before he or she is considered well adapted to community life.[7] Occupational therapy personnel are responsible for assessing the patient's basic potential and teaching primary skills in ADLs. Such assessments are based on mental and chronological age, and the goals for children and adults differ greatly. Moreover, the methods for teaching these two groups vary considerably.

Self-help and daily living skills training is critical in dealing with attitudes that patients may have formed about their conditions. If they receive adequate instruction and support, routine life may be less burdensome, and self-care skill may be a motivating force for pursuing work and leisure activities.[7] The specific activities are categorized as follows:[8]

1. Grooming
2. Oral hygiene
3. Bathing
4. Toilet hygiene
5. Dressing
6. Feeding and eating

7. Medication routine
8. Socialization
9. Functional communication
10. Functional mobility
11. Sexual expression

Skills are developed in three essential ways. First is the ability to perform tasks independently. Second, assistive devices may be developed to aid the physically impaired in accomplishing such tasks. Finally, other persons within an individual's environment may be trained to assist the patient in the performance of certain tasks. Many disabled persons learn to achieve daily living skills through a combination of these three methods.

Evaluating Physical Daily Living Skills

The first step in any rehabilitation plan is to evaluate the patient's abilities and dysfunctions. Figure 7-2 provides an example of a form that may be followed to evaluate daily living skills. A variety of other **evaluation tools** are available and are used to determine performance definitions.

Independence is the focus of ADLs; therefore, the certified occupational therapy assistant (COTA), working under the supervision of the registered occupational therapist (OTR), must observe and analyze each action. It is not enough merely to identify skills that the patient is unable to perform. How the patient performs the task is equally important, as this determines the level and quality of the skill performance in carrying out selected tasks. The patient may be able to complete some tasks independently, but the evaluator needs to study the "how" very closely and answer the following questions:

1. How long did it take to perform the activity?
2. Did the activity take twice as long as it would for a person of average ability?
3. Did the patient complain of fatigue and need frequent rest periods?
4. Was the patient, despite working steadily, still unable to complete the task because movements were too slow?
5. Which motions are functional, and how do they function?
6. When did the patient first require assistance, and what kind of assistance was needed?

Although terminology often varies, COTAs may report patient needs in terms of the following observations:

- *Stand-By Assistance (SBA):* The patient completes the activity independently, but may lack confidence. The patient may require verbal or physical assistance in completing the activity.
- *Minimal Physical Assistance (Min PA):* The patient requires physical assistance to complete the activity.
- *Moderate Physical Assistance (Mod PA):* The patient requires physical assistance to continue and complete the activity.

Name _____ Age _____

Address _____

Diagnosis _____ Occupation _____

GROOMING	Date	Needs Equipment	Needs Assistance	Needs Minimal Assistance	Needs No Assistance
Comb/brush hair					
Wash hair					
Set hair					
Shave					
Apply make-up					
Trim nails					
File nails					
Manage feminine hygiene					
Brush teeth					
Manage toothpaste or powder					
BATHING					
Shower					
Turn on/off faucet					
Bathe					
Dry self					
DRESSING					
Over shirts					
Button shirt/blouse					
Ties					
Jacket/coats					
Hats/gloves					
Zipping					
Putting on shoes					
Tying shoes					
Lace shoes					
Putting on socks/hose					
Pants					
Skirts/slacks					
Dress					
Secure clothes from drawer					
Hang up clothing					
COMMUNICATION					
Read book or magazine					
Write/type					
Speaks coherently					
Comprehends spoken words					
TRANSPORTATION					
Bus					
Drive					
Walk					

Figure 7-2. Daily living skills evaluation. Used with permission of Wayne County Community College, Occupational Therapy Assistant program.

Name _____   Age _____

Address _____

Diagnosis _____ Occupation _____

COOKING	Date	Needs Equipment	Needs Assistance	Needs Minimal Assistance	Needs No Assistance
Peel					
Measure basic ingredients					
Mix					
Follow simple directions					
Follow complex directions					
Prepare cold meal					
Prepare hot meal					
Convenience foods					
Boxed					
Frozen					
Canned					
CLEAN-UP					
Wipe counters					
Sweep floors					
Scour sink					
Wash pots/pans					
Dishes/silver, glasses					
Put away supplies					
Dishes, bowls, spoons					
Find supplies (memory)					
Dusting					
Mop floor					
Make bed					
Change bed					
Wash clothes					
Vacuum					
Clean tub					
Clean toilet					
Windows					
TIME MANAGEMENT					
Planning day					
Planning meals					
Coordinating schedules					
Manage watch					
MONEY MANAGEMENT					
Making change					
Checks					
Paying bills					

Figure 7-2. Continued.

		Needs Equipment	Needs Assistance	Needs Minimal Assistance	Needs No Assistance

Name _____ Age _____
Address _____
Diagnosis _____ Occupation _____

EATING	Date	Needs Equipment	Needs Assistance	Needs Minimal Assistance	Needs No Assistance
Eat with fingers					
Pick up utensils					
Use fork/spoon					
Cut food					
Spread butter on bread					
Use salt and pepper					
Drink from glass/cup					
Open milk container					
Pour from container					
Stir liquid					
Open screw-top bottles					
MOBILITY					
Sit balanced on edge of bed					
Get in/out of bed					
Turn over in bed					
Sit in straight chair					
Rise from straight chair					
Open doors					
Stand unsupported					
Walk					
Walk carrying objects					
Pick up objects from floor					
Independent transfers					
MISCELLANEOUS					
Manage keys					
Manage glasses					
Operate radio or TV					

Figure 7-2. Continued.

- *Maximal Physical Assistance (Max PA):* The patient requires physical assistance to initiate, continue, and complete the activity.
- *Mechanical Assistance:* The patient completes the activity independently with the use of an assistive or adaptive aid.

During the evaluation it is important for the COTA to remember to actually observe the patient in the performance of each task. This gives the assistant an opportunity to monitor the patient rather than to rely on the patient's descriptive statements about how the activity was or will be performed. Such a procedure also provides a more accurate assessment of how the patient will function in the performance of ADLs when he or she no longer is receiving direct care.

The COTA, in collaboration with the OTR, determines the underlying reason or reasons for lack of independence in ADLs, such as muscle weakness, lack of coordination, poor balance, or visual perceptual deficits. Short-term goals should focus on improving functional impairment, whereas long-term goals should emphasize independence of function in the activities.

Case Study 7-1

The patient is unable to dress himself. He lacks trunk balance and has limited shoulder range of motion. Short-term goals would center on improving balance, thus freeing the upper extremities for functional activities, while allowing trunk range and "righting" and increasing range of motion at the shoulder joints. This will allow more reaching and extending movements. The result will be improved physical function, thus allowing the patient to focus on the long-term goal of achieving greater independence by improving skills in ADLs where deficits exist.

Adaptations in Physical Daily Living Skills— Definition and Purpose

The physical ADLs have been enumerated in the early part of this chapter. They may be defined as those daily activities necessary for fulfilling basic needs, such as personal hygiene and grooming, dressing, feeding and eating, use of medications, socialization, functional communication and mobility, and sexual expression. In every aspect of life—play, leisure or work—daily living needs act as both prerequisites and corequisites to accomplishing everyday routines.

The COTA, under the supervision of the OTR, evaluates patient's abilities to perform daily living activities and identifies deficiencies and strengths. The COTA may assist the OTR in the establishment of goals for the treatment plan and the methods that will be used to accomplish these goals through acceptable levels of activity. Patients and their families are informed about the occupational therapy treatment plans and are encouraged to participate in the rehabilitation/habilitation process. A variety of methods are used to teach skills, including verbal instruction, demonstration, and visual or verbal cues.[9] More information on specific teaching techniques may be found in Chapter 8.

The need for independence in daily living skills is often more acute for the physically disabled population. The need to eat, dress, work, recreate, and manipulate the environment generally does not diminish for the individual, although he or she is limited in physical abilities. The person with a disability learns to perform necessary daily living tasks by adapting the surrounding environment through manipulation of those elements within his or her control. This manipulation may take many forms, including:

1. Assistive aids
2. Adaptive equipment
3. Energy conservation techniques
4. Work simplification skills
5. Effective time management
6. Positioning
7. Designs to eliminate barriers
8. Vocational modifications

These techniques entail using the environment in creative ways to fulfill tasks that are easy for the physically able.

Beyond environmental concerns, a patient's functional impairments, such as spasticity and rigidity, may contribute to an inability to perform daily living tasks. These functional impairments are attributable to various pathologic diseases and disorders. The combination of functional impairment and environmental barriers cause a need for change in the patient's daily routine through adaptation. They compel the patient to rethink or relearn otherwise simple activities commensurate with the changes in abilities.

Spasticity may result in the following:
1. Joint motion limitation
2. Muscle weakness/paralysis
3. Motor ataxia/sensory ataxia
4. Lack of trunk control/balance
5. Athetoid/tremorous movements
6. Impaired cognition
7. Concentration/attention span

Rigidity may cause the following:
1. Contractures/deformities
2. Decreased physical tolerance/endurance
3. Sensory impairment
4. Impaired visual perception
5. Impaired coordination
6. Motor/sensory/kinetic apraxia

Assessing the Need for Assistive/Adaptive Equipment

Assistive/adaptive equipment is often the key to independence for the person who is disabled. Not only can it assist in improving the quality of life for the patient, but it can often help to restore the patient's sense of dignity and self-esteem through newly found independence.

Several important factors should be considered before recommending, constructing, or ordering adaptive aids for patients. Cost, design and maintenance are three of the primary considerations (see Chapter 15).

Cost. The following questions must be answered: Is the recommended item covered as reimbursable in the patient's insurance plan? If so, what percentage of the cost will be covered? If not, what is the maximum amount the patient can afford? Is it less expensive and more feasible for the occupational therapist or assistant to construct the item than to purchase it?

Design. The following questions must be answered: Will the recommended item serve more than one purpose? How durable is the item (especially if it will be used frequently)? Is it attractive as well as functional? Is the item easy to use or wear, or is it too cumbersome? Is the patient embarrassed about using the device? (If so, it may not accomplish the intended purpose.)

Maintenance. The following questions must be answered: If the item requires repair or replacement, can a local vendor fulfill this need? Can the patient make minor repairs or adjustments? Can the device be cleaned easily?

Adaptations in Treatment Implementation

Many assistive devices are available to help the patient with various functional impairments, such as muscle weakness, paralysis, joint limitation, or poor grasp. Although too numerous to list in detail, the more common items are illustrated in Figures 7-3 and 7-4.

Grooming and Hygiene. Grooming and hygiene include the skills of bathing, oral hygiene, toileting, hair and nail care, shaving, application of cosmetics, and other health needs.[8,10] When the patient is unable to perform tasks without assistance, an assessment for the potential use of the adaptive equipment should be made. The following aids are commonly used to improve independence in grooming and hygiene: long-handled bath brush, hair brush, scrub sponge, hand mirror and shaver, built up handle on toothbrush and comb, tube squeezer, electric razor holder, deodorant/shaving cream dispenser handle, suction denture brush, toilet tissue dispenser holder, raised toilet seat, toilet and bath safety rails, bath seat/chair lift, tub chair, hand-held shower nozzle, and rubber tub mat.

Dressing. The skill of dressing includes the ability to choose clothing that is seasonal and occasion-appropriate, remove it from a storage area, and don it in a sequential fashion, including use of special fasteners and adjustments.[8] Dressing instruction usually begins with dressing the disabled side first and undressing it last.[10] Clothes that are loose-fitting and open are recommended for easy wear. Some of the common adaptive equipment used for dressing tasks include long-handled shoe horns, sock aids, dressing sticks and reachers; stabilizing botton hooks, Velcro or clip shoe fasteners and elastic laces, one-handed belts, zippers and trouser pulls, and Velcro fasteners, elastic waistbands, and suspenders.

Feeding and Eating. Feeding includes the skills of setting up food, use of appropriate utensils and dishes, the ability to bring food or a beverage to the mouth, chewing, sucking, swallowing, and coughing to avoid choking.[8,10] The patient must be alert; proper body positioning is critical. It may be necessary to instruct the patient in sucking, chewing and swallowing. Some of the more common types of adapted equipment used to increase functional use of feeding utensils include long-handled, lightweight, or swivel spoons; forks with built up handles or triangular finger grips; plastic handle mugs with pedestal cups and other modified drinking utensils; splints with palmar clips; straw holders; scoop dishes; plate/food guards; suction plates; rubber mats; weighted utensils; rocker knives; ball bearing and offset suspension feeders; and universal cuffs and splints.

Medication Routine. Medication routine may be defined as the ability to obtain medication, open and close containers, and take the prescribed amount at the specified time.[8] Adaptive devices may include enlarged, easy-to-open containers or a divided container with medications placed in specific compartments with time noted when they should be taken.

Socialization. Socialization is defined as one's skill in interacting appropriately in contextual and cultural ways.[8] Adaptive equipment may include proper positioning devices to allow greater comfort and ease in social situations and slings that are made of fabric to match or complement clothing, thus improving self-image. In addition, a number of the adaptations listed under functional communication, such as the telephone, assist in promoting greater socialization in some cases.

Functional Mobility. Mobility includes the ability to move physically from one position or place to another. Such movement includes bed mobility; transfers to and from bed, chair, toilet, tub, and automobile; wheelchair mobility; ambulation; and driving.[8,10] Some of the common adaptive equipment used to facilitate mobility includes manual and electric wheelchairs, motorized scooters, mechanical and hydraulic lifts, trapeze bars, walkers (which may or may not have bag attachments), canes and cane seats, crutches, transfer boards, elevated chair and toilet seats, and modified vans, cars, and public transportation vehicles.

Functional Communication. Communication includes the ability to receive and transmit information verbally or nonverbally. Adaptive devices used to enhance communication skills include telephones, talking books, tape recorders, computers with printers and Braille writers, typewriters, radios, television, prism glasses, page turners, clip boards, and mouth sticks.[10]

Sexual Expression. Sexual expression has been defined as the ability to "recognize, communicate, and perform desired sexual activities."[8] Adaptive equipment such as pillows may be used to enhance function and increase comfort.

Related Adaptations. A large variety of adaptive devices are available to assist with performing work tasks. They will be discussed briefly here in relation to the specific areas of general object manipulation and cooking.

Object manipulation includes the skill and performance of handling large and small objects such as calculators, keys, money, light switches, doorknobs and packages. To assist the patient in manipulating common objects, positioning splints and other types of adaptive equipment are useful. These devices include tweezers, mouthstick holders/wands,

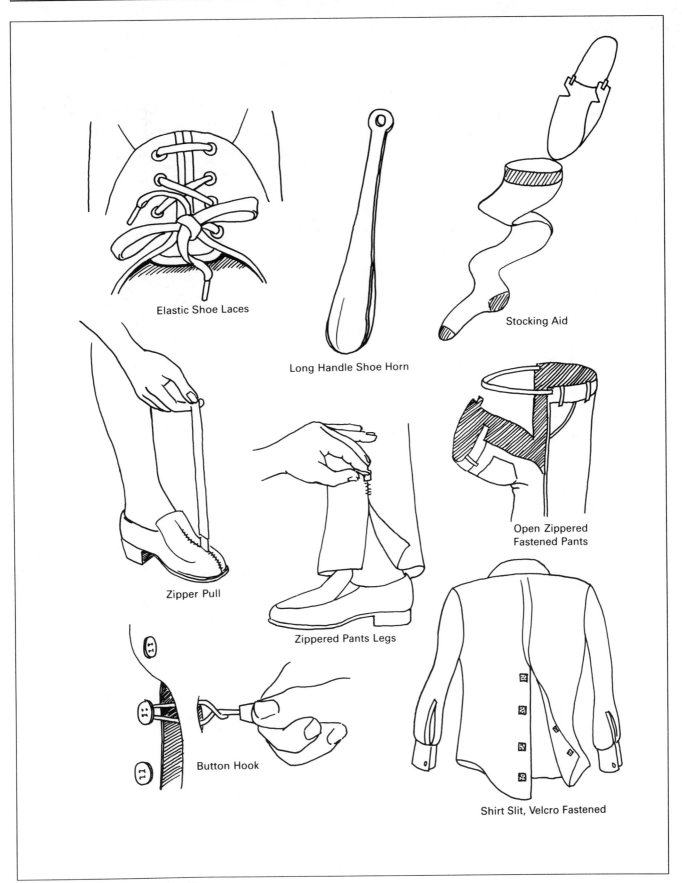

Figure 7-3. Adaptive/assistive dressing aids.

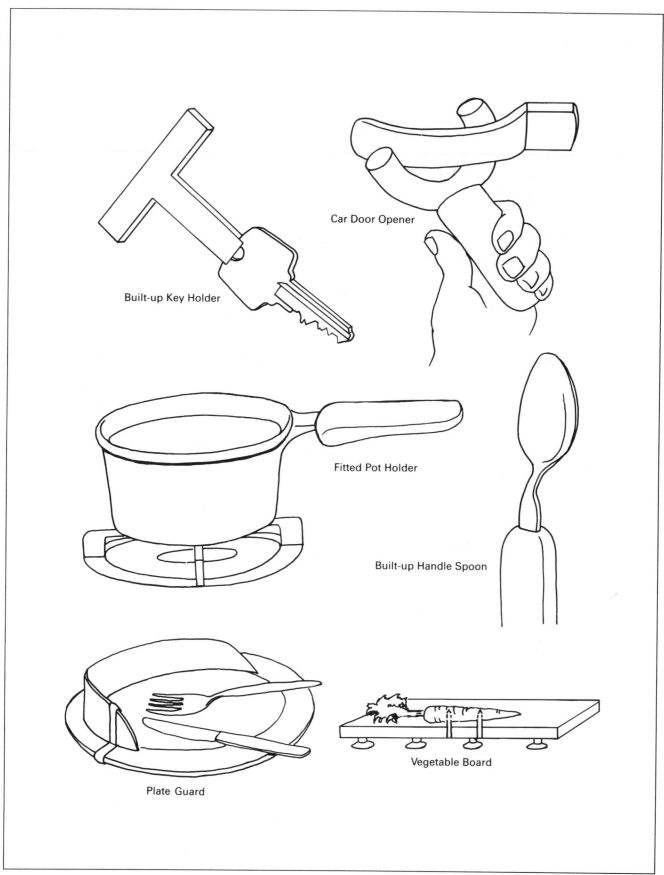

Built-up Key Holder

Car Door Opener

Fitted Pot Holder

Built-up Handle Spoon

Plate Guard

Vegetable Board

Figure 7-4. Adaptive/assistive devices.

light switch extensions/levers, key holders, and door knob extenders and turners.

Physical cooking skills range from simple peeling skills to preparing entire meals. Some of the common types of cooking adaptations are built up handles on utensils, plate guards, rubber mats, fitted potholders, and vegetable boards (see Figure 7-4).

Psychological/Emotional Daily Living Skills

Although this section focuses on the patient with psycho-social/emotional problems, these problems may also be seen in a patient with a physical disability. Conversely, the patient with psychiatric problems, owing to medication for example, may experience difficulty with gross motor, fine motor, and coordination skills.

ADLs for psychiatry are also centered around self-concept, self-identity, and coping with life situations in family, organizational and community involvement. Unlike patients with physical disabilities, individuals with psychiatric conditions have the motor ability to perform the tasks in most cases, but emotional conflicts may reduce the desire or motivation to carry them out. Patients may not attend to personal hygiene and grooming without assistance or verbal prompting from others. Occupational therapy provides a structured setting in which to learn how to take charge of their lives and be responsible for personal actions. Through therapy, the patient is guided in decision-making activities with the assurance that behaviors exhibited can be acceptable. With the contemporary emphasis on community mental health, the COTA is an important team member responsible for contributing to program planning and carrying out day-to-day activities.

The occupational therapy program in psychiatry provides service to the individual whose ability to meet psychosocial needs is impaired. This inability may be demonstrated through socialization, personal self-care, and play. For example, an individual may become disorganized or preoccupied, resulting in an inability to perform some task. The person may be very demanding and hostile, resulting in upsetting relationships with family and peers. The person may withdraw, become fearful, and reject communication.

Treatment begins with a psychosocial evaluation to assess the individual's self-concept, orientation to reality, and ability to communicate with others and to perform life tasks. Determining the patient's level of motivation, maturity, socialization, interpersonal relationships, and ability to cope with frustration and conflicts is another important part of the evaluation. Evaluation tools, techniques and methods used by occupational therapy personnel are the following:

1. Observation
2. Interest checklist
3. Anecdotal notes
4. Cumulative records
5. Rating scales
6. Self-report forms
7. Sociometric devices
8. Psychological tests
9. Standardized tests
10. Interviews
11. History taking

Patients who are referred to occupational therapy in psychiatry may have problems with occupational performance areas for a number of reasons, such as depression, which leaves them with little energy to cope with routine activities. The patient who is out of touch with reality may be unable to cook and eat because of fear that the food is poisoned.

Teaching task skills to patients can be very challenging and offers the therapist and the assistant opportunities for creativity. The most common areas of treatment addressed by the COTA practicing in psychiatry are grooming and hygiene, cooking, time management, socialization and organizational skills. Helping patients learn or relearn skills in these areas can increase their awareness and self-esteem.

Case Study 7-2

A creative COTA responsible for treating an adolescent who was chemically-dependent recently learned the latest fad for painting striped fingernails. The assistant taught this skill to a female patient, and the patient proceeded to teach the technique to her peers. Through teaching the patient a new skill, the therapist developed a closer relationship with the patient that helped her to discuss her problems more openly. The patient's relationships with peers were also improved through this single activity.

Case Study 7-3

A male patient who was in the midst of a divorce was admitted to a hospital for depression. He could not cope effectively because his wife had always taken care of so many of his daily needs. Occupational therapy personnel taught him basic cooking, washing, and cleaning skills. After discharge, the patient informed the staff of his successes, one of which was cooking dinner for six guests.

Program Planning

The reduction in in-patient hospital insurance coverage for psychiatric care influences decisions about the nature of treatment and changes in the therapist's and assistant's roles. These budgetary constraints have caused a rethinking of traditional occupational therapy rehabilitative services and new planning and structuring to assure the most cost-effective delivery of services.

Occupational therapy personnel frequently plan and implement a **group approach** to patient treatment. This approach involves the provision of therapy to three or more people at the same time. Task-oriented groups, which focus on a particular skill or set of skills, are often referred to as daily living groups. The focus may include the following topics:

1. Personal hygiene and grooming
2. Laundry and clothing care
3. Budgeting
4. Personal care shopping
5. Menu planning
6. Grocery shopping
7. Cooking and table setting
8. Kitchen and household safety
9. Home management and housekeeping
10. Seasonal dressing

Within the structure of such a group the leader may use specific methods to assist patients in developing skills. These methods include behavior modification using a token reward system; individual patient contracts regarding goal achievement; or shaping, which uses prompts to promote desired behavior.

Group experiences are also used to provide opportunities for patient interaction while activities are performed. A primary goal is to enhance social interaction skills relative to the patient's potential and the conditions of home and community environments. This overall goal may also include reinforcement of socially acceptable behavior, fostering of effective communication skills, encouraging self-awareness, and strengthening interpersonal confidence.

For example, a patient may be assigned to participate in a group where the members must cooperate in planning a holiday party. Through the planning and decision-making experience, each member learns to recognize the ways in which his or her behavior affects the achievement of tasks and the members of the group. Greater awareness is often gained after the task has been completed and members discuss their observations and feelings openly. Such discussions are often termed *processing the group*. Occupational therapy personnel are skilled in using activities and group process as structures to develop healthy interpersonal relationships. This topic is discussed in detail in Chapter 9.

The patient experiencing problems in reality orientation is an ideal candidate for task and activity experiences. Persons who are unable to distinguish reality are given concrete examples through activities that require the use of the five senses: sight, hearing, smell, touch and speech. The occupational therapy program helps individuals work toward recognizing and reacting to reality in both work and social relationships.

Community Involvement

The profession of occupational therapy is committed to patients returning to their communities and successfully managing life tasks and roles at the end of hospitalization or rehabilitation. The occupational therapist and the assistant may visit the patient's home or workplace to assure that these environments provide adequate safety and sufficient functional freedom.

Many patients do not progress smoothly through mental health care. In some cases it is necessary to provide the patient a longer adjustment period for successful reentry into community life. Community involvement refers to the patient interacting with others and understanding the social norms. Activities must be planned to introduce the patient to more complex scheduling, organizing, and executing of personal daily life activities. These activity experiences may include budgeting time, social role management, independent housing arrangements, and assessing and using community resources. The latter is encouraged by teaching techniques such as how to take a bus, how to use an instant cash machine, and how to follow the rules of organized meetings and to participate in such meetings.[11]

Occupational therapy plays an important role in reestablishing community support systems for patients. Support groups such as family, friends, church, and day program and community centers are important links in the patient's total rehabilitation. The recognition and positive responses furnished by the patient's support systems are crucial to the resumption of life tasks and roles.

PLAY

In medieval Europe, there was no concept of childhood as it is conceived today. Even among some contemporary societies, nearly all community resources are devoted to the business of survival, and little time is allotted to the needs of children. Play as a concept has evolved considerably in the last 20 years. The earlier neglect of play as meaningful activity is perhaps attributable to the perception that it was thought peripheral to the mainstream of individual development. The modern individual views play as an activity engaged in primarily by children.[12]

Play is a difficult concept to define because it is so broad in scope and includes many forms of behavior. However, it may be classified in several meaningful ways, including simple to complex, evolutionary, and developmental. Play can also be dichotomized into the following:[8]

1. Social or asocial
2. Cooperative or competitive
3. Imitative or original
4. Repetitive or novel
5. Overt or covert
6. Active or passive
7. Organized or spontaneous
8. Peaceful or boisterous

Scholars define play in various ways. As a process, play lies at the core of human behavior and development.[12] Play is an intrinsic activity done purely for its own sake rather than as a means to an end. It is spontaneous and voluntary, undertaken by choice and not compulsion. Play involves enjoyment and activity that leads to fun.[12] One author suggests that play is what children do when they are not eating, sleeping, resting, or doing what parents tell them to do. The preschool child's play is "serious business." It is his or her work; a means of discovering the world.[13] In 1916, a Swiss scientist, Karl Goes, proposed that play is the way children rehearse roles they are destined to fill in adult life. Play gives us permission to make mistakes.[12] Scholars emphasize life preparation, recapitulation, and surplus energy in explaining play activities. Although these notions have changed in recent years, they are still considered important features of play. Contemporary researchers focus on the spontaneous, voluntary, active and pleasurable aspects of play.[14]

It is generally accepted that play makes a substantial contribution throughout life and affects every aspect of human behavior. This view presumes that adults play and that such activity involves both work and recreational activity. These activities serve both conscious and psychological purposes.[14]

How Play Contributes to Development

Play contributes to physical, intellectual, language, social, and emotional development.

Physical Development. Play is closely associated with physical development at all ages. Infants respond by squirming and wiggling their bodies when adults play with them. As toddlers, their play involves gross motor activities such as climbing, running and jumping. Sports become important during middle childhood, with football, basketball, and swimming being common activities. Physical ability finds an outlet in play, and such activities lead to further refinement of physical ability.

Intellectual Development. As a form of symbolic expression, play can be a transitory process that takes the child from the earliest form of sensory-motor intelligence to the operational structures that characterize mature adult thought. Because play is cummulative, it has both immediate and long-range effects on development. Play leads to more complex, sophisticated cognitive behavior, which affects the content of play in a continuous, upward spiral. In the cognitive domain, play functions in four ways:[14]

1. It provides access to more avenues of information.
2. It consolidates mastery of skills and concepts.
3. It promotes and maintains effective functioning of the intellectual abilities through the use of cognitive operations.
4. It promotes creativity through the playful use of skills and concepts.

Language Development. Language and play are mutually reinforcing. Where play preceded the advent of language play, it formed a language embodying symbolic representation. Hence, some scholars suggest that the ability to represent objects, actions, and feelings in symbolic play is paralleled by a corresponding ability to represent those phenomena in language.[12]

Social Development. The primary goal of childhood is to allow socialization into active and productive adult roles in the culture. When social relationships pose problems for children, play is often a way to prevent frustrations and act out possible solutions without fear of reprisals. In learning and practicing socially desirable behavior, such as cooperation and sharing, the child uses play as a foundation for adult behavior.

Emotional Development. Much of the social learning occurring in childhood involves a balance between individual needs and the demands of social behavior. Play is an important medium for learning this balance, and children deprived of play will find it difficult to adapt to social demands in the future.

Types of Play

Play can be classified primarily as *physical* or *manipulative*. In physical play, action and boisterousness are the focus. The child attempts to gain control over the environment in manipulative play. Two additional types of play are *symbolic play* and *games*. Symbolic play includes pretending, make believe or fantasy play, and nonsense rhymes. Pretend play is exhibited as early as 18 months of age. It increases steadily with age into middle childhood and then disappears. Children rarely engage in pretend play after puberty; instead, they daydream.[12] When play is governed by rules or conventions, it is called a game. Games have two important characteristics: 1) They involve mutual involvement in some shared activity; and 2) the interactions are identified by alternating opportunities to play, repetition, and succession in chances to play.[12]

In a classic study in 1932, Mildred B. Parten observed the play of children in nursery school settings. She identified six types of play, based on the nature and extent of the children's social involvement:[15]

1. *Unoccupied play:* Children spend time watching others.
2. *Solitary play:* Children play with toys and make no effort to play with others.
3. *Onlooker behavior:* Children watch other children play but make no effort to join in.
4. *Parallel play:* Children play alongside other children but not with them.
5. *Associative play:* Children interact with each other, borrowing or lending material.

6. *Cooperative play:* Children integrate their play activities, and group members assume different roles and responsibilities.

Psychologists believe play contributes to childhood development. In 1952, Piaget emphasized the importance of exploration and play behavior as vehicles of cognitive stimulation. Ultimately play allows children to develop a sense of self-identity and objectivity. More information on the work of Piaget may be found in Chapters 5 and 8.

Play is an essential phase in childhood. It is critical to healthy development and useful to the individual and society in explaining roles. Play activities are a key to developing sound minds and bodies. Table 7-1 shows some of the play activity behavior patterns from ages six months to six years.

Different developmental disabilities such as mental retardation, cerebral palsy, or disorders characterized by difficulties in organizing and interpreting incoming stimuli (such as learning disabilities) may result in the level and proficiency of the child's play skill being directly related to mastery of a specific domain. A child may be unable to become involved in all of the many social interaction skills of play such as sharing, taking turns, asserting self, recognizing the feelings of others, and showing awareness of rules. Without the acquisition of these social skills, many forms of play (such as competitive play, small group play, and social play) cannot occur.

The relationship of psychomotor skills to play skills is also interdependent. Without the development of certain gross motor, fine motor, and coordination skills, the child will have difficulty engaging in midline hard play, object play, frolic play, or exploitive play (see Chapter 5). Perceptual skills are needed to fully participate in imaginative play, pretend play, dramatic play, means-end play, or creative play.

Children's play skills are related directly to behavior they have learned. Their proficiency, interaction, and understanding of how and why to carry out play activities is based on mastery of developmental stages.

Case Study 7-4

Jason. Jason is a shy, withdrawn four-year-old boy of African American heritage. He weighed two pounds, five ounces at birth and was born 3.2 months premature. His mother was a cocaine addict and had pneumonia at the time of delivery. Jason has been placed under protective custody by the Michigan Child Protection Services agency since age two and one-half years because his mother and father, both drug addicts, were unable to care for him properly.

The child has lived with foster parents for two years. He appears to be very attached to these people who have provided him with excellent care, but who have also unnecessarily indulged him. They have no other children and have petitioned for formal adoption.

At age three, Jason was diagnosed as having cerebral palsy with moderately involved spastic quadriplegia. Before diagnosis, the child's foster mother observed that Jason appeared to be "slow" and did not use his hands and arms, particularly the right, to reach out and grasp during normal ADLs or while playing with toys. He was referred to occupational therapy to develop skills in daily living activities, including head, trunk, and extremity control; feeding; and dressing: Lack of motor functioning interfered with play skills, so the following activities were used to address the problems: therapy balls, coloring, bead stringing, pull toys, computer games, obstacle course games, barrels to climb on or roll in, soft and lightweight foam toys, and inflatable toys. Emphasis was placed on dyadic or small group play activities and games requiring interaction with peers.

Progress was slow but steady. Jason used his right upper extremity to reach and was able to grasp some objects. Because his cognitive functioning was within normal range, he was accepted in the public school system in a traditional classroom setting.

LEISURE

As individuals progress from childhood to adulthood, activities once described as play become leisure activities. Leisure is an integral part of a balanced American lifestyle. Just as children learn about themselves and the world through structured activity (play), so do adults. Through work and leisure, individuals learn about themselves and their environment. This learning process is perpetual and continues throughout life.

By the year 2000 life expectancy is anticipated to increase by five to ten years. Alternative work patterns are being proposed to provide greater worker flexibility and to improve the quality of life. The quality of one's life is determined by, among other factors, the combination of work and nonwork activities. Numerous studies have shown how repressive working conditions and impoverished social environments create a meager existence for many workers.[16] The quality of life is greatly influenced by leisure activities.

Leisure is a subjective term. Individuals define leisure by their perceptions, taking into consideration their values and cultural orientation. One commonly used conceptualization in sociology literature is leisure as discretionary time. That is, leisure is the time remaining after the basic requirements of subsistence (work) and existence (meeting daily needs) are met.[17] Leisure may also be viewed as "nonwork activity" engaged in during free time.[18] Actually, leisure is not a category but rather a style of behavior that may occur in any activity. For example, one can work while listening to music, thus providing a leisure aspect.[19] Leisure is free time where content is oriented towards self-fulfillment as an ultimate

Table 7-1
Play Activity Behavior Patterns

Typical play activity behavior patterns of children from 6 months to 6 years are indicated in the following chart.

AT SIX TO SEVEN MONTHS

He holds toys and plays actively with a rattle.
She looks at herself in a mirror, smiles, vocalizes, and pats the mirror.
He watches things and movements about him.
She can amuse herself and keep busy for at least 15 minutes at a time.

AT NINE MONTHS

He bangs one toy against another.
She imitates movements such as splashing in the tub, crumpling paper, shaking a rattle.

AT TWELVE MONTHS

He responds to music.
She examines toys and objects with eyes and hands, feeling them, poking them, and turning them around.
He likes to put objects in and out of containers.

AT EIGHTEEN MONTHS

She purposefully moves toys and other objects from one place to another.
He often carries a doll or stuffed animal about with him.
She likes to play with sand, letting it run between her fingers and pouring it in and out of containers.
He hugs a doll or stuffed animal, showing affection or other personal reaction to it.
She likes picture books or familiar objects.
He scribbles spontaneously with a pencil or crayon.
She plays with blocks in a simple manner—carrying them around, fingering and handling them, gathering them together—but does not build purposefully with them. It takes many trials before she can make three or four stand in a tower.
He imitates simple things he sees others do, such as "reading" a book or spanking his doll.

AT TWO YEARS

She likes to investigate and play with small objects such as toys, cars, blocks, pebbles, sand, water.
He likes to play with messy materials such as clay, patting, pinching and fingering it.
She likes to play with large objects such as huggies and wagons.
He can snip with scissors but is awkward.
She imitates everyday household activities such as cooking, hanging up clothes. These are usually activities with which she is closely associated and things she sees rather than remembers.
He plays with blocks, lining them up or using them to fill wagons or other toys.
She can, with urging, build a tower of six or seven blocks.

AT THREE YEARS

He pushes trains, cars, fire engines, in make-believe activities.
She cuts with scissors, not necessarily in a constructive manner.
He makes well-controlled marks with crayon or pencil and sometimes attempts to draw simple figures.
She gives rhythmic physical response to music: clapping or swaying or marching.
He initiates his own play activities when supplied with interesting materials.
She likes to imitate activities of others, especially real-life activities.
He likes to take a toy or doll to bed with him.
She delays sleeping by calling for a drink of water or asking to go to the bathroom.

AT FOUR YEARS

In playing with materials such as blocks, clay, and sand, the 4 -year-old is more constructive and creative. Such play is often cooperative.
He uses much imagination in play and wants more in the way of costumes and materials than formerly.
She draws simple figures of things she sees or imagines, but these have few details and are not always recognizable to others.
He can cut or trace along a line with fair accuracy.

Table 7-1
Play Activity Behavior (continued)

AT FIVE YEARS

She plays active games of a competitive nature, such as hide-and-go-seek, tag, and hopscotch.
He builds houses, garages, and elaborate structures with blocks.
She likes dramatic play—playing house, dressing up, cowboy, spaceman, war games—and acts out stories
    heard. This is more complicated and better organized than at age **4**.
He uses pencils and crayons freely. His drawings are simple but can usually be recognized.
She enjoys cutting out things with scissors—pictures from magazines, paper dolls.
He can sing, dance to music, play records on the phonograph.

AT SIX YEARS

The 6-year-old can learn to play simple table games such as tiddly-winks, marbles, parchesi, and dominoes.
He likes stunts and gymnastics and many kinds of physical activity.
She wrestles and scuffles in a coordinated manner with other children.
At this point the play interests of boys and girls are different.

---

end. This time is granted to the individual by society when he or she has complied with occupational, family, spiritual and political obligations.[19]

Leisure is progressive rebirth, regrowth, and reacquaintance with oneself, renewing, refulfilling, and recreating.[20] It should be compatible with physical, mental, and social well-being. Most scholars agree that leisure is characterized by a search for a state of satisfaction. This search is the primal condition of leisure. When leisure fails to give the expected pleasure, when it is not interesting, "it is not fun."[21] There are two dimensions of leisure: the satisfaction inherent in the activity itself and the relations of the activity to external values, or social well-being.[20]

In 1960 Dumazedier[19] identified periods of leisure, including the end of the day and during retirement. During such times, leisure covers a number of structured activities connected with physical and mental needs defined as artistic, intellectual, and social leisure pursuits, within the limits of economic, political, and cultural conditions in each society.

Purpose and Function

The fundamental purpose of leisure is to provide an opportunity to develop talents and interests. Leisure also meets the following needs:[20]

1. Belonging
2. Individuality (through interests and abilities that distinguish the individual)
3. Multifunctional purposes in behavior (Some activities offer a wide dimension of function.)
4. Multidimensional effects of behavior (Some activities serve additional persons in society at the same time they serve the participant.)
5. Activities and created objects as projections of the person (providing expression of feelings, projection of self-knowledge and objects for future pleasure)

Classification

There have been many attempts to classify leisure. In a study of leisure in Kansas City in 1955 Havighurst[22] distinguished 11 categories:

1. Participation in organized groups
2. Participation in unorganized groups
3. Pleasure trips
4. Participation in sports
5. Spectator sports (excluding television)
6. Television and radio
7. Fishing and hunting
8. Gardening and country walks
9. Crafts (sewing, carpentry and do-it-yourself)
10. Imaginative activities, music, and art
11. Visits to relatives and friends

Developmental Aspect

Leisure patterns are also related to developmental tasks and issues individuals face at different stages in the life cycle. In many cases, these tasks and issues will be shaped by preoccupations, culture, and needs at each stage.[23] Because infants cannot distinguish between obligatory and nonobligatory activity, it is doubtful whether the concept of leisure is relevant to them. Socialization through play, however, influences the child's ability to cope in interpersonal relationships and is the beginning of adult leisure behavior.[24] Leisure activities help to socialize adolescents to adult attitudes and roles.[26] During adolescence, leisure time activities are an important preoccupation. Activities may represent an extension of a school subject or may be extracurricular. Among young adults, leisure is important for marital satisfaction, as it provides an environment for personal communication, sharing of experiences, and family cohesiveness. These joint activities encourage interaction and shared commitments.

Work and family continue to be the dominant themes in early maturity (ages 30 to 40). Leisure activities in this category are often home- and family-centered and provide a means of increasing the growth and stability of marriage and the family. At full maturity (age 45 to retirement), leisure activities may become less home and family centered, as there are fewer family responsibilities in many instances. There often are increased economic resources to provide opportunities for more evenings out, travel, and other less home-oriented leisure.

Leisure and Retirement

Individuals sometimes need to rediscover or develop new leisure interests as work diminishes and retirement approaches. Retirement can result in a relinquishment of social involvements. Leisure can provide a context for autonomous decision-making and social integration with meaningful other persons whose support and encouragement is very important to life cycle transition at old age.[23]

Because of improved medical science and social welfare, more people are living long past retirement age. Prime predictors of retirement adjustment are adequate retirement income and retired friends with whom to share leisure time. The loss of income, rather than employment, accounts for the negative retirement effects for many. Activities that build skills and interests of preretirement should provide a foundation of personal adjustment and life satisfaction after retirement.[23]

How do elderly people use the time freed from work? Time budget surveys have demonstrated that leisure takes most of the spare time enjoyed by the elderly, even more time than the personal, household, and family care activities. The amount of leisure activities increases with age. Eighty percent of those age 65 and over have at least five hours of leisure time per day according to Dumazedier.[19]

Retired persons often face the problem of what to do with extra time. The problem may affect men more because women may find that retirement from their responsibilities is replaced, to some extent, by activities related to their grandchildren.

The impact of retirement is considerably different between social classes and cultures. Men in professional occupations are often able to continue some form of work after official retirement. This is less possible for those in blue-collar or service occupations. Middle class women who reach retirement status are more likely to be members of voluntary organizations than working class women. Among Americans, church is an important and approved medium of social activities and entertainment for the elderly. The church is a place to meet and relate with friends. In addition to ministering to spiritual needs, the church sponsors activities such as bazaars, dinners, bowling teams, travel clubs, special lectures, and picnics as well as other activities that constitute a rich offering of social opportunities.

The influence of preretirement leisure activity patterns on retirement planning and attitudes toward retirement was investigated by two occupational therapists. Sixty male retirees were surveyed to determine the degree of preretirement planning and the type and extent of leisure participation before and after retirement. The results showed that a high degree of preretirement leisure participation correlates with a high degree of preretirement planning.[25] If the patterns that predict satisfaction among retirees can be identified, they can be used in activity planning to structure the healthful use of time for retirees. Further, if one or more characteristic activity patterns can be associated with retirement satisfaction, then occupational therapy personnel could implement preretirement programs accordingly.

Recreation

Recreation is a term often used to suggest leisure. In its literal sense, re-creating is seen as one of the functions of leisure—that of renewing the self or of preparing for work. Thus recreation is characterized by the attitude of a person when participating in activities that satisfy, amuse, direct, relax or provide opportunities for self-expression. It is generally associated with arts and crafts, outdoor activities, hobbies, literary activities, culture, clubs, and other organized groups.[26]

Leisure Activities

The physically disabled and patients with mental illness have a need for leisure. Today these individuals participate in nearly every sport and craft activity and also engage in other forms of leisure such as drama, dance and music. Participation in these activities is both enjoyable and therapeutic. Persons with physical disabilities are recreating more and more with the nondisabled, thus integrating into the mainstream of society. The need for adaptations often dictates that many disabled train and compete with others of similar functional abilities, particularly in sports.

Occupational therapy personnel are not recreation specialists; however, OTRs and COTAs are adaptation specialists and are often called on to evaluate the need for adaptation with a particular leisure activity. In many instances the patient is more skilled at the activity than the OTR or the COTA; however, as adaptation specialists, occupational therapy personnel can adapt equipment and teach compensatory movements so that the patient can engage in the leisure task as independently as possible. This could range from instructing the visually impaired to thread a needle to adapting a tripod for the photographer in a wheelchair. The following questions should be considered in making adaptations:

1. *Cost:* How much can the patient or family afford for the adaptation needed?
2. *Use:* How frequently will the equipment or aid be used? Does the frequency of use justify the cost?
3. *Expense:* What expense will be required each time the patient engages in the activity?

4. *Maintenance:* Will the adaptation be primarily maintenance free? Are replacement parts readily available?
5. *Location:* Will the leisure activity be easily accessible?
6. *Appearance:* Is the adaptation so prominent that the patient will be embarrassed to use it, or is the activity so altered that it no longer resembles its original form?

In psychiatry, individual activity patterns are often lost with the onset of mental illness. Because these activity patterns are the expressions of the individual's proper use and appreciation of time, the loss of these patterns can result in reality disorientation with others, the environment and time.[27] Consequently, many patients have difficulty engaging in play and leisure activities. There is also an inability to identify satisfying leisure-time interests. Fidler[27] notes several possible factors that may contribute to these deficits.

1. Limited self-awareness concerning one's strengths, skills, present and past accomplishments, personal goals, beliefs, and values
2. Lack of adequate planning skills
3. Pragmatic barriers to participation, such as locked wards, insufficient finances, lack of transportation, lack of equipment, and lack of opportunity
4. Limited knowledge of resources and how to use them
5. Lack of underlying competencies in sensorimotor skills, cognitive skills, and/or interpersonal skills needed to participate and experience pleasure

The activity histories of many members of the patient population receiving psychiatric occupational therapy treatment generally reveal a sparse repertoire of childhood play experiences on which to base adult leisure experiences. Play is widely recognized as the child's arena for learning and practicing rules and social skills necessary for subsequent roles in school, work and recreation. Play and leisure competencies are developed along with other daily living skills and may, in fact, facilitate the development of other functional roles, such as work.[27]

The patient's use of leisure time can be measured by having the individual complete a schedule of a typical day and a leisure questionnaire. An example of the latter is shown in Figure 7-5. It may be found that a patient's television viewing consumes 90% of leisure time. Exploring patient talents and interests and providing opportunities to experiment with and experience some of them might lead to more gratifying activity patterns.

Goals of Leisure Activity

Leisure activity can assist in developing **psychomotor** and **affective skills,** both of which can lead to helping the patient reestablish his or her role in society. Psychomotor goals include the following:

1. Improve visual perception
2. Improve range of motion
3. Improve muscle strength
4. Improve balance
5. Improve physical tolerance and endurance
6. Improve coordination
7. Increase attention span

Affective goals include the following:
1. Improve self-esteem
2. Improve interpersonal skills
3. Improve social skills
4. Improve communication skills
5. Aid in acceptance of disability
6. Develop friendship/comradeship
7. Improve self-discipline

Case Study 7-5

A "hard driving" professional man, who rarely had any time for leisure was admitted to a psychiatric treatment center with the diagnosis of major affective disorder. While in occupational therapy, he developed an interest in making clay pots on the potter's wheel. The occupational therapy assistant who was responsible for carrying out his treatment encouraged him to continue his work after discharge. She maintained a resource file of community leisure resources and drew on this material to locate a nearby art association that held classes as well as periodic exhibits. By sharing this information with the patient, an avenue was provided for him to continue to pursue his interest and develop a new area of leisure.

A knowledge of activities and interest groups within the community is essential for all occupational therapy personnel who treat patients.

Leisure Task Groups

The use of **task groups** is a common way to treat patients in occupational therapy. The types of patients who could benefit from task groups are the following:

1. A large variety of patients except the very young
2. Those with neurologic disorders or physical or mental impairments
3. Those who need to increase their levels of independence
4. Those with inadequate social skills
5. Those unfamiliar with community resources
6. Those who make poor use of free time
7. Those who have an inability to identify leisure interests
8. Those who have poor leisure planning skills

Common treatment goals for the task groups are the following:

1. To develop knowledge of and skills in using community resources
2. To develop new leisure and interest options

Name _____ Date _____

Ward or Room _____ Age _____ Sex _____

__INSTRUCTIONS__: Put an X before the activities you know and would like to do.
Put an O before the activities you do not know, but would like to learn or take part in.
Write, under "Other," any activities not listed that you would like to do.

QUIET GAMES
_____ Bridge
_____ Canasta
_____ Checkers
_____ Chess
_____ Pinochle
_____ Dominoes
_____ Rummy
Other:

_____ _____

_____ _____

ACTIVE GAMES
_____ Ring toss
_____ Billiards
_____ Horseshoes
_____ Darts
_____ Croquet
_____ Bowling
_____ Basketball

_____ _____

_____ _____

SOCIAL ACTIVITIES
_____ Game nights
_____ Bingo
_____ Parties
_____ Folk dancing
_____ Square dancing
_____ Dancing
_____ Picnics
_____ Trips and tours
Other:

_____ _____

_____ _____

ENTERTAINMENT
_____ Amateur nights
_____ Variety shows
_____ Puppet shows
_____ Quiz programs
_____ Plays
_____ Pageants
_____ Festivals
Other:

_____ _____

_____ _____

_____ Baseball
_____ Boccie
_____ Football
_____ Golf
Other:

_____ _____

_____ _____

DRAMA
_____ Acting
_____ Stagecraft
_____ Script writing
_____ Costuming
_____ Makeup
Other:

_____ _____

_____ _____

NEWSPAPER
_____ Writing
_____ Reporting
_____ Artwork

Figure 7-5. Leisure interest checklist. Used with permission from Wayne County Community College, Occupational Therapy Assistant Program.

3. To increase independent functioning
4. To develop transition skills for readjustment to the community
5. To further develop the ability to make decisions and follow through
6. To demonstrate basic skill in selecting activities for use during free time

Sample Activity Tasks. Trips to places of interest, such as art and historical museums, zoos, theaters, parks, cider mills, shopping centers, and movies, can be planned. Ideas for such trips may be suggested by either the group leader or the participants. A decision may be made by concensus or majority vote. Once a decision has been made, additional procedures or rules may be established by the task group,

Name _____ Date _____

Ward or Room _____ Age _____ Sex _____

INSTRUCTIONS: Put an X before the activities you know and would like to do.
Put an O before the activities you do not know, but would like to learn or take part in.
Write, under "Other," any activities not listed that you would like to do.

MUSIC
_____ Community singing
_____ Quartet
_____ Choir
_____ Chorus
_____ Instrument instruction
_____ Instrument playing
_____ Rhythm band
_____ Orchestra
_____ Listening
_____ Music appreciation
Other:

_____ _____

_____ _____

ARTS AND CRAFTS
_____ Drawing and painting
_____ Leathercraft
_____ Woodcarving
_____ Ceramics
_____ Jewelry making
_____ Shellcraft
_____ Basketry
_____ Weaving
_____ Needlework
_____ Party decorations
Other:

_____ _____

_____ _____

HOBBIES AND CLUBS
_____ Photography
_____ Discussion groups
_____ Magic
_____ Nature lore
_____ Stamp collecting
Other:

_____ _____

_____ _____

_____ Creative writing
_____ Model building
_____ Gardening
_____ Reading
Other:

_____ _____

_____ _____

List other special interests: _____

What kinds of books do you like to read? _____

What kind of movies do you like to see? _____

What kind of music do you like to hear? _____

What kind of songs do you like to sing? _____

How do you spend your leisure time? _____

_____

Figure 7-5. Continued.

depending on the nature of the activity. For example, if the activity of going to a particular movie is decided on, the following rules could be established:

1. Each patient must sign up on the van transportation form in the occupational therapy office.
2. Each patient must be dressed appropriately for the outing.
3. Each patient must be at the van pick-up site at the designated time.
4. Each patient must purchase his or her own ticket and be responsible for obtaining correct change.
5. Each patient must purchase his or her own refreshments and be responsible for obtaining correct change.

Outside Meals. Meals can be planned at restaurants. If the task group decides on this activity, rules 1, 2, and 3 of the preceding would apply. The group may also wish to establish additional requirements which might include learning proper use of a menu, how to place an order, use of correct table manners, use of appropriate tableware, paying the bill and tipping.

Table Games. A number of suitable table games can be chosen. When task group members determine a game or games to be played, a member may volunteer or be appointed to be responsible for obtaining the needed supplies and equipment. Another group member could be in charge of explaining the rules of the game. Depending on the specific nature of the particular game chosen, additional tasks might include awarding prizes to winners or teaching the game to nongroup members.

Kitchen Activities. Kitchen activities can involve many tasks depending on the scope of the activity. Some of these might include planning the menu, obtaining the necessary supplies and equipment, making copies of the recipes to be used, inviting guests, cooking, table setting, serving, and clean-up. Some of the rules that could be established include the following:

1. All patients will wash their hands thoroughly.
2. Patients working with food will wear hair nets.
3. Everyone in the group will be responsible for carrying out at least one task.

After each group activity, the group leader or leaders can discuss the event with the patients in the task group. Topics should include positive and negative aspects, with patients being given constructive feedback on their behaviors. All members also should have an opportunity to discuss their personal feelings. More information on task groups may be found in Chapter 9.

Case Study 7-6

John. John was 30 years old when he was referred to the occupational therapy department after surgical removal of a brain tumor. He had been living in a group home before the surgery and had worked as a factory foreman up until the previous year. He began having seizures, which ultimately interfered with his job responsibilities, and he was terminated from his position.

Family members reported that John withdrew from social and physical activities after learning of his tumor and losing his job. He became extremely depressed. After an occupational therapy evaluation, the following goals were established in collaboration with the patient:

1. Develop social skills necessary for active community participation after discharge from the hospital
2. Demonstrate independence in ADLs and productive occupation
3. Exhibit improved self-esteem and feelings of self-worth

4. Demonstrate increased personal involvement in leisure activities
5. Demonstrate increased ability to structure leisure time
6. Provide evidence of ability to use resources to aid in transition from hospital to community

The COTA responsible for supervising John's treatment activities in relation to leisure goals used a supportive and flexible approach, offering John encouragement and reassurance as appropriate. Among other activities, the patient participated in a number of day trips, very reluctantly at first. He enjoyed the parks and particularly the beautiful fall colors of the trees. The COTA provided him with a city map and assisted him in locating parks near his home. She also pointed out the availability of guided nature hikes. John took his family on one of these hikes during a weekend leave from the facility.

As John became involved in meaningful activities, including leisure, his depression disappeared and self-esteem improved. He became interested in community activities again and expressed a desire to return to the cider mill as well as a museum he had visited with a patient group.[28]

Included in Appendix B is a list of recreational organizations for disabled individuals located throughout the United States. Many can provide the names and addresses of individual contacts in the patient's community.

WORK

In 1909 R.C. Cabolt, a professor of medicine at Harvard University, wrote an article entitled "Work Cure," suggesting that work is best of all psychotherapies. In a later book, *What Men Live By,* he discussed the relationships among work, play, love and religion and called for a balance among them. He believed work caused greater physical and emotional health. The relationship between a healthy body and work is also suggested throughout occupational therapy literature. Work can provide a source of satisfaction and emotional well-being.

Occupational therapy views work as skill in socially productive activities. These activities may take place in the home, school, or community and include home management, care of others, educational pursuits and vocational activities.[8]

Public opinion surveys reveal that work, in addition to its economic function, structures time, provides a context in which to relate to other people, offers an escape from boredom, and sustains a sense of worth. Moreover, work affects the individual's freedom, responsibility, social position, attitude, mental capacities, achievements, friends, self-concept and "chances in life."[20] As one writer suggests, work is not a part of life, it is literally life itself.

Studs Turkel[29] wrote that "the job" is a search for working Americans to find daily meaning as well as "daily bread" for recognition. Turkel clearly recognized the linkage between mental health and meaningful work, pride in accomplishment, recognition, hunger for beauty, and a need to be remembered by "the job."

Significance of Work

Work provides an opportunity to associate with others. Through membership in work organizations, individuals gain a fundamental index of status and self-respect. The relationship to work influences one's use of time and leisure, the nature of the individual's family, and the state of one's mental health.[30]

The importance of work is pervasive; it determines what is produced, what is consumed, how individuals live, and what type of society is created and perpetuated.[30] Human motivation ranges beyond the drive for satisfaction of essential and discretionary materialistic needs. Higher needs must be satisfied to approach the fullest potential of human existence through the activity of work.

Parker[21] categorized life space as the total of activities or ways of spending time. In considering the various definitions of work and leisure, to allocate all the parts of life space either to work or to leisure would be a gross oversimplification. It is possible to use the exhaustive categories of work and nonwork, but it is still not possible to draw a line between the two categories. Parker analyzed the 24-hour day in five main groups:[21] 1) work, 2) working time, 3) sold time, 4) semileisure time, and 5) leisure.

When analyzing life space, work is usually identified with earning a living, even though work has a wider meaning than employment. Homemaking, parenting and child care as well as the student's work of achieving an education are examples.

Apart from actual working time, most people have to spend a certain amount of time traveling to places of work and preparing for work. At least part of the traveling time may be regarded more as a form of leisure than as work related, such as time spent reading the newspaper or a book, knitting, or chatting with fellow travelers. Other activities related to working time involve husbands and wives sharing in household tasks that were considered to be solely "women's work" in the past, voluntary overtime or having a second job, reading related to one's job while at home, and attending work-related conferences and meetings.

Parker's use of the term *sold time* refers to meeting the person's physiologic needs. The satisfaction of these self-care needs includes sleeping, eating, bathing, eliminating, and sexual activities. Beyond the time necessary for reasonably healthy living, extra time spent on these tasks may become a leisure activity, such as eating for leisure, or attending to one's appearance before going to a party.

Domestic work such as making beds, caring for a pet,

gardening, and odd jobs in the home are examples of semileisure tasks. Semileisure arises from leisure, but represents the character of obligations in differing degrees. These obligations are usually to other people but may be to pets, homes, and gardens as well.

Leisure is free time, spare time, uncommitted time, discretionary time, and choosing time.[21] It is time free from obligations either to self or others, a time to do as one chooses.

Analysis of life space based on the majority, those who are employed full time, would be incomplete. Those who do not work at full-time paid positions must be considered as well. People in these groups include housewives, prisoners, the unemployed, and, in some instances, the rich.

For example, the life space of a prisoner is much more constricted than that of the average citizen in terms of both time and activity. Although some prisoners are employed outside the prison, the choice of work is severely restricted and the motivation for it is rather different. Insofar as some prison work may be more or less voluntarily undertaken to relieve boredom or satisfy a physiological or psychologic need to work, it may resemble the "work obligation" of the average citizen.

Doing housework is often the housewife's work. When compared with the husband's paid employment, it usually offers less scope for interest and less social contact. There is no real difference between work obligations and the responsibilities of the household.[21]

Many unemployed individuals develop feelings of uselessness and may be driven to occupy themselves with trivial tasks and time-filling routines. They lose the companionship and social support of co-workers. Lack of money produces a restriction on the range of leisure activities, thus narrowing the scope of life experiences. The retired are similar to the unemployed, except that absence of employment is normally planned and permanent.

Worker Satisfaction

The highly productive economy of the 1970s reduced the moral value of work. There is much discussion today about worker dissatisfaction. Although the degree of job satisfaction differs, studies reveal that substantial numbers are dissatisfied with their jobs because the job does not meet their need for self-actualization, that is, their chance to perform well, opportunities for achievement and growth, and the chance to contribute something personel and unique.[31] Scholars have identified six elements that bring satisfaction on the job:

1. Creating a product that reflects the individual's input
2. Using skill
3. Working wholeheartedly
4. Using initiative and having responsibility
5. Mixing with people
6. Working with people who know their job

The most desirable work-related outcomes are as follows:
1. To feel pride and craftsmanship in one's work
2. To feel more worthwhile
3. To be recognized and respected by others
4. To require little direct supervision
5. To have contact with others in the same type of work, both on and off the job

Women and Work

The American family has undergone many changes in recent years. One significant change is the increase of women working outside the home. Women now represent nearly 46% of the national labor force.[33] If one spouse must stay home to care for the children, however, it is almost always the wife who does so.[21] In interviews with housewives in one community study, some women thought that leisure came when all the household chores were done and children were in bed.[20]

Growth of the female work force can be traced to many factors, which include the increasing availability of contraceptives, a preference toward smaller families, inflation, a rising divorce rate, an increasing number of equality-oriented college women, expansion of the service-oriented economy, and changing attitudes toward careers for women.[31] Although a greater number of women are employed outside the home, a majority are in low-paying occupations or in service industries. Like homemakers, they teach children, care for the sick and prepare food.[32]

Types and Phases of Work

Aristotle believed that there were two types of work: bread and labor, or work for the purpose of subsistence; and leisure work, or labor that was interesting in and of itself. In today's society, individuals do not work solely for economic self-interest, but also because work is psychologically necessary. Work is important to human dignity. The majority of the poor do not want to remain idle and accept welfare. Eighty percent of the labor force say they would work even if they did not need the income because work keeps them occupied and healthy. Without it, they would feel lost, useless and bored.[33]

Sociologists and psychologists identify five work phases in life:
1. Preparatory—usually school
2. Initial—first employment
3. Trial—a period of job changing as the worker tries to find work which is attractive
4. Stable—usually the longest period when there are relatively few changes in occupations
5. Retirement

One test of the importance of work in the lives of individuals is found in the activities of retired persons. Less than 20% of men drawing Social Security benefits retire to enjoy leisure. Almost three fourths of these retirements are involuntary due to the employer retiring the worker or the worker being forced to retire because of poor health.

Occupational Therapy and Work

In occupational therapy, work and related skills and performance may be defined as the functional ability and proficiency needed to carry out the task of productive activity. The occupational performance area of work may be further defined and categorized according to *Uniform Terminology*, Second Edition, published by the American Occupational Therapy Association. Work activities in the area of home management include the following:[8]
1. Clothing care
2. Cleaning
3. Meal preparation and cleanup
4. Shopping
5. Money management
6. Household maintenance
7. Care of others

Work activities centered around the care of others include providing physical care, communication, nurturance, and activities that are age-appropriate for one's spouse, children, parents or significant others.[8] Educational activities are also defined as they relate to the student's participation in a school environment, including school-sponsored activities such as field trips and work-study programs.[8] The final category presented in this document is vocational activities. These are categorized as vocational exploration, job acquisition, work or job performance, and retirement planning.[8]

Nelson[6] has said that the concept of activity includes "activity as form" and "activity as action." Action is that part of the activity concerned with one's actual performance of the activity, that is, the specific operations needed to carry out the activity, whether it be work, play/leisure or ADLs. Activity as form denotes the cultural expectations or general procedures an individual would follow in order to do the activity well. The term *function* describes activity of form.

Because skill and performance are functional abilities, occupational therapy personnel must concentrate their efforts on a thorough analysis of the patient's functional abilities, along with his or her affective skills. Such an analysis could assist in determining the feasibility of the patient's chosen work. More information on activity analysis may be found in Chapter 17.

Function can be divided into the following categories: physical tolerance demands, sensory/perception, motor, daily living skills, cognition, and affective demands. Subcomponents of each of these are enumerated in Table 7-2.

The occupational therapy assistant, under the supervision of and in collaboration with the occupational therapist, must relate each functional ability to the impact it will have on a patient's work, whether at home, in an office, or in the community. The interrelatedness of skill to the work task must be determined.

Table 7-2
Work Behavior Skills

Physical Tolerance and Demands	Sensory/Perception	Motor
Work pace/rhythm	Color discrimination	Finger dexterity
Standing tolerance	Form perception	Manual dexterity
Sitting tolerance	Size discrimination	Coordination:
Endurance	Spatial relationship	eye-hand
Performance with repetition	Ability to follow visual instruction	eye-hand-foot
Muscle strength	Texture discrimination	fine motor
Walking	Digital discrimination	gross motor
Lifting	Figure-ground	bimanual
Carrying	Form constancy	bilateral
Pushing	Visual closure	Use of hand tools
Pulling	Parts-to-whole	ROM:
Climbing	Shape discrimination	stopping
	Kinesthesia	kneeling
		crouching
		crawling
		reaching
		Balancing

Daily Living Skills	Cognition	Affective
Self-care:	Numerical ability	Attendance
personal hygiene	Measuring ability	Punctuality
grooming	Safety consciousness	Response to:
dressing	Care in handling work and tools	praise
eating/feeding	Work quality	criticism
object manipulation	Accuracy	assistance
Mobility:	Neatness	frustrating situation
transfers	Attention span	Relationship with:
travel (mode of)	Planning/organization	evaluator
transportation	Ability to follow:	co-worker
Communication:	verbal instruction	Work flexibility
with peers	written instruction	Attitude toward work
with supervisor	Retention of instruction	Behavior in structured setting
writing	Work judgment	Ability to work independently
dialing phone	Ability to learn new task	Initiative
talking on phone	Orientation	
typing		(In psychiatry, also observe for additional pathologic behavior.)

Used with permission from Wayne County Community College, Occupational Therapy Assistant Program.

Relationship of Work to Physical Disability

Whether a homemaker or a plumber, managing everyday tasks can be difficult for anyone; but for the individual with a physical disability, the need for good management and organization is essential to success. Evaluation and training for these skills can be assessed both formally and informally. Much valuable information can be obtained when the individual completes daily living skill tasks, as well as through interviews with the patient and significant others, such as close family members. Table 7-2 identifies skills that may be assessed.

Of concern to the COTA are the following questions, which must be answered before planning and implementing an occupational therapy program to meet the patient's needs in relation to home management and child care:

1. What is the extent of the patient's handicap, and what is the subsequent functional loss?
2. What is the apparent cause of the functional loss? (eg, sensory, judgment, range of motion limitation)?
3. What role in homemaking and child care did the patient have before the disability?

4. What financial resources are available to the patient for task assistance?
5. What are the patient's goals for independence?

Other principles must also be considered in planning an occupational therapy treatment program. These include:

1. *Energy conservation*—includes work simplification and time management needs for adaptive/assistive equipment including carts, chairs, and utensils
2. *Barrier free design*—ranges from simple adaptations such as removing scatter rugs, to kitchen modification of shelves and cabinets, to use of a microwave oven, to redesigning doorways, entrances, and bathrooms
3. *Physical abilities*—includes reaching, stooping, bending, balancing, walking, standing, sitting, pushing, pulling, lifting, coordination, and speed
4. *Sensory awareness*—such as temperature, proprioception, and kinesthesia
5. *Cognition*—includes attention span, judgment, organization, and memory
6. *Family expectation*—total independence or independence with assistance
7. *Community resources*—home-delivered meals, catalog shopping, child care

The COTA should stress to the patient the need for organized, planned activities. Every step saved and energy conserved is to the individual's advantage. Simulated tasks should be practiced in the occupational therapy clinic as frequently as possible before discharge. Numerous resources are available. For example, when working on home management tasks, a detailed reference, giving step-by-step guidelines for many tasks is the *Mealtime Manual for People with Disabilities and the Aging*, compiled by Judith Klinger, OTR.

Psychosocial Implications

The emphasis when working in psychiatry is quite different from that in the physical disability setting. Rather than stressing psychomotor abilities the focus is on the affective domain. Goals may include some of the following:

1. Demonstrate the ability to develop interpersonal relationships (which the patient may have lost as a result of illness or may never have acquired)
2. Exhibit improved self-esteem
3. Provide evidence of development of decision-making skills (by encouraging individual responsibility)
4. Exhibit increased skill in socialization
5. Demonstrate adequate skills in areas such as budgeting, time management, purchasing and menu planning

The hospitalized patient may never have worked, may be temporarily unemployed, or may be deprived of the work role due to the illness. The occupational therapy clinic offers a work area where the patient can learn new skills and develop existing ones. In work adjustment programs, tasks are chosen to promote and teach work skills to allow the patient to function at an optimum level. These skills might include the ability to follow written and oral directions, sustain attention to tasks, or organize work according to priority.[34] The structured activity or craft task group may be used to assist patients in learning skills as well as to assess their readiness to return to life activities such as work or school.

SUMMARY

This chapter provides information on the areas of occupational performance: daily living skills, play, leisure, and work skills, which are the primary foundations of the profession of occupational therapy. Each section focuses on theories, principles, and adaptations; illustrative case studies are provided to explain the importance of these activities in the individual's life. The goal is to assist the reader to understand not only the individual areas but also to appreciate their relationship to each other.

Daily living skills are a prerequiste for the other areas. These basic skills must be mastered before the individual can be well adapted to community life. The focus is on independence, as well as on improving the quality of the patient's life, and to assist in restoring a sense of dignity and self-esteem for many through new-found abilities.

Play as a process lies at the core of human behavior and development. It is an intrinsic activity done purely for its own sake rather than a means to an end. It is spontaneous and pleasurable, voluntarily selected, and actively engaged in. Play activities lead to more complex and sophisticated cognitive behavior. They promote creativity, enhance social and emotional development, and make a valuable contribution to the growth of the individual.

Although we live in a work-oriented society, leisure, a natural outgrowth of play, fulfills many significant human needs. It can relieve tensions, strain, and boredom that has become so much a part of modern technologic society. Leisure or discretionary time greatly influences the quality of people's lives.

Work is presented as skill in socially productive activities and, in addition to full-time employment, includes home management, care of others, educational activities, and vocational activities. It provides the individual with a source of satisfaction and emotional well-being.

Skills in ADLs, play/leisure, and work, coupled with a healthy balance among these, assist individuals in meeting their needs, adapting to society, assuming their occupational roles, receiving gratification, and reaching self-actualization.

Acknowledgments

The editor wishes to thank Louise Fawcett, PhD, OTR for her assistance in preparing the play case study and LaDonn

People, MA, OTR for overall editorial and content suggestions and general assistance with many phases of the preparation of this manuscript.

Related Learning Activities

1. Develop a card file of community resources for a variety of play and leisure activities.

2. Working with a peer, develop a leisure activities program for a group of men aged 16 to 22 who are wheelchair-bound patients in a rehabilitation hospital.

3. Make a chart in which to list all of the activities engaged in on a recent weekday according to the following categories: ADLs, work and leisure. List times of day at half-hour intervals along the left side of the chart. Evaluate these data in terms of overall balance among the activities by answering the following questions:

   a. Do you need to make some changes?

   b. Do you need to gather more data?

   c. Did you consider the time spent in rest and sleep?

   d. How does the completed chart compare with the way you spend time on weekends?

4. How do occupational therapists and assistants manipulate the environment or components of a task for a physically disabled patient? How is this accomplished for a person with psychosocial problems?

References

1. Havighurst R: Social roles, work, leisure, and education. In Eisendorfer C, Lawton, MP (Eds): *The Psychology of Adult Development and Aging.* Washington, DC, American Psychological Association, 1973, p. 805.

2. Cynkin S: *Occupational Therapy: Toward Health Through Activities.* Boston, Little, Brown, 1979, p. 6.

3. Reed K, Saunderson S: *Concepts of Occupational Therapy.* 2nd Edition, Baltimore, Maryland, Williams & Wilkins, 1983, p. 9.

4. Rogers J: Why study occupations? *Am J Occup Ther* 38:47, 1984.

5. Mosey AC: *Activities Therapy.* New York, Raven Press, 1973, p. 7.

6. Nelson D: *Children with Autism and Other Pervasive Disorders of Development and Behavior: Therapy Through Activities.* Thorofare, New Jersey, Slack Inc., 1984, p. 38.

7. Deloach C, Greer B: *Adjustments to Serve Physical Disability: A Metamorphosis.* St. Louis, McGraw-Hill, 1981, pp. 94-109.

8. *Uniform Terminology for Reporting Occupational Therapy Services.* Rockville, Maryland, American Occupational Therapy Association, 1989.

9. Shillam L, Beeman C, Loshin M: Effect of occupational therapy intervention on bathing independence of disabled persons. *Am J Occup Ther* 37:744, 1983.

10. Hopkins H, Smith H (Eds): *Willard and Spackman's Occupational Therapy,* 6th edition. Philadelphia, JB Lippincott, 1983, pp. 900-901.

11. Bradlee T: The use of groups in short-term psychiatric settings. *Occup Ther Mental Health* 3:47-57, 1984.

12. Chance P: *Learning Through Play.* New York, Garner Press, 1979, pp. 4-24.

13. Stone J, Church J: *Childhood and Adolescence.* New York, Random House, 1966, pp. 108-112, 150-156.

14. Yawkey T, Pellegrin A: *Child's Play, Developmental and Applied.* Hillsdale, New Jersey, Lawrence Erlbaum Assoc, 1984, pp. 343-360.

15. Parten MB: Social participation among pre-school children. *Journal of Abnormal and Social Psychology* 27:243, 1932.

16. Cherrington D: *The Work Ethic, Working Values and Values That Work.* New York, Amacom Press, 1980, p. 262.

17. Murphy J: *Concepts of Leisure.* Englewood Cliffs, New Jersey, Prentice-Hall, 1981, p. 26.

18. Kraus R: *Recreation and Leisure in Modern Society,* 2nd edition. Santa Monica, California, Goodyear Publishing, 1978, p. 40.

19. Dumazedier J: *Sociology of Leisure.* Amsterdam, Netherlands, Elsevier Publishing, 1974, pp. 62-71.

20. Kaplan M: *Leisure in America, A Social Inquiry.* New York, John Wiley and Sons, 1960, pp. 28-37.

21. Parker S: *The Future of Work and Leisure.* New York, Praeger, 1971, pp. 25-30, 58.

22. Havighurst R: The leisure activities of the middle-aged. *Am J Sociology* 63:152-162, 1957.

23. Teaff J: *Leisure Services with the Elderly.* St. Louis, Times Mirror/Mosby, 1985, pp. 43-56.

24. Yoesting D, Burkhead D: Significance of childhood recreation experience on adult leisure behavior. *J Leisure Rec* 5:25-36, 1973.

25. Orthner D: Leisure activity patterns and marital satisfaction over the marital career. *J Marriage Fam* 37:91-102, 1975.

26. American Association for Health, Physical Education and Recreation: *Guidelines for Professional Preparation Programs for Personnel Involved in Physical Education and Recreation for the Handicapped.* Washington, DC, Bureau of Education for the Handicapped, US Office of Education Department, Education and Welfare, 1973, p. 5.

27. Fidler G: *Design of Rehabilitation Services in Psychiatric Hospital Settings.* Laurel, Maryland, Ramsco, 1984, p. 51.

28. Berry J: *Activity Therapy Services.* North Billerica, Massachusetts, Curriculum Associates, Inc., 1977, p. 150.

29. Turkel S: *Working.* New York, Partheon Books, 1974.

30. Best F: *The Future of Work.* Englewood Cliffs, New Jersey, Prentice-Hall, 1973, p. 1.

31. Zander J: *Human Development.* New York, Alfred A. Knopf, 1981, pp. 344-355.

32. Gross E: *Work and Society.* New York, Thomas Y. Crowell Co., 1958, p. 25.

33. Evans R: *Foundations of Vocational Education.* Columbus, Ohio, Charles H. Merrill, 1971, p. 103.

34. Minnesota Occupational Therapy Association: *Description of Occupational Therapy Services,* Minneapolis, Minnesota, Minnesota Occupational Therapy Association, 1972, pp. 15-23.

The Teaching/Learning Process

M. Jeanne Madigan, EdD, OTR, FAOTA
B. Joan Bellman, OTR

INTRODUCTION

Occupational therapists and assistants teach every day. They teach the "whats," the "hows," and even the "whys" of everyday living. They have an additional task because they must teach persons who have cognitive, emotional, or motor problems or a combination of all three. In addition to identifying the assets and limitations of patients and evaluating whether patients have accomplished goals of independent functioning, occupational therapy personnel use teaching/learning principles. These principles enable their patients to accomplish tasks they were not able to perform due to birth defects, social problems, illnesses, or injuries.

For example, consider the case of Lottie, a 29-year-old woman, who is mentally retarded. She was institutionalized all her life, but has been discharged to a sheltered home situation with a court-appointed guardian. Assessment findings indicated that she was ambulatory and cooperative but highly distractable. Lottie held a spoon awkwardly, spilling food on herself and the table. She could don clothes but could not button small buttons or tie a bow. She was able to manage toileting independently, but needed assistance in hand-washing in terms of turning the faucet on and off and drying her hands. Hand function patterns were normal only for gross cylindrical grasp; thumb opposition and wrist stabilization were poor. After discussing the patient with the guardian, the registered occupational therapist (OTR) indicated that the first goal to be addressed in occupational therapy treatment was to improve independent eating. The certified occupational therapy assistant (COTA) was assigned to work with Lottie to help her achieve this task.

In this scenario, the COTA can be identified as the instructor or teacher and the patient as the learner. The teaching/learning problem then becomes threefold:

KEY CONCEPTS

Connectionist approach

Cognitive approach

Gagne's learning types

Bloom's learning domains

Conditions affecting learning

Characteristics of the learning task

Occupational therapy teaching process

1. What is the best way to teach the patient to feed herself?
2. What methods will best facilitate this learning process?
3. What is the process called learning?

Learning has been defined as a relatively permanent change in behavior resulting from exposure to conditions in the environment.[1] Although this definition implies observable events, learning cannot be observed directly, and it is difficult to know what has happened within the learner. However, one can find out whether the learner has acquired the knowledge by posing a problem that requires an individual to use the knowledge then observing if the learner can accomplish the task.

The **teacher's role** is to help the learner to change behavior in specified directions. To do this effectively, the teacher must not only know what is to be taught, but also the methods that will facilitate the desired changes. The first section of this chapter briefly discusses theories of learning; the second section presents some conditions that aid or impede learning; the final section outlines steps in the teaching process that are helpful when working with patients.

THEORIES OF LEARNING

There are two main theoretical approaches to learning: *connectionist* and *cognitive*. A brief overview of these two positions is given to provide better understanding of the various techniques associated with them. Information for this section has been drawn from the writings of Travers,[1] Biehler,[2] Hilgard[3] and Hill.[4]

The Connectionist School

Connectionism is also known as *reductionism, associationism,* and *behaviorism*. In this school, learning is considered to be a matter of making connections between stimuli and responses. A response is any item of behavior, and a stimulus is any input of energy that tends to affect behavior. A simple illustration would be a child who eagerly reaches for a cookie on seeing the cookie jar. An earlier "handout" from the jar brings forth memories of delectable tastes.

Ivan Pavlov was the first to study learning under highly controlled experimental conditions. In one of his earliest experiments, he gave a dish of food to a dog a few seconds after a bell was rung. After many repetitions, the dog salivated at the sound of the bell even though no food was given. This **conditioning** process was referred to as *classic conditioning,* that is, tying a reflex to a particular stimulus so that a desired response can be triggered at will. It should be noted, however, that if the bell was rung too many times without food being presented, the response tended to disappear (become extinct). Once conditioned, the dog tended to salivate to almost any similar sound. To prevent indiscriminate salivating, Pavlov repeatedly rewarded the dog with food only after the bell sound but never after similar sounds.

John B. Watson popularized Pavlovian theory in the United States by conducting experiments demonstrating that human behavior could be conditioned. He also did much to establish the tradition of objectivity and the concern with observable behavior in psychology, and thus became known as the founder of behaviorism.

Edward L. Thorndike conducted experiments using a hungry cat in a cage that had a door with a release mechanism and food outside the cage. After repeated attempts to get at the food, the cat hit the opening mechanism by chance. After repeated trials, the cat learned to make the correct response (hitting the release mechanism) almost immediately. Thorndike concluded from this trial and error process that learning consisted of making connections between stimuli and responses and that repetition was essential to learning.

Following these traditions, B.F. Skinner conducted experiments with rats and pigeons in which he shaped their behavior by reinforcing the action he wanted with a reward. This process, the learning of voluntary responses, is termed *instrumental conditioning* and is highly dependent on the consequences of the response. Skinner referred to the process as *operant conditioning* to emphasize that a person can operate on the environment to produce an event or cause a change in an event. Instrumental conditioning involves trial and error during the learning process, but the response must be rewarded if it is to be repeated. If a response produces positive **reinforcement** or removes negative reinforcement, it will be strengthened; if negative reinforcers are produced or if positive reinforcement is removed, the response will not be repeated and behavior will be extinguished. Secondary reinforcement (such as gold stars or smile stickers) will also strengthen the behavior. Reinforcing a desired response every time it occurs is described as following a schedule of *continuous reinforcement*. When the number of responses between reinforcement varies, *intermittent reinforcement* is being used. It has been found that the fastest, most efficient learning occurs with continuous reinforcement, but learning is less readily extinguished when intermittent reinforcement is used.

Shaping is the process of changing behavior by reinforcing responses that approximate the desired response. At first, any behavior that is close to the desired response is rewarded. Gradually, only those responses that more nearly resemble the desired response are rewarded.

Behavior modification consists of reinforcing desirable responses while ignoring undesirable ones. A reinforcer may be food, praise, opportunities to perform a favorite activity, or tokens to be traded in for prizes or privileges.

Skinner applied what he discovered to the field of teaching by inventing teaching machines and programmed instruction methods. He maintained that to promote effective learning a teacher must divide what is to be learned into a large number of very small steps and reinforce the successful accomplishment of each step. By making the steps as small and gradual as possible, the possibility of errors is low, and therefore the frequency of positive reinforcement is high. The basic techniques of deciding terminal behavior and then shaping behavior have been used by some educators to develop instructional objectives used to structure learning experiences, the mastery learning approach, and performance contracting.

Thus, many educational practices in use today are derived directly or indirectly from operant conditioning techniques based on Skinner's and other behaviorists' research and theories. It is also the basis for the occupational therapy practitioner's practice of breaking down activity into component steps, praising successful accomplishments of patients, and being sure that a patient masters one process before going on to the next. It is also one of the reasons that occupational therapists and assistants grade activities. For more information on these topics see Chapter 17.

The Cognitive School

Cognitive theories, also known by the terms *gestalt, field theory* and *discovery approach,* are concerned with the perceptions or attitudes that individuals have about their environment and the ways these cognitions determine behavior. This school of thought was developed in reaction to the researchers who accepted only measurable behavior as experimental evidence and who were preoccupied with physiologic concepts. Early cognitive theorists emphasized whole systems in which the parts are seen as interrelated in such a way that the whole is more than the sum of its parts. They also studied the ways in which cognitions are modified by experiences.

At about the same time that Thorndike was developing his laws (1920s), a group of German psychologists began experimenting with chimpanzees. Wolfgang Kohler put a chimpanzee named Sultan in a large cage with a variety of objects, including sticks. Sultan discovered that he could use a stick to rake things toward himself. One day, he discovered that he could use a small stick to reach a long stick which, in turn, he used to rake a banana that was outside his cage and too far away to reach with the short stick. This "learning" involved a rearrangement of a previous pattern of behavior. It was a new application of a previous activity. This example is the essence of learning as viewed by a cognitive or field theorist: the perception of new relationships. Rather than learning by conditioning or trial and error, the problem was solved by gaining insight into the relationship between the objects. It should be recognized, however, that Sultan's previous experience with the essentials of the problem was

necessary in order for the insight to occur.

Kurt Lewin provided an important link in the development of cognitive-field theory. He used concepts from mathematics and physics to devise a system of diagramming behavioral situations, which he called the field of forces. He also defined life space, which he said consists of everything that influences a person's behavior (objects, goals, and barriers to those goals, for example). He and his followers believe that individuals behave not only because of external forces to which they are exposed, but also as a consequence of how things seem to them, what they believe them to be.

Edward C. Tolman's "cognitive map" or *sign theory* forms a bridge between strict behaviorist and gestalt theories. He said that human learning depends on the meaning that individuals attach to situations or objects in their environment. While concerned with observable evidence, Tolman hypothesized that numerous intervening variables existed between the situation and the resultant behavior; learners vary their responses according to conditions as they know them. Thus, experience is the underlying factor in insightful and cognitive learning.

Jean Piaget believed that a person organizes and adapts sensory information through two basic mental operations: assimilation and accommodation. In **assimilation,** incoming information is perceived and interpreted according to existing schema that have already been established through previous experience. **Accommodation** is the changing of existing schema as a result of new information. Piaget described four stages of cognitive development. During the first, *sensorimotor,* which begins at birth, children form the most basic conceptions about the material world. They learn the relationship of objects to each other and themselves. The *pre-operational* stage, which begins at approximately two years of age, is that stage when children are conscious of their existence in a world of permanent objects that are separate from themselves, and they realize the causal effects between them. Behavior is still directly linked to what the child perceives and does at the time. During the *concrete operations* stage, beginning at seven years, children's thinking is no longer restricted to physical objects. They are able to make inferences from verbal information that are linked with movement or other information. In the final stage, *formal-operational,* beginning at 11 years, children develop adult abilities and characteristics. They can deal with words and relationships, solve problems involving manipulation of several variables, intellectually examine hypothetical ideas, and evaluate alternatives (see Chapter 5).

Jerome Bruner, who regards learning as a rearrangement of thought patterns, stresses the importance of structure and of providing opportunities for intuitive thinking. He believes that emphasizing structure in teaching makes the subject more comprehensible, more easily remembered, and more able to be transferred. Believing that knowledge is a process rather than a product, Bruner developed techniques for teaching by the discovery method that include the following components:

1. Emphasizing contrast
2. Stimulating informed guessing
3. Encouraging active participation
4. Stimulating awareness

Proponents of the **discovery** or **reflective method** of teaching also believe that too much exposure to lectures, texts, or programs tends to make a student dependent on others and minimizes the likelihood of the individual seeking answers or solving problems independently.

Thus, learning can be considered to be either an accumulation of associations (connectionist school) or the perception of new relationships (cognitive school). Depending on which theory one adheres to, the teacher would use quite different techniques to instruct another person. It should be noted, however, that some theorists feel that rigidly adhering to a single theory is wrong and that, depending on what one wishes to teach, one should make selected use of the techniques based on different theories.

D.O. Hebb proposed two basic periods of learning: primary learning and later learning. *Primary learning* begins at birth and continues until about age 12. It consists of sensory events that impose new types of organization through classic and instrumental conditioning. *Later learning* is conceptual and involves patterns whose parts are familiar and have a number of well-formed associations. Using this line of reasoning, one could conclude that much of adult learning requires few trials unless confronted with situations in which there has been no past experience. Somewhat along this same line, Robert Gagne identified eight progressively complex types of learning:[5]

1. *Signal learning*—an involuntary reflex is activated by a selected stimulus
2. *Stimulus-response learning*—voluntary actions are shaped by reinforcement
3. *Chaining*—individual acts are combined and occur in rapid succession
4. *Verbal association*—verbal chains acquired by connecting previously acquired words and new words
5. *Discrimination learning*—varying responses to verbal associations as what is known becomes more numerous and complex
6. *Concept learning*—response to things or events as a class
7. *Rule learning*—combines or relates chains of concepts previously learned
8. *Problem solving*—combines rules in such a way that permits application to new situations

Gagne believed these kinds of learning are hierarchical and, therefore, the more advanced types of learning can take place only when a person has mastered a large variety of verbal associations based on a great deal of stimulus-response

learning. According to this theory, it would be important for the occupational therapy assistant to have some knowledge of a patient's background so that he or she could select the most appropriate type of learning for that particular individual. It also suggests why it is so important for all children to have many experiences to form the foundation for higher levels of learning, particularly for those who may be restricted physically or mentally due to disease or injury.

Another quite different classification of learning was proposed by Benjamin S. Bloom and his associates. They classified all learning into three domains: cognitive, affective and psychomotor. Categories of the cognitive domain areas follows:[6]

1. *Knowledge*—remembering ideas, material, or phenomena
2. *Comprehension*—understanding material and being able to make some use of it; includes translation, interpretation, and extrapolation
3. *Application*—being able to use correct method, theory, principle, or abstraction in a new situation
4. *Analysis*—breaking down material into its constituent parts and detecting relationships of the parts and the way they are organized
5. *Synthesis*—putting together elements and parts to form the whole in a way that constitutes a structure not previously in existence
6. *Evaluation*—making judgments about the value of ideas, methods and materials

Although the cognitive domain deals with remembering, using something that has been learned by combining old and synthesizing new ideas, the affective domain deals with a feeling tone, awareness, appreciating, etc. Categories in the affective domain are the following:[7]

1. *Receiving* (attending)—being aware, willing to receive and attending to certain phenomena
2. *Responding*—actively attending to a phenomenon by acting, which implies willingness and satisfaction in the response
3. *Valuing*—internalizing a phenomenon and accepting it as having worth; preferring it and being committed to it
4. *Organization*—building a value system that is interrelated
5. *Characterization by a value or value complex*—acting consistently in accordance with internalized values and providing a total philosophy or world view

Bloom and his associates[6] identified the psychomotor domain as including muscular or motor skill, manipulation of material and objects, or some act that requires neuromuscular coordination. However, they did not go on to develop a classification or taxonomic system for it. A number of individuals have proposed schemas that have not received the wide acceptance accorded to the two previously outlined taxonomies. However, since the psychomotor domain is of great importance in occupational therapy because many of the profession's concerns relate to neuromuscular actions, it is important to consider some classification of this domain. Harrow classifies the psychomotor domain as follows:[8]

1. *Reflex movements*—includes segmental, intersegmental, suprasegmental, and postural reflexes or movements that are involuntary in nature and are precursors of basic fundamental movement
2. *Basic-fundamental movements*—includes locomotor, non-locomotor and manipulative movements
3. *Perceptual abilities*—includes kinesthetic, visual, auditory, and tactile discrimination as well as coordinated abilities
4. *Physical abilities*—includes endurance, strength, flexibility and agility
5. *Skilled movements*—includes simple adaptive skill, compound adaptive skill and complex adaptive skill
6. *Non-discursive communications*—includes expressive and interpretive movements

These classifications could aid in planning learning experiences for teaching skills and activities to patients by identifying levels of ability and specifying graded objectives in one or more of the three domains. Since they are all hierarchical in nature, the occupational therapist would have to assess the patient to be sure that a previous level is in good order before attempting subsequent ones. For example, patients should not be expected to apply a principle before they can recall it and know what it means; nor should they be expected to respond to the therapist if they have not attended to the therapist.

CONDITIONS THAT AFFECT LEARNING

What individuals bring to the learning situation in terms of personality traits, motivation and general background has an important influence on what they are willing to learn, what they can learn, and how efficiently they will learn it.[9]

The basic motivation for learning is found in the human being's normal tendency to explore and make sense of the environment. Gradually, this general exploratory tendency is differentiated in terms of specific needs, interests, and goals, so that individuals are motivated to learn some things but remain relatively uninterested in others. If curiosity is discouraged or punished, as it may be by some parents or societies, the natural inclination for learning is greatly dulled. If what is to be learned bears little relationship to the learner's immediate interests and purposes, motivation may have to be induced by manipulation of rewards and punishments.

An individual's frame of reference (assumptions and attitudes) determines in large part what one sees and learns. The range of information that will be meaningful; the way new material will be interpreted; and whether the task is perceived as a challenge, a threat, or of no importance, depends on the individual's perception of self and the world.

Usually an individual is eager to tackle learning tasks when they are seen as related to needs and purposes and appropriate to one's competence level. On the other hand, an individual usually tries to avoid those tasks that appear of little value or with which he or she feels unable to cope. For some persons, a vicious cycle may develop in which, feeling inadequate, they force themselves into a learning situation with anxiety and trepidation; they expect to do badly and they do. The resulting negative feedback then reinforces their concept of inadequacy.

A learner must also be able to tolerate immediate frustration in the interest of achieving long-range goals. Preoccupation with inner conflicts, a high level of anxiety, feelings of discouragement and depression, and other maladaptive patterns can also seriously impair one's ability to learn.

CHARACTERISTICS OF THE LEARNING TASK

Coleman[9] outlined four characteristics of the learning task itself that influence how it should be approached and how easily it can be mastered.

Type of Task

Motor skills usually require time and practice to train the muscles to function with the desired skill and coordination (an example would be learning to hammer a nail or doing a range of motion test). Meaningful verbal information results from intensive sessions, with a focus on relationships leading to the quickest learning and best retention (an example would be for the teacher to relate new information to something similar the student already knows). Unrelated data often require a spaced drill for material that must be memorized (an example would be learning the origins and insertions of muscles).

Size, Complexity and Familiarity

Generally more material needs more time, although less time is needed for meaningful material than for unrelated data that must be memorized. Added complexity tends to increase the time required for study and understanding, but may be offset if the learner is familiar with the material in a general way and has adequate background for organizing and understanding it (in this case, the teacher should try to relate new concepts to what the learner already knows).

Clarity

The less clear the task, the more time and effort needed to master it (here, the teacher should point out the essential elements of the task or the thing to be learned).

Environment

Things that make learning more difficult include disapproval by one's peers, unfavorable study conditions, lack of essential tools or resources, severe time pressures, and other distracting life demands. Ways to enhance learning include using a well-lighted, well-ventilated study place, which is free of distractions; getting an overall view of the task; and organizing the task in terms of key elements. Long-range retention is encouraged by distributed study, periodic review, and tying new material in with previous learning and real life situations. Knowing these principles should give students very helpful clues to make their study time more effective. You will be learning many things in your classes that you must not only know for the final examination, but also remember next semester because it is the foundation for later coursework. You will also need to use the knowledge for your fieldwork experiences, the certification examination, and work itself. Therefore, long-term retention is the goal of this learning.

Little is known about how previous learning affects the ease with which individuals can understand and master subsequent learning. The available evidence indicates that some transfer will occur if there are identical elements in the two learning situations or if they can be understood in terms of the same general principles. Transfer of learning seems to depend on the learner's ability to perceive the points of similarity between the old and the new information.

The return of information individuals receive about the progress or outcome of their behavior (feedback) not only tells them whether they are proceeding satisfactorily, but also serves as a reward or punishment. Learners can modify or adjust responses on the basis of feedback. Motivation, self-confidence, and learning efficiency (not having to unlearn errors) are all facilitated by frequent feedback. Praise and progress toward desired goals reinforce what has been learned and motivate further learning.

THE OCCUPATIONAL THERAPY TEACHING PROCESS

Once the patient has been evaluated and the goals of treatment specified, it is necessary to identify what is to be taught and how to teach the patient in order to best accomplish these goals. Using principles from the theories discussed in the previous sections of this chapter, the teaching process steps are outlined and applied to specific patient treatment situations.

Teaching Process Steps

The following **teaching process steps** must be carried out in the order in which they are discussed.

State Learning Objectives. Identify what the patient needs to learn. This step can be done with a great deal of specificity or in more general terms. Using Lottie, whose case was briefly discussed in the beginning of this chapter, as an example, the learning objectives could be stated as follows:

1. "Within three weeks the patient will be able to scoop applesauce with a spoon from a bowl and place it in her mouth without spilling any sauce on self, table, or floor, seven out of ten trials."
2. "The patient will be able to feed self without spilling."

It is fairly obvious that the first objective leaves no room for guessing what exactly is to be accomplished and how the outcome is to be evaluated. A new therapist or assistant may find it useful to explicitly state all objectives in similar detail until it becomes second nature to think in these terms. If one is using a behavior modification approach, it is necessary to be even more specific in identifying what the present behavior is and what are the incremental steps between that and the target behavior. This will allow reinforcement to be applied for each small behavior that represents a movement toward the desired behavior change.

Determine Content. What exactly is to be taught? In the preceding example, the motor skills of grasp, bringing the spoon to the mouth, and removing food from the spoon with the mouth must be taught. Activities related but not included in the objective as it is stated are selection of the proper eating utensil, cutting food, drinking from a glass, and using proper table manners.

Identify Modifications Necessary for the Particular Patient or Group. In planning this step, it is important to refer to the history and assessment of the patient to determine whether any physical, mental, or sociocultural findings require adjustment of methods or adaptation of equipment that will be used. The most basic consideration to assist in determining what to teach and in selecting appropriate methods to use is the patient's **developmental level.** The term developmental level refers to the process of growth and differentiation when compared to others. One will have little success teaching a two-year-old an activity that requires the neuromuscular coordination of a four-year-old, or, in the case of Lottie, using abstract reasoning with a retarded adult who is still in the pre-operational stage.

It is also important to consider the physical limitations such as loss of mobility, coordination, sight, and hearing. The presence of pain or use of medications that affect the patient's functioning must also be considered. Educational and socioeconomic levels may require the teacher to adapt the general language and the technical terms used.

Lottie is functioning at a preschool level in many ways. It would be important to use simple words and short sentences when giving her directions. Because of her grasp and prehension difficulties, a spoon handle could be built up to facilitate grasp strength and control. Using a spoon, a bowl and applesauce at first is desirable because it is easier to get the applesauce onto the spoon and less likely to spill than peas on a fork. Use of the sauce will provide a greater chance for success early in the process. As Lottie gains skill, more difficult foods and other utensils can be introduced.

Break Activity/Process into Small Units of Instruction.
In the learning objective in the example, numerous skills will need to be learned, including the following:
1. Grasping the spoon
2. Scooping the food onto the spoon
3. Bringing the food to the mouth
4. Holding the spoon so the food does not fall off
5. Inserting the spoon in the mouth without knocking the food off the spoon
6. Removing the food from the spoon with the teeth and lips
7. Closing the mouth so that food does not dribble out
8. Chewing food with the mouth closed

What seems like a very simple activity actually has at least eight separate skills that will need to be taught and combined to accomplish the original objective.

Assemble Materials. To prevent delays in the process, it is important to gather all equipment and supplies that will be needed to complete the activity. If the teacher is planning to use learning aids such as diagrams, printed instructions, or samples, they should be prepared in advance. As with the learning activity itself, these materials should be modified to be appropriate for the patient or group.

Because the learning objective in Lottie's case consists of psychomotor skills, and since she is functioning at the pre-operational stage of development, visual aids would probably only confuse her. The materials needed for this activity are few. However, if one were teaching a patient copper tooling, it would be important to think through all of the steps and ensure that the necessary supplies were on hand so that the project could be carried to completion.

Arrange Work Space. Set up the table or whatever area is to be used so that needed materials are conveniently located. If the patient is easily distracted, however, anything that is not being used at the moment should be kept out of sight. Ensure that the patient is comfortable and uses good posture to minimize fatigue. Lighting that illuminates the work area but does not shine in the patient's eyes is important. Lighting is a critical concern for someone with failing eyesight. The person instructing must assume a position in relation to the patient that will be the most advantageous to demonstrate, assist and observe, being careful not to obstruct the patient's view of the task or activity. Usually, sitting next to the patient is preferable. In this way the work will be at the proper height, angle and perspective. When teaching a group, one must assure that all participants can see what is being shown. Lottie is easily distracted; therefore, it would be important to try to reduce visible objects and eliminate sounds in the area that may divert her attention from what is being demonstrated or displayed.

Simulate as closely as possible the conditions under which the patient will have to carry out the activity. If circumstances between the learning situation and the "real" one are very different, the patient may not be able to transfer the learning, even though he or she can accomplish the task perfectly in the treatment setting.

Prepare the Patient or Group. Try to determine if the patient is ready to learn by asking the following: Is the patient alert? Is the patient paying attention to the person in the teaching role? Does the patient appear interested in what is to happen? Concerns, anxieties, or other emotions may divert the patient's attention and make it difficult to concentrate on what is being taught. The therapist or assistant may need to deal with these matters or to make a referral to another discipline to attend to them before the patient is fully ready to learn.

Does the patient need basic skills or knowledge before learning can proceed? Learning will be more successful if it can be tied to some familiar elements. Does the patient know what is going to happen and the purpose of the activity? Instruction will be more easily grasped and retained if the patient knows why he or she is doing the activity and feels that it is something needed or wanted. For example, Lottie wanted to be like "other people," which included not having to wear a bib. This was her ultimate aim—no spilling, no bib!

Present the Instruction. Once the activity has been broken into small component steps, the next phase is presentation of the first step. Begin by securing the patient's attention. Tell the person what you are going to do and what you expect him or her to do. If diagrams or other visual aids are being used, point out the salient features. Demonstrate the first step accompanied by a verbal explanation that emphasizes a few key words that provide "word pictures," cues to the action or important signals to watch for. In this way the instructor is provid-ing input through two senses, sight and hearing. Repeat the step and observe whether the patient seems to understand. Ask questions that will indicate the level of comprehension. Point out precautions or common errors to avoid. When teaching a motor skill to a patient who is very young or has limited cognitive skills, it may be desirable not only to demonstrate but also to physically guide the patient through the action (an example would be to place the patient's hand on the spoon, place your hand over the patient's hand, and guide the individual through the correct action several times; this will allow the patient to "get the feel" of the correct movement).

Have the Patient do a "Tryout". Ask the patient to proceed with the activity independently. If working with an object, give it to the patient and do not assist in the task at hand. If help is needed, repeat the verbal cues. Have the patient repeat the step several times, gradually decreasing the cues until he or she is doing it independently without any assistance. Correct any errors immediately so that the patient does not learn the incorrect method, as it will be difficult to unlearn the wrong way before relearning the correct way. In Lottie's case, self-feeding had been accomplished in a very sloppy manner, so it will be difficult for her to overcome a set habit pattern and to learn a new way of eating.

Observe whether the patient gives nonverbal clues that he or she understands or does not understand; the individual may not want to admit confusion. Invite questions. Allow the patient to perform independently several times to provide assurance that the individual knows the correct procedure and did not just happen to do it correctly by chance. Offer sincere praise for correct work. Look for indications of fatigue, pain, or waning attention. A rest or redirection may be necessary.

Lottie was eager to please others and so responded well to praise when she accomplished one of the component skills. Good performance was also rewarded by adding new foods that she liked, especially ice cream.

Evaluate Performance. Decide how many times, how far apart, and in how many different circumstances the correct performance should be observed to assure that the patient has mastered the skill or skills that have been taught. Carry-over will be greater if the patient has repeated the activity several times and made it a habit.

If the activity is composed of several steps, present each one, making sure the patient has learned one step before going on to the next. Retention will be aided if each previous step can be practiced as each new step is added.

The therapist and assistant should ask themselves the following questions:

1. Does a caretaker need to be instructed in the particular process to increase the likelihood that the activity will be done correctly when the patient returns to the ward or home?
2. Does the patient have a sense of accomplishment?
3. Is the activity accomplishing the desired effect or goal?

The following brief case study is presented as a contrast to the profile of Lottie; it presents quite a different teaching/learning situation:

Case Study 8-1

Mildred. Mildred is a 57-year-old woman with a diagnosis of degenerative joint disease. She complains of low back pain when performing many household chores. She lives at home with her husband, who is receiving disability benefits because of a heart condition. He is unable to assist with heavy housework. Mildred is of average intelligence but has a high level of anxiety about keeping her home neat and clean. She is also afraid of pain. The occupational therapy goal was to enable Mildred to perform household work within a tolerable level of discomfort.

In this case, the COTA identified the learning objective: "The patient will apply principles of body mechanics and energy conservation to carry out household tasks." The content includes, for example, 1) the correct method of lifting heavy objects and 2) reducing the amount of bending and stretching. Because this patient has a high school education, is of average intelligence, and has no limitations other than the arthritis for which she is receiving treatment, no special modifications in teaching methods are necessary.

The COTA prepared charts that illustrated each principle. The principle was printed at the top of each chart and a stick-figure diagram showed how the principle is applied in a particular cleaning or cooking task. The COTA discussed each principle with Mildred, pointing out how the illustration of the figure in the diagram made use of the principle. She then demonstrated several times how to perform the task correctly, noting precautions. Next, she asked Mildred to perform the same task, correcting errors as soon as they occurred. Mildred was asked to repeat the task until she could carry it out correctly three consecutive times.

Because the objective was to have the patient apply the principles rather than just learn specific techniques, the COTA could not conclude instruction at this point. She continued by asking Mildred to identify a chore that she did in her home that could be accomplished by using the principle that she had learned. At first, Mildred was at a loss to associate the principle with another task, so the COTA asked her to describe how she washed clothes. When Mildred described carrying the clothes basket from the bedroom to the washing machine, the COTA suggested that she could use the principle of lifting objects by keeping her trunk erect, bending at the knees, and holding the object (the clothes basket) close to her body. Mildred showed recognition that this task used the principle. The COTA again asked Mildred how the same principle could be used with another, closely related task. Mildred identified carrying a scrub bucket of water. A similar process was used in identifying chores that required the patient to bend and stretch and, as a result, Mildred has altered how she carries out many household tasks. For example, she rearranged her cabinets and cupboards so that commonly used items would be within easy reach.

She now uses a long-handled feather duster to dust her bookcases and china cabinet, and cleans the kitchen and bathroom floors with a sponge mop with a squeeze attachment at midshaft on the handle.

Once Mildred had mastered a principle (by correctly doing the task during the treatment session and identifying another task that used the same principle), she was directed to incorporate it into her home routine. She was also asked to look for ways to use the same principle with other chores. During the next treatment session, the COTA asked Mildred to list the tasks that she had identified since the last treatment session and to demonstrate how she applied the principle taught during the previous session. In this way, the COTA determined that the patient had understood the principle and could easily apply it to her everyday functioning. As Mildred demonstrated that she understood and was using a principle, the COTA introduced additional ones. She made up a little booklet with principles and diagrams so that Mildred could refer to it and continue to modify tasks in the future.

It should be noted that the COTA used some of the same teaching principles with Mildred that she used with Lottie (eg, immediate correction of errors), but other techniques were not necessary. Praise of work well done and use of extrinsic rewards were not necessary because Mildred understood what was being accomplished, and the ability to keep up her house according to her standards while suffering less pain was reward enough. The COTA was able to use the modified discovery approach by having Mildred reason out how she could use the principles she had learned. This meant she would be able to apply the principles daily and not have to rely on the COTA to teach her the modified method for every task she needed to carry out.

SUMMARY

Much of what occupational therapy assistants hope to accomplish through their treatment relates to patients actively carrying out certain activities as independently as their condition permits. Thus, the COTA becomes a teacher, the patient must become the learner, and the treatment planning process must include consideration of the most effective and efficient methods to facilitate the learning process.

Knowledge of how learning occurs and of conditions that aid or impede learning will improve the COTA's ability to help patients change their behavior in specified directions identified through evaluation and goal selection. Two main approaches to learning are connectionist theory and cognitive theory. The former, a result of Pavlov's classic conditioning experiments, proposes that learning is a matter of making connections between stimuli and responses; careful

attention to reinforcing desired responses will result in accomplishing behavioral changes. Cognitive theorists, on the other hand, regard learning as a perception of new relationships. Emphasis is on providing the basic knowledge and structure of a subject and motivating the learner to actively explore and discover concepts related to the subject at hand.

These views are shunned by some individuals who maintain that neither of these theoretical views adequately explains all learning. They propose a hierarchical progression of learning, which uses different teaching methods for different levels and domains of learning. Other important considerations include the learner's previous experiences, motivation to learn, and personal and environmental conditions that aid or hinder the learning process.

Related Learning Activities

1. Use the following scenario to plan learning experiences and methods: The long-term goal for a group of five patients is to improve interpersonal social skills. The short-term goals are learning to take turns, to share materials, and to respond appropriately to one another.

Make two separate plans, one using the connectionist school of learning approach and the other using the cognitive school approach. List differences and similarities.

2. Select a craft activity and prepare a plan outlining how you would teach it to a classmate or a peer. Be sure to consider all ten steps in the teaching/learning process.

3. Using the plan developed in item two, teach a classmate or peer the craft. Ask the person to give you feedback on the teaching session.

4. Select a different activity than the one used in item three, and prepare a plan for teaching it to a group of six classmates or peers. Again, use the ten steps, but be sure to adjust your plan to accommodate six different individuals instead of one. Present the activity to the group and have them critique the experience.

5. Make a chart illustrating the steps in making a pizza.

References

1. Travers RMW: *Essentials of Learning,* 4th edition. New York, Macmillan, 1977.
2. Biehler RF: *Psychology Applied to Teaching,* 2nd edition. Boston, Houghton Mifflin, 1974.
3. Hilgard ER, Bower GH: *Theories of Learning,* 4th edition. Englewood Cliffs, New Jersey, Prentice-Hall, 1975.
4. Hill WF: *Learning,* 3rd edition. New York, Thomas Y. Crowell, 1977.
5. Gagne RM: *The Conditions of Learning,* 3rd edition. New York, Holt, Rinehart & Winston, 1977.

6. Bloom BS (Ed): *Taxonomy of Educational Objectives Handbook I: Cognitive Domain*. New York, David McKay, 1956.

7. Krathwohl DR, Bloom BS, Masia BB: *Taxonomy of Educational Objectives Handbook II: Affective Domain*. New York, David McKay, 1964.

8. Harrow AJ: *A Taxonomy of the Psychomotor Domain*. New York, David McKay, 1972.

9. Coleman JC: *Psychology and Effective Behavior*. Glenview, Illinois, Scott, Foresman, & Co., 1969.

Interpersonal Communication Skills and Applied Group Dynamics

Toné F. Blechert, BA, COTA, ROH
Nancy Kari, MPH, OTR

INTRODUCTION

Understanding oneself and learning how to live and work with others in satisfying relationships are goals for healthy living. Occupational therapy personnel teach skills that lead to improved interpersonal relationships. The teaching and reinforcement of these skills can happen within a one-to-one relationship or within a group setting. The registered occupational therapist (OTR) makes this choice based on the patient's needs and skill levels.

Working effectively with people, whether on a one-to-one basis or within a group, requires that the occupational therapist and the certified occupational therapy assistant (COTA) develop specific intrapersonal and interpersonal skills. Intrapersonal skills are related to developing a clear and accurate sense of self. These skills allow the individual to cope effectively with the emotional demands of the environment. Interpersonal skills are communication skills that help occupational therapy personnel to interact effectively with a variety of people. One must be able to identify, assess and strengthen skills in both areas. These skills are prerequisites to group work.

Group work is an effective and powerful medium for planned change in occupational therapy treatment. The group creates an environment that enhances the individual's abilities to gain new insights and increased self-awareness. Within a therapeutic group, a controlled environment is carefully designed to provide opportunities for patients to identify and practice specific skills. Members establish peer relationships that can support and

KEY CONCEPTS

Intrapersonal and interpersonal skills

Group role functions

Group norms

Group growth and development stages

Leadership preparation, attitudes, and approaches

Activity qualities and examples

strengthen self-confidence and encourage risk taking. Members can experience conflict and personal struggle in a supportive setting. When resolution occurs, a heightened sense of affiliation with others emerges. In this way, the occupational therapy group becomes a "living laboratory" where members learn about themselves in relation to others.

It is strongly recommended that all entry-level occupational therapy personnel begin group work under the supervision of an experienced therapist. Co-leading a group provides an opportunity for the beginner to learn and refine group facilitation skills. Team leading is also a benefit to group members, as it provides role models of appropriate interaction. This chapter offers a summary of the key factors involved in effective intrapersonal skills, interpersonal communication and applied group dynamics.

INTRAPERSONAL AND INTERPERSONAL SKILLS

The establishment of a relationship among the therapist, the assistant and the patient is the first step in the process of facilitating any change in a therapeutic setting. Specific skills in effective communication and skills related to forming helping relationships are discussed in detail in later sections. These are prerequisites to effective group leadership. Their importance cannot be overemphasized.

A COTA must first develop the skills to relate to others on a one-to-one basis. This level of interaction is defined as a *dyad*. People are relating when each is responding to the other as a person instead of an object. An example of the latter would be to say, "Hello, how are you?" when passing someone on the street without stopping to hear the reply. Relating to another individual as a person involves time, interest, energy and interpersonal skill. The ability to relate effectively to another is an art that can be learned and improved with experience and practice.

An effective COTA demonstrates four characteristics: self-awareness, self-acceptance, awareness of others, and the ability to communicate that awareness.[1] A person need not develop these competencies in sequence; they are singled out as important attributes. A COTA needs to achieve and integrate all four areas. One cannot become self-aware and accepting in isolation. These abilities are developed and refined simultaneously through interaction with others.

Self-Awareness

The ability to recognize one's behaviors and emotional responses is **self-awareness.** As one plays and works with other people, personal strengths and weaknesses emerge. Feedback is received from others and from the environment. Self-concept emerges from this dynamic, continuously developing process of interaction. Self-concept refers to the individual's overall picture of self. Both positive and negative qualities are a part of this self-concept. The more experience one has with others, the clearer the picture becomes. Accompanying these pictures is a set of judgments and evaluations of one's self that have been accumulated over a long time. Examples of these judgments include competent or incompetent, effective or ineffective, and intelligent or dull. Feelings about self come from these evaluations and judgments. These feelings help form self-esteem. Self-esteem can be influenced by many feelings including guilt, confidence, shame, and security. Self-concept and self-esteem usually remain relatively stable but can fluctuate at times. For example, one may feel basically good about self but feel embarrassed or shameful about a specific action.[2]

For the COTA to communicate and relate effectively with the patient, he or she must have an awareness of self and an acceptance of individual limitations and strengths.

Self-Acceptance

Acceptance of one's own feelings is an important step in gaining self-respect. When a person dislikes himself or herself, feelings of worthlessness may occur and interfere with personal growth; however, people often make their greatest strides in personal growth just when they begin to see themselves realistically and recognize their limitations.[1]

Part of self-acceptance is learning to understand the difference between self-concept and self-ideal. Self-ideal refers to the way one would most like to be seen by others. Self-ideal may differ considerably from one's true self-image. Self-acceptance does not mean that a person is resigned to his or her self-image. It means that one does not dislike oneself. There is a recognition and acceptance of strengths, limitations, and the feelings that accompany these.

Awareness of and acceptance of one's own feelings enable a person to express those feelings more openly to other people. Verbal expression of feelings helps one gain a fuller understanding of them, as well as emotional relief. Openness, when appropriate, is a positive signal to others that can create opportunities to develop more meaningful interpersonal relationships.

Awareness of Others

To be highly sensitive and responsive to another person's feelings is to be **sentient.** Sentience is a quality that is difficult to describe. The COTA who learns to be keenly aware of the feelings of other people is more likely to gain the trust and cooperation of patients as well as co-workers. Sentience enables the COTA to enter empathetically into the lives of others. This does not happen on an intellectual level; instead, it occurs on a feeling level. One must behave in such a way that the patient can feel the concern being expressed. When the patient senses this interest and caring, a bond is created.[3]

People are motivated to take action and make changes in many different ways. Healthy people have need-satisfying environments, supportive friends and family, and energy reserves. Those who are suffering from emotional or physical trauma are sometimes lacking these supportive elements. Through affiliation with a sentient individual, a patient may receive the support and energy that is needed to make positive changes.

Demonstrating Acceptance and Awareness

Although it is important to have a clear understanding of oneself and of others, this alone is not sufficient to establish a therapeutic relationship. The purpose of a therapeutic relationship is to facilitate change and collaborative problem solving while maintaining or promoting the patient's autonomy. To accomplish this goal, the effective COTA must be able to communicate awareness of others. In a therapeutic environment the therapist and assistant assume a variety of important roles. For example, he or she may be a catalyst creating challenges for the patient, a solution giver, a resource person, or a process helper by assisting the patient to identify his or her own needs and choose appropriate solutions. These roles are all legitimate and necessary to facilitate change. In the initial phases of the relationship, however, the most important role is that of the listener. It is essential to clearly understand the patient's point of view and to be able to communicate understanding. This goal is achieved most effectively through active listening. There are a variety of listening responses; some are actually blocks to communication, whereas others enhance understanding. The following four common responses can become barriers to communication in initial patient relationships.

Giving Advice. One way that people try to be helpful is by *giving advice.* Many times people do not really need or want advice at all. They have already thought through options and may even have the problem solved. What they need instead is a listener who can demonstrate true understanding. Giving advice tells a person that the primary interest is in the content rather than in the feelings expressed. Here is an example:

Patient: I'm worried about telling my friends I've been in the hospital for treatment. I don't know if I want to tell them I've decided not to use drugs anymore.
Assistant: The way I would handle that is to be as clear about it as possible. Make an announcement as soon as you are back in school that you are through using drugs.

In this situation the assistant ignores the feeling of concern expressed by the young patient. The response might imply a lack of confidence in the patient's ability to find his or her own solution. Although COTAs may need to assist the patient by giving advice at some point, it is an ineffective response when the individual is trying to communicate a feeling.

Offering Reassurance. Another common response in conversations is *offering reassurance.* Reassuring another person is usually well intended but can limit further communication. When one gives reassurance, the person talking tends to feel that he or she ought to discontinue discussing the problem. This can minimize the uncomfortable emotion expressed by the patient. Here is an example:

Patient: I feel so confused and overwhelmed now, I don't know where to start.
Assistant: Don't worry so much; things always work out in the end.

In this example, offering reassurance is a kind of emotional withdrawal from the patient. It does not acknowledge the feelings expressed. Encouragement and assurance are often important verbal responses in a therapeutic relationship. Reassurance used as a response to another's expression of a feeling is not effective.

Diverting. A third response choice, referred to as *diverting,* involves relating what the patient has said to one's own experience.[4] This is sometimes done in an effort to communicate understanding, or it can be used to change the subject when the topic of conversation becomes uncomfortable. Sometimes people find it difficult to talk about topics such as anger, death, divorce, or violence because they create an inner tension. Changing the subject or shifting the focus of the conversation may reduce tension, but it does not communicate to the patient that the message has been heard. Here is an example:

Patient: One of my biggest problems right now is feeling so lonely. That is worse than going through the divorce itself.
Assistant: I know how you feel. My sister just had a divorce and she talks about that often. She's joined a ski club though, and is meeting all kinds of people. Do you like to ski?

In this example, the focus of the conversation is shifted by the assistant to his or her own experience; therefore, the assistant is not making a clear response to the feelings the patient has shared. The patient may feel as though the message had not been heard.

Questioning. A fourth response that is sometimes used ineffectively is *questioning.* To try to understand the details of an individual's situation, the COTA might ask questions that relate more to the facts than to the feelings expressed. Although it is important to have a clear picture of the patient's situation, excessive questioning or responding with an immediate question can limit the patient's opportunity to clearly describe the experience. In this regard, questioning is not a useful response to another's expression of feelings. Here is an example:

> *Patient:* The doctor told us our daughter's problems are caused by rheumatoid arthritis. We were so hoping it was just growing pains.
> *Assistant:* How old is your daughter?

The question asked by the assistant in this example does not respond to the emotion shared by the patient.

ACTIVE LISTENING—NONVERBAL AND VERBAL COMPONENTS

Active listening is a term given to a set of skills that allows an individual to hear, understand and indicate that the message has been communicated. It is an effective listening response. Active listening is a necessary component in the relationship between the COTA and the patient. It is fundamental to effective communication and basic to the occupational therapy process. Active listening enables the assistant to understand more objectively and accurately the meaning of the verbal and nonverbal messages communicated by the patient. It is important and sometimes difficult to achieve a balance between too little and too much listening. However, if the therapist and the assistant do not understand the meaning of the messages communicated by the patient, inappropriate treatment goals and treatment activities may be chosen. If the interview or treatment session is entirely unstructured and the therapist or assistant "listens" to whatever the patient wishes to say, valuable and expensive treatment time may be lost. Active listening on the part of a COTA is a combination of the verbal and nonverbal behaviors and skills that communicate an attitude of acceptance. These are discussed in terms of the following nonverbal components: appropriate body posture and position, eye contact, facial expression, and a nondistracting environment. Paraphrasing and reflection are also important elements in this process.

Body Posture and Positioning

The most effective body posture includes facing the patient in an open, relaxed manner and leaning forward slightly. Arms should not be folded across the chest; legs should not be crossed. Tightly crossed arms and legs can be interpreted by the patient as rigidity or defensiveness.[5] Extraneous body motions such as swinging legs or tapping

fingers do not indicate a relaxed posture and should be avoided. It is better not to sit behind a desk but to position oneself directly across from the patient. In an occupational therapy clinic it is acceptable and often desirable to use a table during the interview. In this instance sit across from or beside the patient. Optimal communication usually occurs when the participants are three to five feet apart.[6] Cultural differences may dictate variations. It is always useful to watch for and respond to nonverbal cues given by the patient regarding a comfortable distance for communication.

Eye Contact

An effective listener maintains good eye contact with the speaker. Eye contact is thought to be an effective way of communicating empathy.[7] Avoiding another's eyes in an interaction can communicate disinterest, discomfort, or preoccupation.[6] At the same time, staring intently can make the speaker uncomfortable. It is important to look directly at the patient without staring.

Facial Expression

One's facial expressions are an important component of non-verbal communication. A frown, a smile or raised eyebrows send a specific message to the other party that indicates disapproval, approval or questioning.

Environmental Considerations

To actively listen to another, the interaction must take place in a nondistracting, pleasant environment. It is important to hold group sessions or dyadic interviews in quiet, uncluttered areas. Avoid interruptions from others or the telephone. It is sometimes useful to use "Do Not Disturb" signs and to ask that telephone calls be held.

Paraphrasing and Reflection

Two verbal techniques related to active listening include paraphrasing and reflection. **Paraphrasing** is repeating in one's own words the verbal content of the message received. **Reflection** is a summary of the affective meaning of the message and may include the patient's verbal and nonverbal communication. These techniques are used to ensure understanding by checking the accuracy of the message received. A paraphrasing response might begin with "Do you mean that. . ." or "I understand you to say. . ." and then rephrasing the content of the message. Message content includes information about an event or situation: who, what, when, where, how. The affective meaning is the accompanying feeling or emotion that is stated verbally or implied in nonverbal cues. It is important to listen to both aspects of the message. The following patient statements are provided as examples:

> *Patient 1:* I haven't had time to get used to the idea that I'll soon be leaving, and I'm scared to death of this change.

In this example, "I haven't had time to get used to the idea that I'll soon be leaving" is the content because it provides information about the situation. "I'm scared to death" is the affective message because it describes the emotion.

> *Patient 2:* I'm disappointed with the way this turned out. I guess I didn't read the directions thoroughly.

In the second example, "I'm disappointed" is the feeling response and, therefore, the affective message. "I didn't read the directions thoroughly" is the content because it describes the "what" in the situation.

When the patient does not directly state how he or she feels about the situation just described but expresses this nonverbally through body movements, facial expression, or tone of voice, the assistant can reflect what the patient may be feeling by naming an emotion. To practice using reflection as a listening tool when the patient does not directly state the feeling one can 1) listen for the feelings inferred by the overall tone of the message, 2) observe patient body language, or 3) ask, "How would I feel?" Putting oneself in another's place allows one to guess another's reaction. This technique is sometimes helpful but it must be remembered that each person's response is unique.[4] Following are examples of a COTA's response to the feelings implied by the patient:

> *Patient 1* (an elderly woman who recently moved to an apartment): When my husband was alive he did everything for me. Now not only do I have to take care of things myself, I have no one to talk to.

The assistant recognizes that the patient is feeling lonely.

> *Response:* It must be an empty feeling to suddenly find yourself without your spouse.

> *Patient 2* (a patient who is recovering from severe burns over the upper half of her body. The patient's hair is gone and she is trying on the wig for the first time. She adjusts and readjusts the wig. Finally she says): There, I can almost stand to look at myself again.

The assistant observes the patient's frustration and depressed manner and thinks that the woman feels unattractive, anxious and depressed.

> *Response:* This recovery period must be a very difficult time for you. I can tell your appearance is important to you and that you are anxious to look yourself again.

> *Patient 3* (a woman whose ten-year-old daughter is having trouble in school states that): Nancy has never

had problems before. She seems discouraged, and her teacher appears disinterested in her.

The COTA thinks the patient is expressing anxiety or concern about her daughter and anger or frustration with what she thinks is the teacher's disinterest.

> *Response:* It's worrisome to see your child struggle, and it's irritating when the teacher doesn't seem interested.

OTHER IMPORTANT COMMUNICATION COMPONENTS

Other components of effective communication incorporate both verbal and nonverbal responses. These include communicating respect, warmth and genuineness.

Communicating Respect

The COTA must be able to effectively communicate respect to the patient. Respect means to believe in the value and the potential of another person. When respect is communicated, a person feels more capable of self-help. Attention must be focused on the patient's interests and needs instead of the therapist's concerns. The COTA attempts to help the patient meet his or her needs without dominating the situation or the patient.

Communicating respect involves the process of affirmation. To affirm means to reinforce the worth of an individual. This process allows the patient to begin to value himself or herself. The COTA must develop the capacity to recognize quickly the strengths in the patient, and these must be communicated to the patient whenever possible. A sense of timing is needed, however, because sometimes patients are not ready to hear their strengths and the feedback may be threatening. Communicating respect is associated with the ability to communicate personal warmth and genuineness.

Communicating Warmth

Warmth is the degree to which the therapist communicates caring to the patient. Warmth by itself is not adequate for developing a therapeutic relationship or for assisting someone in problem solving; however, it can facilitate these positive outcomes.

Warmth may be demonstrated in tone of voice, facial expression, or other body language, as well as in words and actions. Touching, for example, is an effective way to communicate concern and empathy. Touching a patient's hand or shoulder may offer reassurance, approval or encouragement. It is important to remember, however, that not all people like to be touched, and in some situations touching may be contraindicated.

Communicating Genuineness

Genuineness, also termed *authenticity,* is a human quality that greatly enhances communication and the establishment of therapeutic relationships. Individuals who communicate genuineness respond in an honest, unguarded, and spontaneous manner. This means the therapist is willing to appropriately share reactions to what she or he experiences within a group or dyadic relationship. The ability to communicate genuineness as well as respect and warmth through effective use of listening skills, body language, and feeling centered messages enables the COTA to give and receive feedback in a responsible manner.

FEEDBACK

Giving and receiving feedback are important interpersonal skills necessary for the COTA when working with groups.

Giving Feedback

The purpose of giving another person feedback is to describe as specifically and objectively as possible one's perception of another's behavior. It is essential that therapists and assistants know the guidelines for responsible feedback, because they must frequently teach this skill or serve as role models when working with groups. Following are five rules for responsible feedback:[8]

1. Feedback represents an individual perception. It is therefore necessary to own what is said by making "I statements."

Response 1: I'm upset when I see you come late to work as you did this morning.
Response 2: We're all getting frustrated with your frequent tardiness.

Note that the second response is general in that it tries to represent everyone's reactions. This kind of statement is not responsible and can leave the receiver feeling defensive. The message can also be distorted.

2. Be specific rather than general; give examples of the behavior described. It is often difficult to respond accurately to a broad, nonspecific statement.

Response 1: When you came in the room just now you slammed the door. I feel upset when you express your anger that way.
Response 2: You are always going around expressing your hostility by banging things and slamming doors. I'm tired of it.

Phrases such as "you always" or "there you go again" are too general and become blaming statements. It is difficult not to react defensively to feedback worded in this way.

3. Be descriptive rather than evaluative. This means that the behavior should be described rather than labeled. Avoid making judgments about another's behavior, as this is also likely to elicit defensiveness.

Response 1: I heard you speaking to your friend in an abrupt manner. I thought you were not responding to his question seriously and it bothered me.
Response 2: I've always thought you were too flippant, and when I heard you speak to your friend like that, I thought you were a fool.

The words "flippant" and "fool" are labels and imply a judgment in this example.

4. Give feedback as soon as possible after the specific event occurs. This technique is called *immediacy.* Giving feedback immediately avoids problems caused by built-up feelings, which are often expressed out of proportion to the incident if they have been held back for a long time.

Response 1: I feel frustrated and uneasy today because I don't know where you stand. You said nothing during this session.
Response 2: This is the third week you have sat here and not made a response. I'm getting frustrated with you, and I don't trust you at all.

Because giving feedback requires risk taking, group members are often reluctant to state how they feel at the time. The second response is much angrier than the first and, therefore, harder for the receiver to hear. The assistant needs to help group members express feelings as they arise; this helps the group build trust.

5. After giving feedback, check to see that the feedback has been heard accurately. This is a critical part of the feedback process. To do this one might say, "I want to make certain you understand what I've said, could you tell me what you've heard?"

Responding to Feedback

Receiving feedback is one way people learn how they are perceived. It is a valuable tool in making behavioral change. Because giving feedback to another person requires risk taking, it is necessary to avoid misunderstanding. When feedback is given, the receiver should indicate what message was heard. It is not necessary to decide immediately what to do about it, but the person giving the feedback needs to know that the message was heard accurately. The receiver might say, "I don't know how I feel about what you've just said, or what I'll do. I need some time to think this over. This is what I heard you say to me. . ."

Giving and receiving feedback in a group can initially create tense situations because of the risk taking involved, and it is a skill many people do not have. It is a necessary part of learning about oneself and making change. COTAs can help facilitate this process by teaching the skill using the guidelines listed in the preceding discussion. It is useful to provide groups or individuals with specific activities that elicit and reinforce these skills.

UNDERSTANDING HOW GROUPS WORK

A group is three or more people who establish some form of an interdependent relationship with each other. In occupational therapy groups, the activity usually provides the common ground for these relationships. This definition, however, does not include that human quality that is brought to an effective group by the leader and group members. This quality helps provide each individual with a sense of belonging and sharing which in turn facilitates and reinforces learning. The word *community* is also used to describe the desirable outcome of member relationships. Implied in this definition is *union with others*. At their best, groups form true communities in which members are able to give and receive support and insights, which in turn encourage personal growth. To achieve this degree of group cohesion, the COTA must understand how groups work.

Group process refers to how members relate to and communicate with each other and how members accomplish the task. Group process might be described in terms of the way the group solves problems, makes decisions, or manages conflicts that arise. This process perspective of group assumes a holistic view that describes how different group functions fit together to determine the ongoing development of the group. To better understand how groups work, the following characteristics will be considered: group role functions, group norms and developmental group stages.

Group Role Functions

Analysis of individual roles assumed within a group is one of the most familiar ways people use to understand how groups work. Bales[10] suggested the presence of two main areas in all groups based on types of communication that describe the particular behavioral roles: task roles and maintenance or group-centered roles. **Task roles** refer to those behaviors that facilitate task accomplishment. **Group-centered roles** refer to those behaviors that enhance relationships among members. The COTA needs to be versatile in the roles that he or she assumes during group work. Role flexibility refers to an individual's ability to take the action necessary to accomplish a task and, at the same time, maintain cohesiveness in the group. Balancing task and group-centered roles is an important goal for effective group work. In examining a group with a definite leader, one finds that the leader initially assumes multiple roles. As groups mature, leadership is distributed among the members who are able to play the following functional roles: task roles, group-centered roles and **self-centered roles.**

Task Roles. Task roles are concerned with the accomplishment of the group task. Following is a summary of group task roles:

1. *Initiator/Designer:* This role involves starting the group and providing direction. The person who assumes this role plans activities and suggests learning experiences.
2. *Information Seeker/Information Giver:* This role is assumed by asking for or offering facts related to task accomplishment.
3. *Opinion Seeker/Opinion Giver:* The member who assumes this role asks for reactions from others or states his or her own beliefs and values.
4. *Challenger/Confronter:* This role involves asking for clarification about what is communicated. A member who assumes this role also raises issues that are being avoided in the group.
5. *Summarizer:* The member who acts in this role stops the group occasionally to state what is being accomplished. This role serves to keep the group on track.

Group-Centered Roles. Group-centered roles are concerned with keeping the group together by maintaining relationships and satisfying the members' needs. The most important of these roles are the following:

1. *Encourager:* The member who assumes this role is meeting the esteem needs of individuals in the group by offering praise in response to what members do or say.
2. *Gate Keeper:* This role involves facilitating and regulating communication by spreading participation among the members. It involves drawing out quiet members and managing conversation monopolizers.
3. *Tension Reliever:* The member who assumes this role is sensitive to the frustration level of self and others. It is a role involving the use of appropriate jokes, kidding remarks, or suggestions for compromise that dissipate anxiety or hostility in the group.
4. *Harmonizer:* This role is focused on the feelings group members may have. The harmonizer demonstrates caring by naming feelings, thus acknowledging their importance. Harmonizing can help promote positive relationships among group members.

Self-Centered Roles. The roles just described are considered *functional* because they support task accomplishment and the people within the group. Other roles are considered *nonfunctional* because they interfere with group process. These roles are termed self-centered.

Self-centered roles are common in groups and occur because an individual is primarily concerned with satisfying his or her own needs and lacks the adaptive skills needed to function effectively. It is necessary for the COTA to learn to recognize and deal with these roles, which interfere with individual and group progress.[9] Some of the most common self-centered roles include the following:

1. *Withdrawer:* This member does not participate in the activity or discussion at any time. A person may withdraw because of feelings of insecurity, fear of rejection, anger, or lack of interest. A distinction should be made between a withdrawer and an active listener. The listener may be quiet for a time while absorbing information. The active listener does not remain passive for the entire session. To help a member who is withdrawn, the COTA may sit next to him or her, ask open-ended questions, take time at the beginning of the session to establish a greater comfort level among members, or take the individual aside and try to identify the reason for the withdrawal.

2. *Blocker:* This individual may consistently raise objections or insist that nothing can be accomplished. A common phrase used by a blocker is "We've already tried this" or "It won't work." To help a person who is blocking progress in the group, the COTA must let the individual know how this behavior is affecting other members and task accomplishment. Direct feedback is necessary and may be provided within or outside the group depending on the skill level of the group members.

3. *Aggressor/Dominator:* This member tries to take over the group by interrupting when others are speaking, deflating the status of others, insisting on having his or her own way, or telling other members what to do. To help members deal with an aggressor/dominator one may provide and encourage feedback by directing the discussion to identify feelings or call for "time out" to discuss what is happening in the group.

4. *Recognition Seeker:* A recognition seeker tries to get the attention or approval of other members in inappropriate ways. He or she may make distracting jokes or comments, engage in "horse play," boast about accomplishments, or seek pity or sympathy. The COTA may be helpful to a recognition seeker by offering approval of the member's strengths and discouraging inappropriate behaviors.

Group dynamics research is clear regarding the outcome of self-centered behaviors. Initially, considerable leader and group effort is directed to the member who behaves in the manner(s) described previously. If the leader or group perceives that there is a reasonable chance of changing the behavior this effort may go on for some time. If, at some

point, it becomes clear that the inappropriate behavior cannot or will not change, communication toward the individual declines. Group members may begin to exclude the member, and he or she may have to be asked to leave.[10] All members of the group are responsible for dealing with disruptive behavior; however, if the group is unsuccessful, the formal leader must intervene. If issues are not resolved, members may lose confidence and commitment to the group.

Group Norms

Group norms are standards of behavior that can be stated or unspoken. They define what behaviors are expected, accepted and valued by group members. Group norms serve several purposes. They allow groups to function in an organized manner; they define ways in which members respond to conflict, make decisions or solve problems; they help define ways in which members relate to each other and to the leader. They define "reality" for the group. Norms can change as the group evolves and as expectations of member behavior changes. Those attempting to understand how groups work must carefully examine group norms. Sometimes it is useful for the members to identify their own group norms and to determine whether or how these norms should be changed. In this way, implicit norms, or those that influence member behavior but are unspoken, can be made explicit. Some examples of implicit norms might include manner of dress, attitudes toward authority, or group response to change.

The group leader can influence group norms when the group is forming. The norms that the COTA encourages influence the behaviors that will lead to trust, group cohesion and goal attainment. Norms that might be facilitated by the COTA include the following: 1) Each member is valued, 2) expression of feelings is important, 3) making mistakes is expected, and 4) disagreement is desirable. A group that demonstrates these qualities creates a social support system. This quality is important in a therapeutic setting. Social support systems consist of meaningful, often long lasting, interpersonal ties that one may have with a variety of groups of people. A system like this may be found at home, church, or other settings where friendships form. The people in these groups think and behave in accordance with shared values and offer each other support and assistance when needed.

Social support systems are crucial to an individual's well-being. They serve as a buffer to stress in one's life. The effects of exposure to difficult situations can be minimized by social support; conversely, the effects of stress will often be made worse if these systems are not in place.

Group Growth and Development

A third consideration in learning about how groups work is understanding the developmental phases of group life.

Researchers who study groups agree that common, predictable, sequential and developmental stages emerge as the group matures. Group phases are best observed in closed groups in which membership is stable over time. These stages often overlap, and earlier stages may be repeated with the introduction of new tasks or change in membership. For this reason, some theorists describe group evolution as a developmental spiral.[11]

Many theorists have studied and described phases of group development. Bales[12] describes three stages: orientation, or defining the problem/task; evaluation, or how the group feels about the task; and control, or how the task will be completed. Tuckman[13] summarized the literature available on group development and determined four stages:

1. *Forming* deals with orientation issues of coming together.
2. *Storming* represents conflict and power struggles that relate to the issue of control.
3. *Norming* is the stage in which members determine how they will relate to one another.
4. *Performing* represents how the task will be accomplished.

It is important to use a developmental frame of reference when working with groups. This approach can help give meaning to events occurring within the group and can assist the leader in choosing an appropriate intervention.

For the purposes of this discussion, two dimensions of group development will be examined. Mosey's developmental framework lists and describes levels of group interaction.[14] Those groups are parallel group, project group, egocentric cooperative group and mature group. A group at any one of these levels, if together long enough, can also mature. The predictable maturation phases possible for each group are named by the authors as initial dependence, conflict, and interdependence.

Initial dependence describes the first phase of group maturation. Members are concerned about their place within the group. Feelings can be manifested in different ways depending on the developmental level of the group; however, each newly formed group, regardless of developmental level, experiences an initial dependency phase.

The second phase of maturation within each level is characterized by some **conflict** and struggle. The important issue in this phase is control—control of self and control of others or of the environment. This struggle is a necessary and normal part of group development. It should be recognized and encouraged because learning usually requires some degree of labor. It is necessary for groups to experience and resolve this issue before interrelatedness is achieved.

The final phase, **interdependence,** emerges through successful resolution of control issues. This stage is characterized by a high level of affiliation. Members relate at a deeper interpersonal level. It is at this point, when members experience a sense of community with each other, that greater risk taking can occur, thus enhancing the opportunity for greater personal growth. The potential for learning and behavioral change may vary among patients, especially those with cognitive limitations; but even in low level groups, the opportunity for this phase of interdependence is present.

APPLICATION TO DEVELOPMENTAL GROUPS

This section details the application of interpersonal communication skills to various groups. Specific examples are provided to illustrate the developmental progression in terms of level of independence and interpersonal competence of participants. Emphasis is placed on characteristics of the group as well as leader preparation, attitude and approach. Qualities and examples of various group activities are also delineated. It is important for the reader to have an understanding of the following basic concepts:

Leader preparation refers to those activities the group leader completes prior to convening the group to assure that it will run smoothly. Examples include learning as much as possible about the group members and their goals; reviewing instructions and gathering materials for group activities; and arranging the environment to assure maximal interaction.

Leader attitude and approach refers to the affective qualities exhibited by the leader to enhance overall group effectiveness. Examples include showing warmth and genuineness by greeting each member of the group by name; establishing structure, consistency and routine as required by the level of the group; and acting as a role model for effective behaviors.

Activity qualities and examples refers to the selection of group activities that have attributes that will assist group members in achieving their goals. Types of activities include mosaic tile work with limited supplies to encourage sharing; quilt making to encourage cooperation; and planning and implementing a party to encourage consistent interaction over time.

The Parallel Group

The first and most basic group in terms of independence and interpersonal competence of the members is the parallel group. There are usually five to seven members who work side by side but on individual projects. The leader assumes total leadership and responsibility for meeting the group members' needs for security, love and belonging, and esteem while assisting them with their activity.[14] Treatment goals of this group are to develop work skills, experience mastery over a simple task, and develop basic awareness of others. Craft projects are designed to offer opportunities to meet these goals.

At first, the group members exhibit anxiety and total dependence on the leader(s). Members may express uncertainty about why they are together, appear passive, laugh nervously, or seem confused. The activity presented in the parallel group provides a means of focusing a person's attention away from self and onto other objects in the environment. The conflict phase in a parallel group is seen in the patient's struggle for control over the materials, tools, and the process of the task. For mastery to occur, the COTA must make certain that activities provide a manageable challenge. To do this, the occupational therapy assistant serving in this role must have a clear understanding of each person's limitations. Mastery must be strongly reinforced as the patient works.

Interconnectedness or **community** can occur even at this group level if the COTA helps to create the connections among members. One way to achieve connections is to have individuals work on similar kinds of projects.[14] As the assistant helps patients recognize their success, self-esteem begins to build. A reinforced sense of self enables a person to begin to experience others.

Another means of providing individual identity to group members in a parallel group is through *sentient role recognition*. The COTA, serving as a group leader, learns to observe members carefully and to recognize and reinforce personality qualities that may have brought the individual recognition at one time. The leader may notice evidence of nurturing qualities, sociability, or a sense of humor in particular members. Once identified, the personality quality may be described to the patient in positive terms and its use directed. For example, a patient with nurturing qualities may be asked to sit next to a new member and told that his or her warmth and manner would make the new person feel more comfortable. If this quality is recognized by the patient and has given meaning and uniqueness to his or her self-concept, it will be strengthened by providing a special role for that person in the group.

It is ideal to work with an occupational therapist, sharing leadership responsibility and providing members with a parental team. OTRs and COTAs, working together as a complementary team, model appropriate and caring interaction skills.[15]

Leader Preparation, Attitude and Approach. Before the group arrives, it is important for the COTA to attend to the following:

1. Know as much as possible about the individuals beginning the group to provide members with meaningful activities.
2. Preplan and organize the activities and instructions carefully so that energy is used most efficiently during the group itself.

After group members arrive, the leader is responsible for carrying out the following tasks with particular attention to affect and attitude:

1. Greet each member individually and use names frequently (name tags are visual reminders).
2. Project warmth, friendliness, and calmness through facial expression, words, and actions to promote comfort and trust.
3. Provide consistency in approach and routine through assignment of permanent seating and storage space for each individual.
4. Explain the purpose of the group and the activity.
5. Give clear and structured directions.
6. Sit down and spend time with each individual.
7. Stimulate members to perform at their highest level by offering activities that provide a manageable challenge with help from the leader.
8. Offer approval and recognition of members' efforts as well as their completed projects.
9. Establish a nurturing milieu. The leader's ability to demonstrate a warm, caring attitude is important. Meaningful objects present in the environment can also be helpful. Sometimes serving food or beverages can create this feeling of hospitality.
10. If members become disruptive, take them aside for feedback.
11. Encourage interaction among group members by expressing and modeling concern if individuals are absent or ill.
12. Direct positive use of personality strengths to create opportunities for interaction.

Activity Qualities and Examples. The following activity qualities and examples must also be given consideration by the group leader. Activity length depends on the attention span of the members (from 15 minutes to 45 minutes in most cases). Efforts should be made to structure the activities to minimize the need for personal decision making and to assure success. Equally important, activities should be meaningful and have a recognizable end product or provide a sense of identity. With this goal in mind, the COTA should provide projects that do not require heavy concentration, as this allows the opportunity for participants to develop an awareness of others in the group. Most any craft can be adapted to meet the needs of the parallel group. Examples include textile stenciling, mosaics, simple leather work, needlecraft, papercraft, simple weaving, copper tooling, and ceramics.

Project Group

A project group requires higher level social and work skills. The larger group is broken down into subgroups of two and three people and a short-term task requiring some interaction and sharing is provided. Member interaction is secondary to the activity and primary interest is in task completion.[14]

The dependence phase of the group presents itself in much the same way as the parallel group. Members view the group leaders as protectors and authorities who define limits and goals and satisfy needs. The COTA allows this dependence but begins to encourage reliance on others.

The conflict emerges as dependency shifts from the leader to peers in the subgroup. Members may struggle as they attempt to establish trust in other members and cooperate in the shared activity. Members may seek out the leader for help instead of working with their partners. Some individuals may express dissatisfaction with the activity and the ability of peers. Members may appear overwhelmed by the task.

Interrelatedness begins to occur as the patients' sense of community encompasses the small work group. Patients are now able to share completion of the task, but this group level still will rely on the group leader or leaders to create connections or at least strengthen them through questions, comments and summarizing activities. For example, after completion of a subgroup activity, a sharing session may be used to display completed projects. Members could be asked to name those with whom they worked. Each subgroup could be given a symbol or name to help members identify themselves as a member of a team. A short and competitive game between "teams" could be encouraged at the end of each session to reinforce the concept of belonging.[16]

Leader Preparation, Attitude and Approach.   The following approach should be taken:

1. Gently encourage members to rely on others in the group.
2. Answer some questions but redirect questions to other members when possible.
3. Help members examine ideas and problems by asking pertinent questions.
4. Assist individuals in asking for help from partner or group by helping them to phrase questions.
5. Reinforce positive behaviors and relate them to *successful task completion.* (At this level the activity provides a concrete reference.)
6. If members appear overwhelmed, restructure a specific part of the activity and offer repeated contact and support.
7. If individuals in the group display negative behavior, intervene; help identify the problem and suggest possible solutions.
8. If negative behavior is persistent and if it interferes with task completion, remove the person from the group to discuss the problem.

Activity Qualities and Examples.   The projects should be short-term, lasting from 20 minutes to one hour. At first, projects should have easily divided components so that cooperation and contact is not constantly required among members. The following activities can be used at this level:

    planning menus
    "no bake" cookies
    stir and frost cakes
    simple dips for snacks
    pizza
    making holiday or other decorations
    assembling party favors
    decorating bulletin boards
    potting plants or planting a terrarium
    making collages
    making mobiles
    dyeing eggs
    making ice cream
    games, including relays
    team bowling
    cards

Egocentric Cooperative Group

In the egocentric cooperative group, members work together on a long-term activity requiring substantial interaction, cooperation and sharing. Members are primarily self-centered at this level and are able to recognize and verbalize their own needs. Members are beginning to identify the esteem needs of others because of a developing awareness of the effect of their behavior on individuals in the group. The members begin to assume responsibility for selecting, planning and implementing the activity.[14]

The dependence phase will be seen as ambivalence. Members may exhibit heavy reliance on authority at times and then shift to an attitude of disregard. Although this tendency is sometimes difficult for the therapist or assistant to deal with, it may be regarded as a positive behavioral sign, as it signals the members' growing sense of self.

Conflict occurs within individuals and externally among members as the group struggles with the increased complexity of the activity and the interpersonal demands of the expanded group. Competition will be evident. Some individuals may have difficulty following established norms and may arrive late or ask to take frequent breaks. This testing behavior is an attempt to identify boundaries, and the COTA must offer guidance, identify feelings, and stress each individual's value in the group. The group leader must avoid power struggles and yet reinforce cooperation and adherence to the rules, as they pertain to successful task completion and interpersonal relations.

To help this group achieve interrelatedness or community, one must assist members in understanding what occurred as they worked together. Work time may be followed by discussion that focuses on the behavioral strengths that have enhanced group progress and also on the group norms that have been established.[14] A sense of community can be identified when individuals receive recognition from other members.

Leader Preparation, Attitude and Approach. The following steps should be taken:

1. Reinforce autonomy by demonstrating respect and concern for the feelings and rights of each individual through direct verbal statements and acknowledgment of contributions

2. Provide structure as the group begins by clarifying directions or plans for each session.

3. Assist the group in establishing implicit and explicit norms by clarifying behavioral expectations, modeling desired behaviors, and complimenting positive behaviors observed in peers.

4. Assist members in recognizing the progress they are making by asking individuals to describe their own strengths and weaknesses after the activity is over.

5. Manage conflict between members by facilitating understanding of one another's perspectives.

6. Help members discuss whether they feel accepted and appreciated because they are learning to recognize esteem needs in others.

7. Model empathy and concern for the feelings of members.

8. Encourage members to provide support for each other.

9. Provide members with a decision-making process that encourages participation by all. Brainstorming or taking turns can be used as procedures.

10. Provide constructive feedback within the group because members are learning how their behavior effects others.

Activity Qualities and Examples. Activity time may be expanded to 45 to 60 minutes, and the task may take more than one period to complete. Activities should require consistent interaction among all members. The following are some examples:

newspaper layouts
planning and implementing parties
planning picnics or outdoor cooking activities
refinishing furniture
painting murals
planning and presenting skits and videotaping the performance

Cooperative Groups

The cooperative group is most often homogeneous; that is, members share similarities of age, sex, values, and interests.[16] Because of these likenesses and the members' increasing ability to identify and articulate their own needs, they begin to recognize the multiple needs of other people as well. At this level the task becomes secondary and a vehicle for interaction. Interpersonal relationships become the primary focus.

Initially members will depend on the leader(s) for structure, support and guidance as new group roles are learned

and trust is established. Members will need help in identifying and responding to the needs of others as well as expressing positive and negative feelings. Members will also depend on the COTA to help maintain cohesiveness.

Conflict occurs as members attempt to learn the balance of task and group-centered roles. Some members will see conflict or disagreement as bad and will need help in understanding that disagreement is a positive element and a sign of growth.[17] Members must learn to deal with conflict as it occurs and then to give and receive feedback responsibly. At this level, members are capable of learning many new communication skills but may have difficulty as they practice new roles and behaviors.

Affiliation potential is very high as members experience a stronger belief in themselves. Individual strengths are validated by others, and members begin to feel accepted and understood. In this phase, members are able to share leadership and a sense of equality, which strengthens bonds among people. Members are able to identify problems, propose solutions, and have an improved sense of how the group as a whole functions. The group begins to deal openly with conflict and members experience cohesion. Warmth and caring are evident even when members disagree.

Leader Preparation, Attitude and Approach. The following steps should be taken:

1. Assist members in establishing trust with one another by modeling openness and a willingness to be vulnerable. (This means that the COTA should openly admit shortcomings and mistakes to the group.)

2. Ask the group to decide what new skills members would like to learn.

3. Clarify the purpose of the group by emphasizing that although participation in the task is essential, the purpose of working together is to learn group and communication skills.

4. Offer skill building resources to the group and provide structure and information as necessary.

5. Monitor verbal and nonverbal communication to facilitate processing when the activity is over.

6. Encourage risk-taking behavior.

7. Provide group with activities that teach group processes such as problem-solving, decision-making, and conflict management.

8. Assist members in taking on new leadership roles.

9. Provide activity choices that encourage the development of ability to give and receive feedback responsibly.

10. Provide encouragement and suggest activities or assignments for members to practice new skills outside of the group.

11. Teach members how to process their own group.

12. Disengage self from the authority position as affiliation emerges.

Activity Qualities and Examples. A variety of suggestions may be offered to the cooperative group so that members may plan and implement an activity that could last through multiple periods. The process of choosing and planning the project provides an excellent opportunity for learning. It is useful to provide suggestions of shorter term tasks intermittently so that newly learned skills can be applied and gratification is immediate. This process reenergizes the members. The following are some examples of long-term cooperative projects:

banner design and construction

quilt making

plays and talent shows

outdoor gardening

camping trips

Among the short-term cooperative projects that may be used occasionally are activities such as meal preparation, writing a group poem, designing a group symbol, and planning an outing.

Mature Groups

Mature groups function at the highest interpersonal level. They are heterogeneous, meaning that members vary in age, sex, values, interests, and socioeconomic or cultural background. Individuals able to function at this level are comfortable with a variety of people and are flexible in performing group roles. This is a skill level attained by healthy people and may be difficult to achieve in a hospital or rehabilitation setting. A COTA may more likely encounter a group at this level in a community setting, such as adult education groups, senior citizen centers, and neighborhood and special interest groups.

Dependency on occupational therapy personnel or any appointed leader will be minimal even in the initial meetings of this group. There may be an expectation that the COTA will make necessary physical arrangements for the meeting place or initiate discussion.

Members may experience conflict or ambivalence toward acceptance of increased responsibility and leadership roles. Issues related to the use of personal power may arise as members attempt to discover the extent of their influence over each other. Members struggle as they learn to draw on their own assets more consistently and look inward for answers rather than relying on others. Another phase of conflict may occur when the group loses members or comes to closure. This occurrence may cause the members to return to a brief dependency phase as they experience disequilibrium. These tensions usually last only briefly.

Members develop a strong social support system and experience a satisfying sense of community with others. Genuineness is evident in the sincere communication patterns. Openness and honesty become established group norms. Members respect and value each other. Each individual feels a sense of worth and importance in the group.

Individuals feel deeply understood owing to empathetic communication. Risk taking occurs as members challenge each other and gain new personal insights leading to fuller awareness and social integration. Group members at this level not only accept diversity but seek it out and enjoy gaining new perspectives of self through understanding difference.

Leader Preparation, Attitude and Approach. The following approaches are appropriate:

1. Facilitate formation of group and establish a conducive environment for meetings.
2. Relinquish leadership and allow the group to be self-directed.
3. Become an equal member of the group.

Activity Qualities and Examples. The group will determine its own direction and will choose activities related to the purpose of the group. As an activity specialist, the COTA will serve as a resource person to the group. Some possible activity categories would include the following:

community service activities

academic/intellectual activities

creative thinking/problem-solving activities

self-help activities, such as grief encounter groups and parenting

CONCLUSION

Although group phases and characteristics are somewhat predictable, every group develops a unique process and profile. Occupational therapy personnel seldom find a group that fits the developmental levels exactly as they have been described. These descriptions are intended as a guide in assessing individual and group levels and for planning appropriate activities to encourage growth.

A patient group is more likely to become cohesive and contribute to one another's growth if the members have been selected for their ability to function at a particular level. Too much variance in the members' abilities will interfere with individual and group progress.[17]

Many patients will never function at the cooperative or mature levels. It is important, however, to recognize that through the effective use of interpersonal and group skills, the COTA can assist even low-functioning groups to achieve a measure of interrelatedness or community. This sense of belonging will help satisfy basic needs, develop adaptive skills, and contribute to maintenance of physical and emotional health.

Groups that function at the higher developmental levels present more complicated patient issues, behaviors and interactions. Entry-level COTAs need to work with groups

Table 9-1
Roles and Functions of Occupational Therapy Team Members in Group Work

Task	OTR	COTA
Screening	Determine appropriate screening information; initiate referrals; interpret findings; document recommendations	Collect information from patient, family and other resources; report findings to supervisor
Assessment	Determine patient's level of ability in cognitive, psychological, social and sensory areas; determine appropriate group level	Determine dyadic and general work ability through interview, observation and structured tasks

Collaborative Roles

Task	OTR	COTA
Treatment planning	Plan patient's placement in a specific group and examine profile of the total group, including such factors as ages, backgrounds, interests and treatment goals. Collaborate with patients to set individual goals for each group member. Explore task and activity options. Analyze component parts of activity choice. Consider environmental factors to provide a meeting room and seating that satisfies the physical and security needs of the patients. Determine the role, attitude and approach of team members, maximizing the use of personal strengths. Document the overall plan.	
Treatment	Introduce the activity; explain the purpose of the activity and reinforce individual goals. Engage the group; assume leadership roles as determined by the group level. Process the group; enable the members to achieve the maximum amount of learning from the group experience by providing time at the end of the session to discuss problems that occurred as members worked together; discuss progress the group is making, feelings related to problems and progress, and reaffirm or establish new group goals.	
	Summarize and analyze each patient's progress; document response to program; reassess and modify program	Document patient performance as directed; assist in determining need for program change

over an extended time to develop and refine the necessary skills. Forms appropriate for use by a COTA in assisting with the assessment of patient work and social skills, as well as patient exercises, may be found in Appendix C.[14,18]

Entry-level personnel are advised to seek supervision and guidance from advanced clinicians. Table 9-1 provides an outline of the roles and functions of OTR and COTA team members involved in cooperative group work.

SUMMARY

This chapter described the need for COTAs to be interpersonally competent. To become competent, one must gain an awareness of self and others and be able to demonstrate that awareness through the use of verbal and nonverbal communication skills. Active listening, a necessary communication skill used to help establish therapeutic relationships, was described.

A general knowledge of group leadership roles, group norms, and the maturation phases of small groups helps the COTA develop a basic understanding of how groups work. This information can be applied to the use of groups in occupational therapy treatment. Groups used in this context can help the patient develop self-esteem, work skills and interpersonal competence.

Mosey's developmental group levels identify group characteristics related to patient skill levels. Maturation phases of the group at each of the levels were described to help the COTA recognize group and patient issues. This information allows the appropriate choice of an activity as well as structuring it to appropriately challenge group members. A skilled group leader will be able to help a group at any developmental level to work toward some form of community, also referred to as relatedness. The leader must allow for an initial dependency and help members resolve the personal struggles and interpersonal conflicts as they arise within the group. From the successful resolution of these experiences, members are able to risk interaction on a deeper, more personal level. Group cohesion is strengthened, and members then have greater opportunities for insight and personal growth. Interpersonal skills are thus improved.

Related Learning Activities

1. Attend a small party and spend some time observing nonverbal forms of communication. Identify those that enhance communication and those that do not.

2. Invite a small group of people to your home to plan a shower, a birthday party, or other social event. Practice leadership skills and roles appropriate for a cooperative group. Determine the factors present or not present that would allow mature group functioning.

3. Working with a peer, volunteer to conduct two short-term craft groups for children who are mentally retarded. Establish both parallel and project groups using the same activity. Co-lead both groups and seek feedback about your effectiveness.

4. Role play a conflict situation with peers. Identify your strengths and weaknesses in this situation.

5. View a segment of a television "soap opera," involving three or more people, with a small group of peers. Identify and discuss functional and nonfunctional group roles noted.

6. Identify ways that a COTA group leader can effectively interact with a group member who is demonstrating the behavior patterns of a blocker.

References

1. *Basic International Relations: A Course for Small Groups.* Atlanta, Georgia, Human Development Institute, 1969, pp 15-21.
2. Miller F, Nunnally E, Wackman D: *Couple Communication: Talking Together.* Minneapolis, Interpersonal Communication, 1979, pp 144-145.
3. Curran CA: *Counseling Learning.* New York, Grune & Stratton, 1979, pp 20-27.
4. Bolton E: *People Skills.* Englewood Cliffs, New Jersey, Prentice Hall, 1979.
5. Smith-Hannen SS: Affects of nonverbal behavior on judged levels of counselor warmth and empathy. *J Counseling Psychology* 24:87-91, 1977.
6. Cormier WH, Cormier LS: *Interviewing Strategies for Helpers—A Guide to Assessment, Treatment and Evaluation.* Monteray, California, Brooks Cole, 1979, p 44.
7. Hasse RF, Tepper D: Nonverbal components of empathetic communication. *J Counseling Psychology* 19:417-424, 1972.
8. *Basic Interpersonal Relations—Book 2: A Course for Small Groups.* Atlanta, Human Development Institute, 1969.
9. Miles M: *Learning to Work in Groups,* 2nd edition. New York, Teachers College, Columbia University, 1981, pp 241-245.
10. Bales RF: Task roles and social roles in problem solving groups. In TM Newcomb, EL Hartley (Eds): *Readings in Social Psychology,* 3rd edition, New York, Holt, Rineholt & Winston, 1958.
11. Sampson DD, Marthas MS: *Group Process for Health Professions.* New York, John Wiley & Sons, 1977.
12. Bales RF: Adaptive and integrative changes as sources of strain in social systems. In AP Hare, EF Borgatta, RF Bales (Eds): *Small Groups.* New York, Alfred Knopf, 1955.
13. Tuckerman BW: Developmental sequence in small groups. *Psychol Bull* 63:384-399, 1965.
14. Mosey AC: *Activities Therapy.* New York, Raven Press, 1973.
15. Napier R, Gershenfeld M: *Making Groups Work.* Boston, Houghton Mifflin, 1983, pp 108-109.
16. Hopkins HL, Smith HD (Eds): *Willard and Spackman's Occupational Therapy,* 5th edition. Philadelphia, JB Lippincott, 1978, pp 293-295.
17. Loomis ME: *Group Process for Nurses.* St. Louis, CV Mosby, 1981, pp 101-109.
18. Fidler G: The task oriented group as a context for treatment. *Am J Occup Ther* 1:43-48, 1969.

Individualization of Occupational Therapy

Bonnie Brooks, MEd, OTR, FAOTA

INTRODUCTION

One of the foundations of occupational therapy theory is that humans have a need to be active and participate in various occupations. Occupation is essential for basic survival and optimal mental and physical health. **Occupation** is also an integral part of survival and a basic drive of every person. Within this individual frame of reference, a person's activities and occupations enable him or her to function as a central part of a larger whole. It is the difference between existing and actively participating. Participation and optimal functioning within a person's environment provide an individual with feelings of purpose and self-esteem throughout his or her life span.

What does the word occupation mean? To those in occupational therapy, it means engaging in purposeful activity. Occupations are effective in preventing or reducing disability and in promoting independence through the acquisition of skills, as the following examples illustrate:

1. The occupation of a preschool child with a disability is learning the motor skills necessary to enter school.
2. The primary occupation for a young adult may be planning for a career or vocation.
3. Occupation for others may be providing for financial security through employment, which may require a variety of activities.
4. Occupation for an individual with serious cardiac problems may include learning to conserve energy while doing daily activities.
5. An occupation for the elderly may be prolonging participation in rewarding activities and maintaining personal independence.

ESSENTIAL VOCABULARY

Occupation

Individualized

Self-image

Phobia

Climate

Community

Economic status

Customs

Traditions

Superstitions

Disruptions

Prevention

KEY CONCEPTS

Uniqueness of the individual

Internal environment

External environment

Sociocultural considerations

Impact of change

Disuse syndromes

Misuse syndromes

An occupation may require a variety of activities and skills. For example, the occupation of self-care includes the activities of bathing, shaving, dressing, and feeding, each of which requires varying degrees of skill in gross and fine motor coordination and judgment.

Occupational therapy is the art and science of directing an individual's participation in selected tasks to restore, reinforce, and enhance performance. Occupational therapy facilitates learning of skills and functions essential for adaptation and productivity, for diminishing or correcting pathology, and for promoting and maintaining health. The word occupation in the professional title refers to goal-directed use of time, energy, interest and attention. Occupational therapy's fundamental concern is developing and maintaining the capacity to perform, with satisfaction to self and others, the tasks and roles essential to productive living and mastering self and the environment throughout the life span.[1]

Three main types of occupation are necessary for the achievement of optimal performance and quality of life: activities of daily living, work and leisure. These areas are discussed in greater depth in Chapter 7. Acquiring and maintaining skills in these areas enable a person to interact successfully with the environment. Activities and skills also enable a person to engage in a variety of occupations that result in the establishment of the individual's lifestyle.

Occupational therapy provides service to those individuals whose abilities to cope with tasks of living are threatened or impaired by developmental deficits, the aging process, physical injury or illness, or psychological and social disability.[2]

Intervention programs in occupational therapy are designed to enable the patient to become adequate or proficient in basic life skills, work, and leisure, and thereby competent to resume his or her place in life and interact with the environment effectively. With these goals in mind, this chapter focuses on case studies and examples of how occupational therapy intervention can be **individualized** in relation to the environment, society, change and prevention.

CASE STUDIES IN INDIVIDUALITY

The profession of occupational therapy recognizes that the level of optimal function to which a patient may aspire is highly individual and determined by all of the circumstances of the individual's life.[3] No two patients are alike, even if they are the same age and have identical problems or disabilities. Intervention programs should be individualized and focus on the **uniqueness** of the individual. To understand the multitude of factors that create an individual lifestyle, a description of John and Darlene follows. They will be referred to later in this chapter to illustrate various content areas.

Case Study 10-1

John. John is a 24-year-old obese man. He smoked two packs of cigarettes a day for four years and recently quit. He appears in good health.

Family Information

John is the oldest of three children. His sisters, aged 19 and 21, are away at college. His mother is 53 years old and in good health. His father is 57 years old and has high blood pressure. Three years ago the father experienced two severe heart attacks and was hospitalized both times. The following year the father had three minor attacks. He had generalized weakness and has been very depressed; however, he exhibited significant improvement recently.

Vocational Information

John graduated from college two years ago. He returned home to manage the farm because of his father's illness. The crop farm is located 25 miles outside a rural town in southern Minnesota. Employment opportunities were very limited for John in that particular region of the state, and he had just accepted a job to work as an accountant in Duluth. He plans to move there in four months.

Leisure and Socialization

During the winter, John watches television a great deal and plays cards. Recently, he decided to take half-hour walks twice a day to lose weight. In the summer, John plays softball on a local team, goes swimming, and meets socially with friends.

Case Study 10-2

Darlene. Darlene is a 35-year-old woman in good health. She is slightly underweight because of constant dieting.

Family Information

Darlene is an only child. She was married for five years, lived in California, and divorced two years ago. She had no children. Her mother is 62 years old and her father is 65 years old and retired. They are healthy and travel extensively, spending most of their time in Florida. Darlene lives in her parent's home located in a wealthy suburb of New York City.

Vocational Information

Darlene worked for a short time prior to her marriage at age 27. Before that time she took classes at a local college periodically and worked in her father's office part-time. Darlene completed a computer course three years ago and now works as a full-time programmer for a moderate salary. She pays no expenses while living in her parents' home; however, she does buy groceries and presents for her parents periodically. Her parents recently decided to sell their home and move to a condominium in Florida.

Leisure Information

Darlene is very active. She goes out every evening and frequently takes weekend trips. She is very fashion-conscious, often attending fashion shows, and identifies shopping as a major interest. After shopping sprees, she and her friends frequently go to art galleries or the theater. Darlene belongs to a health spa, racquet ball club and country club. She enjoys golf and swimming.

John and Darlene have been introduced to provide a context to examine some of the factors that have impact on the development of their present lifestyles. These include the effect of the environment, sociocultural aspects, local customs and economic implications. All of these factors must be considered to gain an understanding of an individual's current lifestyle, who they are, what roles they have, what they want and expect, and what they need.

ENVIRONMENT

A person's environment is comprised of all of the factors that provide input to the individual. The environment includes all conditions that influence and modify a person's lifestyle and activity level. Environmental considerations vary significantly in complexity. They can be as simple as climate, geographic location, or economic status or as complex as considering the sociocultural aspects of traditions, local customs, superstitions, values, beliefs and habits.

Every individual has two environments that constantly provide input: internal and external. These environments are so closely integrated in an individual's life that it is often difficult to consider them separately. Both internal and external environments must be considered in designing treatment intervention that will allow a person to function at maximum capacity. This coordinated approach is the essence of total patient treatment in occupational therapy.

Internal Environment

One method of separating the internal and external environments is by considering the physiologic feedback provided by the various body systems. This feedback is the body's way of informing a person of his or her ability to respond to the daily requirements of the external environment.

Some common examples of this feedback occur when an individual has not had enough sleep the night before or has eaten something that was not agreeable. Often, there is a generalized feeling of unresponsiveness of the body. This commonly happens before the development of a cold or flu. It can be a temporary condition (such as muscle cramps, indigestion, or premenstrual syndrome), or it can be a warning signal of early symptoms of disease such as diabetes or ulcers.

Moods and emotional states can be considered parts of an internal environment that influence the way a person responds to the external environment. Depressed persons frequently respond more slowly to their environment and may decrease social activities. Some may further restrict the environment by remaining at home.

A person's mood is often the direct result of something that has occurred in the external environment. Grief is an internal reaction that can result from the loss of a loved one through death, divorce, or the termination of a relationship. Euphoria and states of elation and happiness can result from a promotion, salary increase, falling in love, or inheriting money. These moods affect an individual's ability level and daily occupations.

Moods and emotional states can also be totally unrelated to the external environment. Some people complain of loneliness. These feelings can persist even when a person is with a group of people he or she knows. Such individuals complain of shallowness in relationships and interactions, and can feel lonely even in a crowd.

Self-image is another example of previous feedback from the external environment that creates an *internal set* or environment. These internal environments can exist long after the external environment has changed. One can encounter a person who has lost a significant amount of weight and yet still feels "fat" and dresses to camouflage weight that no longer exists. Conversely, others may gain weight and dress as they did when they were thin. Persons who have been demoted from high authority positions or have changed jobs to assume lesser positions may still present themselves as authority figures and dress accordingly. They maintain the same nonverbal body language that they had in their previous status. Periodically one encounters an individual who graduated from college 30 years ago and still wears a Phi Beta Kappa key in an effort to maintain a self-image that was appropriately achieved three decades before.

Phobias are yet another example of adverse internal environments. They are defined as abnormal fears or dreads and are as illustrated in the following case:

Case Study 10-3

Mrs. Anderson. Mrs. Anderson is 45 years old, married, and the mother of two children, aged 13 and 17. Her husband's job as an industrial consultant requires periodic travel for up to four consecutive weeks at a time. He is generally at home one week at a time between trips.

Approximately eight years ago, Mrs. A began to decline social invitations from friends when her husband was at home. She would excuse herself for some minor or nonexistent complaint or say that their time together was so limited that they needed to be alone as a family. Eventually, she reached the stage where she encouraged her husband to attend events without her because of headaches.

Mrs. A no longer liked driving the car. She complained about heavy traffic, crowded grocery stores and rude clerks in department stores. She located a small grocery store that would deliver orders, and she began buying mail-order clothing. Cosmetics and other items were ordered through door-to-door distributors. Her family became concerned and began encouraging her to go for rides or have an occasional dinner out. Mrs. A was very uncomfortable and obviously in a state of anxiety. Finally she simply refused to leave her home.

Mrs. A was exhibiting symptoms of *agoraphobia,* a Greek term meaning fear of the marketplace which, in current usage, refers to a fear of open or public places. In all probability, her agoraphobia had occurred as a result of previous environmental feedback; however, once the condition developed, it then became an internal environment affecting her occupation and effectiveness as a member of her family unit.

External Environment

The external environment is comprised of a number of factors, including climate, community and economic status. One of the most obvious external environmental factors is the **climate.** Some climates are warm or cold for most of the year and offer extremes in temperatures and weather hazards during several months. Many regions experience four seasons. In general, spring and fall are periods of transition. Whereas winter and summer exhibit extremes in weather such as floods, hurricanes, tornadoes, or blizzards. Individual responses to climates and weather conditions vary. Many people dislike the winter months and restrict their activities. It is very common for some people to gain weight during these months and then lose the added pounds when the weather permits them to resume their outdoor activities.

The Effects of Climate on John and Darlene. The impact of winter weather is greater for John than for Darlene. Darlene's work and leisure activities occur within a much smaller geographic area than those of John. Her suburban environment offers a variety of transportation options. The winter months impose more restrictions on John. This period of snow storms and icy conditions usually limits his transportation, which in turn restricts his opportunities for socialization. During severe weather, John restricts his leisure activities to watching television and playing cards, and he frequently gains weight during this period.

Summer also affects John more than Darlene. Although Darlene experiences some changes, these have minimal impact on her activity level. John's farm work requires heavy labor as soon as the soil is workable, beginning with the first sign of spring and continuing well into the fall. He completely changes his leisure, recreation, and social activities, which include playing on a softball team, swimming and meeting with friends.

Case Study 10-4

Special Splint Consideration. A patient living in Georgia was required to wear a basic cock-up splint. During his monthly visits to the clinic, his splint always needed significant adjustments. It was discovered that he would frequently leave the splint on the back shelf of the car. The internal temperature of the closed car in a hot climate was excessive. The splint had been fabricated from a low temperature material, which tended to change shape in the high heat. A new splint was made from a heavier material that would withstand high temperatures, thus solving the problem.

Severe cold can also affect the selection of splinting materials. Some are made of plastic, which can become brittle and shatter on impact in extreme cold. Metal braces and splints can also be very uncomfortable in extreme temperatures. Special attention should be given to lining the splint to protect the skin that comes into contact with the device.

Community

Another important environmental consideration is the type of **community** in which the person lives. There are three basic types of communities: rural, urban and suburban. Each type has different characteristics that can affect an individual's occupations, activities and lifestyle.

Rural communities have small populations distributed over large geographic areas with a somewhat denser population near the town center. Resources can vary greatly in rural communities. Public transportation is often extremely limited or nonexistent. Social activities often revolve around community groups (such as Rotary and Lions Clubs) and socials and dinners sponsored by churches and schools.

Urban communities contrast sharply with rural areas. They are densely populated in small geographic areas. There is usually a variety of public transportation such as buses, taxis and subways, and a wide range of resources are available. Material goods (such as groceries, clothing and furniture) and services (such as car repair and medical care) must be selected from a wide variety of options. Urban areas may still offer activities designed by community members and groups; however, these represent a much smaller component of the overall offerings. There is usually a wide variety of leisure activities to choose from, including theater, museums, dance, galleries, concerts and sporting events. Crowding affords individuals anonymity and privacy in contrast to the rural communities where individuals seem to know each other and come into contact with one another more frequently.

Suburban communities are often a blend of their rural and urban counterparts. They are less densely populated than cities and have larger lots for homes, parks and some recreational activities. Public transportation is somewhat limited but is generally available. Necessary services are available; however, there are fewer options from which to choose than there are in cities. Fewer choices exist for leisure activities compared with those in the core city, and contact with neighbors and other community members is variable.

The Effects of Community on John and Darlene. John is well known in his small farming community. His neighbors know that he completed college and returned home to help his father. John knows the grocer, auto mechanic, drug store clerk, dentist and physician personally.

Darlene shops and receives necessary services in a variety of places and therefore does not know many of these people personally. She knows the names of two women who work in her favorite boutiques. Personalized service and recognition can be status symbols if deliberately developed.

Economic Environment

The economic environment of the community and the **economic status** of individuals must also be considered. Values and standards vary greatly and affect occupational therapy treatment, as shown in the three case examples that follow.

Case Study 10-5

Susan. Susan was 16 years old when she was diagnosed as having juvenile arthritis, which was affecting her right hand. The rheumatologist referred her to occupational therapy to have a splint fabricated, which would block metacarpophalangeal (MCP) flexion of all four fingers. A variety of splints were presented to the patient and her family. All were visually unacceptable. The patient agreed to wear the "ugly" splint when she was at home, but adamantly refused to wear it in public. Her family supported her in this decision, even though they understood the medical benefits that could be achieved by a regular wearing schedule. The parents requested that the occupational therapist work in collaboration with their local jeweler to design something more attractive.

Working with the jeweler, the OTR designed rings for each finger, which were connected by chains to a large medallion on the back of the hand. The medallion was then connected by chains to a snug, wide bracelet. The design proved to be highly workable, although not ideal medically. The final product was made of 14-carat gold and studded with rubies and pearls. The patient wore it constantly and several of her friends requested similar jewelry. It seemed that the "splint" had become a status symbol in her social group.

Case Study 10-6

Mrs. K. A diagnosis of rheumatoid arthritis had far reaching implications for Mrs. K, a 36-year-old woman employed as a bank clerk in a small community. Weight bearing had become very painful, and a total hip replacement and bilateral knee surgery had been recommended.

Several months before the diagnosis was made, persistent pain and stiffness had forced Mrs. K to give up her job in the bank, even though her salary was important to maintain the family's modest standard of living. She had allowed her health insurance coverage to lapse and was in the process of applying for coverage under her husband's policy when her condition was diagnosed. As a result, she was denied coverage.

Mrs. K was referred to occupational therapy for homemaking training and self-care activities before surgery. The evaluation revealed the need for a variety of adaptive equipment, including a wheelchair and a ramp to access her home. She also needed a commode, as the only bathroom was upstairs. A utility cart would be needed for basic kitchen activities.

When these recommendations were presented, Mrs. K began to cry. She explained that the family had already remortgaged their home to pay for her medical bills and the planned surgery. There was no money for the necessary equipment. She felt that in less than a year she had gone from being a contributing member of society to becoming a burden on her family. She was worried about the effects of financial stress on her husband and her inability to care for their two small children. The mere mention of possible sources of community assistance brought a fresh flood of tears.

The COTA working with Mrs. K had grown up in a small community and knew how important it was for people to maintain their pride and sense of self-worth. She also knew that friends and neighbors would welcome the opportunity to help Mrs. K and others like her who might need assistance. She suggested to the occupational therapist that they contact the local Kiwanis and Lions Clubs to propose the development of a community adaptive equipment bank. She also recommended that Mrs. K be asked to serve as coordinator of the equipment bank, receiving requests from physicians and family members, arranging for purchase and delivery of equipment, and maintaining records and inventory. The occupational therapist approved the plan, which was put into action within two weeks. Mrs. K was pleased to have an opportunity to use her office and managerial skills and to have the use of the equipment until she recovered from her surgery.

Case Study 10-7

Mr. J. Mr. J had recently experienced a stroke with resultant right side hemiparesis and severe disarthria. He also exhibited overt personality and behavioral changes and was very hostile. Mr. J was a very wealthy, prominent public figure. Once he had been medically stabilized, he refused to stay in a hospital room and instead rented a penthouse suite in a hotel across the street from the hospital.

An occupational therapist received a referral to evaluate the patient's functional level and to begin remediation treatment including self-care activities. When seen for the initial evaluation, a male companion was feeding Mr. J a sandwich. Although eating a sandwich is a one-handed activity, he preferred to be fed.

The evaluation began with a discussion of Mr. J's functional level with his companion. The companion explained that he had signed a two-year contract to see to all of Mr. J's basic needs. While providing neuromuscular and other remediation treatments, occupational therapy intervention also included treating the patient indirectly by advising and training the companion in transfer techniques, dressing techniques, and identifying one-handed activities. The occupational therapy assistant was primarily responsible for carrying out this aspect of the program.

SOCIOCULTURAL CONSIDERATIONS

Many communities contain diverse ethnic groups. People from the same cultural background have common traditions, interests, beliefs and behavior patterns that give them a common identity. Frequently these individuals tend to cluster in geographic areas to preserve their customs, values, traditions, and (at times) their native language. The ethnic neighborhood can be viewed as a society within a society. These clusters or environs provide individuals with opportunities for perpetuation of their culture and lifestyles.

Some cultures are *matriarchal,* or female controlled, whereas others are *patriarchal,* or male controlled. The roles and performance expectations of the oldest, middle or youngest child can also vary among cultural groups. In some societies, the number of male children may determine the financial security of the parents in later life.

Customs

A **custom** is a pattern of behavior or a practice that is common to many members of a particular class or ethnic group. Although rules are unwritten, the practice is repeated and handed down from generation to generation. Cultural implications can have a significant impact on designing occupational therapy intervention techniques that enable a person to function at his or her maximum in the specific environment, as shown in the following case study:

Case Study 10-8

Mrs. F. Mrs. F was a 61-year-old Italian woman who had recently had a stroke. Her primary residual deficit was mild, right-sided hemiparesis. Mrs. F was also slightly disarthric and difficult to understand, as her native language was Italian.

When she returned home from the hospital, Mrs. F was depressed, unmotivated, and not interested in beginning any

activities of daily living. When cooking activities were suggested, she became very upset and burst into tears. This behavior was discussed with one of her sons, and it was discovered that the entire family routinely gathered at the parents' home for Sunday dinner. Mrs. F greatly enjoyed this custom. She made all of her own pasta and canned home-grown tomatoes for sauce. She did not want her daughters-in-law to bring food or assist too much in meal preparation. Convenience foods and ready-made pastas had never been used, and the suggestion was totally unacceptable to the family.

In occupational therapy at the rehabilitation center, Mrs. F was encouraged to regain her cooking skills, which required some minor adaptations. Her family bought her an electric pasta machine since she was no longer able to knead and roll her own pasta. Her heavy cooking pots were replaced with new, lightweight styles.

Once Mrs. F regained her cooking skills and resumed a role that was very important to her, she became receptive to relearning other aspects of daily living skills.

Traditions

Traditions are inherited patterns of thought or action that can be handed down through generations or can be developed in singular family units; they also may be perpetuated through subsequent generations. Many families develop their own special traditions during holidays, birthdays, vacations, and other occasions.

Customs and traditions may also occur on a daily basis and can be highly individualized. Their origin may be unknown and not related to any particular sociocultural custom or event, as illustrated by the following case:

Case Study 10-9

Mr. W. Mr. W, who is 50 years of age, was admitted to the Veterans Hospital with a diagnosis of multiple sclerosis. He was confined to a wheelchair and exhibited severe weakness of the upper extremities. His wife was 45 years old and they had six children all living at home who ranged in age from four to 16 years.

In occupational therapy, Mr. W participated in dressing activities, bathing and transfer techniques and was actively experimenting with a variety of adaptive equipment that would assist him in returning to his previous employment. Although he was a very quiet, nonverbal person, he seemed highly motivated and always carried through on any requests made as a part of his treatment.

When the occupational therapy assistant suggested that he begin shaving techniques, Mr. W said that it simply wasn't necessary and told the assistant not to worry about it. The COTA reminded him of the accomplishments he was making in independent living skills and pointed out that this was one more activity in which he could achieve independence. He acquiesced and went along with the program to please the COTA. One day, when Mr. W had successfully shaved himself, the COTA asked him if he didn't feel better shaving independently. Mr. W replied that "it felt okay"; however, in his family it was a tradition for the wives to shave their husbands. Mr. and Mrs. W felt that this daily activity reaffirmed their commitment to each other and was a daily declaration of their devotion.

Superstitions

Superstitions can be difficult to identify and define. They can be customs, traditions, and beliefs of a very small population that may be geographically localized. They can also be highly individualized and border on mental or emotional pathologic states. Webster defines them as "beliefs and practices resulting from ignorance and fear of the unknown."[4] They are also viewed as a statement of trust in magic. Superstitions are further defined as irrational attitudes of the mind toward supernatural forces.

It can be very difficult for occupational therapy personnel to deal with superstitions. It may be easy for a therapist or an assistant to point out how "ridiculous" superstitions are and to present facts that disprove such "ignorant" notions. The personal environment, standards, values, traditions and beliefs of the COTA and OTR can, at times, be in direct conflict with those of the patient. Occupational therapy personnel must realize that the ultimate goal of occupational therapy is to return the individual to his or her lifestyle with all of its implications. The following case illustrates this point.

Case Study 10-10

Mrs. C. Mrs. C is an 82-year-old woman who was admitted to the hospital with severe circulatory disturbances in her left leg. This condition resulted in surgical amputation of the lower left extremity.

The patient was referred to occupational therapy for generalized strengthening activities, cognitive stimulation, and reality reorientation. Although she frequently did not know where she was, past memory appeared to be intact. Mrs. C presented herself as a very pleasant person with a warm, personable manner.

During one of her initial treatment sessions it was noted that she wore a small bag of coins tied tightly around her right thigh with several strips of gauze. When the occupational therapist questioned her about this, she explained that the bag of coins "kept evil spirits away" and made a person happy. She elaborated further saying that she had always worn the bag on her left leg, but since the doctors had to remove that leg, she would now have to tie it to the right one. This situation had not been noted during prior medical examinations, as Mrs. C always removed the bag when she disrobed.

Occupational therapy intervention consisted of introducing a six-inch wide cohesive, light woven, elastic bandage, applied lightly on the thigh, with the small bag of coins attached with a safety pin. This solution was accepta-

ble to Mrs. C. She also reported that all of the other family members also observed this practice. Therefore all 12 family members were also instructed in this new method.

Values, Standards and Attitudes

Values, standards and attitudes are other aspects of an individual that develop through environmental transaction and influence lifestyle. These facets of a person's life usually result from feedback received from other people within one's work and leisure environments, as well as from the individual's sociocultural and economic status and self-image. They are very personal and become an important part of a person's internal environment. The presence of disease or injury can be very disruptive and require reassessment of all aspects of an individual's life and lifestyle, requiring some temporary or permanent adaptations. It is important for occupational therapy personnel to use intervention techniques that can be adapted to minimize the stresses that occur when the patient's values, standards, and attitudes are in jeopardy or must be compromised to some extent. Two case examples are presented to elaborate on these points.

Case Study 10-11

Mr. H. Mr. H, a 50-year-old farmer living in a rural community in Indiana, had sustained a nerve injury to his left wrist. When his wrist was maintained in 50° hyperextension, he could perform most prehension patterns and his hand was functional.

All standard splints were unacceptable to Mr. H, who stated that he would "feel like a sissy" and wouldn't wear any of them in front of his friends. The solution was to fabricate a splint from a tablespoon, which was bent and angled to the correct medical alignment. The spoon was then riveted to a wide leather wrist band. Mr. H wore the splint daily and enjoyed joking with his friends that he was "always looking for a meal." This adaptation was the change that convinced the patient to wear the appliance.

Case Study 10-12

Mrs. B. Mrs. B was 60 years old when she had a stroke, which resulted in left hemiparesis. She had slight subluxation of the left shoulder. Shoulder subluxations are very common, as the pull of gravity on the paralyzed or weakened limb frequently causes the ligaments surrounding a joint to stretch and the head of the humerus to pull out of the socket. Hemiplegic arm slings are almost always recommended to prevent this condition. These slings are very noticeable and not very attractive.

The patient was a very well-dressed, fashion-conscious woman of financial means. She frequently met with friends for luncheons and other social gatherings at her country club. Wearing the sling was an embarrassment for her. The solution involved adapting a leather shoulder bag to wear on these occasions. The bag was strong and large enough to support her forearm, and the strap was adjusted to a length that would support the humeral head in the shoulder joint. A wooden handle was attached to the bag, which maintained Mrs. B's wrist in hyperextension and held her thumb in opposition.

Consideration of these individual values and self-images enabled the occupational therapist to use everyday objects to fabricate necessary medical appliances in a form that was acceptable to both of the patients and compatible with their lifestyles.

Each occupational therapist and assistant has values, standards and attitudes that may be in direct conflict with those of the patient, thus making it difficult to work with some individuals as noted in the example that follows.

Case Study 10-13

Mr. S. An occupational therapist was working one-half day per week in a very small, rural general hospital. When she reported for work she found four treatment requests for one patient, Mr. S. Two were referrals from physicians requesting immediate initiation of feeding and toileting activities. There were also memoranda from the Director of Nursing and the Hospital Administrator requesting the same services. Mr. S had been admitted for prostate surgery. He refused to use the toilet in his room, preferring instead a small, rectangular, plastic-lined wastepaper basket.

The patient was seen for an initial evaluation during the lunch hour. The meal consisted of cube steak with gravy, mashed potatoes, carrots, and a dish of sherbet. Mr. S used no utensils; he ate with his fingers and licked up some foods. This behavior, together with his lip-smacking and belching noises, was in total violation of the therapist's standards and values, as well as those of two female aides who cleaned up the food scatterings on the bed.

Limited information was available in Mr. S's medical record. In addition to the problems discussed previously, nursing notes indicated that his behavior was that of a very hostile and angry person. It was difficult to determine whether Mr. S was experiencing mental changes that required psychiatric intervention, whether his behavior was a reflected form of his personal lifestyle, or whether a combination of both was involved. Intake records revealed that Mr. S refused to state his age or financial status.

Since there was no social worker available, the occupational therapist was requested to gather additional information from neighbors and the community. Mr. S was described by his neighbors as an antisocial recluse. He had lived for at least 40 years in a large old toolshed on the back acres of a farm, which was a long distance from town. There had been windows in the building; however, he had covered them with roofing material many years ago. His home had

no electricity or running water. He was always piling up wood and rubbish, so the neighbors felt certain that he had some sort of stove for cooking and heating.

The therapist visited a small grocery store nearby to see if Mr. S bought food there. It was learned that he had indeed shopped there as long as the elderly owners could remember. Mr. S would slip a grocery list under the door and specify when he would pick up the items. He always paid in cash and requested that no females be present when he came to the store. He would talk with the male owner and periodically try new products that he recommended. If the owner's wife or other females were present, Mr. S would slip in the back entrance, grab his groceries, pay, and leave hurriedly. With this information, the therapist made the following changes when she returned to the hospital:

1. A male orderly was assigned to the patient.
2. Mr. S was informed that he could eat in any manner he chose; however, he would have to change his own linen. (He began to cover himself with a large towel when eating and folded it neatly when finished).
3. A portable commode was placed in his room. (He liked it and stated that he had disliked the coldness of the toilet seat and the loud rushing of water. He also disliked two females taking him to the bathroom).

If Mr. S had recently developed this lifestyle, intervention techniques may have been different. When a therapist or an assistant encounters a lifestyle that has existed for over 40 years, it requires different consideration. At times it can be difficult to understand how persons living in the same general environment respond in such highly individualized manners.

CHANGE AND ITS IMPACT

Changes in lifestyles, roles and activity levels occur throughout the life cycle. Normal changes are expected at various ages. For example, a child is expected to walk and talk at a certain age, and a young adult is expected to begin a career when he or she has completed the necessary education.

Changes can be self-imposed or superimposed on an individual. Self-imposed and superimposed changes and their resulting influence on the individual can occur over a prolonged period or they can be very sudden. The length of time and timing of such change have an impact to varying degrees on lifestyles, roles, self-image and activity levels.

Retirement, whether self-imposed or superimposed, is a change that affects most aspects of a person's life. Many professionals are becoming involved in preretirement planning. These programs are designed to help people consider the various aspects of their life and plan ahead. The emphasis is on all important areas, not just financial planning.

Stress

The potential for stress is inherent with any change. Individuals react very differently to what appears to be the same stress situation. People who have explored different environments and adapted to change may have some sense of mastery over their environment. They can recall and apply previous actions and thoughts that either worked successfully or were ineffective. This provides them with more resources and information to plan an action and respond appropriately.

John and Darlene: Follow-up. Both John and Darlene will be experiencing significant changes in their environment. These changes will effect their activities, roles and lifestyles. John's decision to relocate in Duluth is a self-imposed change. He has given a lot of thought to this decision to move and start a new career. This cognitive planning has prepared him for the changes in his environment, new roles, and a markedly different lifestyle from the one he has established on the farm.

Darlene's future change has been superimposed on her by her parent's decision to move. She must now identify and evaluate alternatives and make a decision. She could locate a place of her own or move to Florida with her parents. These two alternatives offer very different considerations in terms of finances, employment, social status, and activities, as well as the total physical environment.

As these changes occur, they will create stress for both John and Darlene. Individuals who have made significant changes in the past often find that they can draw on these past events in terms of future decision making and adjustment.

Severe Disruptions

Disruptions are sudden changes in a person's environment that require immediate attention and response. They are usually superimposed on an individual. Disruptions can be as simple and temporary as a common cold or loss of a job, or as complex and permanent as a stroke or death of a loved one. Most disruptions are high stress situations for the individual directly affected, and they can also directly affect and cause stress for other persons in the individual's environment.

Case Study 10-14

Michael. Michael, a mentally retarded young man functioning at about a five-year-old level, had a severe disruption when his parents were in an automobile accident. Due to multiple injuries they both sustained and the length of time needed for rehabilitation, it was necessary to move Michael from his home to an institution. Michael's reaction to this abrupt change was evidenced by withdrawal and frequent tantrums. The OTR at the facility visited the parents in the hospital to gain information that might assist in helping Michael to adjust to his new environment. She learned that Michael had particular food preferences and favorite television programs and enjoyed hearing short bedtime stories. Other details of his daily routine were discussed. The therapist then made the appropriate changes in Michael's daily regimen, and Michael discontinued his tantrums and began relating to others again.

Case Study 10-15

John. John was recently discharged from the hospital after his involvement in a tractor accident. The tractor had overturned and his left arm was almost completely severed. John also experienced a head injury and was comatose for five days.

John was seen in occupational therapy for reality orientation, daily living skills, and instruction in stump care. When first seen, he was confused, his speech was slightly impaired, and his left arm had been surgically amputated just above the elbow. John is right-handed.

John was pleasant, highly motivated, and exhibited a good sense of humor. Several of his friends came for regular visits, as did his family. He would show them some of his one-handed activities and talk about what he would do when he got his new prosthesis.

He exhibited much improvement during his five-week hospitalization. John was no longer confused and his speech was almost normal. His stump had healed well, and a prosthesis had been ordered. He became independent in most self-care activities and used minimal adaptive equipment. John and his mother were instructed in stump massage and wrapping techniques. At the time of discharge John needed minimal assistance with these activities.

John's accident had a profound effect on his parents. His father had difficulty accepting the appearance of his son's missing arm and seemed to blame himself for the accident. He became very depressed and cried about his son being disabled for life. John's mother appeared exhausted from the daily drives to the hospital. She seemed to feel burdened with the needs of her son and her husband, who both required so much help and attention.

As John developed his ability to perform self-care activities, his parents were encouraged to attend occupational therapy sessions. They soon began to realize that he would be independent again. John's mother observed some of her son's struggles to learn to perform various self-care activities. As a result, she decreased the amount of assistance she had been providing, offering verbal encouragement and praise instead. After watching John engage in various activities, his father seemed more accepting of his son's disability. He became intrigued with adaptive equipment and spent hours with John discussing devices he could invent. His depression began to subside.

The family minister visited John and also attended a treatment session. He said that the neighbors were working the farm while John's parents were at the hospital. The occupational therapist explained that John would need to be seen as an out-patient three times a week for an extended time. She indicated that this was very difficult and exhausting for the parents, as the hospital was 60 miles from their farm. The minister said that other church members would be happy to provide transportation twice a week so that John's parents could return to their work at home.

Case Study 10-16

Darlene. Darlene had been admitted to a hospital several months ago. She had been cooking when grease caught fire and exploded. She had first-degree burns on the lower left side of her face and neck, the dorsum of her left hand, and distal third of her left forearm. There were possible second-degree burns on the anterior portion of the left glenohumeral area and upper arm.

The patient received occupational and physical therapy on an out-patient basis for exercises and activities to maintain range of motion at the shoulder. The first-degree burns healed very quickly, and the skin was only slightly pink, which was barely noticeable. The second-degree burn areas were healing and would not require skin grafting.

When seen in occupational therapy, Darlene was wearing a scarf draped across the lower third of her face and a long-sleeved blouse. She adamantly refused to remove the scarf due to her disfigurement. She also refused to believe that there were no visible markings on her face and neck. This situation was discussed with her parents who indicated that Darlene was seeing a counselor.

The accident had occurred about six weeks after Darlene had moved to Florida. She was just beginning to explore the area and establish new relationships. Since her release from the hospital, she had refused to go anywhere and stayed in her room when her parents entertained guests. Darlene's parents felt guilty whenever they went out and left her alone. It was also awkward for them to have friends at their home.

The occupational therapist contacted the counselor and recommended a referral to vocational rehabilitation. Eventually, Darlene was encouraged to work part-time and assist a boutique in opening a central office. Darlene convinced them to purchase a computer. She is now a partner in the firm, has her own apartment, and no longer wears scarves or feels deformed.

Case Comparison of Change. In comparing the cases of John and Darlene, it is important to note that John was still at home when the disruption occurred, whereas Darlene had just changed her environment. Darlene had no friends and no job and was not familiar with the area when her accident occurred. The only constant element in her environment was her parents, who were also in the process of change and adjustment to their new surroundings.

John and his parents had a strong support system in their community. The people knew of their problems and offered their help in a variety of ways. Fortunately, John was comfortable with his role in the family, the community, and working on the farm. He had been apprehensive about moving to the city and working regular hours on a new job. He knew what was expected of him in his home environment. He could work toward achieving familiar roles, lifestyles, and activity levels before exploring a new environment.

On the other hand, Darlene was not only adjusting to a new environment, but was also entering a new role with her parents. When she had first moved back home, her parents traveled a great deal. Her presence at home was quite independent of them. They appreciated the fact that her presence made the home look "lived in," and she was also available if anything went wrong. This arrangement had been mutually beneficial. Now she was simply living with them. Darlene's disruption occurred at a time when her stress was paramount in relation to the external environment, and the potential disfigurement was an assault on her self-image and her relationship with the external environment.

John's body image and internal environment was also disrupted. Although he was concerned about his appearance, his values and standards placed a priority on performance. He had made achievements while in the hospital and knew he would be independent again with the prosthesis. Although the changes brought about by John's disruption seemed more severe than Darlene's, both individuals required therapeutic intervention to resume successful performance in their environments and to successfully adjust to change.

PREVENTION

Humans strive to achieve a balance between their internal and external environments. This is an ongoing process occurring throughout an individual's life span. This same principle can be applied to the structure and function of the human body. No body part, system, or organ functions in isolation. Physiologically, the body works to achieve a homeostatic balance among all of its parts. It is of the utmost importance to remember that any change in the structure or function of one part results in a corresponding impact or change of other parts.

At times, the change in the structure or function of a part may have a healthy and positive influence on another part. For example, a person who begins an exercise program may increase the strength and range of motion of a muscle group; improve vital capacity; and increase heart rate, general circulation, and activity tolerance. Changes in the structure and function of a part can also result in pathologic responses of other areas. Such responses are usually referred to as misuse or disuse syndromes. Health care personnel need to be knowledgeable about these syndromes to include prevention techniques in their treatment programs.

Prevention may be defined as taking measures to keep something from happening.[5] It is a global subject that has numerous components, which must be considered. In health care fields these include adequate environmental shelter and safety; preventive health care (such as inoculations and regular medical checkups); a diet that provides adequate nutrients; moderation in the use of alcohol; abstinence from tobacco; regular exercise; and (particularly in occupational therapy) a healthy balance between work, play/leisure, self-care, rest, and sleep activities.

Many studies confirm that activity is necessary to the well-being of an individual. Activity enhances health and promotes mental abilities, while reducing stress. It provides individuals with feelings of self-control and mastery of their environment, which is necessary for self-satisfaction.

Studies have also documented the impact of inactivity on an organism. Complications arising from inactivity are called hypokinetic diseases and are a direct result of inactivity or lack of use of a part. Hypokinetic diseases are more commonly referred to as disuse syndromes.[6]

Disuse Syndromes

Many disuse syndromes are preventable and reversible; however, some become irreversible. Prolonged inactivity without preventive intervention can create disuse syndromes or secondary complications, which can lead to morbidity. When prevention measures are not initiated, these common disuse syndromes frequently become secondary complications that can be more disabling and life threatening than the primary diagnosis or disability.

A primary disability is the presenting diagnosis and the direct result of pathologic change or injury. Secondary complications are frequently created by the primary disability. These complications can be the result of superimposed activity restrictions that occur as a direct result of the disease process or injury. Examples include the patient who must spend weeks in traction due to a back injury, or the depressed, suicidal patient who must be kept under constant surveillance on a small locked unit.

Prolonged disuse is inherent in a multitude of different diagnostic categories. It is important for health care team members to recognize this problem and to initiate appropriate prevention and health promotion techniques. Consider the individual whose primary diagnosis is a stroke with paralysis on one side of the body. If preventive techniques are not initiated within a few weeks, secondary complications can develop, such as bed sores (decubitus ulcers), contracted joints, deformities of upper and lower extremities, urinary tract infections, and incontinence. Mental health may also deteriorate as evidenced by withdrawal, dependence and depression.

The health problems that result in inactivity or disuse of a part are caused by a variety of conditions and demands. Some of these include the following:

1. Pain resulting in a protective response
2. Loss of sensation
3. Enforced bed rest
4. Restricted activity due to a primary disability, such as cardiac precautions or recent surgery
5. Immobilization of a part due to casts or braces
6. Mental disorders that result in activity level changes or self-imposed decreases in range of motion
7. Limited activity due to cultural or vocational requirements

Some restrictions are temporary and resultant complications can be reversed in a short time. A broken arm or leg that is immobilized in a cast may restrict a person's activity level until the cast is removed. Normal function usually returns after a short period of generalized weakness and decreased range of motion. Physical therapy and occupational therapy personnel frequently treat such individuals and assist in reversing any disuse limitations as quickly as possible.

Ten Disuse Syndromes

Most of the disuse syndromes discussed can be prevented by three simple, physical intervention techniques: active exercise, passive exercise or range of motion, and frequent changes in position. These physical intervention techniques will be effective only when combined with psychological considerations.

In the area of psychosocial dysfunction, it is important to provide a variety of activities within the interest area and ability of the patient. Efforts must be made to provide opportunities for decision making and control over elements of the environment. Maintaining communication with family and friends is another important factor. More specific information on the diagnostic categories and techniques outlined may be found in the case study chapters in *Practice Issues in Occupational Therapy,* SLACK Inc.

Prolonged restrictions and permanent changes require specific, ongoing intervention techniques to prevent the following ten most common disuse syndromes.

Decubitus Ulcers. Decubitus ulcers are areas of tissue necrosis (cell death) due to prolonged pressure. The ulcers frequently occur in bedridden and paralyzed patients. They usually occur around large bony prominences such as the trochanter when the patient is in a side-lying position. They can also occur around the ischial tuberosity from prolonged sitting and around the sacrum from maintaining a supine position for prolonged periods.

Prolonged pressure in these areas results initially in a red or blistered area. These areas become discolored or black and eventually the necrotic tissue sloughs off, leaving a deep open ulcer. Decubitus ulcers can be prevented by frequent changes in position and the use of special mattresses and chair pads.

Muscle Atrophy. Muscle atrophy is the diminution of muscle mass due to disuse. The two major types of atrophy are *denervation* and *disuse*. Denervation atrophy occurs when a muscle has lost its nerve supply. This is a normal physiologic reaction to some conditions and is not preventable or reversible. In contrast, disuse atrophy is preventable and usually reversible. This type of atrophy takes place when a muscle has not been contracted for a period of time. The muscle fibers gradually diminish in size and maintain the length required in their position. They lose their elasticity. Volitional contractions can occur as well; however, the involved muscles are usually very weak.

Joint Contractures. Contractures of the joints are brought about when the soft tissue surrounding the joint shortens due to a decrease in range of motion. If a joint is not moved through its full range of motion for a prolonged time, the contracture can be irreversible or require surgical intervention. These are usually referred to as "frozen" joints. Complete contractures do not exhibit increased range of motion, even when the area is anesthetized.

Orthostatic Hypotension. This condition is caused by a rapid fall in blood pressure when assuming an upright position. It is usually caused by blood pooling in the abdominal area and the lower extremities, which is a result of the loss of elasticity of the blood vessels. Persons who have been confined to bed for three or four days frequently experience dizziness or weakness when they first stand up. However, if a patient is maintained in an upright position after a prolonged recumbent position, brain damage and death can occur. People with quadriplegia and other patients are frequently placed on tilt tables and the upright position is assumed by degrees over a period of time.

Phlebothrombosis. This disuse syndrome most frequently occurs in the lower extremities from lack of motion or prolonged positioning. The stasis of blood in the circulatory system can allow the development of a venous thrombosis (vascular obstruction), which can become a pulmonary embolism, an often fatal condition.

Pneumonia. Another complication of prolonged disuse is pneumonia; it is frequently seen in bedridden persons. The decrease in vital capacity leads to an accumulation of fluid in the lungs, which causes congestion. Many persons die of pneumonia as a secondary complication of enforced or prolonged bed rest.

Osteoporosis. This metabolic disturbance can occur with immobilization. When the muscles do not pull on their origins or insertions, the bones begin losing their matrix and excreting minerals, and become porous and brittle. Osteoporosis can be painful and render a person susceptible to fractures. Calcium is the most common mineral excreted by the bone. The abundance of calcium in the system can lead to the development of stones in the urinary tract.

Kidney and Bladder Stones. These conditions can be brought about as the result of disuse syndromes. One causative factor is the overabundance of calcium circulating through the body. This problem is frequently compounded by the high calcium content of hospital diets. The patient who is in a prolonged supine position may have urine pooling in the kidneys and bladder, which encourages the development of stones.

Incontinence. Incontinence is a common complication of disuse from a prolonged supine position. It can be a result of decreased gravitational "push" against the sphincters of the urethra and colon, which, under normal circumstances, elicits sphincter contractions that permit control of elimination of body wastes.

Psychological Deterioration. The condition of psychological deterioration is perhaps the most devestating disuse syndrome. Prolonged inactivity can be catastrophic to some individuals. These persons frequently exhibit loss of appetite, decrease in communication, and lethargy. They appear to have "lost the will to live." The many personality changes that lead to psychological deterioration depend on the individual and range from withdrawl to aggression.

Misuse Syndromes

Any change in the structure or function of a part can result in the misuse and abuse of other parts. While disuse syndromes affect other body parts and systems, misuse syndromes usually occur at the primary site of assault or abuse. Some misuse syndromes develop as a result of leisure activities, some are work related, and some develop in response to a change in another body part.

Complications from leisure activities were observed during the sudden popularity of video games, which resulted in a medical condition commonly referred to as "Atari thumb." This condition is actually the development of tendonitis of the thumb due to excessive use. Tennis elbow is another example of a misuse syndrome.

Work-related conditions are very common. People who install carpet frequently have one enlarged knee. This is due to the accumulation of calcium in the knee that is used to strike the carpet stretch hammer. The quadriceps of the same leg may also be more developed than those of the other extremity.

Functional changes require special consideration. Occupational therapists and assistants frequently work with persons who have difficulty reaching a standing position from a seated position. This condition can be due to the normal aging process, arthritis in the hips and knees, or pain and other medical problems in the lower extremities. Many of these individuals have a "favorite" chair in their home. These chairs are frequently large, overstuffed, and have a bottom cushion that provides support from the sacrum to just behind the knees. These chairs may also support the calves of the lower legs and maintain the knees in 90 degree flexion. This position makes it difficult, if not impossible, for most people to easily assume a standing position.

Persons experiencing this difficulty usually put excessive strain on their upper extremities. They commonly form a tripod pattern with their thumbs and first two fingers and then push on these small joints to lift their body weight. Prevention of this misuse syndrome in the hand can be accomplished by providing instruction in using the entire length of the forearms to bear the body weight. If grab bars are available, it is important for occupational therapy personnel to instruct these individuals not to grasp the bars with their hands but rather to loop the entire forearm around the bar and then pull up.

In addition to analyzing self-care and other daily activities, the OTR and COTA may need to investigate the patient's daily use of tools, appliances and accessories. It may be necessary to check something as simple as a handbag or purse that the individual routinely carries, as these vary greatly in style, size, weight and types of closures.

Mrs. B, the stroke patient previously discussed in this chapter, agreed to use an adapted shoulder bag instead of a sling. When Mrs. B visited the occupational therapy clinic on an outpatient visit, the COTA asked her about the adapted purse. Mrs. B stated that it was effective and added that her husband also appreciated the added convenience of having her carry such extra items as his camera, extra film, maps, and tour guides when they went on their frequent day trips. The occupational therapy assistant instructed Mrs. B to keep her purse as light as possible and suggested that Mr. B purchase a separate carrying case for his equipment.

The examination of the type of purse carried by a person with arthritis can be critical in preventing damage to the joints of the upper extremity. Unfortunately, this consideration is frequently overlooked.

There is no existing list of common misuse syndromes comparable to those for disuse syndromes. Misuse and abuse problems and the potential for developing misuse syndromes need to be identified on an individual basis. These problems and preventive measures are identified through the therapists' and the assistants' knowledge and understanding of the interrelationships of the various body parts and through a thorough knowledge of the components of task and activity analysis as they relate to the individual's values and lifestyle.

SUMMARY

It is much easier for health care personnel to treat arthritis, a hand injury, a personality disorder, a suicide attempt, or an amputee than to treat the *whole* person. The latter requires knowledge and insight about the individual's development, values, lifestyles, environments, self-images, roles, and activities in planning and implementing purposeful and meaningful therapeutic intervention programs.

The goal of occupational therapy is to return the person to his or her environment with the skills necessary to resume previous occupations and roles. Occupational therapy is concerned with the quality of life, which is determined by the individual and his or her environment. The relationship between humans and their environs goes far beyond the simple stimulus and response theory. A total transaction occurs between the individual and the external and internal circumstances that make up the person's unique environment.

To effectively treat a person and not a disability, all members of the profession must know the sociocultural, economic, psychological and physical aspects and view them in relation to the standards, values and attitudes of the patient's total environment. Occupational therapists and assistants are performance specialists who design and implement highly individualized developmental, remediation and prevention programs.

Related Learning Activities

1. Identify some of the customs, traditions or superstitions in your family and discuss how they might affect therapy.

2. Working with a peer, compare and contrast how your plan for therapy might be different in each of the following instances:

Patient Condition	Patient Environment
arthritis	well-to-do matron bag lady
stroke	rancher in Texas accountant in Chicago
depression	Cambodian refugee American suburban housewife

3. Discuss common misuse and disuse syndromes with a classmate or peer. Determine what intervention techniques are likely to be most effective.

References

1. The Philosophical Base of Occupational Therapy. American Occupational Therapy Association Resolution #531, April 1979.
2. Reed K, Saunderson S: *Concepts of Occupational Therapy,* 2nd edition. Baltimore, Maryland, Williams & Wilkins, 1983.
3. American Occupational Therapy Association Council on Standards: Occupational therapy: Its definition and functions. *Am J Occup Ther* 26:204-205, 1972.
4. Guralnik DB: *Webster's New World Dictionary,* 2nd College Edition. New York, Simon and Schuster, 1982.
5. *The Doubleday Dictionary.* New York, Doubleday, 1975.
6. Kielhofner G: *Health Through Occupation.* Philadelphia, FA Davis, 1983, pp. 98-99.

Section III
TECHNOLOGY

Video Recording

Small Electronic Devices and Techniques

Computers

As a profession, we have entered an age of rapid technologic advances that impact on the delivery of occupational therapy services. The use of video recording continues to make new inroads as a tool for evaluation, treatment, patient education, record keeping and leisure enjoyment. The lightweight portability and high-quality picture of today's camcorders have added a new practical tool for occupational therapy personnel. Simple, inexpensive microswitches, easily purchased or constructed, allow individuals to interact actively with their human and mechanized environments in ways never thought possible. This single basic electrical component has afforded patients many new opportunities for achieving greater independence. The invention of the microcomputer and a wide variety of peripheral input and output devices has greatly influenced the profession and the individuals we serve. It has allowed people with performance deficits to achieve many goals both in occupational therapy treatment and in their personal lives. It has, in many cases, revolutionalized our society. The microcomputer has also greatly improved our management and communication systems by greatly reducing the time necessary to collect and process data and produce reports.

It is important for the reader to focus on specific technologies in terms of developing new skills or enhancing existing ones. After content related to basic applications is mastered, one should explore the numerous opportunities for applying technologic concepts in management and system development in health care. As we find increasing ways to use technology in occupational therapy practice, we must heed the words of Dunford who stated, "Traditional occupational therapy skills must be the basis for a practical approach to using technical aids."

Video Recording

Azela Gohl-Giese, MS, OTR

INTRODUCTION

Recent advances in technology have allowed video equipment manufacturers to market systems that are so automated and easy to operate that practically anyone can produce a video product of reasonable quality. This development has allowed occupational therapists and assistants to create ways of adapting the media for individual patients and groups.

This chapter focuses first on the video recorder as a machine. A simplified explanation of the mechanical aspects is presented, and diagrams illustrate the relationships between input and output devices. Next, the use of video recording to provide a historical library is presented. Historically referenced tapes can be of great value to the educator, researcher, and writer, as well as occupational therapy personnel involved in day-to-day treatment activities. Some recordings may "sit on the shelf" for years, whereas others that present education topics to the patient, parent, or family may be used daily. Standard treatment procedures that are used frequently can be taped for use with patients as well as new staff members as a part of the orientation process. A videotape library will be commonplace in every occupational therapy clinic in the future.

The use of video recording as a mirror that reflects an objective view of the subject on camera is then considered.[1] The intent is to provide immediate feedback to an individual or a group as to how they performed or reacted in a particular situation during a specific time interval. Replay of the videotape can assist in recalling the actions that took place as well as the feelings that may be associated with these actions. In a group situation the replay will assist in focusing the group so that the critique will be based on input from everyone. These recordings are generally not cataloged and stored.

Occupational therapy staff members seeking specific, objective feedback on skills such as interviewing or supervising can replay a videotape at their convenience, in privacy if desired. This approach can be an effective way to improve skills. Camera shy people may have difficulty using video for this purpose; however, the fact that the tape can be erased instantly may give them added comfort in using this medium for self-evaluation. It need not be an embarrassing experience.

KEY CONCEPTS

Recording principles

Maintenance and problem solving

Production techniques

Developing an historical library system

Objective recording of behavior

Projective tool applications

Creative uses

Future applications

The fourth part of this chapter describes the use of video recording as a projective tool. Segments of commercial television such as "soap operas" and news broadcasts may be used as a part of the treatment milieu. Psychodrama techniques may be added to tailor the roles of particular characters in the television program to the patient's real life situation. The psychodrama skit may also be taped for later viewing and discussion. Finally, video recording is presented as a tool for creating. The intent is to emphasize the human quality of creativity and encourage the patient to use video for this purpose. Future trends in the creative use of video recording are explored along with the importance of keeping abreast of new technologic advancements.

THE MACHINE

Over the last 20 or more years, video recording has evolved from an amateur's nightmare to a fairly common leisure activity. In the past, it seemed that only a person with a degree in electrical engineering could possibly cope with the technical maze of connecting a video camera, recorder, monitor and microphone system. Today, because of the tremendous advances made in automating video recording equipment, a person who is familiar with a 35 mm still camera and with making adjustments on a commercial television set, may feel fairly comfortable using a video camera and recorder after minimal instruction. There is a standard electrical connection system for operating video equipment. Once this basic system is understood, extra enhancements, such as use of a character generator for titles and dubbing in background music on a second audio channel, can be tried when more professional recordings are required.

The following neurologic analogy is used to provide a basic understanding of the video recording system. Consider the camera as the eye and the microphone as the ear picking up environmental sounds and actions that become **input** and travel via cables, which are the nerves of the system. The cables connect directly to the videotape recorder and store the information on tape just as the brain stores information in memory. When **output** is needed, the "play" button on the videotape recorder is depressed and the recorded information is sent to the television monitor via an output cable. Three basic principles must always be followed when using video recording equipment:[2]

1. The camera and microphone must be connected to the input terminals of the recording unit.
2. Output cables are connected to the output terminal of the recorder and the input terminal of the monitor.
3. When taping a commercial television program, the monitor is providing input; therefore, it is connected to the input terminal of the recorder.

The diagrams in Figure 11-1 show specific connecting patterns for four different uses of video equipment. Either commercial power outlets or batteries may be used.

It should be noted that the camera and the microphones provide input only. When one or both of these pieces of equipment are being used, the "record" switch on the videotape recorder must be turned on to record the information on tape and view it on the monitor. Newer camera models have built-in microphones with a fairly long range; thus the camera cable contains both the audio and video connections. When connecting the various components of the system, it is important to apply firm pressure, but never force. If force seems necessary, it is likely that an improper connection is being attempted. Consult the operation manual for possible errors in the procedure.

The quality of the video recording is determined when it is being produced. There is little that can be done to improve a flawed or inferior recording while it is being viewed on the monitor, no matter how sophisticated the monitor's tuning system may be. Therefore, at the time of recording it is important to check and recheck the functioning of the camera, recorder and monitor. By making a short "trial" tape and viewing it on the monitor, the following common problems can be avoided:

1. Poor color or black-and-white contrast
2. Improper focus
3. Inadequate lighting
4. Inaudible or unclear sound

By checking the monitor for proper contrast and "sharpness" of images, the camera can be adjusted for both focus and level of light. In some environments it may be necessary to use auxiliary lighting. Sound problems can generally be solved through the use of extra microphones and the elimination of background noise such as traffic, air conditioning, and fans. It takes several practice sessions to successfully accomplish all of these tasks and develop the skills necessary to produce a quality tape.

Video equipment in current use is designed for either a VHS or Beta cassette tape format used on a video cassette recorder (VCR), with the VHS type being the most popular. Care must be taken to use the proper size and mode of recording material that fits the specific video recorder available, as the various formats are not interchangeable. For example, a $3/4$-inch videotape cassette cannot be used on a video recorder that is designed for $1/2$-inch tape. Once the correct tape is selected, it is fairly simple to insert the cassette into the machine. When the tape is in place and the camera is connected to the recorder, the recording process may begin.

Lighting

It is important to evaluate the **lighting** in the room where the videotape is to be produced. Before recording a trial tape, the following steps should be taken to assure adequate

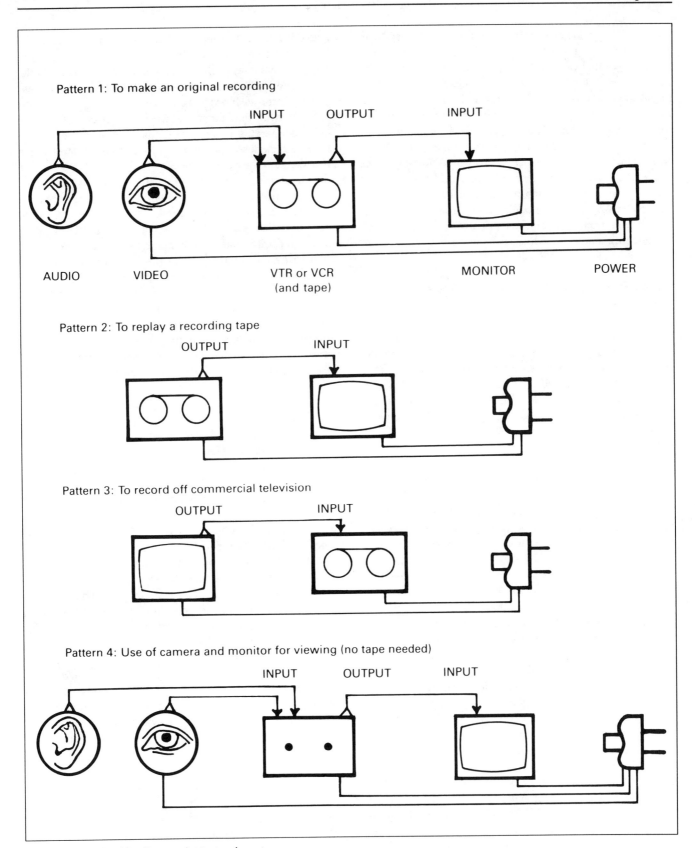

Figure 11-1. Relationship of input and output equipment.

lighting. The subjects should be positioned so that their faces are not in a shadow. If there is bright sunlight, the camera should be placed so that the light comes from behind. Never point the camera lens into the sun or other bright light, as this can cause damage. Most clinic settings that have fluorescent lighting provide adequate illumination for videotaping. If other lighting is needed, auxiliary lamps can be used to "bounce" light off a wall or the ceiling. Place these lights so that the stands or shades do not appear on camera. Producing an outdoor videotape can be particularly difficult due to the wide range of light and shadow. Camera lens filters may provide a partial solution in this situation. Seek advice from a factory representative or a local audiovisual consultant about which style filter works best on the particular camera you are using.

Other Environmental Considerations

The more isolated the environment selected for making a videotape, the less likely background noise and interruptions will interfere with the production. It is advisable to close windows to help eliminate noise from traffic and aircraft, unplug telephones, and turn off fans and air conditioning units. Post a sign on the door or doors that states "Video Taping in Progress—Do Not Disturb!" Interruptions of any kind can mean that the work must be retaped. When a very professional tape is required, it is best to use a soundproof video studio.

Arrange all furniture and equipment that will be needed in the production to assure that the camera can be moved about the area with ease. Consider the location of electrical outlets to be used for the camera and other video equipment. If the placement of electrical cables is likely to interfere with the tape production, battery power should be used.

Focusing and Timing

The key to good videotape production is focus and timing. Most video cameras have "zooming" power. This literally means that the lens is capable of quickly moving very close to the subject for a close-up view. Many new users of a video camera will overuse this technique, which tends to distract or tire the viewing audience. It is better to try to provide a mixture of varying distances and angles, using the zoom technique occasionally for emphasis or a detailed close-up picture, to help keep the viewer interested in the subject. Record what is being communicated by the subjects both orally and physically as the person may be saying one thing, but body posture or action may be conveying a different or conflicting message. It is important for patients to see such incongruence to develop self-knowledge and to improve communication.

Timing is also essential for keeping the viewer's attention. It is important to maintain a balance; moving the camera too fast will result in the viewer missing the action; moving too slowly may cause the viewer to be bored and some important action may be missed. As you move the camera, keep the motion as smooth as possible. Avoid sudden stops and starts as the videotape will appear jerky when it is shown.

Supporting the camera securely on a tripod allows the camera operator to have both hands free to focus and move the camera smoothly about the room. There is also less danger of dropping the camera or being bumped. The one great advantage of having a small, portable camera is the flexibility of moving quickly into a narrow space or at a specific angle to the subject for a special shot. A tripod does not allow that motion in most cases. The trade-off is safety and smoothness for accuracy and immediacy.

If written material, such as titles, is included in the tape production, focus the camera on each line of print from four to five seconds to give the audience sufficient time to read the message. When in doubt, add an additional second or two. Chances of maintaining viewers' attention are better with too much time rather than not enough. Above all, try to maintain a professional approach and avoid reminding the viewer that the producer was a clever person with a brand new camera.

Portability

The elements of videotaping described to this point are standard, regardless of the brand of camera used; however, there is a great deal of difference in the degree of **portability,** or ability to be moved easily from place to place, among the various models of videotape production equipment. Heavy-duty systems tend not to be moved about too much except on carts made especially for that purpose. Portable video recorder units weighing as little as 25 to 30 pounds come in "packs" that have harness-type straps that secure them to the waist and shoulders in much the same manner as a camper carries a backpack. The lightweight cameras have various types of hand grips and shoulder rests, which provide some added stability. Their disadvantage is that they tend to be easily dropped, bumped, or shaken beyond the normal limits. For these reasons, mechanical adjusting needs to be made on a regular basis to assure proper functioning. Care must be taken to evaluate what measure of use the equipment is to withstand before investing in new equipment.

The **camcorder** is one solution to the portability problem. All functions of the video recording process are combined in one package—camera, microphone, recorder with cassette tape, miniature monitor, and battery power option. The same principles of video production presented previously apply to this video format. Although the camcorder is relatively lightweight and portable, a tripod should still be used for a precision quality production. Figure 11-2 shows a composite model of the camcorder.

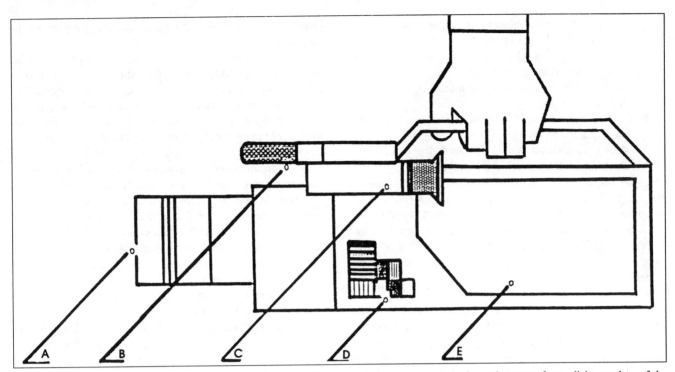

Figure 11-2. Camcorder. A. Zoom lens; B. Microphone; C. Electronic viewfinder; D. Control panel (power, focus, light regulator, fader, record/review);   E. Cassette tape holder.

Maintenance and Related Problem Solving

Like any other precision tool, a video camera and recorder require a certain amount of **maintenance** to operate properly. Use of dust covers and storage in a clean area make it unnecessary to clean the vital parts of the equipment before each use. Excess dust can scratch videotape. The operation manual gives precise instructions on specific areas to be cleaned and frequency of cleaning to assure long-term service. For example, if you notice that the picture on the monitor seems "grainy" or distorted, it may be caused by an accumulation of dust and dirt on the recording heads of the video recorder. Follow the operator's manual instructions carefully when cleaning. If this technique does not solve the problem, the distortion could be caused by using a tape that was recorded in a different timing format. For example, if the video recorder being used is designed for two-hour tapes, it will not play a tape recorded in a four-hour format.

It is advisable to document when the equipment is cleaned, as well as when it is sent out for professional repair or maintenance. Information on the replacement of parts and other adjustments should be noted together with costs and may well serve as justification for replacement when necessary.

Videotapes last longer if they are stored in closed cabinets in an area where the temperature is moderate and the humidity is low. It is best to set the tapes on edge rather than flat so that the tape does not become distorted by binding to the edge of the container.

PRODUCTION TECHNIQUES

Developing Scripts

Once the user has made several short video recordings, preferably in varying environmental settings with both group and individual subjects, a taping "layout" or a **script** must be developed to explain exactly how the equipment will be used to maximize the best of its unique qualities in the production.

Initially, one must determine the objectives for using videotape recording: Why is it essential to have a visual record of the situation? Would an audiotape and still photographs or slides be just as effective? If not, then lay out a general plan to determine what equipment is to be used, where it is to be placed, and when it should be moved. Try to anticipate how the events will unfold and generate ideas on possible events so the camera operator knows what is important and what might occur. The latter is a particularly important aspect in the recording of group interactions. Realistically, all group actions cannot be recorded; however, fewer surprises will occur if careful planning takes place before the actual videotaping. The following is an example of a segment of a production script for a videotape on the topic of learning to knit:

Production Title: "Learning to Knit".
Initial Camera Location: Five feet from table and title easel.
   1. Zoom in on title for five seconds.
   2. Film presenter from waist up during introduction.

3. Zoom in on specific pieces of equipment as they are described, then back to presenter.
4. Move camera to the left and behind the presenter to demonstrate "casting on stitches."
5. Maintain this position throughout this segment, using zoom initially.
6. Change camera angle to show one or two students practicing the technique.
7. Move from presenter to students as dialogue occurs.

A videotape on this or other craft techniques can be a valuable aid in student learning. The tape can be viewed at the student's convenience, perhaps in a media center. The program can be designed to allow the student to look at one or two segments and then stop the tape to practice the required skills before moving to the next step. The student may watch the tape again, before a test, to review the material.

It is important to note that the script for the camera operator is different from a dialogue script. The latter reads in much the same way as the script for a play and is used for productions where factual interchange is the primary objective rather than spontaneous conversation. This script should also be prepared in advance and rehearsed with the participants. Once the script is finalized, the camera cues can be added directly to the dialogue pages, the goal being to give the camera operator as much information as possible to ensure a good quality production. Figure 11-3 presents an example of how a dialogue script may be written.

Since activity analysis is such an important aspect of occupational therapy, a student who is absent when this information is discussed can view the tape at a later time, thus gaining information that may not have been recorded in notes borrowed from a classmate.

Editing, Tape Reuse and Tape Transfer

Although it is fairly simple to do "add on" editing at the end of a tape, most individuals who need more sophisticated editing take their tapes to a professional studio, as most health care facilities do not have the necessary equipment to do a professional job.

Videotape can be reused by simply recording over it. As the new material is recorded, the recorder automatically erases the material that was on the tape before. The number of times this can be done successfully depends on several factors, including the original quality of the tape, the age of the tape and the number of times a tape has been used.

Both occupational therapists and occupational therapy assistants can be involved in making videotapes, depending on their individual interests and skills as well as the particular needs of the department. Helpful resouces for information on both the mechanical and production aspects of video recording are listed in the bibliography.

As technologic advances continue to improve the video recording process, new formats will be marketed. Fortunately as part of this development, techniques are available to transfer existing tapes to these new formats. When replacing video equipment, it is important to keep the old recorder until all tapes that are to be retained can be transferred from the old format to the new.

Other General Considerations

Policies for honoring patient's rights of freedom and **confidentiality** (ie, the maintenance of secrecy regarding entrusted information) apply to video recording. Each occupational therapy department should have a written policy and necessary consent and release forms on file and available to patients. The policy should outline the specific instances where videotaping will be used as a therapeutic technique, as well as the conditions under which the tapes are used for other purposes, such as student education. Some facilities require that all patients sign a consent and release form before participating in any video projects, whether used internally or externally by the facility. The right of the patient not to be videotaped must always be respected.

CAMERA CUES:	DIALOGUE:	
4 feet from teacher	Teacher:	"Knitting is frequently used as a treatment modality in occupational therapy. What are the major therapeutic strengths of this activity?"
Move to student A	Student A:	"I think knitting is relaxing now that I've learned how to do it. It might be a good activity for an anxious patient."
Move to student B	Student B:	"I agree, but my field work supervisor said that knitting could be used only in the clinic, where the patients are closely supervised. This surprised me—it looks pretty harmless."
Move to teacher Zoom in on yarn and needles	Teacher:	"While yarn does indeed appear harmless, a depressed, suicidal patient might use it to braid a noose. Knitting needles can be used to inflict personal injury."

Figure 11-3. Sample dialogue script. Production title, *Activity Analysis of Knitting.*

THE HISTORICAL LIBRARY

One of the most common uses of video recording is to make a permanent audiovisual record of the treatment of a patient over time. Due to the complexities of some treatment regimens, a visual record is essential in recording the patient's progress or lack of progress. It is a way of objectively documenting the changes and improvements that have been gained and those that have not. In some pediatric programs, a videotape record is made at regular intervals over several months or in some cases several years. Thus all pertinent details of work with the child are documented. If the therapist's memory fades, the recording maintains a firm image. A written record usually accompanies the tape and serves as a sequential index of the recorded content. The tapes are then cataloged using a convenient library system for efficient retrieval.

The key to the effective use of a videotape library is the accuracy of the index. A good index includes not only the title, producer, and date but also a detailed listing of the location of specific categories and events on the tape. These categories are referred to as "time locations." The critical measure in determining accurate time locations is to check that the timing gauge is on zero at the beginning of the recording session. Once the tape is running, begin a recorded log of the general categories and significant events. Such information will allow the user to locate quickly a particular segment when needed. When viewing the tape again, return the time gauge to zero before beginning. If tapes are frequently used in this way, an automatic time gauge can be purchased.

Occupational therapy personnel are also using videotapes to record evaluation procedures. If the same person is repeating the evaluation, the previous assessment can be reviewed to duplicate the procedures accurately. If a different person is doing the procedure, viewing the tape will help ensure consistency in administering the evaluation.

This video recording technique was used to establish rater reliability while using a checklist of behaviors designed for a research project.[3] A number of videotaped sessions were produced showing an occupational therapist testing children individually. The tapes were then viewed later by occupational therapists who were asked to observe the children being tested and record their observations on the checklist. Using the videotaped programs as part of this research allowed participants in the research project to contribute over time at different locations. They did not have to be present at the actual time or place of the testing. More important, all viewers were observing the same testing situation, thus assuring a more valid research procedure.

Holm[4] describes another use of video recording in which information was taped to be used at a specific time in a treatment program when the patient is ready for it. For example, a patient can view a tape of another patient engaged in an activity. By viewing another patient engaged in the activity, instead of watching a nondisabled therapist demonstrating it, the patient may show less resistance to attempting an unfamiliar or difficult task. A number of different tapes can be available in the clinic for this use. If new tapes are made on different patients on a regular basis, the library will be current and aid in a variety of patient informational and motivational needs. Holm also describes the use of video in providing an orientation for patients who will be having a new experience or feel uncomfortable with attempting an activity. The therapist filmed the environment in which the activity was to take place and then showed it to the patient as a means of "rehearsing" before the actual experience. This technique allowed the patient to visualize where and how to approach the unfamiliar, thus reducing anxiety and even discovering some of the enjoyable aspects of the activity.

A certified occupational therapy assistant (COTA) added another dimension to patient viewing of a videotape on home care programming by engaging the family to watch the same tape. As a result, the family members were less apprehensive about their responsibility for patient care and more enthusiastic about the patient's return home.[5]

Columbia University's program in occupational therapy also produced a videotape about home care programming. The tape consists of assessments used to evaluate levels of function for the elderly, as well as examples of group activities that will assist older adults in accomplishing the developmental tasks of aging.[6]

Another common reason for developing videotapes is for staff in-service or continuing education.[7] The Minnesota Occupational Therapy Association, Continuing Education Committee is building a library collection of videotapes for this purpose. The project was given impetus when the public service department of a local television company agreed to provide free use of their equipment and recording studio. The committee had to furnish the videotape, script and actors. Several videotapes on topics such as feeding techniques and wheelchair adaptations have been completed and are available to therapists and facilities for a modest fee to cover postage and handling. This educational method is particularly helpful for occupational therapy personnel residing outside of metropolitan areas where continuing education opportunities may be less available.

This educational service demonstrates one of the advantages of using video recording rather than 16mm film production. A video product may be produced at less cost and more quickly because the processing time is shorter, requiring only the time necessary to record the tape. The advantage of 16mm film over videotape is that the film provides sharper color distinction. The structure of film may also provide a better slow-motion mechanism because it can be moved forward one frame at a time, a feature not possible with videotape.

The educator in the classroom or the clinic can access many tape libraries nationwide. Often these libraries are found at larger universities, which may furnish catalogs of their current holdings upon request. Usually the tapes are available in more then one format, and the exact type required must be specified when ordering.

A MIRROR OF BEHAVIOR

The video camera is often compared to an eye focusing in on the action. Just as a famous individual, because of his or her degree of notoriety, can detract the viewer from the content of a television interview, the presence of a video camera in an occupational therapy clinic can detract from what would otherwise be spontaneous action. Until the subjects being taped have become comfortable with the camera and less aware of its focus on them, viewing of their actions must be tempered somewhat when interpreting the scene on the monitor.

Add to this predisposition the historical situation for most people in middle-class society; they have watched television for many hours during their lifetimes. The content viewed and the normal viewing environment will surely have an impact on how seriously they view the monitor in a therapeutic situation. If they have maintained a regular schedule of watching certain quiz shows and situation comedies, their participation in a videotaped psychodrama as part of a psychiatric occupational therapy treatment may not make a lasting impression. They may view television as primarily fantasy that can be turned on and off. Such individuals may also "turn off" a display of their anguish or hostility as they view the playback of the psychodrama. For the most part, television is passive. Nothing is required of the viewer except to select the channel and make slight tuning adjustments from time to time. This passive viewing pattern is difficult to alter due to long-term conditioning and the fact that most individuals see television as a form of entertainment.

Cater[8] suggests the presence of an additional conflict for the television viewer who happens to be left-brain dominant in mental development. Such individuals show resistance to taking the television media seriously, as it is a type of media that appeals more to the right hemisphere of the brain. It does not fit into the intellectually analytical thinking of the left-brained viewer. Thus, from a therapeutic standpoint, the right-brained individual may be more adept than one who is left-brain dominant at using **video feedback,** the information received objectively via the camera and tape. If the video feedback can be structured in a sequentially analytical manner using propositional thought, the left-brained person perhaps also will become engaged in using video feedback therapeutically.

A simple measure that helps patients reach a comfort level with this media is to demonstrate how easy it is to erase the tape used in the treatment session. Knowledge of this fact can aid the patient in relaxing and being spontaneous during the videotaping. Although few patients request erasure of a tape, knowing that erasure is possible provides continuing reassurance. Once patients recognize the value of the feedback, their anxiety over the recording is reduced. Engaging the patient in the mechanical control of the video equipment provides a sense of control over what is going to take place in the therapeutic session. The patient who feels in control is likely to make a greater investment in and commitment to changing behavior or risking new behavior. With the availability of instant replay, the patient is able to receive immediate feedback on what effect his or her behavior has in relation to the human and nonhuman environment. They also gain a perspective of how their behavior was seen by others viewing the tape.

Engaging the Viewer in the Results

Although the recording process is basically the same, the reasons for making the video recording and the manner in which the tape is viewed may differ considerably. The following examples of six situations offer methods for actively engaging the viewer in the results shown on the tape.

Example One. The video recording of a staff member or a student who wants to improve a skill, such as interviewing a patient or administering a patient evaluation, may be set up at his or her convenience. Once the tape has been made, the individual can review it at a later time either privately or with a colleague who has agreed to review the performance. By allowing these two options, the individual is able to choose the one with which he or she is most comfortable. The tape does not make any judgments; the person being taped controls how the tape will be used. Once the person has viewed the first taped experience, some confidence will be gained, and the next taping is much easier to accomplish.

Example Two. The complex situation of using video feedback in a group therapy session can be invaluable to the group. The technical aspects of filming should be accomplished with ease and in the most unobtrusive manner possible. Using two cameras and two operators is ideal because it significantly reduces the amount of camera movement. If a second camera cannot be used or operators are not available, consider having group members take turns being the group observer and operating the camera. This alternating of tasks allows the individuals to continue in their roles as group members while also contributing to the collection of objective feedback that will be shared with the group at the appropriate time. Using this type of system frees the group leader to address the immediate needs of the members as they occur. It should be noted, however, that it is best to have a nongroup member operate the equipment. An occupational therapist or an occupational therapy assistant is ideal to run the camera because he or she possesses knowledge of group process and dynamics.

Placement of the camera or cameras should minimize distraction. The type of action to be focused on should also be discussed. Usually the group's action provides clues that may suggest what should be emphasized. Because of the size of some therapeutic groups, it may not be possible to tape all activity and dialogue. Larger groups generate more background noise that may effect the clarity of the sound track. Adding extra auxiliary microphones and a second group observer may assist in providing accurate feedback.

Example Three. One form of video feedback that has been found invaluable to parents is viewing taped therapy sessions of their children. Often parents find it difficult to believe that their child acts differently in an environment away from home. With the help of tapes made over a period of weeks or months, insight may be gained as to how the child is behaving and the degree of progress that is being made to improve inappropriate behaviors. The tapes may also show the parents how specific reinforcement techniques can be used with the child at home. Since progress may be slow or very minimal at times, a tape may provide contrast if viewed again at a later time. Occupational therapy personnel have noted that the use of videotape can be an effective way of obtaining support from parents during the treatment of their child. The University of Colorado School of Nursing has developed videotaped "packages" to help parents, families and professionals who care for handicapped and at-risk infants. These include six training tapes for use on home video cassette recorders, accompanied by self-instructional lessons.[9]

Example Four. Video feedback may also be used to motivate patients to make behavioral changes on their own behalf. Patients who experience seizures or have behavior disorders may be appropriate candidates for this approach, as they are unable to control themselves and are unaware of what is happening during an episode. By viewing the specific event on videotape with a staff member present for support, the patient can gain insight into what is happening. Patients may be more willing to cooperate with the staff in taking the prescribed medication or attending the group therapy sessions that are often so uncomfortable for them.

Example Five. The use of the video camera and monitor without tape can be of great assistance in presenting information to a group of people, particularly when the content being emphasized requires close-up viewing for comprehension, and a permanent record of the material is not necessary. When demonstrating how to use small tools

such as needles, be sure to focus the camera on the detail so that each member of the audience can see an enlarged view of the proper technique. This method is effective for teaching students the detailed steps in beginning or ending double cordovan leather lacing, for instance. It also could be used to show a group of patients with hemiplegia how dressing techniques can be adapted to the use of one hand or the best methods for paring vegetables unilaterally. Recording on tape may occur at the same time as the viewing, but, as stated earlier, it is not essential unless a permanent record is needed.

If the room being used is too small to accommodate both the audience and the subject and equipment, the camera and subject can be placed in a smaller room, and extension cables can be connected to the monitor or monitors in the larger room.

Example Six. Whereas some people are camera shy, others enjoy being filmed, finding it stimulating and energy generating. This increased patient energy can be used to advantage by filming the patient when he or she is exhibiting appropriate behaviors. Occupational therapy personnel must structure the experience so that the patient does not become overstimulated and lose self-control.[10] Later viewing can serve as a reinforcement and, in many cases, can enable the patient to gain greater confidence and self-esteem in attempting the unfamiliar. Use of such a reinforcement technique can help many to live more enriched lives.

A PROJECTIVE TOOL

In contrast with other aspects of videotaping, when emphasis is placed on more subjective aspects of the medium, the tool may become an effective **projective technique**. Projective techniques may be defined as activities and methods that provide information about patients' thoughts, feelings and needs. As in finger painting and clay modeling, videotaping is pliable, leaving room for personal interpretation. At least three facets of video recording may be a part of a projective technique: soap opera, documentary and psychodrama.

The first and one of the most common video projective tools is the commercial television soap opera serial. This program can be viewed on a daily basis, or prerecorded and shown at a time that is more therapeutically appropriate. It is essential to structure the viewing and discussion so as to involve the patients in an active manner. The highly defensive person may assume an attitude of being passively entertained and be unwilling to become involved in the projective exercise.

The viewing of the program can be structured by providing the group members with carefully constructed questions in advance. Questions may focus on a particular role being portrayed or the patient's reactions to a particular event or situation. One of the advantages of prerecording the television program is that a significant segment can be replayed quickly. This technique aids in uncovering emotional material that some patients may not wish to acknowledge by insisting they do not remember what was being depicted or said. Once the discussion has covered the specific content, the next segment of the program can be viewed. The primary objectives in using this method are to explore the roles and situations the patient identifies with, support any insights gained, and enable the patient to risk a change in behavior.

The plot of the soap opera may play as important a function in the projective process as the identification of a particular role by the patient. When the patient views the program on a regular basis, the questions used to structure the experience may direct the focus to how a situation developed and what actions were being taken to alter the results, which may be healthier for the people involved. The patients may be willing to describe attempts that they have made in similar situations and discuss the degree of personal satisfaction gained from this action. In other instances, the patients will take this new information or approach and apply it to similar situations in their own lives.

By having the entire group watch the same video action, much can be learned by noting the varying perceptions of the individual group members. The leader needs to assure all members that all perceptions are acceptable and that no moral judgments will be made as to the rightness or wrongness of their perceptions. It is helpful to the group to see how differently a given action can be perceived. Gaining an appreciation of this fact may allow viewers to expand their knowledge, their communication skills, and their sense of self-worth.

The use of video as a projective technique relies heavily on the cognitive ability of the viewer. However, the technique may be adapted to various levels of maturation and functioning by the questions formulated by the OTR and the COTA who may serve as co-leaders. This adaptation begins with the careful selection of the program to be viewed, the questions to be addressed, and the methods for processing the patients' projective reactions throughout the discussion. There is no substitute for effective group facilitation on the part of the therapist and the assistant. Neither the viewing of the video nor the questions asked can, in and of themselves, bring about a therapeutic experience.

Psychodrama, a technique in which patients dramatize their daily life situations, has proven to be an effective adjunct to soap opera viewing. A patient who has just viewed a particular scene may wish to personalize it by requesting the special fellow group members to play roles. The psychodrama is also videotaped and replayed for discussion. When this method is used, patients are often more attentive and curious about viewing themselves and their personal vulnerability, rather than watching a professional actor or actress on the monitor. This curiosity is a part of assessing body image and self-image, as well as congruency and incongruency. It provides another example of how video can serve as an effective projective tool.

A second format produced by commercial television and useful to occupational therapy personnel is the news or documentary broadcast. Although the technique used is similar to the one used with a soap opera, the content of the news is more conducive to helping the patient relate to the world at large rather than being solely occupied with one's inner self. It is advisable to create a degree of structure to assist the patient in meeting the main objective of relating to the societal realities presented through discussion of current events. The use of predetermined questions or a viewing guide outline encourages involvement in both viewing and discussion. Observing the patient's responses to the news program can provide information relative to cognitive and affective levels as well as values. Such observations of responses, together with other information, may serve as measures of appropriate adapted behavior. It also may be a way of determining whether a patient is approaching the time of hospital or facility discharge.

A TOOL FOR CREATING

A vital part of most occupational therapy programs is facilitating the patient's needed behavioral changes. The key to making these changes in behavior is the internal motivation of the individual. Creativity is individual and requires a certain freedom of space and time. When the elements of change and creativity are combined in treatment planning, the patient can be involved in the therapeutic process. Through such involvement in a creative endeavor, verbal and nonverbal communication takes place among the patient, the activity and the therapist.

Occupational therapy personnel are often challenged to introduce activities that will motivate the patient to become actively involved. Creative activities are attractive to many because they offer the creator total control of the materials used as well as a tangible product. If external limits are imposed, creativity can be stifled or lost.

Using the activity of making a videotape as a medium for creative expression may communicate information about how the patient sees the world. The impressions of a paraplegic individual who will be in a wheelchair for the rest of his or her life can be very different from those of a neurotic patient who has many unresolved societal and environmental fears. The simplicity of operating many types of video equipment makes this activity feasible for most age groups except the very young. Although staff instruction and supervision are generally required, once initial learning has taken place, the individual can often proceed with a fairly high degree of independence, focusing energy on the creative process and product rather then on the equipment. When the videotape is completed, it may reveal significant information about the patient that can be used as a communication tool to affect the behavioral changes needed to achieve a more productive and meaningful life.

Goldstein[11] describes the use of video production by individuals and groups. The staff members served as consultants in the use of the equipment and provided structure in the activity process as need arose. The communication that resulted during the production of the video recordings provided important information for therapeutic intervention. Each patient was experiencing a different level of self-confidence; some were intimidated by the equipment, whereas others wanted to control the camera. Several of the adolescents in this group were able to use the taping experience to better adapt to the treatment institution and eventually make some behavioral changes. The staff also gained insight into some hospital procedures that were improved as a result of this treatment project.

An elderly population that may not have "grown up" with television increasingly depends on it to meet social needs. The Mount Sinai Medical Center received grant funding to assist in addressing the problem of isolation felt by the elderly, such as those living in an apartment complex in East Harlem.[12] By means of a cable television system, each resident's television set was connected to a service that accessed an unused channel exclusively for the tenants in the 20-story high-rise apartment building.

The grant program provides a number of television services, one of which is resident-produced programs. Residents were involved in the overall program early in its development by videotaping group discussions about the living conditions and social activities of the apartment complex. The initial shyness of some participants was overcome, and soon about 100 residents had appeared on camera. It should be recognized that it often takes longer for the elderly to become comfortable with handling the equipment, as they did not have exposure to this technology at a young age.

One group project featured several residents demonstrating their favorite recipes, and another focused on discussion of growing up in early America. As involvement increased, so did the number of residents viewing the special channel. By becoming regular viewers, many also participated in the health care program offered under the grant sponsorship. This program was designed to reduce the health care costs of the elderly through televised and other mass media health care education.

During the next stage, resident involvement was individual. Because videotapes featuring the elderly were not that readily available for rent or purchase, the taped programs were designed to show individual residents engaged in interviews, leisure time activity demonstrations, tenant news broadcasts, and a health tips program. Once the recording was made, the resident could watch it in the privacy of his or her own apartment. Residents could also visit the studio during the recording sessions.

The elderly have many lifetime experiences to share, and this sharing enhances the quality of their life within their environments. Video recording provides a vehicle that the elderly can use to communicate to others the social riches and skills they have gleaned throughout their lives.

The use of video recording for creative purposes need not be restricted to patient or client populations. This media has great potential for the student in the classroom. Many educators who previously required that all assignments be prepared in either an oral or written form are recognizing the value of making a videotape. Since increasing numbers of curricula have access to video recording equipment, students may be given the option of making a videotaped presentation as a creative approach to completing assignments such as case studies or research projects.

Case study video productions may dramatically contrast normal and abnormal behavior and conditions. Role plays may be used if actual patients are not available to participate. The effective production and use of a short, ten-minute video presentations can often convey a stronger and more accurate message than a 10- or 15-page paper.

Researchers are finding that videotape is a valuable method for documenting their findings. This medium has helped to demonstrate specific research methods and assists those conducting research to duplicate previously completed studies. Information that may have been overlooked in studying the written research report is often found when the video recording is viewed.

FUTURE TRENDS

As the communication industry makes even more rapid advances, technology continues to have a strong and everchanging impact. For example, in the past ten years competition in the marketplace has caused the demise of the Beta format for videocassettes and the videodisk system. What has emerged is the VHS video cassette format, the camcorder, and a "sleeper"—the video laser disk system. The technology for recording video laser disks is not yet available to the general consumer, but it will soon be in great demand as the process doubles the video resolution, producing a much sharper image, and it has superior audio reproduction.

In the not too distant future, the increased development and expansion of video technology will provide the general population with many new services that are seen now in their early stages of development at mass media and technology fairs. For example, communication systems for every household may include video-telephones connected directly to frequently used services such as the bank, supermarket, department store, and primary health care provider. When considering the latter, it is feasible to predict that the annual physical examination by a physician may be conducted in the privacy of one's home by means of a combination of video, telephone and a microcomputer system connected to a health center. Medical history, current symptoms if any, and other pertinent data can be entered into the computer. Simple electronic devices will automatically record temperature, heart rate and blood pressure and interactive video will allow the individual to talk with the physician. If additional diagnostic tests or services are required, the monitor will display these along with times they can be scheduled, thus automatically making appointments and printing a list of them for the individual.

The home health care delivery system may be dramatically different in the future. For example, occupational therapy personnel could gather some screening and evaluation data through a computerized questionnaire and an interactive video system that would allow discussion of work, play and self-care skills and problems. The individual could move a small video camera about the house that would assist the occupational therapist in making an initial evaluation of the environment. Other health professionals will also be using video techniques and "video visits" as a supplement to actual home visits. Such measures should ultimately result in reduced health care costs and increased efficiency in service delivery.

As more and more families find that economic pressures require both parents to be employed, the responsibility for day-to-day child care will be placed in the hands of people other than the parents. As this trend increases, young parents are increasingly concerned that they do not have sufficient influence on their children during their formative years. Occupational therapists and assistants may become much more involved in the well community in the areas of normal child development and child care. Their services could include the use of videotape and computer programs that address topics such as the roles of parents and ways to develop "quality time" activities with their children. Programming may enable the parents to view the current relationships they have with their children and contrast them to other approaches and options. This technique may provide one method to individualize the child-parent relationship and offer resources when problems occur.

Another aspect of child development that could be addressed is the lack of quality commercial television programming for the toddler and preschool child. There is a good market for occupational therapy personnel to apply their knowledge of child development and related developmental life tasks and activities to create new programs. Programming that engages the child in active viewing and learning, some-

what like that presented on public television, is needed. Adding a parent education and interactive video discussion segment to each presentation would allow both the parents and the child to gain from the viewing experience.

The development of sophisticated satellite relay systems for video signal transmission has aided in the advancement of space science. It has made a particular impact on mass media coverage of events worldwide, which are presented regularly to the public. Of equal importance is the way this technology can be used to improve the quality of life for the handicapped. Resourceful individuals asking the question "how" will continue to find new applications when assessing individual patient needs.

SUMMARY

Each of the functions of video recording described can play an important role in the delivery of occupational therapy services. Assessing the patient's situation, treatment planning and implementation, reevaluation, and discharge planning provide numerous opportunities to use this medium. The ways that video recordings can be used—as an historical reference, a spontaneous feedback mechanism, a projective instrument or a creative experience—all address the components of the occupational therapy process. The examples of specific uses of video recording are intended to challenge occupational therapists and assistants to adapt the techniques to fit the needs of the populations they are serving.

The future of video recording applications for occupational therapy is virtually unlimited at this time. As technologic advances are made, it is imperative that members of the profession seek this new knowledge and develop the skills necessary to help the physically and emotionally handicapped to maximize their potential and improve their quality of life.

Related Learning Activities

1. Discuss some of the positive and negative influences on patients' needs when using video recordings.

2. What are some of the problems inherent in using video equipment? What preventive maintenance measures can be taken to eliminate these problems?

3. Outline factors to be considered when deciding whether an occupational therapy department should purchase new video equipment.

4. Plan a video tape production for the purpose of orienting physicians, residents and interns to the goals and objectives of occupational therapy. Outline all of the taped segments that should be included and write a script to be used with each.

5. Practice using a camcorder or other video camera to make a short film. Have someone experienced in this medium critique your work.

References

1. Fletcher D: Video: Is it too technical for occupational therapists? *Br J of Occup Ther* 30:272-274, 1987.
2. Lewis R: *Home Video Makers' Handbook.* New York, Crown, 1987.
3. Bauer BA: Tactile sensitivity. *Am J Occup Ther* 31:357-361, 1977.
4. Holm MB: Video as a medium in occupational therapy. *Am J Occup Ther* 37:531-534, 1983.
5. Rudolph M: Lights! Camera!—OT collaboration produces video for stroke patients. *OT Week* (February 16): 16-17, 1989.
6. Miller P: Life skills video produced at Columbia U. *OT Week* (May 6): 3 1986.
7. Milner N: Rehab foundation's videos are aids for OTs. *OT Week* (May 21): 12-13, 1987.
8. Cater D: The intellectual in videoland. *Saturday Review* 12: 12-16, 1975.
9. Smith A: Videos instruct care of at-risk infants. *OT Week* (July 23): 6, 1987.
10. Heilveil I: *Video in Mental Health Practice.* New York, Springer, 1983.
11. Goldstein N: Making videotapes: an activity for hospitalized adolescents. *Am J Occup Ther* 36:530-533, 1982.
12. Wallerstein E: Television for the elderly—a new approach to health. *Educational and Industrial Television* (April): 28-31, 1975.

Small Electronic Devices and Techniques

Mary Ellen Lange Dunford, OTR

INTRODUCTION

Patients with severe physical handicaps and multiple disabilities often have limited interaction with others and with their environment. Modern technology and advanced technical aids have revolutionized many areas once restricted for persons with handicaps. Powered wheelchairs and adapted automobiles provide independent mobility. Communication aids allow independent oral and written communication. Environmental control units offer access to the operation of lights, radios, coffee makers and other electrical appliances. Sophisticated instructional devices for teaching educational skills to the severely physically and cognitively disabled are now available.

Technologic advances have provided versatile opportunities for the disabled to exercise control within their environment, to live and work semi-independently, to communicate, to learn, and to be constructive, contributing members of the community. Technology has created new avenues of therapeutic intervention for health care professionals and educators who work with the handicapped. The use of electronic aids is a relatively new phenomenon in occupational therapy. It presents a challenging treatment modality as well as a valuable evaluation tool.

One of the electronic components being used to adapt devices for the handicapped is the **microswitch.** A microswitch is a small on/off lever switch. When combined with the appropriate circuitry, it can be used to replace common on/off switches found on battery-operated devices such as toys and tape recorders. Instructions for the construction and therapeutic use of a Plexiglas pressure switch operated by a microswitch are described later in this chapter.

ESSENTIAL VOCABULARY

Microswitch

Method of activation

Feedback

Effectiveness

Efficiency

Tracking time

Selection time

Accuracy of response

Repeatability

Interfaces

Splitting a wire

Soldering

Scanning

KEY CONCEPTS

Evaluation process

Selection of control site and switch

Switch effectiveness factors

Interface and assistive device selection

Basic technical procedures

Specific switch construction techniques

Safety precautions

Treatment applications

EVALUATION PROCESS

Traditional occupational therapy skills must be the basis for a practical approach to using technical aids in treatment sessions. An assessment of each patient and his or her individual needs is essential and the first step toward incorporating electronic devices into the practice of occupational therapy.

A patient's needs can first be assessed through a brief and informal interview with the patient and his or her family. An interview will identify the needs and establish objectives to be accomplished with microswitch technology. For instance, a patient with a spinal cord injury may want a switch fabricated to operate a microcomputer or an environmental control unit, whereas the parents of a handicapped child may want to have their child use switches to play with toys that he or she is not able to operate with conventional switches.

The patient evaluation also includes an assessment of physical limitations and functional abilities such as mobility, communication and object manipulation skills. Sensorimotor components that include range of motion, muscle tone, reflex integration, gross and fine motor coordination, developmental skills, strength, endurance and sensory awareness are also assessed. Other aspects of the evaluation include the cognitive and psychological areas such as intelligence, cognitive development, motivation and attitude.

Positioning and seating considerations for the patient are important in the evaluation process. Secure and stable positioning is necessary to enhance learning and skill development.

Patient evaluations should be a team effort. Input from other health and educational professionals working with the patient can provide valuable information and insight. Ideally, a team should include an electrical engineer or a rehabilitation engineer to provide consultation about electronic aids, devices and systems. While this practice may be rare in most occupational therapy work settings today, engineers will play a major part in the therapeutic application of electronic technology in health care professions in the immediate future. Currently, it is recommended that the registered occupational therapist (OTR) be responsible for the overall evaluation procedures, whereas either the therapist or the certified occupational therapy assistant (COTA) could be responsible for the fabrication and use of electronic devices in treatment sessions.

Control Site

When the evaluation of the patient is completed and it has been determined that a microswitch adaptation is an appropriate measure, a control site for switch activation must be selected. A control site is defined as an anatomic site with which the person demonstrates purposeful movement.[1] The location of control sites can be divided into three general anatomic areas: the head and neck, the trunk and shoulders, and the extremities.

Individual control sites from the head and neck include the head, chin, lips, tongue, mouth, eyes and isolated facial muscles. The trunk and shoulders, when used as control sites, offer gross movements such as rolling; lateral tilting; and shoulder elevation, depression, retraction, and protraction. Specific control sites for the extremities include elbows, arms, hands, fingers, legs, feet and toes.

Each site being considered for switch activation is assessed for range of motion, strength and ease, and amount of control. Once the site has been chosen, the method of activation is determined. The **method of activation is** defined as the movement or the means by which a control site will activate a switch.[1] For instance, elbow extension, lateral head movement, or some type of external device such as a headstick or a mouthstick may be used.

Selection of a Switch Control

Commercial and handmade switches can be extremely simple or highly complex. Switches vary greatly in their versatility. The following are some of the general characteristics to consider when choosing a switch: feedback, weight, size, shape, safety, mounting and positioning, stability, durability, adaptability, portability, reliability, appearance, simplicity, warranties, and availability and ease of part replacement.

Three types of **feedback** are provided from a control switch:[1]

1. *Auditory feedback*—the noise the switch makes when it is activated
2. *Visual feedback*—the movement of the switch when it is activated
3. *Somatosensory feedback*—the texture of the surface of the switch, the force required to activate the switch, and the position of the patient's body when the switch is operated

The feedback provided can enhance training and the patient's successful use of the specific switch.

The weight and size of a contol may also need to be considered. Small, lightweight controls are easier to mount and to transport from place to place. Large and heavy controls can be awkward, but they also offer the advantages of having more surface area, thus requiring less motor precision for activation. These larger switches might be used by children with cerebral palsy.

Safety is a critical factor in the use of switches. They *must* be both physically and electrically safe to operate. Physical safety refers to the materials used to make the switch. Sharp edges and rough materials that irritate the skin must be avoided. Electrical safety is not a significant concern when the switches are connected to low-voltage, battery-operated toys and devices; but it is a concern when they are connected to commercial electrical outlets such as those found in the home or treatment facility. When using handmade switches with electrical outlets, it is important to be sure they are properly grounded. An electrical or rehabilitation engineer should check the switch, the mounting, and the grounding before using it with a patient. If the patient drools frequently, a common problem with children, be sure to keep the switches well covered or mounted in a position that will prevent them from becoming wet.

Mounting and positioning of the switch are as important as the positioning of the patient for the most effective use. Frequent documentation of positions and mounting techniques used during the assessment can be useful during later training sessions. Specific patient responses such as spastic movements also should be recorded, as they may interfere with the switch placement.

Stability and **durability** are also important characteristics to consider. A switch must be sturdy and able to withstand reasonable use. In some instances, modifications will need to be made to protect the switch. A switch that is adaptable can be modified as the patient's needs change. This is especially important when working with children as they grow and change.

The degree of portability of the switch is another important consideration. If a patient operates several devices or uses the switch in different seating arrangements, the switch may need to be moved from one place to another, or multiple switches may need to be constructed.

A switch must work when the patient needs it. To help ensure reliability of the switch, standard and easily replaceable components should be used in constructing handmade controls. It is a good idea to make a second switch for use as a "back up" in emergencies.

The physical appearance of a switch is an important element for many patients. It should be cosmetically pleasing and not overly noticeable. Handmade switches should be as simple as possible and not "over designed." Consider warranties and the availability of repair services for commercial switches used.

Evaluation of Switch Effectiveness

Technical research documents the need to evaluate the **effectiveness** and **efficiency** of a switch.[1] Evaluative measures include the speed of response, accuracy of response, fatigue and repeatability.

Speed of response can be assessed related to two performance components: tracking time and selection time. **Tracking time** is the amount of time needed for a patient to move from a resting position to activation of the switch. **Selection time** is the time needed to operate two switches or two functions of a switch. An example would be the amount of time required to activate a dual switch system for a Morse code communication device. Special computer software programs that come with an "adaptive firmware card" are available that will assist in tracking of progress.

Accuracy of response is estimated from the percentage of errors and correct responses recorded during the tracking and selection times. These percentages and the speed of response provide crude estimation of the degree of accuracy. Poor speed or accuracy are generally related to one or more of the following factors:
1. Switch feedback
2. The weight and size of the switch
3. Positioning of the individual
4. Mounting and positioning of the switch
5. The individual's inability to respond and manipulate the switch

Reevaluation, making the appropriate modifications, and monitoring are necessary to improve the patient's performance.

Fatigue is assessed by making comparisons between the speed of responses and the accuracy percentages recorded at the beginning of a training session and at the end of the session. **Repeatability** refers to the ability of the patient to repeat the performance over a specific period of time. It can be assessed by making comparisons between the speed of responses and the accuracy percentages documented at different training sessions over a designated time period.

Case Study 12-1

The following case study illustrates the use of evaluative measures to select a switch for a boy with cerebral palsy, a spastic quadraplegic. An initial interview with his parents identified the child's need for a microswitch. The parents wanted a means for their child to communicate, to play with toys, and to have some control over his environment.

Since the child attended a public school, various evaluations were administered by speech, psychology, education, and physical and occupational therapy personnel. The child was nonverbal with normal intelligence. An occupational therapy assessment indicated severe physical limitations. Increased muscle tone and neurologic impairment significantly delayed motor development. The patient lacked functional use of his extremities, and trunk and head control were very limited.

The child was positioned in a customized seating system built by a local carpenter. His head was chosen as the control site for the switch. The patient had minimal side-to-side head movement, and thus head turning to either side was determined as the method of switch activation.

Two commercial microswitches (round pressure type, DU-IT Control Systems Group, Appendix D) were chosen as the most desirable. They were lightweight, small in size, easy to mount, durable, and provided a "click" for auditory feedback. Mounting was accomplished by gluing pieces of Velcro to the back of the switches and attaching strips of counter Velcro to the headrest of the child's wheelchair. The switches were positioned so that as the child turned his head to either side, his cheek bone brushed against a switch and activated it.

The switches were interfaced with two battery-operated toys and tracking time trials were taken for each switch. The first four trials required 30 to 35 seconds for each switch activation. Selection time, the time needed to operate both switches, was approximately 95 seconds. Accuracy of response (the correct number of switch activations) was 60% (six activations in ten trials) for the switch mounted on the right side. The switch mounted on the left had an 80% accuracy of response. Speed of response increased and accuracy of response decreased after the first four trials, indicating that fatigue interfered with performance.

On the basis of this information, adjustments were made in the position of the headrest angle, and the position of each switch was changed slightly. Records of speed of response and accuracy percentages were compiled during the next six treatment sessions. Speed of response decreased and accuracy increased, indicating that the switches appeared to be working efficiently for the child.

Repeatability was seen as the patient was able to improve and repeat his best performance level over several weeks. Eventually, the child was able to use the two switches to operate a computer, an environmental control unit, and a Morse code system for written communication.

Selection of Interfaces and Assistive Devices

Completion of the evaluation process should result in a recommendation for a switch that can be operated efficiently by the patient, based on performance abilities and limitations. Assistive devices and switch interfaces are determined after the switch has been selected, and the patient has been trained to use the switch.

The operation of electronic assistive devices requires the use of switch interfaces. **Interfaces** are electrical circuits that connect switches to the assistive devices. With the appropriate interface, switches can be used to operate microcomputers, environmental control units, communication systems, and battery-controlled devices.

Various interfaces may be purchased through manufactur-ers or handmade interfaces can be fabricated. Purchasing controls for assessment and training can be expensive, as numerous products are available, and it is difficult to know exactly what to buy to get started. When doubtful about purchasing a particular switch, it may be beneficial to make one first for experimentation. A resource list of supplies, equipment and related information appears at the conclusion of this chapter.

BASIC PRINCIPLES OF ELECTRICITY

Electricity needs a pathway of circuits to conduct energy. The pathway of circuits for the operation of battery-operated devices consists of a power source (the batteries); an on/off microswitch; and the toy, light, tape recorder or other device.[2]

When the microswitch is closed or turned on, it completes the electrical pathway and allows the electricity to flow from the battery to the device, thus turning it on, as illustrated in Figure 12-1. When the microswitch is open or off, the electricity is not allowed to flow from the battery so the device is not turned on, as shown in Figure 12-2.

To construct a Plexiglas pressure switch, three basic electrical components must be purchased: the subminiature microswitch, the subminiature jack, and the subminiature plug. The subminiature microswitch is the on/off lever switch, and the subminiature jack and plug are the two counterparts that make up the electrical connection between the switch and the interface. Either subminiature or minia-ture jacks and plugs can be used; however, the different sizes are not interchangeable and must match in size to fit together correctly. Subminiature components are not as readily available as miniature parts. It should be noted that when using a tape recorder, the subminiature plug will fit directly into the remote control jack on the recorder, and an interface is not necessary. Detailed instructions for making a switch will be provided later in this chapter.

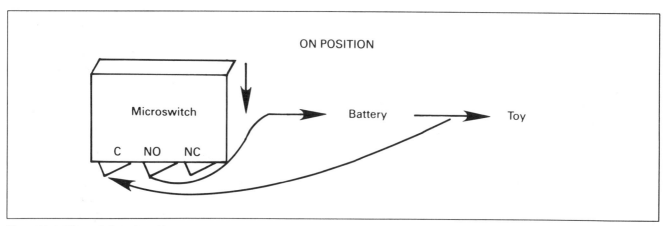

Figure 12-1. Microswitch "on" position.

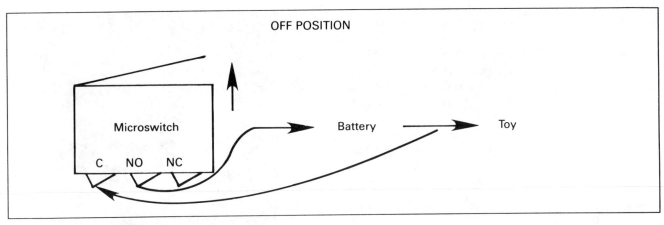

OFF POSITION

Microswitch

C   NO   NC

Battery

Toy

Figure 12-2. Microswitch "off" position.

TECHNICAL PROCEDURES

The technical procedures necessary to construct switches include splitting a wire, stripping a wire, and soldering.

Splitting a Wire

To **split a wire** means to separate the two strands of the wire. Each strand is coated in plastic. With either wire cutters or scissors, the two strands are cut and separated as shown in Figure 12-3. Care must be taken to avoid penetrating each plastic strand so as not to expose the wires.

Stripping a Wire

To strip a wire means removing the plastic coating from a segment of the wire. If wire gauges are marked on the wire stripper, both strands of the wire are placed in the 22-gauge hole, which is the size recommended for projects described in this chapter. The jaws of the stripper are placed about three inches down from the end of the wire. The wire stripper handles are gently squeezed together and quickly pulled up to remove the plastic coating. Care must be taken, because if the wire stripper is squeezed with too much force, the wires may be cut off. If this

should happen, the procedure should be tried again.

Several varieties of wire strippers may operate differently from the one just described. The wire gauge is not marked on some, and it is necessary to adjust a bolt and set the cutter for the size of the wire. Once the plastic coating has been cut, the wire is placed in a separate hole marked on the stripper to pull off the plastic coating.

Soldering

Soldering is the process of fusing two pieces of metal together to facilitate the passage of electricity between them. The following procedure should be followed:

1. Some wires, plugs, jacks and other electrical terminals may need to be cleaned with steel wool.
2. After the wire is threaded to the terminal, hold the parts with pliers or tape them to the table. A small table vise may also be used if the components become very hot and it is difficult to hold them while soldering.
3. To solder, first heat the wire and terminal parts at the same time by holding the soldering iron tip firmly against them. (Be patient until both the wire and terminal are hot.) When both parts are hot, touch the

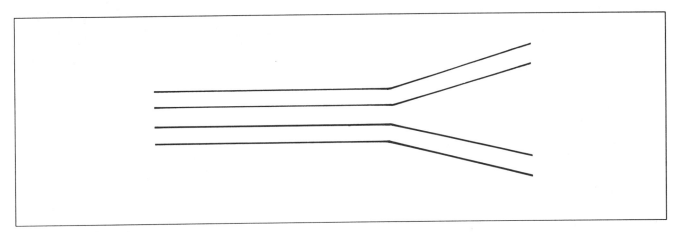

Figure 12-3. Splitting a wire.

rosin core or electrical solder to the connection. The solder should melt and flow evenly to coat the surfaces. Hold the soldered parts in a stable position until cool. If the parts have not been heated enough, the joint will lump. This is known as a cold solder joint and will make a poor electrical connection. If this occurs, simply reheat.

4. Use caution. The soldering iron must be used carefully. It becomes extremely hot and can cause severe burns and ignite fires. Avoid overheating the switch itself, as high temperatures can damage internal parts.

Instructions for Making a Plexiglas Pressure Switch Using Subminiature Components*

Basic Materials
- 2 pieces of Plexiglas each cut to $5^1/_2 \times 3$ inches
- 2 sheet metal screws, No. 6 diameter and $^3/_4$-inch long
- 3 wooden strips cut from $^1/_2$-inch thick pine stock: one piece cut to $5^1/_2$ inches in length by $^1/_2$-inch width and two pieces cut to 2 inches in length $\times$ $^1/_2$-inch width
- 1 spring that will fit under the screw head and is 1-inch in length; the tension of the spring is the individual's choice depending on the amount of strength the user can exert (it's a good idea to have a variety of springs on hand)
- 1 lever-type on/off microswitch
- 1 subminiature plug (miniature can be used)
- 1 22-inch piece of 22-gauge speaker wire

Other Supplies and Equipment. Rosin core or electrical solder, soldering iron, super glue, masking tape, electrical tape, hand drill, screwdriver, wire stripper/wire cutter, knife or taped, single-edge razor blade, needle nose pliers, awl, needle file, varnish, and sandpaper. The assembled switch is shown in Figure 12-4.

Instructions
1. Sand the edges and corners of the Plexiglas until smooth.
2. Sand all surfaces of the wood strips until smooth.
3. Varnish the wooden strips and allow to dry overnight.
4. Glue the $5^1/_2$-inch strip of wood along the $5^1/_2$-edge of one of the pieces of Plexiglas with super glue.
5. Split 2 inches from both ends of the 22-gauge speaker wire with a knife or a taped, single-edge razor blade.
6. Strip about $^1/_2$- to $^3/_4$-inch of plastic coating off each strand on both ends of the wire.
7. Unscrew the cap from the subminiature plug.
8. Thread the wires through the metal holes of the plug. Thread from the inside through the holes to the

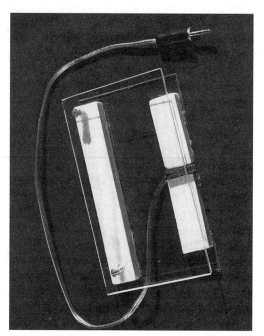

Figure 12-4. Plexiglas pressure switch.

outside. Bend the wires back and trim to $^1/_8$-inch. Be sure to pull through so that the plastic coating touches the inside of the metal hole as shown in Figure 12-5.

9. Solder the wires to the plug. Use only a small amount of solder so that the cap will screw back on. If too much solder is used, the excess can be removed with a needle file.
10. Using a needle nose pliers, bend the two metal prongs at the end of the plug around the plastic coating of the wire passing through that hole. This maneuver helps to hold the wire securely.
11. Screw the cap back on.
12. Test the plug by plugging it into a subminiature jack adapted to a battery-operated toy, or plug it into the remote jack of a tape recorder. The toy or tape recorder needs to have the existing switch mechanism turned to "on." Touch the two wires at the opposite ends together; if the toy or tape recorder turns on, the plug is working properly (Figure 12-6). If the plug does not work, unscrew the cap and check to see if the wires soldered are touching each other. If they are, put electrical tape around one wire and metal prong to keep them separated.
13. Twist and thread the strands of wire on the opposite end of the plug onto the lever microswitch. Thread them from the back of the switch, one through the terminal labled "C" (common) and one through the terminal labeled "NO" (normally open), as shown in Figure 12-7.
14. Solder the wires to the switch and trim off any excess wire.

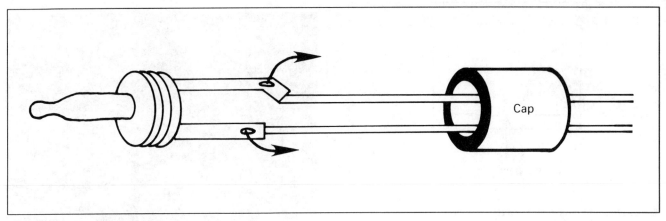

Figure 12-5. Threading wires to plug.

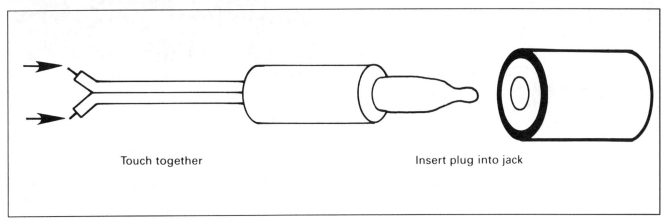

Figure 12-6. Testing the plug.

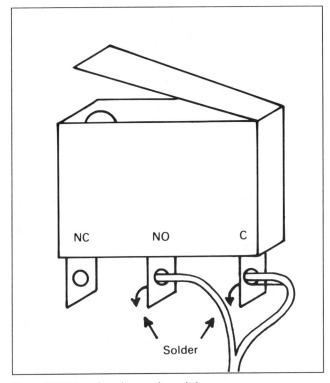

Figure 12-7. Threading wires to microswitch.

15. Test the circuitry again with a battery-operated toy or a tape recorder.
16. Glue the 2-inch strips of wood, one on each side of the switch lever and placed on the opposite edge from the $5^1/2$-inch strip glued earlier. It is best to glue one piece, let it dry 30 seconds, place the lever switch snugly against the glued piece, and glue the second 2-inch strip next to the switch. It is important to note that the microswitch is placed with the "C" terminal facing the inside of the switch as illustrated in Figure 12-8.
17. Drill two $5/32$-inch holes in the second piece of Plexiglas, $1/2$-inch from each edge of the 3-inch side, and $3/8$-inch from the $5^1/2$-inch edge as shown in Figure 12-9.
18. Place the Plexiglas with the holes over the glued $5^1/2$-inch strip of wood. Use an awl or a nail to mark the screw holes on the wood.
19. Cut the spring in half with a wire cutter.
20. Put the screws through the holes in the Plexiglas, slip one piece of spring on each screw (springs under Plexiglas), and screw them into the wood. Tighten the screws so that the tension of the springs keeps the top piece of Plexiglas above and not touching the microswitch.

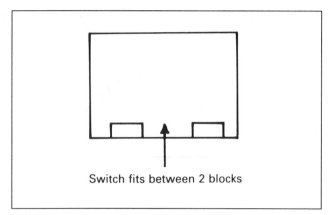

Figure 12-8. Placement of microswitch.

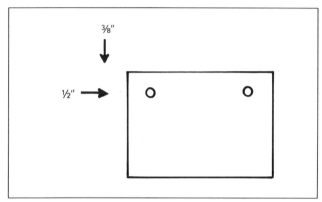

Figure 12-9. Plexiglas hole placement.

21. Retest the microswitch for operation.

This switch can be made either larger or smaller than the specifications given.

Instructions for Making an Interface for a Battery-Operated Device Using Subminiature Components*

Basic Materials
- 1 12-inch piece of 22-gauge speaker wire
- 1 subminiature jack
- 1 small piece of double-stick tape, $^1/_2$-inch by $^1/_4$-inch
- 2 small pieces of copper tooling foil, cut slightly smaller than the double-stick tape.

Other Supplies and Equipment. Wire stripper/cutter, knife or taped single-edge razor blade, soldering iron, rosin core solder or electrical solder, scissors and ruler. Figure 12-10 shows a completed device.

Instructions
1. Using a knife or a taped single-edge razor blade, split 2 inches from one end of the 22-gauge wire and split $^1/_2$-inch from the other end.

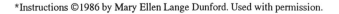
*Instructions ©1986 by Mary Ellen Lange Dunford. Used with permission.

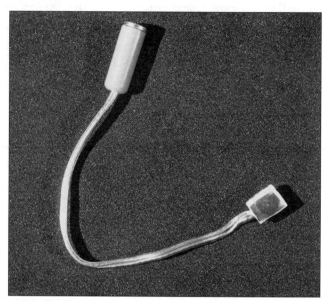

Figure 12-10. Interface for a battery-operated device.

2. Strip about $^1/_2$- to $^3/_4$-inch of the plastic coating off each strand on both ends of the wire. Twist the strands of each separate split piece of wire.
3. Unscrew the cap from the subminiature jack.
4. Thread one end of the split and stripped wire through the metal holes in the jack. Thread from the inside through the holes to the outside. Bend the wires back and trim to $^1/_8$-inch. Be sure to pull the wires through the holes so that the plastic coating touches the inside of each hole as illustrated in Figure 12-11.
5. Solder the wires to the jack; file off excess solder if necessary.
6. Using a needle nose pliers, bend the two metal prongs at the end of the jack around the plastic coating of the wire passing through the hole. This helps to hold the wire securely.
7. Thread the wire through the cap and screw on the cap.
8. Cut a small $^1/_2$- by $^1/_4$-inch piece of double-stick tape.
9. Cut two pieces of copper tooling foil slightly smaller than the $^1/_2$- by $^1/_4$-inch piece of double-stick tape.
10. Place the copper tooling foil pieces on either side of the double-stick tape. The tape acts as insulation and is necessary because the two pieces of copper must not come into contact with each other.
11. Place the $^1/_2$-inch split and stripped wires, one on each side of the copper chip, and solder each wire to it. Be sure that the plastic coating on each touches the end of the copper chip. This keeps the wires from touching each other, as shown in Figure 12-12.
12. Test the interface by using a battery-operated device in this manner: Remove the the cover from the battery compartment and place the copper chip

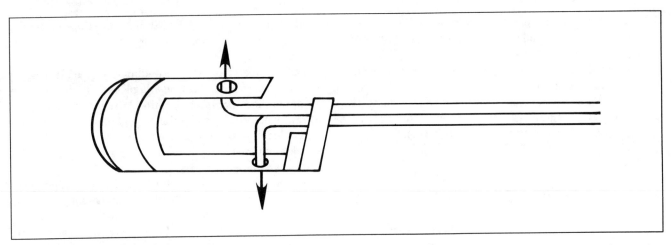

Figure 12-11. Threading wires to jack.

between the two batteries or between a battery and its contact. Turn on the device. It should not run. Connect a microswitch with a subminiature plug to the subminiature jack. Activate the microswitch. The device should work.

Variation. An insulated copper circuit board, cut to the same specifications, can be used to replace the copper foil and double-stick tape. If this option is selected, the wires are soldered to each side of the circuit board. It should be noted that chips made from circuit board are thicker and often more difficult to fit into a battery compartment. Foil-constructed chips are more flexible and fit compartments more easily, but they often break and will wear out faster than chips made from circuit board.

SELECTION OF TOYS AND BATTERY-OPERATED DEVICES

Toys provide valuable learning and growing experiences for children. Switches combined with toys encourage and motivate handicapped children and provide opportunities for them to play alone or with peers and actively participate in learning situations.

When purchasing battery-operated toys, it is important to select the ones with on/off switches. Check the battery box to be sure there is room for insertion of the copper chip from the interface. Some battery boxes are so small that once the batteries are inserted, there is not enough room for a small copper chip.

Toys that provide movement are very stimulating for children. Some action toys have a "bump and go" movement; they accelerate forward until they bump into a boundary or object and then reverse direction. Toys that are safe, durable, and colorful; make noises; and have lights are good choices for handicapped children. Some favorites

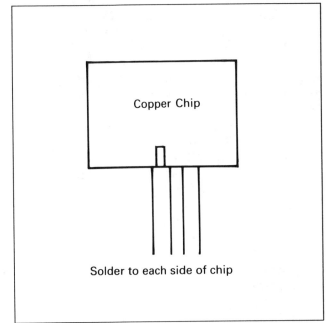

Figure 12-12. Placement of wires.

include small trains or engines, police cars with sirens, and animal characters that play musical instruments.

In addition to toys, small battery-operated fans and vibrators can provide sensory stimulation. Flashlights and other battery-powered light devices can be used for visual tracking and visual stimulation activities.

Tape recorders are also useful. Favorite songs and tunes, voices, and noises can be recorded and used as a play activity or as a reinforcement for correct performance. For example, a handicapped child who correctly moves an electronic car through a simple maze might be rewarded with a short taped segment of a favorite song, which is activated when the car reaches the final point. When using a tape recorder with a switch that has a subminiature plug, an interface is not necessary. The subminiature plug fits directly into the remote control jack on the tape recorder.

Toys that have more than one control switch and radio-controlled toys are difficult to adapt and require sophisticated wiring. *More Homemade Battery Devices for Severely Handicapped Children with Suggested Activities* by Linda J. Buckhart is an excellent resource that provides detailed information on complex toy adaptations. Toys that perform stunts or require a track to run on are not recommended for use with switches because the wires become twisted and break.

SAFETY PRECAUTIONS

When using microswitches and battery devices, it is important to consider the patient's responses and needs. Watch for seizures and signs of boredom, fear or annoyance. Change or stop the activity in response to the patient's behavior.

Low voltage battery-operated devices will not cause an electric shock. They do, however, contain battery acid, so care must be taken to ensure that patients do not put them in or near their mouths.

The type of solder commonly used to join electrical connections contains lead; therefore, never let patients put these soldered parts in their mouths. Exposed soldered areas can be easily covered with electrical tape or electrical solder that is 100 per cent tin can be used.

The switches discussed in this chapter are to be used with battery-operated devices only. When using a tape recorder, run it on the batteries, *not* plugged into an elctrical socket. When in doubt, always consult with an electrician or someone with electrical expertise before using a device with a patient.

TREATMENT APPLICATIONS

The successful use of microswitch controls and other technical devices as treatment activities depends on the abilities and ingenuity of the occupational therapist and the assistant. Hundreds of controls are available, and not all are operated by a microswitch. Joysticks, mercury, toggle, grasp, breath control and voice-activated switches are examples of controls that are not operated by a microswitch. Treatment activities vary depending on the type of switch being used. A joystick can be used to assess a patient with quadriplegia for operation of a powered wheelchair. A mercury switch attached to a patient's head can be used to facilitate head control. The following discussion provides treatment suggestions for the Plexiglas pressure switch.

Tactile stimulation can be provided by placing different textures over the Plexiglas switch. Sandpaper, terry cloth, burlap, lamb's wool, felt and carpet pieces provide an assortment of textures for both stimulation and discrimination.

Battery-operated fans and vibrators provide sensory stimulation. When a pinwheel is placed in front of a fan, it spins and provides a stimulating visual activity. Brightly colored toys and lights can be used to encourage visual localization, tracking and discrimination. Auditory stimulation can be provided by toys that make noise, radios, and tape recorders.

By combining switches with therapeutic handling techniques, positioning of a patient can be maintained or inhibited. To encourage sitting, "on all fours," kneeling or standing, a patient may be placed in the position and required to place weight on the switch. The activity provided through activating the switch diverts attention and motivates the patient to maintain the position. To inhibit excessive or abnormal movement, the switch can be placed so that it turns on when the patient is positioned correctly and turns off with the undesirable movement, thus reinforcing the proper motor response.

Stacking blocks or various objects on the surface of the switch encourages prehension patterns. Squeezing the switch with the fingers to turn it on and off facilitates pincer grasp patterns. Switches can be used to train patients in developing headstick and mouthstick skills. Target areas can be placed on the surface of the Plexiglas and graded in size as skill develops.

Combined with specific interfaces, switches can be used with microcomputers. Computer software programs written to use the technique of scanning must be used with microswitches. **Scanning** is a technique that bypasses use of the keyboard and provides input directly to a cursor or an arrow that appears on the computer monitor. The user activates the microswitch to select specific characters. Microswitches combined with scanning techniques allow computer access for severely handicapped patients. See Chapter 13 for more information on this topic.

The use of switches also can provide leisure and entertainment. Adapted computer software games and modified toys are both enjoyable and educational. These activities offer the opportunity for patients to entertain themselves as well as a means to interact and socialize with others.

In many educational systems, the use of switches is included in the curriculum to teach cognitive skills. Concepts such as cause and effect, object permanence, and other early learning skills can be taught to children with handicaps. For example, a child learns cause and effect by understanding that if a switch is touched the toy will be turned on. Shape discrimination can be taught by placing a switch in a formboard. If the child places the shape in the correct spot, the switch is turned on, activating a reinforcement for the right answer such as a ringing bell.

GOALS AND OBJECTIVES

Switches combined with various devices offer enjoyable, motivating and rewarding activities. As with all other therapeutic activities, the use of switches must be included in the treatment goals and objectives. They must be used with a therapeutic purpose. The following are four examples of goals and behavioral objectives that incorporate switches and devices into treatment sessions for children with severe handicaps.[3]

1. *Goal:* Patient will improve gross motor skills.
   Behavioral Objective: Patient will bear weight on extended arms for at least 30 seconds.
   Procedure: Assist patient into a prone position over a large bolster or ball. Rock slowly forward and place arms and hands on floor. Encourage weight bearing on arms by having patient push pressure switch with both hands. Record length of time for weight bearing on switch.
2. *Goal:* Patient will increase fine motor skills.
   Behavioral Objective: Patient will reach for and activate a pressure microswitch without assistance at least three times out of five trials given.
   Procedure: Position patient in a prone position over a body wedge. Place a toy and switch in front of patient. Encourage activation of the switch.
3. *Goal:* Patient will improve gross motor skills.
   Behavioral Objective: Patient will walk up one step with the assistance of a handrail for three out of five trials.
   Procedure: Place patient's hand on railing. Stand close but offer no physical assistance.
   Alternate Activity: Place large flat microswitch on a step. Encourage patient to step on the step and switch using railing and wall for support. The switch should be attached to a toy and be activated by stepping up.
4. *Goal:* Patient will increase fine motor skills.
   Behavioral Objective: Patient will place four objects into a container on request four of five cosecutive days.
   Procedure: Place a switch in the bottom of a container (dishpan, can, basket, etc.) and attach switch to toy, computer or tape recorder. Give patient a weighted object to place in the container, which is heavy enough to activate the switch. After patient places one object accurately, offer objects of lesser weight so that two, three, or four objects are needed to activate the switch.

SUMMARY

The application of small technical devices in the evaluation and treatment of individuals with severe handicaps is becoming a significant part of health care. Combined with the traditional skills of assessment; use of functional, meaningful activities; and the ability to evaluate performance through the achievement of goals and objectives, this new array of therapeutic intervention techniques offers challenging opportunities for the profession of occupational therapy. There appears to be an increasing need for this technology in many segments of the treatment population. Basic principles of electricity were presented, together with specific instructions for constructing a switch and an interface. Safety precautions and examples of treatment applications were also discussed. Since the role of occupational therapy personnel is not well defined in this area, it is open for expansion and exploration of new ideas and applications. The resource list in Appendix D details sources of supplies and other related information.

Editor's Note

The construction and/or use of the devices mentioned in this chapter may result in harm or injury if not used properly. The Author, Editor and Publisher recommend close supervision and extreme care in working with these materials and cannot accept responsibility for the consequences of incorrect application of information by individuals, whether or not professionally qualified.

Related Learning Activities

1. Construct a Plexiglas pressure switch and an interface.

2. Use the interface and the pressure switch with at least three different toys or devices.

3. What major safety factors must be considered when constructing and using switches and interfaces?

4. How can microswitch devices be used to assist in achieving gross motor goals?

5. How can microswitches assist in teaching cognitive skills?

References

1. Williams J, Csongradi J, LeBlanc M: *A Guide to Controls, Selection and Mounting Applications.* Palo Alto, California, Rehabilitation Engineering Center, Children's Hospital at Stanford, 1982, pp 5-7.
2. Wethred C: *Toy Adaptations.* Toronto, Ontario, Association of Toy Libraries, June, 1979, p 1.
3. Bengtson-Grimm M, Snyder S: *Daily Goals and Objectives Written for Severely Handicapped Using Microswitches.* Clinton, Iowa, Kirkwood School, 1984.

Computers

Sally E. Ryan, COTA, ROH
Brian J. Ryan, BSEE
Javan E. Walker, Jr., MA, OTR

INTRODUCTION

This chapter provides a basic understanding of computers. Large, central computers are discussed; however, emphasis is placed on the microcomputer because of its many uses in occupational therapy management, evaluation and treatment. These small machines have been described as enhancers or amplifiers of human ability.[1] They can assist in many areas such as increasing attention span, developing communication skills, mastering eye-hand coordination tasks, improving sequencing and memory abilities, performing auditory and visual discrimination tasks, problem solving, and controlling their environment. The computer also provides creative outlets through the use of word processing and graphics programs. Both cognitive and creative abilities are used when patients learn to develop their own programs. In many instances, adults with handicaps are finding that their computer skills are creating many new job opportunities and careers that were previously unavailable to them.

Occupational therapy departments are increasing their use of computers in providing patient assessment and treatment, as well as for performing tasks such as maintenance of patient records and generation of reports, budgets, and other word processing and data management projects. Use of the computer also allows access to vast quantities of health care information worldwide.

Microcomputers, also referred to as personal computers or PCs, are small machines that are relatively inexpensive, serve a variety of general purposes, and are easy to learn to use.[2] They do not require a controlled environment or highly specialized installation, and the space requirements are minimal. Many are capable of interfacing with large central computers. Battery-powered, portable microcomputer units can be operated in practically any location.

KEY CONCEPTS

- Basic and auxiliary equipment
- Relationship of input and output devices
- Fundamental programs
- Applications for individuals with handicaps
- Evaluation and treatment implications
- Precautions

ESSENTIAL VOCABULARY

Hardware

Firmware

Software

Byte

Disk drive

Modem

Joystick

Paddles

Mouse

Input

Output

Bulletin board

Networking

Environmental control unit

Central computers, also called *mainframes* or *macrocomputers,* are used primarily in large corporations, health care facilities, educational institutions, and government systems that must process great amounts of data and information. These computer systems can handle hundreds of input/ output terminals at the same time. For example, a corporation might install a terminal at the desk of all supervisors and managers and provide several for the secretarial group in each division. All of these people could be using a terminal at the same time, a system called time sharing. Engineers doing research and statistical analysis at home or at another location would also have terminals connected to the same system by telephone lines.[3]

COMPUTER TERMINOLOGY

To develop an understanding of how a computer works, it is necessary to know the meaning of the following basic terms. Terms and their definitions are presented in an order that identifies relationships among them, rather than in alphabetical order.

Hardware

Hardware refers to the computer and all of its electronic parts. It includes the keyboard, the wires and the electronic components inside the computer case. Hardware is the "brain" of the computer.[1] It is the central processing unit or CPU.[2]

Firmware

The flat electronic cards that occupy slots inside the computer are called **firmware** or boards.[2] They perform functions such as connecting the disk drive to the computer, expanding the computer's memory capacity, and increasing the number of characters that can be displayed across the screen. For example, a computer might come from the manufacturer with a 40 column standard display. By adding an 80 column board, the display potential is increased to 80 characters across the screen which is a great advantage in using work processing programs.

An adaptive firmware card (ACF) allows the use of a variety of different input devices, besides the keyboard, with standard software programs.

Software

Programs that send messages to the computer telling it to perform specific functions are known as **software.** They allow the user to communicate to the computer what needs to be accomplished. Software is stored in the computer's memory on both a permanent and nonpermanent basis. Software program operations are described using the acro-

nyms RAM meaning *random access memory* and **ROM** or *read only memory.*

RAM refers to the part of the computer's memory that receives information and data. The greater the RAM capacity, the greater the amount of information and data that can be stored. When someone describes a computer as "64K" they are talking about RAM. The literal message is that the computer has a random access memory of 64 kilobytes or thousands of bytes of RAM. **Byte** is a term used to measure units of computer memory storage capacity. Another way to think about software is that it gives ideas to the brain in the hardware, the computer.[4] When the computer is turned off, all RAM memory is lost. It is regained by reloading information from a software program (see Disk Drives).

ROM is a permanent part of the computer. Examples of ROM include mathematical computations and programming language such as BASIC (Beginner's All-purpose Symbolic Instruction Code),[2] which are built in to the computer's ROM memory. When the computer is turned off, ROM always remains.[4]

Disk Drives

The **disk drive** is a piece of peripheral equipment controlled by the DOS (disk operating system). It may be mounted directly above the computer in the computer case or it may be a separate "box" connected to the computer with an electrical cable. One of its main purposes is to send messages from a software program to the microcomputer's RAM memory. Some software programs may require the use of two disk drives. The disk drive is also used to save work on disk for future use. A tape recorder may be used in place of a disk drive; however, it is a much slower process and increasingly fewer software programs are available in this format.

Disks or Diskettes

Personal computers currently use hard disks, "floppy" disks, or diskettes for software programs. The latter are circular and made of plastic with a special magnetic coating that allows information to be recorded. The coating is protected by a vinyl envelope. The disk is placed in the disk drive and is activated to send information to the computer memory. This process is called *booting.* If the computer is turned off, the disk must be rebooted to continue the program. Floppy disks must be handled very carefully. Never bend them or touch the "oval window." Be sure that they are not exposed to excessive sunlight, heat, or magnetic sources.[5] Hard disks are made of rigid metal that has been magnetically coated. Although they are more costly than the plastic disks, they are capable of storing much larger quantities of information and allow faster access. Always make an extra copy of all program disks and store them in their protective envelopes in a secure place away from the computer work area.

Monitors

A monitor is another piece of peripheral equipment that is needed to see a display of computer information. The three main types are green screen, black and white, and color. The green shows green characters on a black background and is frequently used for word processing as well as other programs that do not require color. The black and white monitor is used in the same way. Color monitors are the most expensive but are very useful for graphics, games, and a variety of educational programs. A monitor is often referred to as a CRT or (cathode ray tube). A television set may be used in place of a monitor if it is compatible with the computer. If a television set is used, the display will not be as clear as that provided by a monitor. In technical terms, a monitor has higher resolution, which means it displays more lines per inch on the screen.[4] Display peripherals are referred to as terminals or video display terminals rather than monitors when they are a part of a large mainframe computer system.

Printers

Printers are available in four basic types: dot matrix, letter quality, laser, and ink-jet, with dot matrix currently being the most popular for internal daily work and letter quality or laser used for external communication.[4] A dot matrix printer will produce text in a variety of fonts or letter sizes. Many also produce graphics. The quality of the printed material depends on the density of the dots. Printers with high density dot systems can produce printed material that is almost the same quality as that made by a typewriter.[1]

Letter quality printers are most frequently used by people who do extensive word processing and must produce written work of a professional quality. Most of these printers have a "daisy wheel" that produces characters similar to a typewriter.[4] Some models also present excellent graphics.[1] Letter quality printers are more expensive than the dot matrix type.

Laser printers use electromagnetic material and light to reproduce precise images that resemble professionally typeset work. They produce material much faster than a letter quality printer and are more expensive.

Ink jet printers also produce precise characters of a professional quality, with a considerable reduction in operating noise.

Modems

A **modem** is a device that allows computer signals to be sent to and received from other computers over telephone wires. The term modem is a blend word for *modulator/demodulator*. It converts electronic signals received from a computer so that they can be sent through a personal telephone.[1] It also converts information sent from another computer so that it can be received by the initiator. Use of a modem requires a special firmware card in the computer.[4]

Joysticks

A **joystick** is another peripheral device that allows the user to interact with the computer. It basically sends six messages: on, off, up, down, right and left, which are often used with games and elementary educational programs. It operates in the same manner as the computer's arrow keys and can easily be adapted for patients who are unable to control the handle. Methods used include increasing the size of the handle with foam rubber, placing a rubber ball over the handle, or constructing a specialized adaptation with plastic splinting material or plastic pipe fittings available at most hardware stores. A joystick is shown in Figure 13-1.

Paddles

A paddle or a set of two **paddles** may be used in place of a joystick. The paddle uses rotational movements that the computer recognizes and has an on/off switch. Paddles may be adapted in many of the ways described for joysticks.

Mouse

Another common peripheral input device is a **mouse.** This mechanism rolls on a small bearing that electronically guides the cursor on the screen. Its simplistic design often allows individuals with limited strength and dexterity to access the computer.

RELATIONSHIP OF INPUT AND OUTPUT EQUIPMENT

Operation of a microcomputer system requires correct electrical connections and a power source, most commonly a regular commercial current of 110 volts. Follow the directions in the manual *exactly* as they are described when setting up a computer. Figure 13-2 shows a typical work station and the relationship of input and output equipment. **Input** refers to the ways the computer can receive information or how it can be "put in." **Output** refers to the

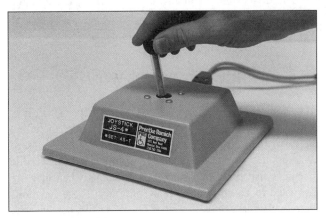

Figure 13-1. A joystick.

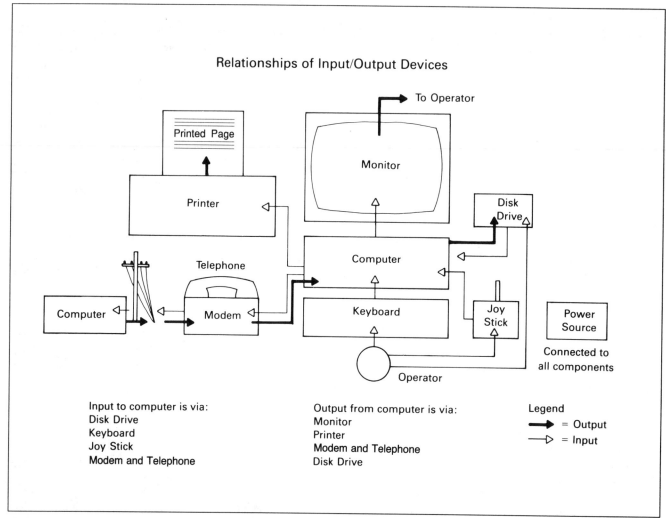

Figure 13-2. Relationships of input/output devices. © S.E. Ryan, 1985. Used with permission.

information that is sent from the computer or "put out."

Input on a microcomputer can be accomplished in a number of ways, including the activation of the disk drive to load a software program and use of a keyboard, joystick, mouse or a modem. In addition to being stored on a disk in the disk drive, output can also be produced by the monitor, the printer and the modem.

HOW COMPUTERS WORK

A complete description of the many aspects of how computers work would require several chapters; therefore, only very basic information on this subject will be discussed as it applies to microcomputers. Computers are versatile machines that perform a variety of functions when they are instructed to do so by a software program. These functions include playing games as well as operating file, spreadsheet, database, and word processing systems. The electronic mecha-

nisms within the computer respond to input from a number of sources and translate the information received into a binary system comprised of zeros and ones. For example, if the user types "MARY" on the keyboard, small electronic components, referred to as microchips, will convert the letter "M" into a binary code of zeros and ones and store it, together with the other input information, in the RAM or random access memory of the computer. The computer's memory might be compared to a block of post office boxes, where "slots" exist to save and categorize information.

To illustrate more clearly some of the computer's functions, the use of a word processing program written in BASIC in a diskette format will be used as an example. The first step is to put the word processing program into the disk drive and turn on, or boot up, the computer and monitor. The program is then "loaded" into the computer's RAM memory. Next, the user removes the word processing diskette from the disk drive and places an initialized "file" diskette in the drive. At that point, information can be entered via the keyboard or another type of input device.

Periodically, as the information is put in, the user can "save" it on the diskette by inputing the correct "save" command and entering a short title so that the information can be easily retrieved if needed. If the computer is turned off before the "save" command is entered, all of the information will be lost. If the user also needs a printed copy or "printout" of the material then the "print" command is used.

If it is necessary to add to the information at a later time, the user simply reloads the word processing program by placing the disk in the disk drive, turns on the computer, replaces the word processing disk with the file disk, and enters the "load" command. Once the information is loaded, additions, deletions and other modifications can be made. As the user continues working on the document, the "save" command must be entered so that all of the revisions are saved on the diskette. More information on the use of word processing is presented in the next section.

FUNDAMENTAL PROGRAMS

Certified occupational therapy assistants (COTAs) who are prepared to practice for the rest of this century and into the 21st century will find using a computer no more of a chore than dialing a telephone or driving an automobile. The "mystery and awe" that sometimes surround use of the microcomputer is gradually disappearing, and it will soon be a tool as common as a video cassette recorder or a microwave oven.

Much of the mystery has revolved around the differences between the concepts of the computer programmer and the computer operator. In the early days of computing, one had to be a programmer because of the relative complexity of computers and the lack of "user friendly" software programs. With the advent of more powerful microcomputers and the tremendous increase in available software, most occupational therapy assistants will be computer operators rather than computer programmers. This change opens up a wide variety of opportunities.

As a computer operator, the COTA may have access by terminal to either a large mainframe computer, such as one used by a hospital, or a microcomputer at a desk or departmental work station. Both can be linked to other computers for information sharing.

Information management is one of the most important features that the computer offers to occupational therapy service programs. With access to an electronic bulletin board or database, occupational therapy personnel will have instant access to information about a variety of health care subjects.

Currently, occupational therapy departments use a computer primarily for administrative purposes; however, use as

a therapeutic tool in patient evaluation and treatment is becoming more widespread. The following four basic computer software programs are in the repertoire of the COTA who is a literate computer user:

1. A word processing program
2. A database manager (DBM)
3. A spreadsheet program
4. A terminal program

Word Processing

A word processor is software that allows a computer to function somewhat like a typewriter. It permits one to compose and edit text; move, duplicate or delete entire blocks of text; check for proper spelling; identify poor writing style; and print the document with data inserted from the keyboard, from files and from a database manager or a spreadsheet.[6]

The word processing program has become one of the most popular programs for occupational therapy personnel. Many of the routine forms necessary for evaluations, progress notes, and discharge summaries can be placed on a computer to avoid unnecessary repetition. Either through the use of a terminal program to access a mainframe computer, or a microcomputer and a printer, the therapist and the assistant can manage more efficiently the information that must be completed for every patient receiving their services. In addition to patient information, letters, reports, patient education documents, public affairs information, and other routine pieces of frequently used printed material can be stored on diskette or in the computer's main core, and quickly called up for easy revision and printing.

Many word processing packages offer added features that may be helpful such as a spelling checker for the poor speller or typist, a thesaurus; a way to link parts of different documents together; or reproduction of forms and mailing labels that are frequently used.

One of the authors worked on a psychiatric ward at Walter Reed Army Medical Center during the 1970s, which allowed all pertinent staff members to record patient chart data on a computer using a word processing program. The individual patient charts were literally maintained on the mainframe computer and hard copies were printed only when necessary. The occupational therapy staff wrote their weekly progress notes at the terminal and were able to have instant access to all data relevant to the patient. Although this program was experimental, it is becoming the norm in many hospitals, nursing homes, and other treatment facilities.

The advantages of using a word processing program over pen and paper or a typewriter become obvious when the use of the program becomes routine. One of the problems with writing a note for a chart is that many therapists and assistants are not gifted writers, and they would like to revise their notes from time to time. Using a pen and a blank progress reporting sheet, the result can sometimes be a sloppy note with error markings or a recopied note. With the typewriter, revisions require either the judicious use of "white out" or the retyping of the entire note. In contrast, the word processing program allows instant revision. By merely moving the cursor—a visual electronic position indicator symbol—back a letter, a word, a line or a paragraph, revisions can be easily made. In addition, entire paragraphs or blocks of information can be moved, edited or deleted before the final note is saved for later storage or retrieval.

Database Manager

Database managers (DBMs) maintain a file or a group of items that are related. A recipe file on small index cards is an example of a noncomputerized database management system.[7] The DBM is another software tool that is being used increasingly in occupational therapy settings. It was created due to the demand for a system to efficiently manage the volume of information created on the computer. A DBM allows access to that information in a predetermined way.

The easiest way to conceptualize a database management system is to think of a personal address and telephone directory. When there is a need to recall the telephone number of an individual named Smith, one goes to the book and looks under the "S" listing. Assuming there are not hundreds of Smiths, the individual is quickly able to gain access to the correct number.

A DBM allows the same type of access, but with considerably more power and speed. For example, if the therapist wants to identify all of the patients in the hospital records with a diagnosis of myocardial infarction who have received occupational therapy services during the last six months, using the more traditional file card or file drawer system, he or she would review all of the occupational therapy records for that period and select or note those patients who met the criteria. Obviously, this task could be long and tedious in a large hospital. On the other hand, if the departmental records are a part of the hospital's mainframe computer system, or if the department has computerized its own files and maintained that information in a database management program, access to the needed data is relatively simple.

A COTA who is seeking this specific information merely enters in the required search parameters:

1. Hospitalization during last six months
2. Treatment given by occupational therapist
3. Diagnosis of myocardial infarction

Depending on the program, such a computer search could take a matter of seconds but no more than several minutes. The information could then be printed out on paper to provide a hard copy. If patients needed to be contacted to obtain information on a posttreatment questionnaire, the computer program would print the mailing labels. If a form letter was being sent, the computer could integrate the names and addresses of each individual in the selected group and repeat the patient's name in the body of the letter, thus personalizing each one.

The database manager can be used to maintain inventories, patient information files, mailing lists, bibliographies, routine treatment techniques, and other collections of data that may be too large to maintain in a simple office filing system. It should be noted, however, that a basic, old-fashioned file card system sometimes may be more efficient. For example, if the database contains fewer than 20 or 30 files, with minimal information in each file, it is much easier to open an address book and get the needed information than to boot up the computer, load the program, call for the data, and read the CRT or wait for a printout.

Spreadsheet Programs

A spreadsheet is a software program that manipulates numbers in the same way that a word processor manipulates words. Electronic spreadsheets organize data in a matrix of rows and columns. Each intersection of a row and column forms a cell that holds one piece of information. The cells are linked together by formulas. When the user enters data to change one cell, the spreadsheet uses the power of the computer to automatically recalculate and alter every other cell linked to the original cell.[8] With the increased emphasis on accountability in health care service delivery, particularly in hospitals, a spreadsheet program can be an invaluable tool for handling the day-to-day maintenance and analysis of numerical data.

The spreadsheet allows the computer operator to perform "what if" scenarios. The program makes it quite easy to project the budgetary effect of adding or eliminating an item or a category or items. Using traditional methods, this information could be obtained only after the time-consuming task of recalculating all of the budgetary figures had been completed.

Information typically needed in occupational therapy departments, such as daily treatment count, staff time sheets, budget, inventory, and other numerically based records, can all be easily maintained on a spreadsheet program. Once the initial format, or template, is established, it can be saved and used repeatedly for subsequent calculations.

Integrated Programs

Advances in technology have produced a variety of integrated software programs that combine a word processor, database, and spreadsheet in one package. Programs may be used simultaneously and information from one mode can easily be transferred to another. This feature is particularly helpful when writing reports that require the insertion of statistical information and other data.

Terminal Programs

A terminal program is a communications program that allows the computer to "talk" with the outside world. It is responsible for instructing the computer to send the characters that are typed through the telephone line to another computer, for establishing and maintaining the connection between the two systems, for making certain that incoming information is displayed correctly on the screen, and for performing other functions to enhance communications.[9] The capability for occupational therapy personnel to communicate with others through a computer system is perhaps the most promising aspect of computing.

One of the problems in a profession such as occupational therapy is that there is an ever-increasing volume of information. Maintaining access to this data through traditional methods can often be a cumbersome and time-comsuming task. The combination of a computer, terminal program, and modem, however, can open up the "whole world" of information on topics such as rehabilitation medicine. The modem, as described earlier, modulates and demodulates the computer's digital signals. Modulation occurs when the modem converts the information coming from the computer into audible sound signals that can be sent over a telephone line. Demodulation occurs when the modem takes the sound signals coming in from a correspondent's modem, converts them into digital pulses, and sends the pulses to the host computer.[9]

Bulletin Boards. Computers are frequently being used for information access. The information can be contained on an electronic **bulletin board.** Much like the corkboard in the office, computerized bulletin boards are established to relay information or send and receive electronic mail between computers. They exist as both private and commercial operations.

These two fundamental uses, gaining or exchanging information, are the primary reasons for using a terminal program. The former is frequently accomplished by contacting commercial networks such as COMPUSERVE, DIAGLOG or the SOURCE. Each of these boards allows one access to a variety of separate electronic databases. Most offer an on-line encyclopedia, the ability to track stocks, access to various news wire services, the ability to select flights and order airline tickets, or shop and do banking electronically. Researchers and consultants have compiled a large database of literature on scientific, medical and engineering subjects. More detailed information on bulletin boards may be obtained through most local libraries or computer centers at colleges and universities.

O.T. SOURCE was established by the American Occupational Therapy Association in 1989. It has three key components: databases, bulletin boards and electronic mail.

Features include a bibliographic search system, product catalog, personnel resource file, calendar of continuing education programs, association meetings and events, and a member question and answer service. More information can be obtained by contacting the AOTA.

Networking. The second use of a terminal program involves **networking,** or electronic interfacing of individuals via their computers to share information, seek answers to specific questions, or just talk with someone electronically. This feature is accomplished either by sending an electronic message to someone (electronic mail) or by simultaneously exchanging information from keyboard to keyboard.

COMPUSERVE, for example, has an online interest section for professionals and consumers interested in medicine. One can send a message to individuals or the general public, which will be answered by anyone accessing the special interest section. On many bulletin boards, conferences have been established to deal with specific subjects. Individuals who happen to be on-line at the preestablished time are able to comment and exchange ideas.

Several bulletin boards have been established specifically for health professionals. Some are operated by universities and medical schools and are quite costly, whereas others are being developed by professional associations or private groups and have very reasonable rates.

With access to a commercial or private board, there is little information that cannot be obtained. The sharing of information among individuals is helping to limit the isolation that occupational therapists and assistants often feel when working in small communities or within highly specialized treatment areas.

When a consultant or a supervising therapist is not on site on a daily basis, a combination of the word processor and a terminal package offers some unique options as illustrated in the following example:

An OTR is employed as an occupational therapy consultant and direct service supervisor at a nursing home. Because she travels to several communities to evaluate patients, communication with the COTA that she supervises at this home is sometimes difficult. The OTR and the COTA have found that using computers makes communication much more efficient. They use electronic mail to send each other messages and other information. For example, when the therapist has completed an evaluation, she sends it to an assistant for downloading and later inclusion in the chart. The COTA can request additional information or provide updates on the patient's progress at any time, and the OTR can access it at home or through her portable computer when away.

COMPUTERS AND THE HANDICAPPED

Small microcomputers offer great opportunities for people with a wide variety of disabling handicaps. In recent years, occupational therapy personnel have been collaborating with rehabilitation engineers and others to develop electronic systems that will permit individuals with handicaps to achieve independence in areas never before thought possible.[10] This is a problem-solving process, based on a comprehensive needs assessment, which results in the design of a system or systems that provide patient-controlled decision making and solutions that assist in achieving many goals. Table 13-1 shows some of the areas of patient rehabilitation that may be addressed.

Environmental Control

The **environmental control unit** (ECU) is an electronic system with sensors that monitors and performs a variety of tasks. This ever-changing technology usually includes a microcomputer and is capable of greatly increasing the independence of even the most severely handicapped individual. A person with a high spinal cord injury is now able to control the position of an electric bed or the operation of a television set, telephone, intercom system, light switches, and electronic door locks through the use of a properly designed environmental control system.

Instead of using the computer keyboard for input, a "suck and blow" tube may be connected that allows the user to send messages consisting of Morse code dots and dashes, which are converted to a form that is recognized by the computer.[11] The computer then relays the message electronically and a task is performed such as dimming a lamp. Voice-activated input systems are also available.

Environmental control systems can greatly enhance patients' independence, as they no longer have to rely on another individual to carry out some of the everyday tasks of living. In many instances they can remain in their own home instead of moving to a nursing home because around the clock care is no longer necessary. This increased independence results in renewed self-confidence and self-esteem.[12] Figure 13-3 illustrates the components of an ECU system.

Enhanced Communication Skills

The microcomputer, coupled with a voice synthesizer, can allow a patient with expressive aphasia to speak. A software program allows the person to simply type in such statements as "I am hungry" or "I want to go to bed" and they will be spoken audibly by the synthesizer so that they can be heard by others in the room. If an intercom system is in place, these messages can also be heard in other rooms. The voice level can be muted for conversations.

A voice synthesizer may also be used to facilitate communication for the blind. Braille "caps" can be placed over the keyboard keys, and the written material is then typed one character at a time and relayed audibly to the user. A Braille printer may also be connected to the system to allow the blind person to go back and review work that has been completed.

Communication does not require use of the alphabet. A young child with cerebral palsy who is unable to spell can interact with others by using a special keyboard overlay that has symbols and pictures. Messages can be sent to the screen and the voice synthesizer by pressing just one key.

For the person who has some knowledge of the alphabet, programs are available that allow programming of complete sentences of up to 250 characters that can be recalled with one or two key strokes. For example, a message that states "I would like to have a hamburger and french fries" could be assigned a simple letter code of "HF"; "I would like to go outside" could be assigned "GO."

People with hearing impairments are able to overcome their communication handicaps by using a microcomputer and a speech analyzer device with a special microphone input system. This device allows them to learn correct pronunciation, accent, and other subtleties of speech patterns. These systems literally allow the user to see the words they are saying by producing a graph on the monitor. The

---

Table 13-1
Suggested Justification and Uses of a Microcomputer in Occupational Therapy

A. Motor Training
  1. Games/programs to train severely handicapped in using specific motor functions
B. Fundamental Skills
  1. Basic cognitive functions such as attention, visual and auditory perception, differentiation and memory
C. Assessments
  1. Test batteries to assess memory functions, intelligence; several standardized assessments are now being computerized
D. Basic Educational Skills Training
  1. Preschool skills building
  2. Pre-reading
  3. Reading
  4. Typing tutors and keyboard skills
  5. Mathematics
E. Basic Living Skills
  1. Money management
  2. Buying and shopping
  3. Foods planning
  4. Job readiness and assessment
  5. Leisure (games designed to enhance motor coordination and learning as well as just fun)

From Rooney JA: Management information systems (MIS): Requesting the system. In Clarke EN (Ed.): *Microcomputers: Clinical Applications.* Thorofare, NJ: SLACK 1986, p 16.

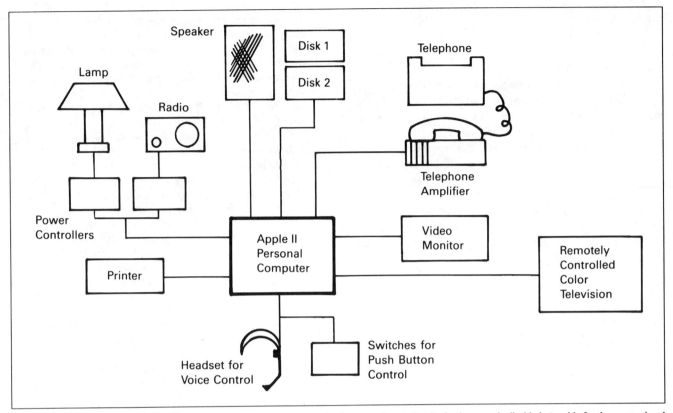

Figure 13-3. Components of an ECU system. From Wambott JJ: Computer environmental control units for the severely disabled: A guide for the occupational therapist. *Occup Ther Health Care* 4:156, 1984. Used with permission.

person repeats the word and tries to duplicate the graph pattern. When the graph pattern has been reproduced exactly as it appears on the screen, correct pronunciation has been achieved. People who do not have hearing deficits are using these programs to assist in learning foreign languages. Programs are also available that teach sign language.

Patients with amyotrophic lateral sclerosis (ALS), or Lou Gehrig disease, can become so disabled in the later stages of the disease that the only motor movements they can perform are swallowing, eye rolling, and raising the eyebrows. Through the development of an electronic eyebrow switch mounted on a special headband that is connected to the microcomputer, the patient can communicate. A software program directs the cursor to scan a group of letters on the monitor screen. When the cursor is on the desired part of the screen, the switch is activated and it becomes the first character in the message. While this is a time-consuming process in the beginning, after some practice, the patient is able to reproduce several words per minute. It is possible for him or her to write informal messages, letters, grocery lists, and other communications and have them reproduced on the computer's printer.

These are but a few examples of the many possible applications. Every day, advances are being made that offer a great variety of both basic and complex communication aids and systems.

Increased Employment Opportunities

People with handicaps are finding that microcomputer skills are "door openers" in the employment market. The ability to use a simple word processing program has allowed the previously unemployed to work at home as typists and free-lance writers and editors. The spreadsheet programs open up many opportunities for work in areas such as accounting, tax preparation and financial planning. Skill in using file programs allows many to fill positions that involve management of inventory systems and other data processing tasks for business and industry. Others who are skilled in the use of graphics and creative applications are finding jobs with advertising agencies and public relations firms.

Shadick[13] wrote about a woman with advanced multiple sclerosis who was able to continue her career as a loan investment advisor at home with a microcomputer, a printer, and a software program that had a spreadsheet and the capability of processing data to predict or forecast future trends. Crystal[14] provided a recent account of a deaf young man who had cystic fibrosis. He developed programming skills in seven different computer languages and is well on his way to a career as a free-lance computer programmer. An article in the *Washington Post* profiles a blind stock broker who uses a microcomputer with a synthetic voice system; *Information Thru Speech* (ITS) allows this account executive to carry out all of his job responsibilities.[15] As technologic advances increase, so will the employment opportunities for individuals with performance deficits.

New Leisure Pursuits

The opportunities for developing new leisure-time pursuits using a microcomputer are virtually endless. The great variety of games that involve one, two, or more players can provide many hours of entertainment and challenge. Programs such as bridge, chess and conversational foreign languages offer education as well as entertainment. Creative abilities can be expressed through the use of word processing and graphics programs. For example, the adolescent with a learning disability who would never have considered creative writing or drawing as a pastime is now able to use a word processing program and a graphics program to write and illustrate original poetry.

OCCUPATIONAL THERAPY EVALUATION AND TREATMENT IMPLICATIONS

Occupational therapy personnel now have a challenging opportunity to use microcomputers for evaluation and treatment of a wide variety of patients. The key to the successful use of computer activities depends on the skill of the therapists and assistants using them.[16] Care must be taken to match the best hardware, peripherals, adaptations and software programs to the needs and goals of the patient. Costs must also be carefully considered, particularly when complex systems are needed.

The following case studies give some specific examples of the effective use of microcomputers in occupational therapy [*Editor's Note:* Please see the information presented in the section on Precautions for Computer Use in this chapter]:

Case Study 13-1

Computer Assisted Rehabilitation for a Patient with Head Trauma. A 26-year-old man suffered a closed head injury in a motor vehicle accident. After treatment in an acute care hospital, he was transferred to a custodial facility with a diagnosis of severe vegitative state based on the Glascow Coma Scale.[17] Two years after the injury, he was admitted to the University of Texas Medical Branch Adult Special Care Unit with left hemiparesis. The patient was then classified as level two severe disability and was oriented to person but was disoriented to the environment. His attention span was less than five minutes. He was without problem solving skills, had severe left-sided neglect, and exhibited an inablility to cross the midline. He had incoordination $1\frac{1}{2}$ inches past pointing and poor dexterity, and all responses were severely delayed. He used a wheelchair for ambulation.

The occupational therapy program included peg and block

designs, range of motion, perceptual tasks, right and left discrimination activities, orientation to time and environment, and activities of daily living. Modalities were used to increase right upper extremity strength and to inhibit hypertonus of the left upper extremity. The patient began to learn bathing, dressing, basic cooking and laundry tasks. He was oriented to the hospital environment, played simple games, and joined in group activities.

Seven months later, computer-generated tasks were added to the treatment plan. A stimulus/response and discrimination software program, which measures latency of response times in averages of computer cycles as well as variance and number of errors, was used for an evaluation tool because of its concrete database. The computer indicates correct responses with an auditory tone so that the patient can receive immediate feedback, and after 15 trials a cumulative score is given.

One discrimination task requires the patient to respond to a 1-inch yellow square and to inhibit a response when a blue square appears. The randomly presented stimuli require the patient to cross the midline visually and to scan the screen, along with eye-hand coordination required to use the keyboard or the joystick. The patient was not trained on these programs to prevent overlearning and thus to ensure an objective evaluation tool.

The computer programs used for training were *Search,*[18] *City Map,*[19] *Driver,*[20] *Sequential,*[21] *Baker's Dozen,*[22] and *Stars.*[23] The cognitive skills required for these programs involve planning, organization, decision making, simple problem solving, attention to details, logical thinking and sequencing. Treatment goals focused on these areas.

On admission the patient had severe deficits in concentration and attention span, which interfered with his functional performance and self-care activities. The computer programs selected for him provided a mechanism for developing his attention span and increasing coordination. A year and a half after admission, the patient was independent in bathing and dressing and required only stand-by assistance for transfers. He was able to integrate visual field information, move his wheelchair through an environment with distractions, and had marked improvement in his ability to delay gratification.

Many computer programs are available for training patients. The programs selected for this patient have resulted in his improvement in activities of daily living as well as cognitive and perceptual skills. Originally diagnosed as severe vegetative state, the patient was reclassified as between severely and moderately disabled.[24]

Case Study 13-2

Computer Assisted Learning for the Child with Cerebral Palsy. Computer assisted learning was used with an 11-year-old boy with cerebral palsy (quadriplegic athetoid type) who is completely dependent for all activities of daily living. His head control, trunk control, and graded movements are all poor. He is nonverbal and uses a Bliss communication system, pointing to the symbols with his index finger. His cognitive abilities are age appropriate and he is a highly motivated person. For mobility, he uses a powered wheel-chair (Figure 13-4).

To address his educational plan objective, "improve written communication skills," the child used a microcomputer, a word processing program, an interface for the computer, and a single switch. The interface converts the input from the switch into audible Morse code signals that provide feedback to the user. A brief activation of the switch results in a single "dot," or "short," of the code heard as a one tone output. A longer activation results in a tone change, and the child can hear by the two tones that he has entered a "dash," or "long" of the Morse code. This code input is converted by the interface and displayed on the computer screen as keyboard characters.

The occupational therapist working with this child has used two types of switch placement. One consists of a plate strapped to his chest, at the top of which, directly below his chin, the pressure switch is placed. He activates the switch by depressing his chin while his arms are secured to his lapboard to provide stability and limited extraneous movement. The other method uses the same switch mounted on his wheelchair lapboard. His right forearm is strapped to a board that elevates his hand approximately two inches to the same height as the surface of the switch. In this manner, flexion of the wrist operates the switch.

Formerly using a head pointer, keyguard, and keyboard input, the child was capable of inputing one word per minute with a large number of errors. Through the use of Morse code, he is now capable of four words per minute with few errors. It is anticipated that his performance will improve as he memorizes the Morse code, as switch operation is mastered, and as input simplification methods (through the use of special interface codes) are introduced.

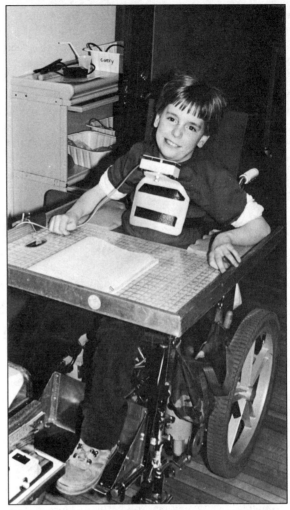

Figure 13-4. Child with cerebral palsy.

PRECAUTIONS FOR COMPUTER USE

Many individuals become so absorbed in the use of computer technology that it can literally consume their waking hours. Such people are often referred to as "hackers." It is important for occupational therapy personnel to carefully monitor the time periods that patients spend working on a computer. Since the lower extremities, trunk and neck often remain in a static position for a considerable length of time, it is necessary to make certain that work breaks are taken at frequent intervals and that proper positioning is maintained while the patient uses the computer. The computer and peripheral equipment should be placed on an adjustable height table to accommodate the individual needs of a variety of users. Adequate lighting must be provided, with glare reduction devices used as needed. Failure to take these measures may result in patients experiencing general fatigue, eyestrain and body aches, particularly in the neck and head.

According to Breines,[25] care should be taken when using computer programs for patients with cognitive and percep-tual disorders. Overemphasis on this treatment medium should be avoided. She has recommended further analysis and points to the problems inherent in using ". . .a two-dimensional tool for the resolution of a problem which derives from a three-dimensional dysfunction requiring peripheral (vision) input. . ."[25]

Breines also notes that furthur investigation is needed regarding the effects of computers for those individuals who are cataract prone or neurologically impaired. She has stated that since bifocal glasses are commonly used by the elderly as well as others, special near vision glasses may need to be substituted for these lenses when doing computer work.[25]

RESOURCES

The wide availability of computer resources may seem overwhelming to the new user. Among the many books on the market, one that is particularly useful to occupational therapy personnel is *Independence Day: Designing Computer Solutions for Individuals with Disability* by Peter Green and Alan J. Brightman.[26] In addition to specific recommendations for particular patient problems, an array of excellent resources are provided. Closing the Gap (see Bibliography) offers publications that are useful to both the new and experienced user of computers. It is also recommended that the reader refer to the "Software Review and Technology" column, a regular feature in the *American Journal of Occupational Therapy*. The bibliography at the end of this book lists additional information sources.

FUTURE DIRECTIONS

As technologic advances continue, opportunities for occupational therapy personnel to use computers will surely expand. The demands of the "information age"[26] will increase our reliance on computer systems to generate the information necessary to carry out everyday management and organizational tasks. For example, the use of bar code scanning, now common in grocery and department stores, will be used in health care settings to input data more quickly and to monitor varying changes more closely.

The Technology Assistance program, established by Congress in 1989, provides funds for states to help "establish programs for education, training, and delivery of assistive devices and services to disabled individuals of all ages."[27] Funding was authorized for $15 million for 1990. The availability of this money will certainly have an impact on our profession and those we serve.

Modern-day inventors, such as Raymond Kurzweil, are providing society with major innovations. Of particular note is Kurzweil's work on voice recognition as a means of computer input.[28] By simply speaking key words to the computer, a report or message can be quickly generated at the rate of 600 words per minute. Originally used by physicians for documentation purposes, this system is now available for health care professionals and their patients.[29] As the demand increases, costs are likely to drop. Kurzweil has stated that the Massachusetts Insurance Commission has ruled that physicians "who use the system are entitled to a reduction in malpractice insurance rates, since a study of reports showed them to be superior from a risk management point of view."[28]

Voice recognition systems are available also for individuals; however, the cost is currently quite high, resulting in limited access.[29]

The use of computer technology as a treatment modality will become even more widespread, as research studies continue to validate its effectiveness. Future research must also focus on identifying precautions and contraindications for specific problems. Work must continue to identify ways in which the use of computers and related devices can serve as a meaningful, goal-directed activity for recipients of occupational therapy services. We must establish standards for practice in all areas of technology as well as in quality assurance.

SUMMARY

Computers have numerous applications in occupational therapy departments. Once the user learns basic operations and related terminology, initial fears are replaced with new challenges. The variety of input and output equipment and devices and software programs available offer numerous opportunities for occupational therapy personnel to use computer technology in administrative tasks as well as patient evaluation and treatment activities. Word processors, databases, spreadsheets, and terminal programs offer ways to accomplish tasks in a much more efficient manner, thus increasing the overall productivity of the department. Small microcomputers offer many new opportunities to individuals with a variety of disabling handicaps. They are often an important tool to enable patients to control elements of their environments, enhance their communication skills, increase their employment opportunities, and develop new leisure pursuits. A great variety of computer systems and software are currently available.

Since use of computer technology is relatively new in the profession, care must be taken to exercise certain precautions, particularly with patients who have cognitive, neurologic, or certain visual impairments. Research must be conducted to further validate the use of computers in rehabilitation in general and in occupational therapy specifically.

Editor's Note
Only the most elementary terminology has been presented to acquaint the reader with basic information. Once one begins using the microcomputer and the many peripheral devices and software programs, efforts should be made to expand one's computer vocabulary and knowledge.

Acknowledgments
Case Study 13-1 was prepared by Ruth Garza, BS, COTA, former employee at the Occupational Therapy Department, University of Texas Medical Branch, Galveston, Texas. Case Study 13-2 was prepared by Mike Meyers, MA, OTR, Michael Dowling School, Minneapolis, Minnesota.

Related Learning Activities

1. Evaluate your skills in using the following programs: word processor, database, spreadsheet, and terminal. Identify areas in which more skill is needed, and enroll in the necessary classes or locate a knowledgeable person who can teach you.

2. Visit an occupational therapy department where microcomputers are used for evaluation and treatment. Prepare a report detailing the following information:

   a. Type of equipment used, including peripherals and input devices.

   b. Diagnostic groups or problems being treated.

   c. Goals being achieved

   d. Precautions and limitations

3. Visit a computer store and try out at least six demonstration programs. Identify programs that might be used in an OT program and specific goals that might be addressed.

4. What are some of the ways a computer could be used (or usage could be increased) in your classroom or clinic?

5. How could a computer be used with patients in a psychiatric setting?

References

1. Gerstenberger L: *The Apple Guide to Personal Computers in Education.* Cupertino, California, Apple Computer, 1983.

2. Doerr C: *Microcomputers and the 3 Rs: A Guide for Teachers.* Rochelle Park, New Jersey, Hayden, 1979.

3. Edwards J, Ellis A, Richardson D: *Computer Applications in Instruction: A Teacher's Guide to Selection and Use.* Hanover, New Hampshire, Timeshare, 1978, p. 13.

4. Sanders WB: *The Elementary Apple.* Chatsworth, California, Datamost, 1983.

5. Poole I: *Apple Users Guide.* Berkeley, California, Osborne/McGraw-Hill, 1981.

6. Robinson D: Word processing guide. *80 Micro Anniversary Issue.* 1983, pp. 28-31.

7. Keller W: The database explained. *80 Micro Anniversary Issue.* 1983, p. 32.

8. Ahl D: What is a spreadsheet? *Creative Computing* 10:S-2, 1984.

9. Glossbrenner A: *The Complete Handbook of Personal Computer Communications.* New York, St. Martin's Press, 1983.

10. Gordon RE, Kazole KP: Occupational therapy and rehabilitation engineering: A team approach to helping persons with severe physical disability to upgrade functional independence. *Occup Ther Health Care* 4:117, 1984.

11. Romich BA, Vagnini CB: Integrating communication, computer access, environmental control, and mobility. In Gergen M, Hagen D (Eds): *Computer Technology for Handicapped.* Henderson, Minnesota, Closing The Gap, 1985, p. 75.

12. Wambott JJ: Computer environmental control units for the severely disabled: A guide for the occupational therapist. *Occup Ther Health Care* 4:156, 1984.

13. Shadick M: Disease was her key to success. *Call A.P.P.L.E.* 10:66, 1983.

14. Crystal B: Computers help the deaf bridge the gap. In *Personal Computers and the Disabled—A Resource Guide.* Cupertino, California, Apple Computers 1984, p. 7.

15. Williams JM: Blind broker takes stock with a talking computer. *The Washington Post,* Monday, July 18, 1983.

16. Wall N: Microcomputer activites and occupational therapy. *Developmental Disabilities Special Interest Section Newsletter.* Rockville, Maryland, American Occupational Therapy Association 7:1, 1984.

17. Caronne JJ: The neurological examination. In Rosenthal M et al (Eds): *Rehabilitation of the Head Injured Adult.* Philadelphia, FA Davis, 1983, pp. 59-73.

18. Anonymous: Search. *Cognit Rehabil* 4:26-27, 1983.

19. Anonymous: City map. *Cognit Rehabil* 2:24-26, 1984.

20. Anonymous: Driver. *Cognit Rehabil* 4:23-24, 1983.

21. Anonymous: Sequential. *Cognit Rehabil* 5:46-52, 1985.

22. Katz R: Baker's dozen. *Cognit Rehabil* 5:42-46, 1984.

23. Katz R: Stars. *Cognit Rehabil* 6:47-50, 1984.

24. Ben-Yishay Y: Cognitive remediation. In Rosenthal M et al (Eds): *Rehabilitation of the Head Injured Adult.* Philadelphia, FA Davis, 1983.

25. Breines E: Computers and the private practitioner in occupational therapy. *Occup Ther Health Care* 2:110-111, 1985.

26. Green P, Brightman AJ: *Independence Day.* Cupertino, California, Apple Computers, 1990.

27. Somers FP: Federal report. *OT Week* 3:60, 1989.

28. Lipner M: Raymond Kurzweil invents his own success. *Compass Readings,* April, 1990.

29. Joe BE: IBM gives voice to computers in rehab. *OT Week* 5:44, 1991.

Section IV
CONTEMPORARY MEDIA TECHNIQUES

Thermoplastic Splinting of the Hand

Constructing Adaptive Equipment

Contemporary media techniques are the focus of this section, which provides the reader with numerous opportunities to acquire new skills or enhance existing ones. Thermoplastic splinting and the construction of adaptive equipment are addressed specifically. Although other topics could have been included, those here are the primary areas in which the COTA should establish competency. Whatever media technique is used, the practitioner must be certain that the procedures are goal directed and are carried out properly and safely to ensure that the patient will derive the maximum benefit.

Thermoplastic Splinting of the Hand

Patrice Schober-Branigan, OTR

INTRODUCTION

The role of the certified occupational therapy assistant (COTA) in the area of splinting may be as varied as the environments in which assistants works. Hand splinting is certainly a technical skill; yet the judgment and knowledge of hand anatomy, biomechanics, and pathology that is required when determining what type of splint to use and for what period of time is considerable. Just as an appropriate splint can *enhance* function, an inappropriate splint cannot only fail in this respect, but may cause *harm*. Therefore, the COTA must work closely with a registered occupational therapist (OTR) to assure that the appropriate splinting is accomplished for an individual patient.

This chapter provides a basic introduction to hand splinting, including historical perspectives, basic principles and purposes, assessment considerations, techniques, and materials. With this background, the entry-level COTA will have some understanding of the many complexities of work in this area of practice. Once necessary knowledge and skills have been demonstrated, the COTA may be assigned to make static splints, such as those presented in this chapter.

The patient with a relatively *unaltered* hand (anatomically) would be best suited for splint construction by an entry-level COTA; making even a simple resting splint for a hand that has been moderately affected by spasticity, injury or rheumatoid arthritis can challenge even the most experienced therapist.

A COTA who works in a setting where a high volume of hand splinting is performed may become particularly adept in this skill. Continuing education, both formal and on-the-job, is essential, as new materials and techniques become available.

HISTORICAL PERSPECTIVES

Splinting has become a commonly used treatment in most physical disability clinics during the past 25 years, in part because of the availability of low-temperature **thermoplastic**

KEY CONCEPTS

Purposes and types

Biomechanical design principles

Construction principles

Construction techniques

Specific fabrication procedures

Impact on role performance

ESSENTIAL VOCABULARY

Thermoplastic

Memory

Functional position

Static splints

Dynamic splints

Joint creases

Deformity prevention

Anatomic arches

Bony prominences

Patient education

materials. These materials are extremely "user friendly," when compared to the old metals, fiberglass, plaster of Paris, and high-temperature plastics.[1-3] Before 1965, when Johnson & Johnson introduced Orthoplast®, therapists and assistants using high-temperature plastics, such as Royalite™, had to use ovens and hot mitts, make repeated fittings, and possibly even use plaster of Paris molds to fabricate what still may have turned out to be cumbersome and less than satisfactorily fitting splints.[2] With the introduction of Orthoplast®, a low-temperature plastic which could be heated in 160° F water, occupational therapy personnel were able to quickly cut and shape material, often with the use of a temporary Ace bandage, directly onto a patient's extremities, with little danger of burning the skin. There was finally a high probability of good fit and appearance, with construction requiring a fraction of the time and effort needed in the past when working with high-temperature plastics.

In the 1970s, other plastics companies introduced competing, low-temperature plastics including, Polyform® and Aquaplast®. The newer materials had similarities, as well as differences, when compared to Orthoplast®. Polyform® contained no rubber, and therfore, did not require the firm stretching that certain types of Orthoplast® splints sometimes required when molding. Polyform® was also a "drapable" material that rarely required the initial Ace bandage wrappings that were commonly needed for work with Orthoplast® to assure that it would conform to contours of the extremity. Unlike Orthoplast®, however, Polyform® had no "**memory**", memory referring here to the ability of a material to return to its orginal flat shape and size when reheated. WFR/Aquaplast® introduced a material that became transparent while warm and also did have memory.

Gradually, more and more materials have been made available, including those that combine some of the qualities of the original rubber Orthoplast® and the stretchy Polyform®. Currently at least six companies produce splint products, with most offering three or more varieties of materials. Each company has competed for a larger part of the splinting market and, in so doing, has tried to develop more easily used materials than those already in existence.

Other technologic advances have helped splint fabrication develop into today's highly regarded modality. The introduction of hook-and-loop products, such as Velcro, has eliminated the need for bulky buckles and straps. Self-adhesive hook-and-loop products, adhered directly onto the splint surface, have also eliminated the need for the majority of riveting that used to be required, once again simplifying the splinting process.

Developments within surgical medicine and the therapy professions have also provided impetus for splinting technique and material development. As hand surgeons and reconstructive burn surgeons began to realize the tremendously important roles that rehabilitative therapies such as occupational therapy and physical therapy could play in assuring optimal postsurgical results, occupational therapy personnel began specializing in these fields. Due in part to the high volume of daily, often complex, and diverse splinting fabrication required of these therapists, more and more innovative designs and construction techniques developed in addition to those developed in the more traditional, long-established clinics by therapists and assistants working with patients having central nervous system dysfunction and arthritis.

In the 1990s and beyond, OTRs and COTAs will find splint fabrication to be not only useful and challenging, but also a highly approachable and effective modality when treating their patients.

BASIC CONCEPTS, TYPES AND PURPOSES

Why Do We Use Splints?

Occupational therapy personnel have always been concerned with the individual's ability to function, and hand use is a critical element. What, in particular, must a hand do to be functional? Perhaps the easiest way to answer this question and to illustrate the components of hand function is to observe your hand as you reach to pick up an object. The majority of the time, your *thumb* will *oppose* your fingers, and your *fingers* will be partially *flexed*. Although we also use our hands for other types of grasp (ie, you may flex your wrist as you reach behind your back, or you may flatten your hand as you smooth blankets on a bed), most of the time this **functional position** is the most critical position in daily activities. Figure 14-1 shows the functional position of the hand.

When individuals experience any kind of disease or injury that threatens their ability to use their hands, we must try to assure them that they will still be able to assume the position of function. A flat hand is not functional for performing *most* activities and neither is a hand that has stiffened into a severely flexed position. The use of splints, together with exercise, engagement in purposeful activities, and rest, is part of a comprehensive rehabilitation program aimed at assuring maximal function. More specific examples are provided later in this chapter.

Types of Splints

Although a wide variety of splints are available, they can be divided into two basic types: *static* and *dynamic*. **Static splints** place and maintain the body part in one position. A static wrist splint does not allow wrist motion. It *holds* the wrist in a functional position as shown in Figure 14-2, which depicts a wrist cock-up splint. These splints may be fabricated from materials, such as plastic, metal, elastic

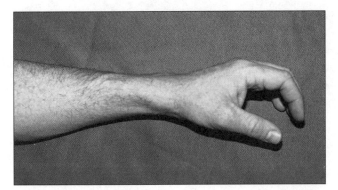

Figure 14-1. Functional position.

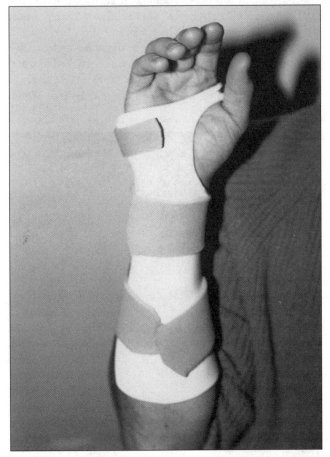

Figure 14-2. Wrist cock-up splint.

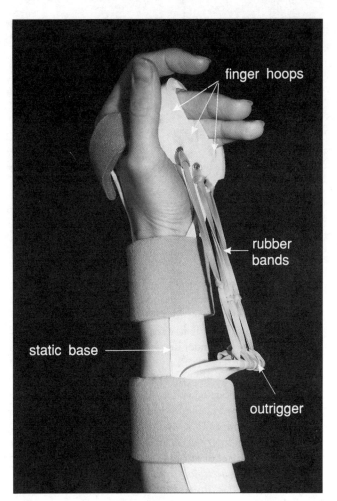

Figure 14-3. Dynamic MP flexion splint.

reinforced with metal, or leather. In contrast, **dynamic splints** allow for movement of the involved part. Usually, a force creates tension on a joint, encouraging extension, flexion or opposition. The part acted on is allowed to move instead of being held in one position. For example, rubber bands attached to leather or cloth loops may pull the metacarpophalangeal (MP) joints into a flexed position as shown in Figure 14-3. Another example is the use of a small spring-activated splint, which may assist in stretching the proximal interphalangeal (PIP) joint that has a flexion contracture into an extended position. Dynamic splints may combine any number of elements, such as a static splint used as a base, an "outrigger" of plastic or wire (see Figure 14-3), rubber bands, finger loops, elastic, rubber tubing, springs, pulleys, hinges and Velcro. Due to the complexity of dynamic splinting, which is beyond the scope of this chapter, readers are encouraged to refer to the references for further information and to consult with therapists who are experienced in this type of splinting.

In most cases, splints are named by the function they serve (ie, "wrist cock-up splint," "resting hand splint," "dynamic PIP extension splint"). Occasionally, names such as "anti-claw splint" as shown in Figure 14-4 or a "thumb spica splint" as shown in Figure 14-5 may need further explanation for COTAs who are inexperienced in working with splints.

Specific Purposes of Splinting

Splints may be used for any or several of the following purposes:

1. *Protection to allow for proper healing.* A physician may apply a bulky plaster splint to a patient's arm immediately after an acute injury such as a fracture or a tendon

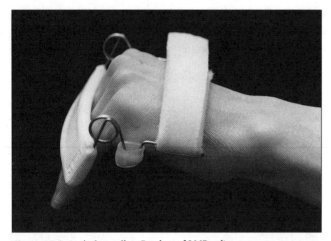

Figure 14-4. Anti-claw splint. *Product of LMB splint company.*

injury. If the physician desires a lighter weight, removable splint, however, the person may be referred to the occupational therapy department for fabrication of a thermoplastic splint. When an injury is not acute, as in the case of carpal tunnel syndrome or tendonitis, which develop over a period of time, the physician is likely to make a direct referral to occupational therapy personnel for fabrication of a splint or fitting of a prefabricated splint. An example is the Freedom Flex® splint shown in Figure 14-6.

2. *Decrease pain.* This often is also a goal of protective splints used after injury or of splints used when joints or soft tissues are inflamed or unstable, as in rheumatoid arthritis.

3. *Increase functional use.* The patient who cannot fully straighten the fingers after a nerve injury may use an "anti-claw" splint during daily activities; this splint serves roughly the same extending function as would the paralyzed muscles. Individuals with quadriplegia may also use functional splints that provide wrist extension and/or finger-thumb opposition. These are referred to as tenodesis splints.

4. *Prevention of deformity and maintenance of range of motion.* Any time a patient is unable to move a joint through its complete range of motion, the use of a splint may be indicated to **prevent deformity** and assist in maintaining range of motion. A person in a coma may have resting hand splints applied as well as lower extremity splints. An individual with rheumatoid arthritis whose MP joints are swollen, inflamed, and stiffened may use a resting hand splint, which places the MP joints in moderate extension, as this motion is typically decreased by rheumatoid disease. Figure 14-7 shows one type of resting hand splint.

Although there are a variety of approaches to splinting for spasticity, whether related to such diverse conditions as cerebral palsy or a cerebral vascular accident, a splint may be used to passively extend the fingers and wrist if the patient has overpowering tone in the flexors. In any of the preceding cases, active assisted range of motion

(ROM) and/or passive ROM exercise would be essential aspects of treatment. The splint would provide an important adjunctive function.

5. *Increase range of motion.* When a joint has limited ROM due to soft tissue tightness or contracture, static or dynamic splints may be used to correct it. Static splints that are regularly *refabricated* to provide increasing, gentle stretch are called *serial* splints. Dynamic splints that have moving parts controlled by springs or rubber bands may also be used and adjusted to provide increasing tension. Of utmost importance is that the tension be applied gently, well within the patient's pain tolerance, and that no adverse effects, such as increased swelling or stiffness, occur. The goal is never to "break loose" shortened or adherent tissue, but instead to gently stretch its fibers and allow the tissue to gradually elongate. In addition, if dynamic splints have outriggers, the line of pull from the cord or rubberband and finger loop unit to the outrigger must be at a right angle in relation to the part of the finger it is pulling (see Figure 14-3).

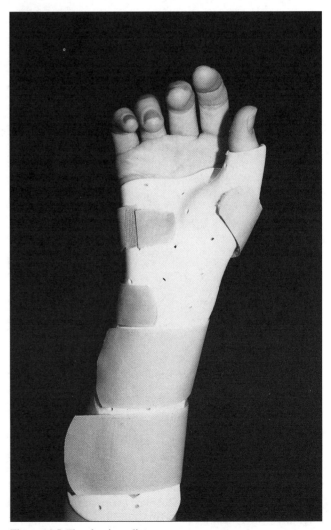

Figure 14-5. Thumb spica splint.

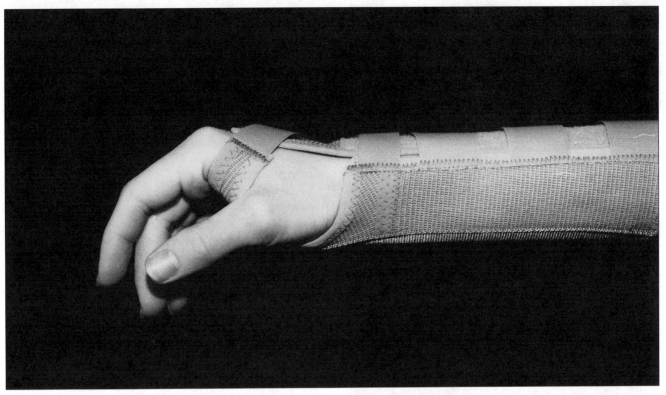

Figure 14-6. Freedom Flex® splint. *Product of Alimed, Inc.*

6. *Scar flattening.* The profuse scarring that occurs after some types of traumatic injury and severe burns may be minimized by proper pressure applied through the application of splints and pressurized elastic garments. As with dynamic splinting, readers who desire more information on this complex subject are referred to references cited in the bibliography.

ASSESSMENT PROCESS

Ideally, use of a splint is simply one part of a comprehensive rehabilitation program, so in most cases when a splinting fabrication order is received, the OTR is also completing a comprehensive assessment of the patient. The COTA may assist in some aspects of obtaining objective data, ie, measuring grip and pinch strength using a dynamometer and a tensiometer, respectively. He or she may also assist in observing and timing the patient's performance during standardized coordination testing, such as the *Minnesota Rate of Manipulation,* or measuring hand volume to monitor edema through the use of a hand volumeter device as shown in Figure 14-8. However, the patient referred to occupational therapy specfically for splint fabrication after an acute injury may be unable to tolerate this type of assessment. In addition, in some cases time and resources may be limited and

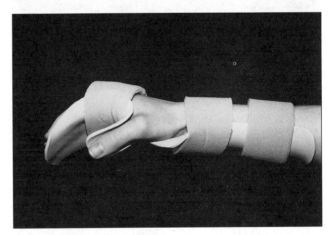

Figure 14-7. Resting hand splint.

completion of a full evaluation during the first visit will not be feasible if adequate time for splint fabrication is allowed. In these situations, the minimal assessment carried out by the OTR would require obtaining the following information:

1. Primary and secondary diagnosis
2. General health/functional status
3. Medical procedures performed, including surgery and exact dates
4. Healing status (if applicable, according to physician)
5. Goal(s) of use of splint(s)
6. Type of splint recommended

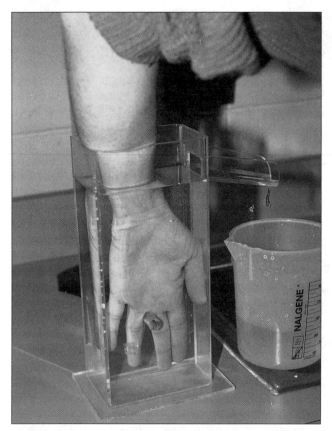

Figure 14-8. Hand volumeter for measuring edema.

7. Splint use requirements—full-time or intermittent (can splint be removed, and if so under what conditions?)
8. Precautions and restrictions
9. Is hand to be *used* with or without splint?
10. Description of location and level of pain, if applicable
11. Description of work duties, if applicable
12. Description of home duties
13. Description of sports and other leisure activities engaged in

Of equal importance, the occupational therapist needs to complete at least an informal examination of the incision (if any), skin status, degree of swelling (if present), sensation and, if possible, range of motion, muscle function, strength, endurance and coordination. If the individual is to wear the splint during specific work, home or sports and other leisure activities, an analysis of the motions required as well as particular tools, materials, and other equipment is desirable. Having the person demonstrate or describe the motions involved in carrying out these tasks is especially important to assure that the splint will interfere as little as possible with task completion.

The attitude of the patient toward wearing a splint and his or her understanding of its purpose is a critical factor. The best splint will accomplish little if the person refuses to wear it.

BIOMECHANICAL DESIGN PRINCIPLES AND RELATED CONSIDERATIONS

A splint should always be made in a way that gives primary consideration to the anatomy of the hand and wrist; the biomechanics, particularly of the involved limb; life tasks; and the abilities of the individual who must wear it. More specific biomechanical design principles are described in the following sections.

Immobilization

Any time a splint is applied to a body part, motion and sensation will be compromised and strength and function may decrease, depending on the length of time it is worn. Therefore, splints should be used only when the physician and the OTR deem them absolutely necessary and only on those parts of the arm or hand that must be immobilized.

Creases of the Hand

If full movement of specific joints is desirable, the splint must be "cut back" or folded over adequately, proximal to those specific **joint creases** (ie, grooves in the skin related to joint movement) as shown in Figure 14-9. For example, a splint that is used to immobilize only the wrist, not the thumb and fingers, should be cut back proximal to the palmar creases (proximal palmar crease for index and middle fingers, distal palmar crease for ring and little

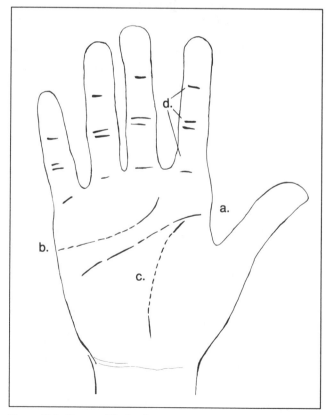

Figure 14-9. Creases of the hand.

fingers). If the thumb is to move freely, the thenar crease should be free.

Arches of the Hand

The human hand has three **anatomic arches:** the distal and proximal transverse arches and the longitudinal arch, as shown in Figure 14-10. The proximal transverse arch refers to the position of the wrist and carpometacarpal joints. This is a more rigid arch than the others and is only subtly visible externally. In contrast, the distal transverse arch refers to the more obvious and flexible arched position of the metacarpal heads that is visible as soon as the fingers are placed in any flexed position such as that shown in Figure 14-11. The long finger metacarpal head is at the highest part of the arch; the other metacarpal heads appear lower on each side. The longitudinal arch intersects the transverse arch longitudinally and is most marked centrally between the long finger MP and the wrist. When considered together, the arches assist hand function by allowing the fingers to rotate toward the thumb and providing a "deepening" of the palmar tissue to assist in securely holding objects in the palm of the hand.

When making a splint, one must be certain that these arches are preserved. The splint shape itself must be "arched" transversely and longitudinally if the patient is to use the hand when wearing it. Splints constructed from thermoplastic materials are particularly well suited to molding of this kind.

Bony Prominences

Bony prominences of the hand (the structures on the surface of bones) have little natural tissue padding and may experience skin breakdown whenever pressure is applied for long periods. The radial and ulnar styloids are two of the most common problem areas. These bony prominences are shown in Figure 14-12. Splints should provide relief over these areas. Taping padding over them before splint fabrication will provide "enlarged" relief areas when the splinting material is

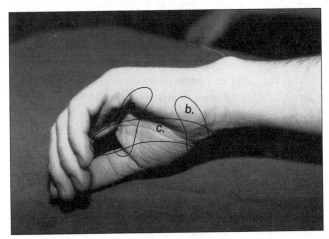

Figure 14-10. Arches of the hand: A. Distal transverse arch; B. Proximal transverse arch; C. Longitudinal arch.

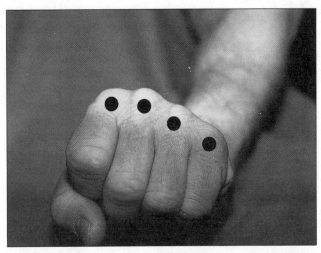

Figure 14-11. Distal transverse metacarpal arch.

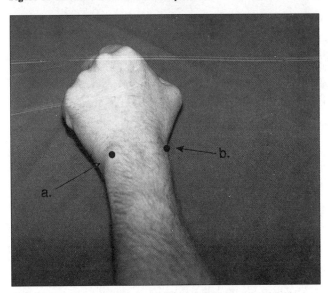

Figure 14-12. Bony prominences. A. ulnar styloid; B. radial styloid.

applied over the prominences. The padding can then be removed from the patient's arm or hand. Once the splint is completed, similar or thinner padding can be adhered to the same areas directly onto the inner surface of the splint. In many cases, however, the relieved areas themselves may provide adequate protection, even without padding.

The 2/3 Principle

Any time a splint must support the wrist or the wrist and digits, the forearm portion of the splint should extend two-thirds proximally up the forearm. This will provide adequate support for the weight of the hand and help prevent the wrist from inadvertently "popping up" out of the splint with hand use.

The 1/2 Circumference Principle

In order for straps to actually have contact with the arm or hand to *secure the splint* and to avoid slipping, the splint material should extend only one-half the circumference of the forearm as shown in Figure 14-13. This curvature also helps provide desirable rigidity to the splint and prevents any need for extra reinforcement, making the splint less cumbersome for the wearer.

Appearance

Splints should be visually acceptable for most individuals to agree to wear them. For example, plastic and strap corners should be rounded, and there should be no fingerprint indentations or ink marks. It is important for splints to be cleaned regularly and worn parts should be replaced or repaired. If dynamic splints have outriggers, they should protrude as little as possible away from the splint, yet still accomplish their goals, ie, flexion or extension.

TYPES OF MATERIALS

With the many advances in modern splinting technology has come greater complexity for occupational therapy personnel in determining which splinting material to select. Names and characteristics of the many materials available can become so numerous that the new practitioner may become overwhelmed. For this reason the following questions must be asked and related information considered to help simplify the decision-making process.

1. *What type of materials are already available in the clinic?* If material sheets are clearly labeled, the COTA can check the chart regarding characteristics (Table 14-1) or read the manufacturer's literature. In addition, occupational therapy personnel are using "1-800" telephone numbers (see Appendix F) to gain timely information. Certainly, observing experienced co-workers and allowing time to practice

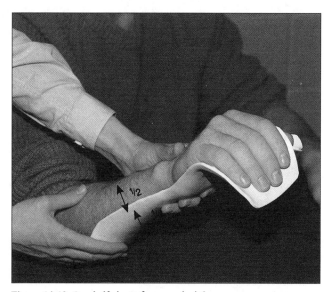

Figure 14-13. One-half circumference principle.

with an unfamiliar material would be most desirable.

2. *What type of splint is needed?* A more rubber-like* material that will not easily lose its shape or fingerprint may be especially good for:

a. the new COTA who may need to repeatedly reform the splint while fabricating it

b. an OTR who is used to stretching, pulling, and wrapping splint materials while forming them

c. an uncooperative patient or one with spasticity

d. a larger size splint with little need for intricate detail

e. a splint that may require a considerable amount of reforming over a period of days or weeks because of edema changes

In contrast, a highly conforming splint material, as described in Type C of Table 14-1, may be indicated in the following situations:

a. the therapist who is adept at draping, working with gravity, and using palms or heels of the hand to avoid fingerprinting

b. the patient is cooperative and does not require significant positioning or repositioning

c. for the burn splint or scar flattening splint when a high degree of detail is desirable

d. times when little need for reforming is predicted and no edema is present

e. construction of smaller splints such as those used for fingers

Some materials that combine rubber-like qualities with conformability are described in the Type B listing found in Table 14-1, and may provide a compromise.

3. *What other factors should be considered?*

Whenever splinting is performed it is also important to answer the following questions:

a. If the splint is to be worn for a long time over palmar surfaces (which may perspire), is perforation needed? Most splinting materials are available in perforated form.

b. Is an outrigger to be fabricated from plastic? If so, one of the more rigid materials may be needed.

c. Is long-term use probable (ie, when a patient has a chronic condition such as rheumatoid arthritis or tendonitis)? Perhaps a smooth, dirt-resistant surface is necessary to withstand frequent or near-constant use.

d. Is the splint very small or does it not require significant rigidity? Perhaps a $^1/_{16}$-inch material would be less obtrusive (check with manufacturers for availability, as standard thickness is $^1/_8$-inch for all material listed in Table 14-1).

e. Is the patient's hand particularly sensitive to touch or pressure or both? A drapable material may require the least therapist or assistant contact.

---

*The material may not necessarily contain *rubber*, but it resembles the rubber-like characteristics of Orthoplast®, which does contain rubber (see Type A in the chart shown in Table 14-1).

Table 14-1
Types of Materials

The COTA is encouraged to become familiar with the manufacturer's literature for any given material. This chart is intended to be a broad comparison of materials (see note 1).

Type A: Rubber-like materials—do not necessarily contain rubber but require stretching and tolerate handling; resist fingerprinting; minimal if any drapability

Name/Manufacturer and/or Supplier	Material Composition	Temperature/Time to Heat	Conformability when Heated	Memory*	Adherence to Self	Finished Product's Rigidity	Finished Product's Surface	Other Notes
Orthoplast® Johnson and Johnson	Isoprene rubber	150°/60 sec.	Requires stretching or wrapping with Ace bandage	Yes	Material should be dry and hot (use heat gun); solvent may enhance	Semi-flexible; requires contouring of edges and/or reinforcement to assure rigidity in finished splint	Absorbent	• Most well-known early thermoplastic • Higher priced than many thermoplastics • May shrink mildly when heated • May yellow with wear/age
Ezeform® Smith & Nephew/Rolyan	Plastic	160°/60 sec.	Requires some stretching; using Ace or firm touch may cause some indentations	Minimal	Dry and hot (may also adhere to lint and towels)	Very rigid	Absorbent	• May soil easily over time
K-Splint III® Fred Sammons	"	"	"	"	"	"	"	"
Synergy® Smith & Nephew/Rolyan	Plastic	"	Requires stretching	Yes	Dry and hot	Mild flexibility	Smooth/non-absorbent	• Available in colors
Ultrasplint® Polymed	"Rubber-like compound"†	"	"	"	"	Rigid	"	
Aquaplast GS (Green Stripe)® WFR Aquaplast Corporation	Plastic	"	Conformable, but least of Aquaplast® products	Yes	Available either in self-adherent (original) or non-adherent, which requires scratching surface or solvent; dry and hot	Rigid	Smooth	• Transparent when heated

Table 14-1

Types of Materials (continued)

Type B: Plastic materials—combine some need for and tolerance of stretching/handling (like Type A "rubber-like" materials), yet also some drapability (like Type C plastic materials)

Name/ Manufacturer and/or Supplier	Material Composition	Temperature/ Time to Heat	Conformability when Heated	Memory*	Adherence to Self	Finished Product's Rigidity	Finished Product's Surface	Other Notes
Polyflex II® *Smith & Nephew/ Rolyan*	Plastic	150-160°/ 60 sec.	Will drape, yet less than Polyform®	Yes	Solvent or scratch finish with scissors before heating; dry and hot	Rigid	Smooth	----
K-Splint Isoprene® *Fred Sammons*	"	"	"	"	"	"	"	---
Customsplint* *Polymed*	"Combination rubber-like/ plastic compound"†	160-170°/ 60 sec.	Will drape, yet less than Precisionsplint®	Some	Dry and hot	"Semi-flexible"†	Very smooth	• A newer material
Aquaplast* Original *WFR Aquaplast Corporation*	Plastic	160°	Highly conformable	Yes	Sticky without special preparation; requires care **not** to adhere inadvertently	Rigid	Smooth	• Transparent when heated
Aquaplast T® *WFR Aquaplast Corporation*	Plastic	"	"	"	Solvent or scratch surface; dry and hot	Rigid	Smooth	• Unlike original Aquaplast®, will not inadvertently adhere to self

Table 14-1
Types of Materials (continued)

Type C: Plastic materials are highly drapable and conformable to details; do not require or tolerate more that mild stretching or handling‡

Name/Manufacturer and/or Supplier	Material Composition	Temperature/Time to Heat	Conformability when Heated	Memory*	Adherence to Self	Finished Product's Rigidity	Finished Product's Surface	Other Notes
Polyform® *Smith & Nephew/ Rolyan*	Plastic	150-160°/60 sec. **Do not overheat!**	Highly conformable, drapable; duplicates contours of hand/body part	Minimal	Solvent or scratch finish with scissors before heating; dry and hot	Rigid	Smooth	---
K-Splint I® *Fred Sammons*	"	"	"	"	"	"	"	---
Multiform I® *Alimed*	"	"	"	Some	Dry and hot	"	"	---
Multiform II® *Alimed*	"	"	"	"	Solvent or scratch; dry and hot	"	"	---
Precisionsplint® *Polymed*	"	"	"	Minimal	Dry and hot	"	"	---
Aquaplast BS® (Blue Stripe®) *WFR Aquaplast Corporation*	"	"	"	Yes	Solvent or scratch; dry and hot	"	"	• Transparent when heated

©1990 Patrice Schober-Brannigan, OTR. Reprinted with permission.
*Memory: Ability to return to original flat shape/size when reheated
†Manufacturer's description
‡Except for Aquaplast BS®, which, unlike the other materials listed under Type C, does have a memory and will return nearly to its original shape/size if reheated.

Rather than deciding that any one material is best, the experienced COTA will discover that different splinting materials require the use of different skills and that individual materials may more easily lend themselves to one type of splint construction over another. When resources are limited or when splinting is only performed occasionally, occupational therapy personnel may prefer to keep a supply of one of the materials listed under Type A or Type B in Table 14-1, as these materials more easily withstand repeated handling without a significant adverse affect on appearance, strength or splint shape.

CONSTRUCTION PRINCIPLES AND TECHNIQUES

Equipment

To ensure the efficient and timely fabrication of a splint, it is essential to have available the correct tools, materials and adequate work space. The following furniture and tools, as shown in Figure 14-14, are necessary:

1. Small table and two chairs for patient and therapist
2. Countertop or table for equipment
3. Electric frying pan or other flat-bottomed pan and a heating device that will allow water to be heated to at least 160° F
4. Thermometer
5. Tongs
6. Heat gun with a funnel (for hard to reach or small areas)
7. Fiskars®-type scissors, preferably one pair for cutting splinting material and one pair for cutting straps
8. Curved blade scissors
9. Utility knife
10. Heavy duty shears for cutting unheated thermoplastic
11. Hole punch
12. Awl

It is also desirable to have access to a sewing machine; a machinist's-type, portable, table-mounted anvil; and a ball-peen hammer.

Supplies for Static Splinting

The supplies specified in the following list should be available:

1. Thermoplastic splinting material

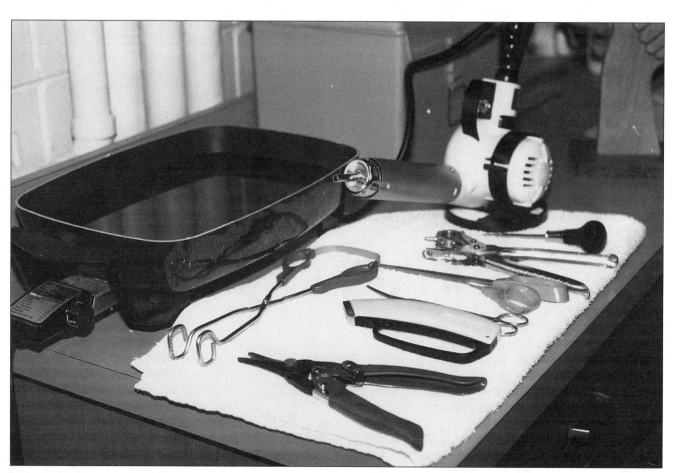

Figure 14-14. Splint construction tools.

2. Straps or rolls of 1-inch and 2-inch hook and loop Velcro
3. Padding (see note 2)
4. Paper towels
5. Ace bandage
6. Tubular stockinnette
7. Needle and thread
8. Rivets
9. Tape
10. Towels

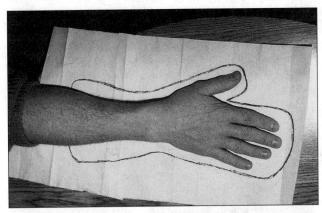

Figure 14-15. Making a pattern for a resting hand splint.

INSTRUCTIONS FOR SPLINT FABRICATION

Resting Hand Splint (Suitable for Someone with Rheumatoid Arthritis)

Materials. The following materials and tools should be located: paper towel, pencil, pen or awl, utility knife or heavy-duty shears, scissors with a curved blade, straps, hook and loop Velcro, Ace bandage (if using Orthoplast®), electric frying pan and thermoplastic material. The author recommends a more rubber-like material that is not highly stretchy or drapable for the COTA who is learning how to fabricate splints (see preceding information on types of materials and Table 14-1). A perforated material may also be desirable (to prevent an accumulation of perspiration) unless particularly rigid support is required. In this case, it may be better to use a plain, nonperforated material for fabrication and then drill several holes as needed for ventilation.

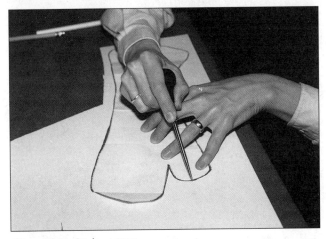

Figure 14-16. Tracing pattern.

Procedure

1. Heat water to 160° F.
2. Trace around hand to make a pattern, adding enough to extend one-half the circumference of the arm, fingers and thumb. If Orthoplast® or another material that shrinks is used, be sure to allow for shrinkage when making the pattern, as excess material can always be trimmed off. Conversely, if the material is likely to stretch, this factor must also be taken into account. The pattern will resemble a mitten. Check to be sure it extends two-thirds the forearm length (Figure 14-15).
3. Trace pattern onto thermoplastic material using a pencil or an awl. A pen is not recommended, as ink may be difficult to remove (Figure 14-16).
4. "Rough-cut" splint out of larger piece of material using heavy-duty shears or utility knife (Figure 14-17).
5. Place into pan—usually about one minute is sufficient for softening. Remove when softened and place on a counter or towel (Figure 14-18).
6. Cut out splint with scissors. If necessary, use smaller pair of scissors with a curved blade to cut thumb web space (Figure 14-19).

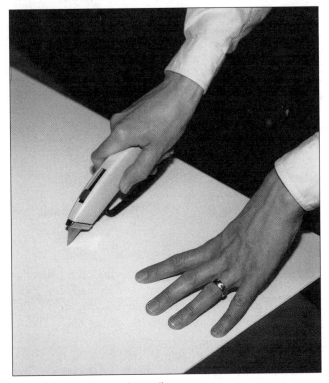

Figure 14-17. "Rough-cutting" splint.

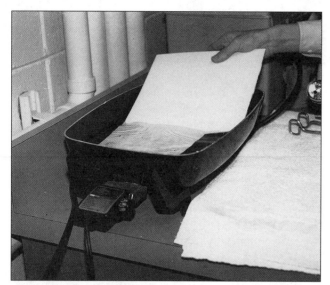

Figure 14-18. Placing material into pan.

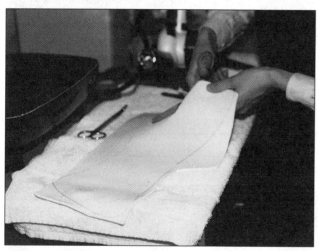

Figure 14-19. Cutting out splint.

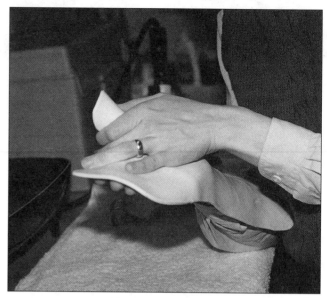

Figure 14-20. Preforming material.

type of material with several fingers or the palms of the therapist's or assistant's hands. Be sure to center it on the hand and arm so that the edge will be stretched around to make the "sides" of the splint. Avoid holding the splint on any one spot for an extended time if the material becomes fingerprinted. Check the position of the hand. Is the wrist in the desired position? Make adjustments as needed. Be sure to smooth the palmar area into the arches of the palm (Figure 14-21).

10. Optionally, gently wrap with an Ace bandage to form the splint if the material requires firm stretching as with Orthoplast®. Assure the thumb web position first; wrap throughout the palm and forearm; if necessary, return for the finger "pan" and thumb "gutter." Use another bandage if necessary. Again, be sure to mold palmar arches (Figure 14-22).

11. When the splint has cooled enough to appear formed, yet is still slightly warm (experience will develop a sense of timing regarding this step), ask patient to pronate arm. Confirm that splint is still centered on arm and adjust as needed. With a pencil or your fingernail, mark the edges of the splint material so that anything in excess of one-half the circumference of the arm will be trimmed. Splint should extend slightly beyond the fingertips and two-thirds of the forearm. Gently remove the splint when it is firm enough not to lose its shape, but still warm enough to trim with scissors. Trim. If necessary, dip edges into hot water quickly before cutting (Figure 14-23). Gently flare the proximal end of the splint so that it does not irritate the patient's forearm.

12. Assure fit on the patient. Gently stretch forearm trough by hand if it is too tight.

13. Round corners on straps near adhesive section (Figure 14-24).

7. Have patient assume functional hand position. Wrist should be in mild extension (15 to 30 degrees), MPs moderately extended (as close to zero degrees as is comfortable). PIPs flexed to approximately 45 to 60 degrees, and DIPs flexed to approximately 15 to 30 degrees; thumb in a gently (not maximally) abducted position from the palm. Have client supinate forearm in this position, if possible (see Figure 14-1; see note 3).

8. Place the thermoplastic material onto your own hand to assist in doing some "pre-forming," unless your hand size is vastly larger or smaller than the patient's. Remember which hand the splint is being made for (right or left)! Let the patient feel the temperature of the material before placing it onto his or her skin (Figure 14-20).

9. Place warm splint onto patient's hand. If the material drapes or stretches somewhat, the supinated position will allow gravity to assist. Work by briefly stroking this

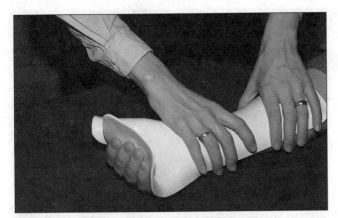

Figure 14-21. Placing of warm splinting material on patient.

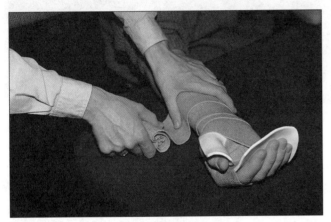

Figure 14-22. Wrapping with Ace™ bandage.

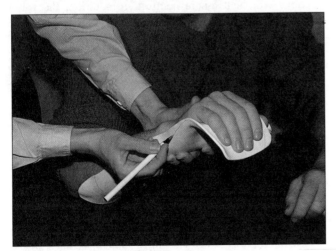

Figure 14-23. Marking splint before trimming excess.

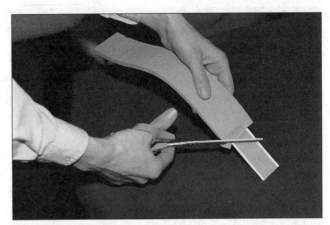

Figure 14-24. Rounding corners on straps.

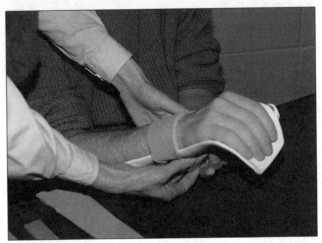

Figure 14-25. Adhering straps to splint.

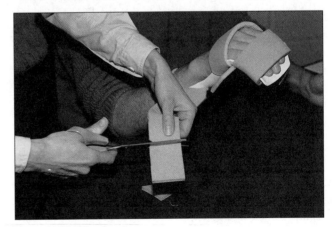

Figure 14-26. Trimming straps.

14. Adhere strap to splint (Figure 14-25).

15. Trim straps (Figure 14-26).

Figure 14-27 shows the finished splint when being worn by the patient.

16. Instruct the patient about precautions for wearing and caring for splint.

17. Check for irritating points (ie, at bony prominences, splint edges, and fingertips) and adjust as needed.

Wrist Cock-up Splint

Before constructing this splint, the reader is referred to the preceding section, "Resting Hand Splint" instructions, for a detailed discussion of fabrication. The following is an abbreviated discussion and assumes some familiarity with the splint construction process.

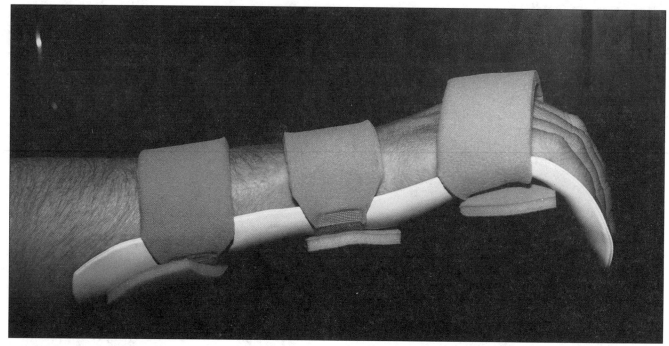

Figure 14-27. Completed resting splint.

Materials. Materials are the same as for the resting splint in the preceding section. A more stretchy, drapable thermoplastic material would be acceptable, although not necessary.

Procedure.

1. Make pattern by tracing around palmar surface of hand and forearm. Extend just distal to the distal palmar creases and lateral to the thenar crease to allow enough material for flaring splint edges. This technique adds strength and comfort (Figures 14-28 and 14-29).

2. Pre-form splint over own hand by flaring and folding over distal portion and thenar aspect (Figure 14-30).

3. Form the splint onto the patient. Be sure it is distal to the palmar creases and nearly clears (is medial to) the thenar crease; radial styloid should be free of pressure; lengths should be two-thirds of forearm. Remember to mold arches (Figure 14-31).

4. Trim edges so that one-half the circumference of forearm and two-thirds the length of forearm are covered by splint.

5. Attach straps.

6. Instruct patient on precautions for wearing and caring for the splint.

7. Check for points of irritation (ie, radial and ulnar styloids, thumb web space, dorsum of hand, and under edges of splint). Adjust as needed.

The finished wrist cock-up splint is shown in Figure 14-32.

SAFETY PRECAUTIONS

Finishing

Splints should be comfortable for the wearer. Adhering to the biomechanical principles presented in the previous sections will help assure comfort. In addition, the splint straps, the splint itself, or, if it is dynamic, its dynamic components should never cut off circulation or cause numbness. Fingertips must never be "blanched" by a splint. Edges should be smoothed.

Adjustments

Splints should be readjusted if they cause "wear" marks that remain on the skin for 15 to 30 minutes after the splint has been removed. Even if a splint is used to increase range of motion, its stretching properties must be carefully monitored and readjusted by the OTR so that stretching is done gradually.

The COTA may be involved in checking a patient's skin to assure that a splint fits properly. If adjustments are required to loosen the splint because of swelling, sometimes one is able to simply stretch the splint by hand without heating to make it wider or more narrow. With some of the more rigid materials, one may wish to use two pair of pliers to assist in stretching, being sure to protect the splint from plier marks by covering the areas with a towel (Figure 14-33).

Sometimes it may be necessary to carefully reheat parts of the splint by carefully dipping an aspect in hot water or by using a heat gun. In using the latter, the funnel may be

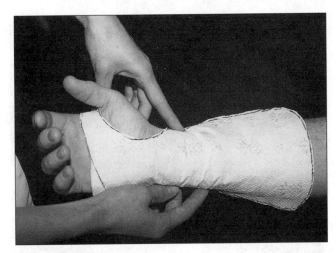

Figure 14-28. Make pattern.

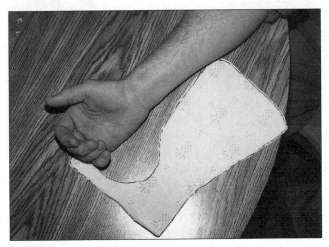

Figure 14-29. Completed pattern.

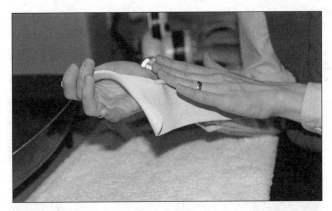

Figure 14-30. Preforming splint.

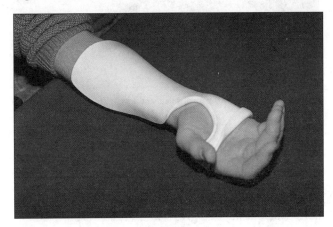

Figure 14-31. Forming splint on patient.

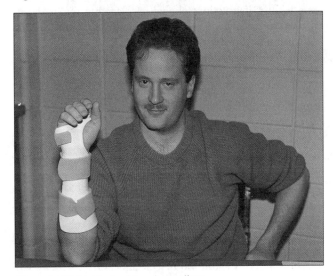

Figure 14-32. Finished wrist cock-up splint.

particularly helpful in directing heat to small areas. Splint straps may need to be repositioned to assure that the splint stays in place. If any of the these adjustments are made and problems are still evident, the splint may require refabricating, and possibly redesigning.

Problems may occur with perspiration or coldness (particularly when splints are worn outside). In these instances, the splints may require ventilation and/or the use of tubular stockinette worn under the splint. Ventilation can be achieved either by using perforated material when fabricating the splint or by punching or drilling small holes in the splint after construction. Holes should always be staggered in their placement to prevent weakening the splint (Figure 14-34).

In general, unless padding is essential for splint comfort and safety and is easily removable (does not stick permanently to the plastic or "gum" onto the plastic), it should *not* be used. Padding also may become rapidly soiled, another reason to avoid its use entirely. A 15-inch piece of tubular stockinette, with a hole cut for the thumb and worn under the splint, may provide a better lining. If padding of more than $1/16$-inch is required, it should be applied under the thermoplastic material as the splint is formed to assure proper fit of the plastic.

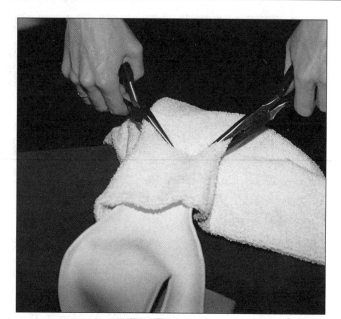

Figure 14-33. Using two pair of pliers and a towel to loosen/enlarge arm trough.

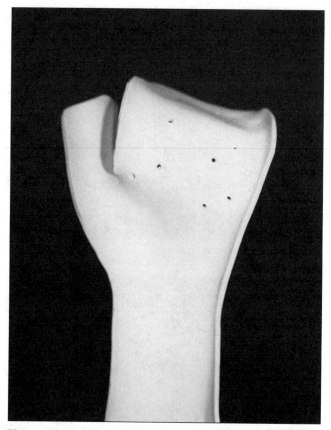

Figure 14-34. Holes punched in resting hand splint to allow for perspiration.

Patient Education

Both patients and their caretakers need to be shown exactly how to apply a splint properly and have opportunities to practice this skill under supervision. Written instructions should always be given, with illustrations if possible. If patients will be using the splint in a hospital or long-term care facility, instructions should be placed in the chart and also at the bedside. A sample instruction form for **patient education** is shown in Figure 14-35.

It is important to check the patient a day or several days after a splint is worn to assure proper fit and application. Even "oriented" patients have been known to experience problems with their splints when they unknowingly applied them upside down!

Patients and their caretakers should always be instructed to remove splints for cleaning and for range of motion exercises, if appropriate. If patients report increased stiffness, pain or edema, which persists after removal of the splint and exercise, the splint-wearing time, fit or design may need to be altered by the OTR.

Another important aspect of patient education is the need to caution patients about inadvertant heating of their thermoplastic splints. A splint left in a closed car on a hot day will be rendered useless if it melts into a flattened mound of plastic. Radiators, hot steam, or any intense heat source may also cause damage.

Other Considerations

No discussion of the topic of safety would be complete without including some specfic precautions that the OTR and COTA should follow in the clinic. They should develop habits of protecting their own hands by keeping sharp tools sharp and using them correctly. Adhesive that accumulates on scissors used for cutting strapping material should be removed routinely with a piece of cloth or gauze moistened with alcohol or a commercially made alcohol pad so that the scissors cut smoothly. Avoid touching hot materials; instead handle them with tongs.

Occupational therapy personnel also need to use good body mechanics, particularly to protect their backs. Rather than bending over to fabricate a splint, sit or kneel at the same level of the patient, as close as possible. The heating pan and cutting area should be on a countertop, to avoid unnecessary bending over a table.

Although chemical areosol sprays are available to speed cooling, occupational therapy personnel who work with splinting materials frequently should consider the risks of regular exposure to these sprays. The extra moments required for cooling without using them can be used for other purposes, such as patient education. Furthermore, if a splinting material requires use of a solvent or bonding agent, the COTA or OTR who is concerned about his or her exposure to chemicals should consider alternatives such as scratching the plastic surface with a pair of scissors before heating for adhering parts, or perhaps, choosing a more easily adhering thermoplastic. If solvents or bonding agents are used, it is important to follow the manufacturer's

NAME: _____

DATE: _____

Your splint was made especially for your hand, per order of your physician. The purpose of your splint is:

_____

_____

It is essential that your splint fit *comfortably* and *correctly*. Improper use could cause problems.

WEARING SCHEDULE

Your splint should be worn:

Daytime:

_____

_____

Nighttime:

_____

_____

PRECAUTIONS

Your hand:

If your splint causes any of the following problems, contact your occupational therapist so that adjustments can be made:
- Excessive swelling
- Severe pain (pain lasting longer than one hour after splint is removed)
- Pressure areas that last for more than $1/2$-hour after splint is removed
- Excessive stiffness

Your splint:
- Keep away from heat or flame. Your splint will burn or lose its shape.
- Cigarettes, hot water, or a closed car on a hot day are to be avoided.
- If any adjustments or repairs are necessary, contact your occupational therapist.

ATTACHMENTS

If your splint is equipped with an outrigger (rubber bands and slings), it is important to remember the following:
- A light, steady pull on your fingers is more effective for stretching stiff joints and safer than a hard pull.
- Slings should not cut off circulation of a finger or cause numbness.
- Rubber bands should provide a gentle stretch that you can tolerate for 20 minutes.
- If you can tolerate your slings for more than 20 minutes (without severe pain, decreased circulation or sensation), they may need to be tightened. Check with your therapist.

CLEANING YOUR SPLINT

- Clean with soap and lukewarm water daily.
- If perspiration is a problem and your hand does not have any open areas, sprinkle with baby powder before applying the splint.

If you have any questions, contact _____

Figure 14-35. Using and caring for your splint. *Developed by Patrice Schober-Branigan, OTR.*

recommendations and precautions regarding skin contact and ventilation. As health care practitioners, occupational therapy personnel should be especially cognizant of preventing occupational hazards.

IMPACT ON ROLE PERFORMANCE

The following brief case studies provide examples of how the use of splints impact on the individuals' role performance.

Case Study 14-1

Mary. Mary is a 42-year-old woman with rheumatoid arthritis affecting her hands and wrists. In addition to her comprehensive rehabilitation program, which includes rest, active range of motion (AROM) exercise, joint protection and energy saving techniques, heat and anti-inflammatory medications, she uses resting splints for her hands and wrists at night. She finds that her swollen MP joints and wrists are more comfortable, and she is able to sleep for considerably longer periods than previously. Although it has not been clinically proven, Mary is convinced that her splints are helping to minimize any deformity that is occurring due to her disease. This is particularly important for Mary's self-image, which is much stronger than when she was first seen by the occupational therapist. By carefully pacing her activities with periods of rest, using joint protection methods, and obtaining assistance for heavy household and yard work, she is able to continue to be actively engaged in her dual roles of corporate attorney and single parent of a 14-year-old daughter. She has also found time in her busy schedule to do volunteer work for the local chapter of the Arthritis Foundation.

Case Study 14-2

Bob. Bob, age 37, has a mild carpal tunnel syndrome of his right hand. His physician does not advise surgery at this time. Bob wears his wrist cock-up splint when his wrist is inflamed. In his position as a paper press operator, the condition does not interfere with his work tasks when he wears his splint, although he does use more shoulder motion with the splint than without it. Bob covers his splint with with tubular stockinette to protect it from dirt and ink. He removes it several times each day on work breaks to do gentle AROM exercises. An avid gardener, Bob has found that if he wears his splint under a work glove, he can continue to enjoy this pastime as long as he limits it to working with soft, well-cultivated soil for one hour or less. Bob continues to carry out the usual household tasks he and his wife have shared during their ten-year marriage.

Case Study 14-3

Susan. Susan, a single, retired accountant, age 63, fell on an icy sidewalk and sustained a Colles' fracture of her left wrist. The bones healed well, and she followed a regular regimen of specific exercise; however, her MP joints have remained somewhat stiff, and she is unable to bend them past 60 degrees active flexion. Her physician and the occupational therapist recommended that she use a dynamic MP flexion splint for 20 to 30 minutes, three to four times each day, followed by AROM exercises and exercises with therapy putty. She reports that the tension on the rubber bands feels gentle when she first puts the splint on, but by the end of each wearing period, her joints feel stretched. Each week, the occupational therapist readjusts the angle of pull, and after three weeks, Susan is now able to bend her joints to 80 degrees. She is beginning to resume her favorite retirement activity of golfing by practicing several times each week on a portable putting green as a part of her home occupational therapy program. In addition, she is now able to do the majority of her household tasks and shopping, the exception being lifting more than 15 pounds.

SUMMARY

This chapter provided a basic foundation of splinting for the COTA. Certainly the advances in thermoplastic technology over the past 25 years have made splinting a more approachable modality for occupational therapy assistants. Splinting principles, both anatomic and biomechanical, form the essential foundation for the assistant as he or she begins to fabricate and use splints. Careful assessment by the OTR/COTA team precedes meaningful implementation of a splinting program. Materials continue to grow in numbers and versatility; as the COTA becomes a skilled practitioner he or she will find that a variety of plastics will work well, as long as one is familiar with their properties and "feel." Furthermore, skill is developed in choosing the optimal material for individual splints and patient needs. Examples of two commonly used splints were illustrated with instructions for fabrication. Safety factors, including precautions, adjustments, and patient education were addressed. The impact of the use of splints on an individual's role performance was outlined in case study examples.

Notes to the Reader

1. Information for the Types of Materials Chart (Table 14-1) was drawn from a variety of sources including Orthoplast®, Smith and Nephew/Rolyan, K-Splint®, Polymed, Aquaplast® et al and Multiform® et al product

information; Schafer A: Splinting materials. *Alimed's O.T. Product News* 1(3):3-3, 1988-1989. Information was also provided by manufacturer's representatives; and the author's experience, which has focused primarily on work with Orthoplast® and the products of Smith and Nephew/Rolyan.

2. Numerous types of padding are commercially available. Personal preference of the therapist or assistant will determine choice. A $1/8$-inch to $1/4$-inch self-adhesive foam, which is easily removed from the splint, and/or a "loop" foam, such as Velfoam®, which can be applied to the splint with small pieces of hook Velcro, are especially practical. A thinner material, such as Moleskin® or Molestick®, may be required occasionally. All distributors of splinting materials also carry a wide variety of paddings, including those used as examples.

3. I prefer to use this "intrinsic minus" position, which gently counteracts the more common "intrinsic plus" imbalance (MP joints flexed maximally and DIP and PIP joints extended) and unstable thumb that commonly occur in rheumatoid arthritis.[4] This splint would not be appropriate for a person with the opposite type of imbalance, an "intrinsic minus" hand, because it would provide no counterbalance.[4] The COTA should confer with the OTR about goals for use of the particular rheumatoid arthritis splint being fabricated.

The modification of the resting hand splint originated at the Occupational Therapy Department of the Mayo Clinic, Rochester, MN, in the late 1970s and early 1980s. I have found this modification especially helpful for thumb comfort for patients with rheumatoid arthritis, while at the same time adding rigidity to the splint, negating the need for reinforcement, even when Orthoplast® is used.

Related Learning Activities

1. Experiment with at least one type of splinting material from each of the groups (A, B and C), as shown in Table 14-1, by making a small shoehorn. Identify problems as well as successes.

2. Construct a simple resting splint to maintain the functional position of the hand for yourself. Ask a person with experience in splinting to evaluate the splint you have constructed.

3. List at least six diagnostic groups or problems where splinting might be used.

4. Discuss important precautions that need to be considered when making splints.

5. List important points that should be discussed with the patient when presenting him or her with a new splint.

References

1. Reed KL, Sanderson SR: *Concepts of Occupational Therapy.* 2nd Edition. Baltimore, Williams & Wilkins, 1983, p. 222.
2. Shafer A: Demystifying splinting materials. *Alimed's O.T. Product News* 1(3):1, 1988-89.
3. Trombly C, Scott AD: *Occupational Therapy for Physical Dysfunction.* Baltimore, Williams & Wilkins, 1977, pp. 281-282.
4. English CB, Nalebuff EA: Understanding the arthritic hand. *Am J Occup Ther* 25:352-259, 1971.

Constructing Adaptive Equipment

Mary K. Cowan, MA, OTR, FAOTA

INTRODUCTION

The term **adaptive equipment** has been used throughout the course of occupational therapy history to describe assistive devices, aides, or pieces of equipment that allow a person with a handicap to participate in a life activity that otherwise would have been difficult or impossible. Although a variety of adaptive equipment is available for purchase, time constraints, budget limitations, and the uniqueness of the specific problem may require the construction of specialized devices.

Adaptive equipment is designed and constructed to assist with solving participation problems in activities of daily living, play or leisure, and work. Of primary importance is the development of appropriate aides that will increase independence in areas such as postural control, positioning, grasping, accessing and hand control, which will ultimately allow active participation in meaningful activities.

This participation will permit the individual to carry out important **life tasks** (activities that must be accomplished for successful living throughout the life span) and roles with a greater a degree of achievement and satisfaction.

Individually constructed equipment may be as simple as using a waxed paper box to hold playing cards or as complex as the design and use of computerized environmental control systems. Whether simple or complex, the focus of this chapter is to acquaint the reader with principles of construction and related applications for solving functional problems.

HISTORICAL USES

Early development of adaptive equipment such as page turners, card holders, and nail boards allowed the person with a handicap to read a book without using his or her hands, to

---

play cards with one hand, and to peel a fruit or vegetable when the person did not have use of a stabilizing hand. Although adaptive equipment was originally developed to provide improved ability to perform activities of daily living and participate in leisure pursuits, it also became commonly used as a term to apply to therapy equipment that helped the person with a handicap develop skills in therapy. Eventually balance boards, bolsters, standing tables, prone boards, and related equipment were designed and used by one or several therapists before they became standard pieces of therapy equipment.

Therapist-made equipment was a necessity for many years and only in recent times have many of these innovations been mass produced, marketed through catalogs, and readily available to occupational therapy personnel. However, this availability does not rule out the need for individually constructed equipment. The unique needs of the individual may require the design and construction of a device that is not commercially available or is too costly to purchase. These situations require the therapist or assistant to use **problem-solving skills** to determine the relationship between the individual's motor skill problem and the life task that needs to be accomplished and then construct a helpful tool to make participation possible. These skills include studying the situation that presents uncertainty or doubt, and arriving at the most likely solution. The process involves definition, selection of a plan, organizing steps, implementing the plan, and evaluating the results.

OCCUPATIONAL THERAPY PERSONNEL ROLES

The *Entry-Level OTR and COTA Role Delineation* describes the certified occupational therapy assistant's role in program planning as it relates to adapting techniques and media and selecting and using therapeutic adaptation (assistive/adaptive devices) under the direction of the registered occupational therapist.[1] As with other areas of treatment, however, close supervision by an OTR is required in situations where "patient conditions or treatment settings are complex (involving multiple systems) and where conditions change rapidly, requiring frequent or ongoing reassessment and modification of (the) treatment plan."[1] Designing and constructing a positioning device for a child with cerebral palsy, based on the theoretical principles of neurodevelopmental treatment, is an example where OTR supervision is required. A therapist with this specialized training should decide if the design and the final product do indeed fulfill the principles and intent of that therapeutic approach. Frequently, the COTA who works closely with an OTR in a complex treatment setting may be the individual with the most knowledge of tools and equipment and, therefore,

the one who will actually construct the needed equipment once the OTR/COTA team has determined the need and type of equipment required.

The COTA working in a setting where chronic conditions are prevalent is continually dealing with recurring functional problems that may not require the OTR's clinical involvement in the adaptive equipment decision-making process. The design and construction of card holders, book holders, and built-up handles on recreational games for people with physical handicaps are examples of situations where the COTA would not require close supervision.

Designing and constructing adaptive equipment, at various levels, can be a collaborative effort between the COTA and the OTR, but it must also be emphasized that the patient or client is the third partner in this collaboration. The individual receiving treatment will often exhibit or describe a problem that creates a need for adaptive equipment. The user gives the therapist or assistant feedback on the fit and comfort. Finally, the user determines the ultimate usefulness of the item by his or her choice to use it or not.

DETERMINING THE NEED FOR ADAPTIVE EQUIPMENT

Whether a piece of adaptive equipment is temporary or permanent, it should meet a **specific need** for the individual. Unnecessary use of specialized equipment has the potential for making any person feel additionally "handicapped." Therefore, it is important for the COTA/OTR team to be certain that the individual meets the following criteria:

1. Unable to complete the task without the use of aides
2. Understands the need for additional equipment
3. Is agreeable to trial or long-term use of the needed equipment

PRECAUTIONS

Whether a device is safe for use is determined during all three stages of the process of development: 1) design, 2) construction, and 3) use.

When designing equipment, safety must be considered so that time in construction is not wasted on a piece of equipment rendered useless later when it is discovered to be unsafe. In this context, **safety** refers specifically to the employment of measures necessary to prevent the occurence of injury or loss of function. Some questions the therapist or assistant should ask during the design phase are the following:

1. Will a breakdown of materials from ordinary wear cause discomfort or injury?

2. Will the shape of the equipment interfere with safe use of any other equipment regularly used, such as a wheelchair or crutches?

When constructing adaptive equipment, safety problems can be anticipated by eliminating rough finishes on wood, metal, or plastic and by sanding all surfaces, edges, and corners smoothly to prevent splinters, cuts, and bruises. It is also important to use nontoxic finishes, particularly for equipment used with children who might be likely to chew on it.

Instructing the patient or client in safe usage of equipment is the final step in making safe equipment. Observing the individual using the equipment and discussing with him or her where, when, and how to use it properly alerts the person to any possible misuse, therefore unsafe use, of equipment made by occupational therapy personnel.

CHARACTERISTICS OF WELL-CONSTRUCTED ADAPTIVE EQUIPMENT

Simplicity in Design

A simple design facilitates the construction of the device and increases the likelihood of it being used more frequently. An example is provided in Figure 15-1, the **Cowan stabilizing pillow,** an adaptive pillow for children who have balance problems when sitting on the floor.[2] The design's simplicity (eight sections of cloth, sewing of simple seams, filling with Styrofoam pellets) makes it possible for others such as therapists, assistants, volunteers, teachers, or parents to make more pillows when recommended for other children (Figure 15-2). The chance of the next item being made improperly is also reduced by having a simple design. Because a small, soft pillow is easily transported and easily stored in a corner of the classroom, both children and teachers will be more likely to use it. If the stabilizing seat had been made from a more complicated design (for example, a metal and leather seat with a backrest), it would be more difficult to make, move, store and use.

Size of Equipment

It is important that the size of equipment be controlled so that it does not become awkward or cumbersome to use. An example of this might be carrying devices for wheelchairs, such as lapboards or trays, armrests, and back pockets. Although anyone in a wheelchair may want to carry large items occasionally, making the tray or pocket too large may make daily use of the wheelchair cumbersome. The **half-lapboard** for patients with hemiplegia shown in Figure 15-3 demonstrates this principle by having a surface large enough to support the person's hemiplegic arm, without having the surface extending out to either side.[3] This thoughtful consideration allows the person in the wheelchair to avoid

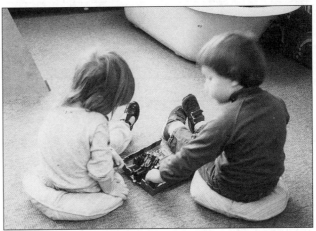

Figure 15-1. Cowan stabilizing pillow.

bumping into objects and people with extra or unnecessary tray extensions, and also allows adequate space to transfer in and out of the chair. (See reference three for specific information on how to construct this equipment.)

Cost of Materials and Construction Time

If a piece of adaptive equipment requires expensive materials, or if it takes a long time to make, the item is no longer **cost-effective.** The hourly wage of the therapist or assistant, as well as the cost of the materials, must be considered. Many hours of therapy time spent constructing one piece of equipment may increase the cost of that equipment to such a point that purchasing a similar item may prove less expensive, as well as a better use of valuable time.

The inexpensive **bolsters** shown in Figure 15-4 are designed for use with children under three years and demonstrate the use of economical materials. Mary Clarke, a COTA in Portland, Oregon, uses vinyl or oilcloth for the covering and lightly rolled newspapers for the interior.[4] The seam on the outside is closed with cloth tape. Larger bolsters can be made by taping empty three-pound coffee cans together, covering them with one-inch foam, and then adding an outside cover of vinyl.[4] She has also used large cardboard tubes from carpet rolls to provide the inner shape of the bolster, adding a layer of foam, followed by a vinyl covering to create the finished equipment.[4] All of these bolsters involve the use of economical materials and require very reasonable construction time. Because the bolsters are inexpensive, they can be provided to many families. In this way, it is possible to leave adaptive equipment in a home, a practice that is often not possible when similar, commercially made but more expensive bolsters are used.

Attractive Appearance

An unattractive piece of equipment, no matter how useful, can interfere with its potential use. People do not like to use equipment that is roughly made or battered from use or that

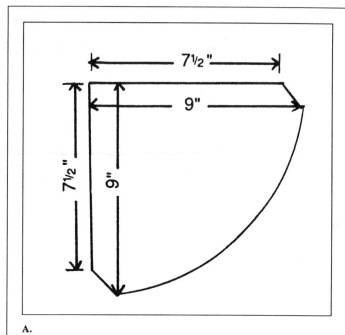

A.

Basic Materials
- 1¼ yards washable upholstery fabric
- Small Styrofoam pellets
- Heavy-duty sewing thread
- Graph paper, pencil and ruler for pattern making
- Pins, scissors and sewing machine

Instructions
1. Using paper, pencil and ruler, make a pattern as shown in Figure A.
2. Cut eight pieces of fabric to pattern specifications.
3. Using heavy-duty thread and a sewing machine, sew four pieces of fabric together to form a circle; repeat with remaining four pieces, as shown in Figure B.
4. Sew the two large circles together, leaving an opening of about four inches.
5. Reverse the pillow so that the finished outside is visible.
6. Stuff the pillow with Styrofoam pellets until it is approximately one-third to one-half filled (this makes it possible for the child to fit snugly into a "nest" of pellets).
7. Top-stitch around the edge of the pillow to finish and close the opening.

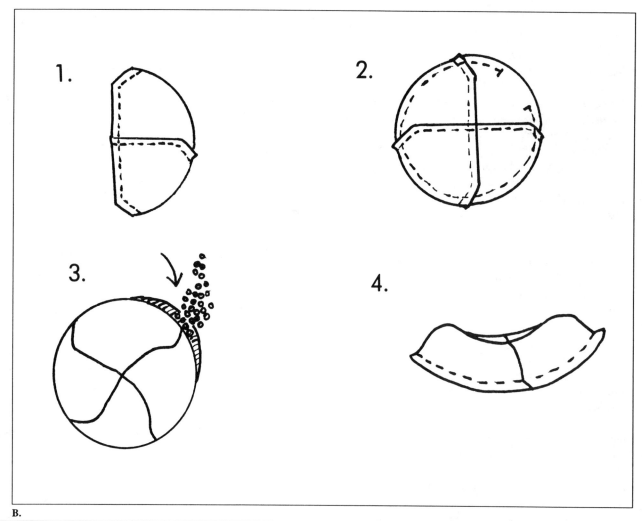

B.

Figure 15-2. Directions for constructing a Cowan stabilizing pillow for children.

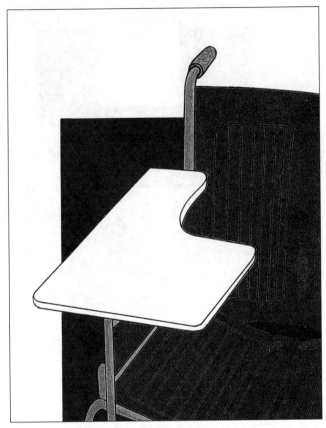

Figure 15-3. Wheelchair half-lapboard. *Adapted from Walsh.*[3]

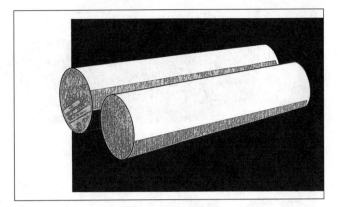

Figure 15-4. Bolsters. *Adapted from Clark.*[4]

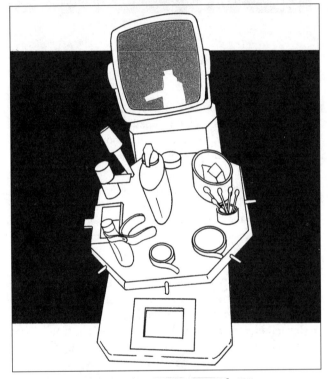

Figure 15-5. Make-up board. *Adapted from Hague.*[5]

has unappealing surfaces. For example, a waxpaper box makes a quick and easy piece of adaptive equipment for the one-handed card player. By covering the box with attractive vinyl wallpaper or other washable, durable material, it is not only useful but pleasant to look at.

Figure 15-5 shows an example of a makeup board designed for use by a women with quadriplegia.[5] It is simple in design and attractive without being medical or therapeutic in appearance and would be a natural addition to a woman's bedroom. (See reference five for specific instructions on how to make this equipment.)

Safety in Use

Although safety as a principle has already been addressed, it is an essential characteristic of well-constructed adaptive equipment that cannot be overemphasized. For example, if a stabilizer for a bowl or a pan used on the stove is not predictably stable, (ie, it can become easily detached from the surface), it serves no purpose. In fact, it complicates the already difficult task of working in the kitchen with the use of only one hand.

Comfort in Use

The comfort of the user is affected by the placement of the equipment when it is used, materials that touch the user's body in some way, and any fit that is required. A handle that requires the fit of a hand grasp or a situation where the body or extremities are resting on the equipment are examples that illustrate the need to consider user comfort. An example of this principle is the foam positioning device shown in Figure 15-6.[6] Because it uses soft foam as a basic material, it appears to be comfortable for long periods of contact with the skin, particularly when the person is immobile. (See reference six for specific instructions on how to make this equipment.)

Ease in Application and Use

The ultimate test of the ease in application and usage principle is to determine if the patient can apply the device

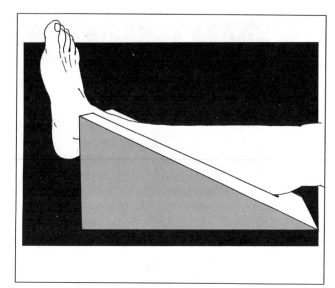

Figure 15-6. Foam positioning device. *Adapted from von Funk.*[6]

to himself or herself independently. If this is not the case, the individual(s) responsible for assisting the patient must be familiar with its proper positioning and use. The knitting device designed for use by a bilateral upper extremity amputee shown in Figure 15-7 is a good example.[7] The piece of equipment requires the use of a C-clamp and wing nuts (both of which the patient can manage with the bilateral prostheses) to attach the device to the table and to tighten or loosen the tension on the yarn. (See reference seven for specific information about how to construct this equipment.)

Ease and Maintenance in Cleaning

Simplicity in the design and choice of materials for any device makes it easier to maintain and to clean. A simple design eliminates corners, holes and crevices that collect debris that is difficult to remove. If the equipment is to be used with people who have infections or are highly susceptible to infection, the construction materials must withstand the intense steam or hot water required for adequate removal of bacteria. Most clinics or schools require that all equipment be washed or cleaned periodically to promote normal infection control. Nonporous surfaces such as plastic and metal are less likely to retain dirt or agents that cause infection, and heavier, porous fabrics that can be washed easily (such as upholstery fabric) are recommended.

DESIGNING ADAPTIVE EQUIPMENT

A Problem-Solving Process

The design of every adaptive device begins with a therapist or assistant and the patient facing a deficit in function together in a thoughtful, problem-solving process.

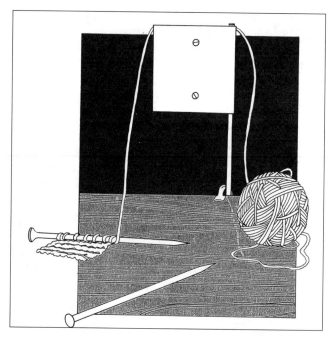

Figure 15-7. Knitting device for amputees. *Adapted from Duncan.*[7]

If the patient is unable to participate in an activity or to attain the position necessary for optimal work or task completion, new methods are tried and catalogs are perused for available equipment likely to alleviate the problem. In some instances, the problem will be solved only by designing a new piece of equipment.

Use of Patterns

Very early in the process of designing equipment, a pattern can be developed to guide the construction process. The Cowan stabilizing pillow (see Figure 15-1) provides a useful example. One quarter of one surface of the pillow was drawn on graph paper to establish the necessary size and shape. The paper pattern was then checked in relation to the patient's body or body part, and any necessary adjustments were made. All of the other examples shown in various figures in this chapter required a basic pattern for construction. The making of a pattern is an important step in the problem-solving process, as it guides the therapist or assistant in estimating size and shape of the piece of adaptive equipment. Errors in the construction phase will be reduced, thus increasing efficiency and reducing the cost of production.

Constructing a Model

Once a pattern has been developed, the next step is to construct the first model of the device. This step allows the patient and the therapist or assistant to discuss and experiment with changes in the design. This first model should be viewed as flexible and malleable, as well a experimental. At this point, the shape of the pattern can be changed, new materials can be tried, and dimensions can be altered.

Redesign After Trials

After any necessary redesign, the patient begins to use the piece of equipment. Some new problems may arise at this stage that inform the patient and occupational therapy personnel of changes that may need to be made. Only through a longer period of trial use can all of the patient's needs in regard to use of an adaptive device become completely clear. In **trial use,** a piece of equipment is repeatedly used in order to assure its effectiveness.

FABRICATING ADAPTIVE EQUIPMENT

Materials

This chapter does not present a complete list of materials and their characteristics for use in fabricating adaptive equipment; however, the following characteristics are examples of those that should be considered when evaluating or selecting materials:

1. *Softness and Pliability of Shape:* necessary for pillows, slings, positioning equipment. Use cloth, canvas or webbing; lamb's wool or "moleskin" for surface coverage; Styrofoam pellets, cotton batton, foam rubber or polyfoam for fillers.

2. *Resiliancy and Pliability of Shape:* needed for positioning devices. Use splinting materials such as Orthoplast™, tri-wall, acetate film, leather, rubber, vinyl.

3. *Strength, Solidity and Weight:* needed for laptrays, wheelchair arm suports, stabilizing equipment. Use wood, metal, hard plastics.

Tools

The materials chosen will determine the tools required to fabricate any piece of equipment. For example, cloth requires scissors and a sewing machine; splinting materials require scissors and a heating device; and the use of wood, metal or plastic requires hand tools or power shop equipment during the construction process. The availability of tools and the therapist's or assistant's skill in using tools contribute to the quality of the finished product.

Finishing

The final step in the construction of equipment is finishing. This step is of primary importance when one considers the emotional impact of equipment use for some patients. Rough or sharp surfaces and edges need to be sanded and rounded. Extraneous threads and uneven seams need to be trimmed and repaired. Finishes such as polyurethane varnish or nontoxic paint need to be applied to wooden objects. Colors selected may be neutral to deemphasize the equipment or bright and colorful to make equipment more attractive. The work of finishing adaptive equipment, like making furniture for a home, merits fine workmanship, with attention to important details, so that the product is both professional and attractive.

PRESENTATION TO USER

Whether or not the user of the designed and constructed adaptive equipment has been part of the collaboration process, when it is completed, the OTR or COTA should review the following information with the patient: 1) purpose, 2) uses, 3) limitations, 4) care and maintenance, and 5) any precautions. Even a young child needs to know that the stabilizing pillow "helps you sit better, or longer" (see Figure 15-1). The adult should know that the half-lapboard shown in Figure 15-3 places his or her affected arm in view to improve body awareness, control swelling, and prevent injury to an arm that lacks sensation. This review of the purposes of the equipment encourages proper use and, therefore, greater likelihood of its success. If the adaptive device is to be applied by another individual (nurse, aide, teacher or parent), the details of proper application and positioning must be presented to avoid any discomfort to the patient and to ensure safe use. On hospital and rehabilitation center wards, in classrooms, and in other community settings where several people assist the individual with equipment use, the placement of a diagram or picture of the equipment properly set up can be attached to the device as a helpful reference.

FOLLOW-UP

Follow-up is the final step of constructing adaptive equipment. Checking with the user about any problems that may have arisen gives the therapist a basis for modifying the equipment or improving its design for optimal function. If a particular device is used by many people, all of them should be followed and the fulfillment of the original purpose of the equipment validated with every patient. Questions such as the following can then be asked:

1. How many individuals have used the equipment?
2. For what length of time?
3. How successfully did it fulfill its purpose?
4. Should any modifications be made?

Compilation of this information will inform the COTA and the OTR who design and construct adaptive equipment whether the equipment is successful. If the equipment is also accepted and used by the patient or patients, it may be timely to share this information with other therapists and assistants through professional publication in journals and newsletters, as the examples provided in this chapter demonstrate.

SUMMARY

Construction of adaptive equipment is addressed within the whole continuum of design and construction that is a part of the occupational therapy process of problem solving. A definition of adaptive equipment is given, together with significant historical uses of such devices. The role of the COTA/OTR team was presented to inform the reader of the areas of supervision, collaboration and independent work. Principles are delineated for determining need, designing, fabricating, presenting the device to the user and follow-up. Important precautions and safety measures are stressed. Examples of well-constructed adaptive equipment are used to illustrate important considerations.

Related Learning Activities

1. List the criteria to consider before making adaptive equipment.

2. Study the characteristics of well-constructed adaptive equipment. Working with a classmate or peer, view at least five pieces of adaptive equipment constructed by therapists or assistants (visit clinics and use journal articles). Determine which characteristics are present and which are not.

3. Construct one of the pieces of adaptive equipment presented in this chapter.

4. Role play the presentation of a piece of adaptive equipment to a patient. Be sure to include the five factors stressed in the chapter.

References

1. American Occupational Therapy Association: *Entry-Level OTR and COTA Role Delineation.* Rockville, Maryland, AOTA, 1981.
2. Cowan MK: Pillow helps keep young OT clients "stabilized." *OT Week* 2(19):5, 1988.
3. Walsh M: Brief or new: Half-lapboard for hemiplegic patients. *Am J Occup Ther* 41:533-535, 1987.
4. Clark M: Unpublished material and personal correspondence, September, 1990.
5. Hague G: Brief or new: Makeup board for women with quadriplegia. *Am J Occup Ther* 42:253-255, 1988.
6. von Funk M: Positioning device has multiple benefits for patients. *Advance for Occupational Therapists* (August 21): 13, 1989.
7. Duncan S: Brief or new: Knitting device for bilateral upper extremity amputee. *Am J Occup Ther* 40:637-638, 1986.

Section V
PURPOSEFUL ACTIVITY AND ANALYSIS

Arts and Crafts

Activity Analysis

The last section may best be described as an integration of the preceding sections. It draws on historically significant principles, values and beliefs of the profession, as well as the core concepts of human development, the components of occupation, and occupational performance areas. Of equal importance are teaching and learning, interpersonal relationships and applied group dynamics, and the individualization of occupational therapy services, which concentrates on factors such as environment, society, change, and prevention. The analysis of activities used for evaluation and treatment requires knowledge and skill that is best drawn from experience in engaging in a wide variety of activities. Through experience one comes to know not only the properties of activities but also their therapeutic potential The chapter on arts and craft offers specific examples of how activities can be applied in therapy.

Activities are universal and are a cornerstone of the profession. As People, Ryan and Witherspoon have stated, developing skill in activity analysis allows the practitioner to "select the most appropriate activity, which is of interest to the patient, relates to his or her life tasks and roles, and provides opportunities for goal achievement."

Arts and Crafts

Harriet Backhaus, COTA

INTRODUCTION

The profession of occupational therapy is concerned with the pursuit of purposeful, goal-directed activity. Among the many activities available, arts and crafts are deeply rooted in our history and continue to be an important treatment modality in many areas of contemporary practice. Just as our early predecessors used tools to construct, create, repair and modify, we continue this tradition as tool users, remembering our past and passing on our heritage to future generations by making artistic and creative objects. The building of a simple, primitive birdhouse or the creation of a magnificent oil painting hold the same degree of value to the person who created it. Each represents the unique interests, knowledge, skills and asthetic interpretation of that individual. Moreover, the completed object offers an opportunity for self-expression and provides another personal link to one's environment. Additional benefits to the patient are numerous and will be discussed later in this chapter.

The use of arts and crafts has been an area of **controversy** in the profession of occupational therapy in recent years. Some practitioners have abandoned these treatment modalities altogether, whereas others have often found a need to defend their use. Those in the latter group might quote Eleanor Clarke Slagle, an occupational therapy pioneer and founder of the profession, who firmly believed in the value of using arts and crafts. She offered an eloquent defense to those who challenged using handicrafts as a therapeutic intervention, particularly during the machine age:

Handicrafts are so generally used, not only because they are so diverse, covering a field from the most elementary to the highest grade of ability; but also, and greatly to the point, because their development is based on primitive impulses. They offer the means of contact with the patient that no other does or can offer. Encouragement of creative impulses also may lead to the development of large interests outside oneself and certainly leads to social contact, an important consideration with any sick or convalescent patient.[1]

KEY CONCEPTS

Historical considerations

Conflicting practitioner values

Contemporary trends in utilization

Activity planning goals

Redefinition of arts and crafts

Rehabilitation applications

Relationships to decision making, work, leisure and social skills

ESSENTIAL VOCABULARY

Controversy

Purposeful activity

Documentation

Criteria of appropriateness

Activity analysis

Therapeutic value

Decision-making process

Difficulty level

Socialization

Work-leisure continuum

The debate over the use of arts and crafts as a method for therapeutic intervention will likely continue well into the 1990s. It will be necessary for each certified occupational therapy assistant (COTA) to examine carefully the historical significance of such endeavors, their contemporary use and interest, as well as future potential, before deciding whether to use arts and crafts as a legitimate tool of occupational therapy practice.

HISTORICAL ROOTS

Purposeful activity, defined as those endeavors that are goal-directed and have meaning to the individual, has, and continues to be, an important cornerstone of the profession. Susan E. Tracy, a nurse who has often been called "the first occupational therapist," noted the importance of activities for the mentally ill.[2] In 1910, some of her ideas were incorporated into the first book on activities titled, *Studies in Invalid Occupations: A Manual for Nurses and Attendants.*[3] It was primarily a craft book and stressed that the action of performing a craft activity was as therapeutic as the final outcome of the craft.

During World War II, occupational therapy schools trained therapists in crafts and occupations. The goal of treatment was to enable the patient to move from acute illness to vocational readiness as quickly as possible. In the late 1940s and 1950s, the profession was challenged by those who favored the medical model, which was becoming evident in other allied health professions. This approach forced traditional crafts to the background, as new treatment techniques were being developed and taught in the curriculum.

Later, some occupational therapy personnel found it increasingly more difficult to include the use of arts and crafts in treatment plans and treatment goals, due to problems with the **documentation** (written records of the patient's health care, including current and future needs) required as justification for reimbursement. As the dilemma became more pervasive, members of the profession continued to look to the sciences for increased credibility and respectability.[4]

CONFLICTING VALUES AND CONTEMPORARY TRENDS

The use of arts and crafts as an occupational therapy treatment modality has become a focal point in our professional literature and discussions. Two questions have arisen:
1. What exactly is the role of arts and crafts?
2. Why has their use decreased?

One answer might be that the therapeutic use of these modalities can be more difficult to document and justify than other structured and standardized activities with more easily reportable outcomes, such as repetition of an exercise or the amount of gross grasp that has been increased. This may be why some occupational therapy personnel view the use of arts, and crafts in particular, as giving a poor image to the profession. Some see the use of these activities as demeaning to the patient, whereas others report that there is not enough space, money or staff to support such programs.[5]

If the use of arts and crafts is indeed so difficult to justify to other members of the profession, to the public, and to third-party payers, what are some of the reasons supporting their use? The answers are complex and multifaceted. For example, many of the skills the COTA may be helping the patient to acquire through treatment can be accomplished by the careful selection of an appropriate activity, which well might include work on an art or craft project. To meet the **criteria of appropriateness,** the activity must fulfill the following factors for the patient:
1. It must be goal directed
2. It must be age appropriate
3. It must have some relevance and purpose

If these factors are not present, the patient may not comply in performing the task(s). For example, it is often difficult for an adult to accept the task of completing a peg board pattern, knowing that the activity was designed for use by a child. Although this activity may sometimes be viewed as necessary, the decision regarding its use should be carefully evaluated.

ACTIVITY PLANNING GOALS

When planning an activity to use in a treatment program, the COTA must consider the following goals/requirements for improving human performance deficits:
1. Attention to task
2. Coordination
3. Strength
4. Perceptual motor
5. Activities of daily living
6. Socialization
7. Leisure interests
8. Self-esteem
9. Time management

Two types of activities can address these goals and requirements. One activity does not produce an end product, such as completing a peg design. The other actvity has a definite end point, such as constructing a project using mosaic tile. Both activities can address increasing coordination and perceptual motor skills, but only one has an end product that represents the work achieved. Making a mosaic tile project can also address a leisure interest, may improve self-esteem and time management, and, depending on the structure of the task, provide some opportunities for socialization. The need to follow detailed steps, such as grasp and release of small objects, and squeeze a substance from a bottle, are also skills needed to carry out activities of daily living. In contrast, the patient who needs to spend a large portion of occupational therapy treatment time working on a peg design repeatedly to increase certain skills may experience frustration. This frustration may be amplified if the individual observes the therapist or assistant quickly removing all of the pegs after the work is completed. Although peg board design duplication does have importance, both as a diagnostic tool and a treatment technique, care must be taken to avoid its repeated use to increase certain skills. Perhaps a more long-term project with an end product should be used, an art or a craft that can provide an alternative to the usual treatment methods.

REDEFINING ARTS AND CRAFTS

Many members of the profession immediately think of traditional projects and kits when the therapeutic medium of arts and crafts is discussed. This is a limited view; one needs to look at many possibilities, such as the art of planning and planting a rock garden, the craft of repairing a leaky fawcet, the art of writing a poem, and the craft of baking cookies. In terms of the latter, much information can be obtained by observing a patient placing cookies on a cookie sheet. For example, size and shape perception can be addressed by observing if the patient makes cookies of uniform size and shape. If the patient puts all of the cookies on one side of the sheet, there may be a visual neglect problem. The same information can be obtained by using a peg board activity, but the bigger question must be answered: Which activity is the most appropriate and will provide the greatest benefit to the patient?

REHABILITATION APPLICATIONS

As stated previously, arts and crafts can be used to complement other activities in the treatment plan. The results of a survey conducted by Barris, Cordero and Christiansen in 1986[5] indicated that crafts were used more frequently in psychosocial occupational therapy treatment programs than in physical disability programs.[6] This practice may result because physical disability rehabilitation tends to rely on the use of strengthening modalities, such as pulley exercises and bilateral sanders and neurodevelopmental techniques. Although occupational therapy personnel in both settings offer treatment for activities of daily living, the physical disability centers tend to view arts and crafts as strictly a leisure pursuit, which is not commonly dealt with.

Once the registered occupational therapist (OTR) has completed an evaluation of the patient, both the therapist and the assistant formulate a treatment plan. The following are examples of some arts and crafts that could be used in achieving treatment goals.

Pediatric Applications

Offer activities to provide opportunities for gross motor manipulation of objects:
- Constructing simple clay slab projects
- Finger painting using palm and forearm
- Kneading and forming bread dough into loaves

Offer activities to provide opportunities for fine motor manipulation of objects:
- Stringing beads
- Constructing pipe cleaner sculptures
- Making mosaic projects with macaroni

Psychosocial Applications

Provide opportunities to make choices or decisions necessary for task completion:
- Leather stamping
- Stenciling
- Original picture painting
- Tile mosaic work

Provide opportunities to follow directions through adherence to clear procedures necessary to complete task:
- Macramé
- Cross stitch
- Basketry
- String art
- Leather lacing

Provide graded cognitive and functional directions to increase attention span and concentration:
- Embroidery
- Weaving on a harness loom
- Stenciling
- Macramé
- Wood kits

Provide opportunities for analysis and problem solving to complete task:
- Handbuilt ceramics
- Macramé
- Weaving
- Tile mosaics
- Wood kits

Provide opportunities to complete specified tasks or subtasks within established time limits:
- Painting
- Knitting or crocheting
- Mosaics
- Slip casting
- Embroidery

Physical Disabilites Applications

Provide activities graded for strengthening:
- Elevated inkle loom with wrist weights
- Sanding wood (for project)
- Handbuilt ceramics
- Leather stamping

Provide opportunites to use fine motor skills:
- Tile work
- Copper tooling
- Jewelry making
- Macramé

It is evident that some art or craft activities can address more than one treatment goal, depending on which aspect of the activity is emphasized. The COTA must always use the process of **activity analysis** to decide if the activity being considered is appropriate, given the goals of treatment and the interests of the patient (see Chapter 17). Activity analysis may be defined as the breaking-down of an activity into detailed sub-parts and steps. The characteristics and values of the activity are examined in relation to the patient's needs, interests and goals. Activities that do not relate to the interests, needs and goals of the patient are not appropriate and should be avoided.

TREATMENT CONSIDERATIONS

When the activity is introduced, the COTA must explain the **therapeutic value** of the particular art or craft to the patient to assure that he or she has a clear understanding of why active engagement in the activity will contribute to improved performance. Therapeutic value refers to the extent to which an activity or experience has potential for assisting the achievement of particular goals. Specific goals must be clearly stated. For example, if the selected activity is macramé, as a means of increasing strength and endurance, the patient should be aware that the problem of decreased strength of the upper extremities will be remedied by working on the project while it is suspended at increasing heights because work is performed against the force of gravity. The amount of time spent knotting the cord could be increased at specified intervals to increase endurance.

From time to time, patients may need reassurance. It is important for them to believe they have the necessary skills to perform the task. The COTA must assure them that the demands of the activity are not greater than their ability to participate.

Relationship to Decision-Making Process

COTAs often treat patients who have difficulty with the **decision-making** process (the process of weighing options in order to reach the best conclusion). These deficits may be the result of head injuries, psychiatric or neurologic dysfunctions, or, at times, prolonged institutionalization. Developmentally disabled individuals may also have a delayed acquisition of skills in decision making. Activities chosen for remediation of these deficits must be graded to accommodate the patient's current level of functioning.

It is important for the COTA to analyze the art or craft to determine the number of steps required, as well as the number of choices necessary to complete the task. A good example of grading a craft for the purpose of improving or developing decision-making skills is ceramics. Molded ceramic projects involve fewer decisions than hand-built projects. Certain steps can be carried out before the patient begins the project, such as pouring the slip into the mold, removing the molded object and cleaning it. In that way only two steps remain: applying glaze and firing. The number of glazes to choose from can be limited if the patient has difficulty choosing colors. As the patient gains greater ability in making decisions, the activity can be graded in complexity accordingly. The following decision making opportunities exist:

1. Choosing the mold to be used
2. Deciding when the project should be removed from the mold
3. Determining what areas need to be cleaned
4. Selecting which glaze(s) should be applied
5. Deciding how long the project should remain in the kiln
6. Determining how the finished project will be used

Alternatively, the patient can make clay sculptures or hand-built pots. The important principle is that the difficulty level of the art or craft used for treatment should increase as the patient's ability increases. **Difficulty level** is the degree of complexity that is required to execute a particular activity or step.

If a patient lacks opportunities to use decision-making skills, due to prolonged institutionalization, an art or a craft activity can be used. Initially, the decision might be choosing the color of paint or yarn to be used from only two possibilities.

Patients may also exhibit better decision-making abilities if they are motivated to participate in the activity. Hatter and Nelson[7] found that the decision of elderly residents residing in a nursing home to participate in a cookie baking task was higher among those who were told that the cookies were a surprise gift to a preschool day-care center than among those who were told to simply join a baking group.

The COTA can provide opportunities to enhance the patient's ability to function in the treatment setting, whether individually or in a group, by knowing his or her decision-making abilities. Allowing too many choices for patients who cannot make decisions adequately can cause disruptions in the treatment session and can be frustrating for both the COTA and the patient.

Relationship to Work, Leisure and Social Skills

Occupational performance areas include work and leisure skills as well as those necessary for self-care. The amount of time devoted to work and leisure changes as an individual matures and ages. The amount of leisure time that a child has is far greater than that of a working adult. Leisure time for a child can be considered play, whereas adult leisure pursuits are considered recreational or diversional and may include arts and crafts. As people age and enter retirement, the amount of leisure time increases again (see Chapter 7).

Socialization skills are needed at each stage of life. These are the skills that enable individuals to establish interpersonal relationships and social involvement. For children, good socialization skills are necessary for making friends at school, carrying friendships over into after-school activities, and to form the basis for later socialization. Often engaging in a craft activity, such as a group finger painting or collage, will strengthen these ties.

For some adults, socialization, work and leisure skills are interrelated (eg, participation in company-sponsored bowling leagues and baseball teams). Many of these adults may find that their ability to socialize changes greatly after retirement because they have not pursued independent leisure activities during their working years. Others, often referred to as "workaholics," are so consumed by their work that they never develop any leisure interests to use in retirement.

Changes in the amount of time spent for work and leisure activities can also be the result of disability or disease. The COTA can help the patient deal with these sudden changes by using information from the initial assessment regarding the individual's work history, leisure interests and social skills to plan a program to address any skills that may have been lost or altered. An important consideration is the disruption in the patient's daily routine and the degree to which the patient can realistically return to that routine. For some, the disruption can be expected to be short-term, such as recovery from a hip fracture. For others, the disruption can be long-term or permanent, as in the case of a cerebral vascular accident, spinal cord injury, or a particular psychiatric condition. The important point is to understand where the patient is in the **work-leisure continuum** (range of activities in which one engages throughout the life span, with varying amounts of time devoted to particular pursuits). To assure a good understanding the following questions should be answered:

1. Do new skills need to be taught, or can existing skills be adapted or modified?
2. Does the patient need to return to some type of meaningful employment, or do other activities need to be found?
3. Does the patient need to improve socialization skills to allow interaction in the workplace or other settings?

COTAs work in numerous settings providing treatment to individuals with a variety of performance deficits. Regardless of the specific treatment facility, the link between work, play/leisure and socialization is an important consideration when planning art and craft activities that are meaningful and appropriate.

Case Study 16-1

Janet. Janet is a 30-year-old married woman who is the mother of two children, ages five and seven years. She has been diagnosed as having leukemia and is an inpatient in the bone marrow transplant unit of an urban hospital. Her family resides in a small town 170 miles from the facility; thus her husband and children are able to visit only on weekends. She has frequently stated how much she misses them and that she feels "very removed and out of touch." It is estimated that Janet will be hospitalized about six weeks.

At initial evaluation, Janet had good strength and endurance. Due to the course of the bone marrow treatment, however, a decrease in strength and endurance could be anticipated. It was also necessary for her to remain active during the treatments.

After receiving chemotherapy and high-dose radiation treatments, Janet did experience decreased strength and endurance, as well as some disruption in concentration skills. The physical therapy department provided a program of exercises and ambulation, and Janet was able to perform light, progressive, resistive exercises and to walk 50 feet.

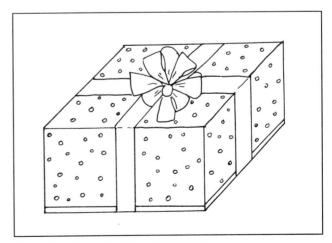

Figure 16-1. Completed gift box 2″ X 2″ X 1″.

The occupational therapy assistant, under the supervision of the occupational therapist, contributed to the planning and independently carried out a treatment program for Janet. The long-term goal was to prevent further debilitation due to the chemotherapy treatment by engaging the patient in vocational and avocational activities. Janet was encouraged to perform her own self-care activities, and she was taught energy conservation techniques to enable her to use her time more effectively and to reduce fatigue. Since she was not able to see her husband and children frequently, the assistant encouraged her to engage in a craft that would provide a meaningful gift for them and also required coordination and endurance.

Several small craft projects were presented to Janet, and she chose to make gift boxes out of wallpaper as shown in Figure 16-1. The boxes would be used to "personalize" small gifts for her family that she could readily purchase at the hospital, such as candy and hair bows. The activity of constructing the boxes would enable Janet to use both physical and cognitive skills, require sitting tolerance, and emphasize fine coordination skills and complex direction following (Figure 16-2).

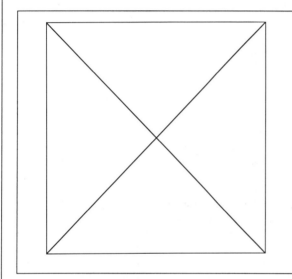

A. Steps 1-4.

Supplies and Equipment
- Wallpaper or other stiff paper
- Rule
- Pencil and eraser
- Scissors

Procedure
1. Measure and mark a square 5 X 5 inches. This is the lid.
2. Measure and mark another square 4 3/4 X 4 3/4 inches. This is the bottom.
3. Cut out the two squares.
4. Draw two diagonals from corner to corner, forming an X on the back of each square (Figure A).
5. Turn each of the four corners toward the center of the X, fold and crease firmly (Figure B).
6. With the corners made in step 5 still folded, turn each "side" of the square in toward the center line, crease firmly and unfold.
7. Completely unfold the square. The creases should correspond to those shown in Figure C.

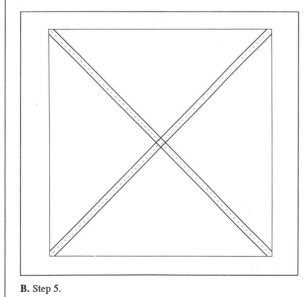

B. Step 5.

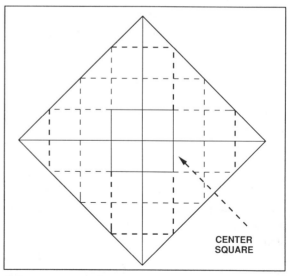

CENTER SQUARE

C. Creases (steps 6 and 7).

Figure 16-2. Directions for constructing a gift box.

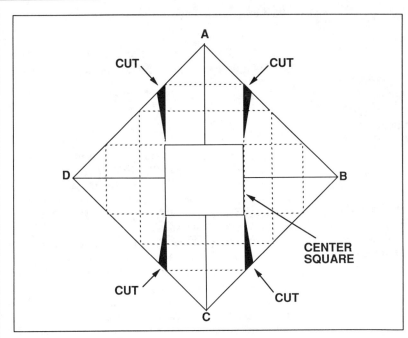

D. Cutting pattern (step 8).

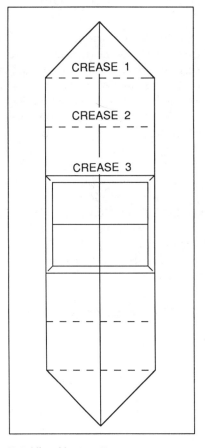

E. Folding sides (step 9).

8. Make cuts from the edge of the square to the corner of the center square formed by the creases. Make two cuts on one side of the box and two cuts on the opposite side of the box (Figure D). Do not make cuts on the adjacent sides.
9. Fold each crease (1, 2, and 3), as indicated by the dotted lines in Figure E, to the center. When the fold is made at crease 3, fold the paper up to form the side of the box.
10. Flip the two "wings" that have been folded up over the box and crease into the bottom. These will form the other two sides of the box. Tuck under folds on adjacent sides to secure.
11. Repeat steps 4 through 9 to complete the other half of the box. The completed box will measure 2 x 2 inches and be 1 inch deep.
12. Ribbon, lace, sequins, feathers, etc., may glued to the box top if desired.

Figure 16-2. Continued.

DOCUMENTATION CONSIDERATIONS

In many instances, the problems occupational therapy personnel have been experiencing in justifying and being reimbursed for arts and crafts as treatment are the result of inadequate or inaccurate documentation. Accurate and thorough documentation is imperative. The goals to be achieved and the skills to be addressed must be clearly stated using appropriate, understandable terminology, consistent with the required documentation format and standards of the profession. Proper documentation of the patient's progress or lack thereof must be made at regular intervals. It is the responsibility of the COTA to inform the supervising therapist of any changes in the level of performance so that the treatment plan can be modified accordingly.

FUTURE IMPLICATIONS

During the last several years, changes in thinking about the old concepts and techniques of occupational therapy have become evident in the literature as well as at presentations and discussions. Many members of the profession feel that the foundation of occupational therapy has been forgotten.[6] It is important to remember that the use of arts and crafts served a necessary therapeutic need at one time, and that a well-chosen art or craft can still be a meaningful form of treatment in keeping with the profession's philosophy of purposeful activity.

SUMMARY

The decision to use arts and crafts in occupational therapy treatment should be made after a thorough review of the patient's history and an activity analysis to assess the appropriateness of the particular arts and crafts being considered. The activity selected should be age appropriate and purposeful; have meaning to the patient in terms of his or her particular needs, interests, and roles; and relate directly to the goals established in the treatment plan. Examples of a wide variety of art and craft activities provide the reader with further evidence of the potential use of these modalities in therapeutic intervention. The importance of relating the activity to decision making and recognizing the importance of work, leisure and social skills in relation to art and craft activities is another primary consideration. Thorough and accurate documentation is essential for reimbursement.

Related Learning Activities

1. Discuss the three criteria for a craft activity to be appropriate for a patient.

2. Make a craft project that you are unfamiliar with. List the specific decisions that you made. How could you increase or decrease the number of decisions required?

3. What other craft activities could have been presented to Janet?

4. Construct the gift box according to the directions provided. Identify areas where difficulties or problems might occur.

References

1. Slagle EC: Occupational therapy: Recent methods and advances in the United States. *Occup Ther Rehabil* 13:5, 1934.
2. Hopkins HL: *Willard and Spackman's Occupational Therapy,* 7th Edition. Philadelphia, JB Lippincott, 1988, Chap 1.
3. Tracy SE: *Studies in Invalid Occupations.* Boston, Whitcomb & Barrows, 1918.
4. Cynkin S: *Occupational Therapy: Toward Health Through Activities.* Boston, Little, Brown, 1979.
5. Barris R, Cordero J, Christiansen R: Occupational therapists' use of media. *Am J Occup Ther* 40:679-684, 1986.
6. Friedland J: Diversional activity: Does it deserve its bad name? *Am J Occup Ther* 42:603-609, 1988.
7. Hatter JK, Nelson DL: Altruism and task performance in the elderly. *Am J Occup Ther* 41:376-381, 1987.

Chapter 17

Activity Analysis

LaDonn People, MA, OTR
Sally E. Ryan, COTA, ROH
Doris Y. Witherspoon, MS, OTR
Rhonda Stewart, OTR

INTRODUCTION

Activity analysis is extremely important in occupational therapy. This process involves the "breaking down" of an activity into detailed subparts and steps, which is a necessary foundation for all activities of daily living, play/leisure and work tasks used in intervention. It is an examination of the therapeutic characteristics and value of activities that fulfill the patient's many needs, interests, abilities and roles. Without such analysis, it may be impossible to use the proper application of activity or to obtain the best treatment results. Skill in activity analysis is critical to determine the validity of the use of activities in occupational therapy assessment and treatment.

The type of activity analysis used will be determined, at least in part, by the individual therapist's or assistant's frame of reference.[1] Such analysis will also be influenced by the use of particular techniques and variations in the use of equipment. While there is no universally accepted method of activity analysis, it is useful to consider the general categories of motor, sensory, cognitive, intrapersonal and interpersonal skills, as well as adaptations.[2] Other considerations should include factors such as the supplies and equipment needed, cost, the number of steps required for completion, time involved, supervision required, space needed, precautions and contraindications. It is also helpful to think of several aspects of experience or functional requirements of the activity and then analyze them in terms of gradability.[3] **Functional requirements** may be defined as components of an activity that require motor performance and behaviors for adequate completion. **Gradability** refers to a process whereby performance of an activity is viewed step-by-step on a continuum from simple to complex, or slow to rapid.

The activity analysis yields the kind of data needed for determining **therapeutic potential** of a particular activity in relation to established patient goals, interests and needs. Therapeutic potential is the degree of likelihood that therapeutic goals will be achieved. As specific techniques and equipment vary considerably for many activities, so will the results of an activity analysis. Once an activity is thoroughly analyzed, it can be adapted for therapeutic purposes.

HISTORICAL PERSPECTIVES

The profession of occupational therapy was founded on the notion that being engaged in activities promotes mental and physical well-being and, conversely, that the absence of activity leads at best to mischief and at worst to loss of mental and physical functioning.[4] Through their activities, human beings show their concern with how to survive, be comfortable, have pleasure, solve problems, express themselves, and relate to others. They come to know their strengths and they fulfill their roles in life. Thus the term occupation, as used in occupational therapy, is in the context of the individual's directed use of time, energy, interest and attention.[5]

Activities being the foundation of the profession, historical definitions and other accounts place a strong emphasis on occupations or purposeful activities.

When William Tuke established the York Retreat in England in the late 1800s, employment in various occupations was a cornerstone of treatment in this facility for mental patients. Review of historical accounts of Tuke's work show that he had spent some time analyzing activities. For example, activities and occupations were selected to elicit emotions that were opposite of the condition; a melancholy patient would be given activities that had elements of excitement and were active, whereas a manic patient would be engaged in tasks of a sedentary nature. The habit of attention was a key element in using activities for treatment.[6]

Among the early pioneers of our profession, history records the work of Susan Tracy in relation to the process of analyzing activity (see Chapter 1). Tracy's work with mentally ill patients led her to believe that remedial activities ". . .are classified according to their physiological effects as stimulants, sedatives, anesthetics. . ."[7] Over time, she analyzed the use of leather projects with patients and identified various components of a specific activity that would measure abilities in areas such as judgment, visual discrimination, spatial relationships, and making choices.[7] In 1918, she published a research paper, "Twenty-five suggested mental tests derived from invalid occupations."[8]

Eleanor Clarke Slagle's work in developing the principles of habit training certainly reflects her knowledge of activity analysis, as she placed particular emphasis on the gradation of activities and a balance among them.[9]

The 1918 principles, established by the founders of our profession, also address aspects of activity that imply an ability to analyze the activity's properties. Emphasis was placed on the qualities of particular activities, with crafts and work-related activities being prominent; games, music and physical exercise were also used.[10]

The terms *employment, labor, moral treatment, recreation, amusement, occupation, exercise,* and *diversion* among others have been used by different writers at various times to describe the forms of treatment used by occupational therapy personnel. The philosophy of the profession also places a strong emphasis on activities (see Chapter 3). Throughout our history, particular properties of activities were also addressed, giving strong roots to our basic belief in the activity analysis process. **Activity properties** are those characteristics of activities (eg, being goal-directed, having significance to the individual, requiring involvement, gradability, adaptability, etc.) that contribute to their therapeutic potential.

Contemporary definitions of occupational therapy are summarized in the 1981 definition of the profession, developed for licensure purposes, which describes occupational therapy as the therapeutic use of self-care (activites of daily living), work and play/leisure activities to maximize independent function, enhance development, prevent disability and maintain health.[11] It may include adaptations of the task or the environment to achieve maximum independence and to enhance the quality of one's life. Implicit in the latter statement is the ability to analyze activities. One must indeed know the particular properties and possibilities of a variety of activities to *adapt the task* to help the patient attain his or her goals. A related point, emphasized by Mosey, is that activities used by occupational therapy personnel include both an intrinsic and a therapeutic purpose.[12] This point is important to consider during activity analysis.

ACTIVITY ENGAGEMENT PRINCIPLES

Occupational therapy personnel must know various types of activities. Some of the **categories of activities** used in evaluation and treatment are the following:

1. Crafts: leatherwork, ceramics
2. Sensory awareness: music, dance
3. Movement awareness: dance, drama
4. Fine arts: sculpturing, painting, music
5. Construction: woodworking, electronics
6. Games: bingo, checkers
7. Self-care: dressing, feeding, hygiene
8. Domestic: cooking, homemaking
9. Textiles: weaving, needlecraft
10. Vocational: rock and stamp collecting

11. Recreational: sports, exercise
12. Educational: reading, writing

For activities to be considered purposeful and therapeutic, they must possess certain characteristics, which include the following:[13]

1. Be goal-directed
2. Have significance to the patient at some level
3. Require patient involvement at some level (mental or physical or both)
4. Be geared toward prevention of malfunction and/or maintenance or improvement of function and quality of life
5. Reflect patient involvement in life task situations (activities of daily living, work and play/leisure)
6. Relate to the interests of the patient
7. Be adaptable and gradable

The selection of appropriate activities for evaluation and treatment of patients must be based on sound professional judgment that is well grounded in knowledge and skill.[13] As activity specialists, occupational therapists and assistants must have strong skills in this area.[14] A thorough knowledge of and experience in analyzing a wide variety of activities is an essential element of this process. The *Essentials and Guidelines for an Accredited Educational Program for the Occupational Therapy Assistant* state that analysis and adaptation of activities is a requirement for entry-level personnel: "Activity analysis should relate to relevance of activity to patient/client interests and abilities, major motor processes, complexity, the steps involved, and the extent to which it can be modified or adapted."[15]

Mosey[12] stresses that purposeful activities cannot be designed for evaluation and intervention without analysis. Dunn[4] states that if activities are to be the core of occupational therapy they must be delineated, classified and analyzed in terms of therapeutic value.

PURPOSE AND PROCESS OF ACTIVITY ANALYSIS

The purpose of activity analysis is to determine if the activity will be appropriate in meeting the treatment goals established for the patient. To analyze an activity with knowledge and skill, it is necessary to know how to perform the processes involved. It is also relevant to know the extent to which the activity fosters or impedes various types of human performance and interaction.

The patient must be receptive to the activity selected. Patients will be more motivated and participate more if their interests, life tasks and roles are considered. In addition, the patient's **functional level** should be considered. The individual may be interested in the activity and it may relate

directly to his or her life tasks and roles, but due to performance deficits, it cannot be accomplished.

The process of analyzing an activity involves breaking it down to illustrate each step in detail that leads to the expected outcome. Consideration must be given to numerous factors that are used to achieve activity completion as shown in examples later in this chapter.

An activity analysis can be helpful when determining the use of an activity for an evaluation or for treatment. When analyzing an activity intended for evaluative purposes, it must be broken down into separate components to determine what opportunities exist to objectively measure what is to be evaluated.[16] For example, as Early[16] points out, when the purpose of engagement in an activity is to measure decision-making skills, the activity selected must provide choices, as well as decision points, to allow it to be useful. She also stresses that occupational therapy personnel must know the exact responses and outcomes that might potentially occur and how they relate to the patient's ability to make decisions. An interpretation of observations of the individual's engagement in the activity (performance) would follow. When the activity is intended to be used for treatment, it again must be broken down into small units to determine which **components** (constituent parts) of the activity will help to achieve the treatment goals, such as to increase range of motion, to improve attention span, or to decrease isolative behavior.

An accurate analysis of an activity allows occupational therapy personnel to select activities that will address the needs and goals of the patient therapeutically. This process also aids in determining the therapeutic potential of specific activities and their purposeful use. The absense of a thorough activity analysis is likely to prevent achievement of the best treatment results.

DEVELOPING SKILLS

Skill in activity analysis is critical to determine the validity of the use of activities in occupational therapy intervention programs. Prerequisite to achieving skill is the ability to understand the basic components of the activity, that is, the fundamental processes, tools, and materials required for task completion. Self-analysis of a simple, frequently engaged in activity, such as bathing, is useful as an initial step. Asking questions, such as the following, is recommended:

1. Why is the activity important to you?
2. What supplies and equipment are needed?
3. What is the procedure?
4. What other factors should be considered?

Once these questions have been answered, look at the information critically to determine if *precise* information was recorded. Recheck to be sure that no important factors were omitted. Ask a family member or peer to also answer these questions. In comparing results, differences in answers emphasize the uniqueness of the individual. Other questions can then be considered, such as how to adapt the activity for persons with various disabilities.

Experience in engaging in a wide variety of activities is also important in building skill, as it allows the certified occupational therapy assistant (COTA) to make comparisons and formulate potential applications based on several possibilities. Practice in using several forms of activity analysis and receiving objective feedback also is as a way to develop skill. Once skill is achieved the COTA can more easily select the most appropriate activity, which is of interest to the patient, relates to his or her life tasks and roles, is within the individual's functional capacity to perform, and provides opportunities for goal achievement.[17] **Goal achievement** is to the accomplishment of tasks and objectives one has set out to do.

RELATED CONSIDERATIONS

Frame of Reference

Occupational therapy personnel use many approaches to analyze activities. The type of activity analysis is determined, at least in part, by the individual therapist's or assistant's frame of reference.[1] For example, if a developmental frame of reference is used, activities are analyzed to determine the extent to which they might contribute to the age specific development and related areas of occupational performance. If gratification of oral needs was a goal of treatment, it would be important to analyze the activity in terms of opportunities for eating, sucking, blowing and encouraging independence, among other factors.[12]

Activity analysis is also influenced by the use of particular techniques and variations in the use of equipment recommended, such as in sensory integration and in the theoretical approaches of Rood, Bobath, and Brunnstrom. Additional information on theoretical frameworks and approaches may be found in Chapter 4.

Adaption

To adapt an activity means to modify it.[16] It involves changing the components that are required to complete the task. Adaptions are made to allow the patient to experience success in task accomplishment at his or her level of functioning. For example, an individual who has had a stroke, resulting in paralysis of one side of the body, will need to use a holding device such as a lacing "pony" or a vice to stabilize a leather-lacing project. A change in positioning of the project, due to loss of peripheral vision and neglect of the involved side, is another important adaption. Although few adaptions

are required in this example, all of the components of the specific activity must be considered for potential changes to increase their therapeutic potential.[16]

Grading

Grading of an activity refers to the process of performance being viewed step by step on a continuum that progresses from simple to complex. For example, a patient might begin by lacing two precut layers of leather together, using large prepunched holes and a simple whip stitch, to make a comb case. Once this is satisfactorily completed, additional challenges, such as the following, could be introduced over several treatment sessions:

1. Use of saddle stitching, followed by single cordovan, and double cordovan lacing, on other short-term leather projects
2. Use of simple stamping, followed by tooling and carving to decorate the project
3. Application of basic finishes, or more advanced techniques, such as antiquing and dyeing with several colors

Activities may also be graded according to rate of time, varying from slow to rapid. An important concept is that the grading of activities builds on what has already been accomplished in progressive stages.

FORMS AND EXAMPLES

Although no universally accepted method of activity analysis exists, the following outline, checklist, and examples are provided to assist the reader in understanding the many diverse and complex factors inherent in the process of activity analysis. Study and use of these materials provides the COTA with opportunities to gain new skills or improve existing ones. Although every effort has been made to make these examples as complete as possible, other relevant aspects could undoubtedly be included. Some of the examples are formated in such a way that they could be filled out and used as protocols for an occupational therapy clinic, thus assuring that all personnel had information about a particular activity and its potential therapeutic uses. Those with limited experience in activity analysis should focus first on the general outline shown in Figure 17-1. From time to time, unfamiliar terminology may be introduced. Definitions may be found by consulting the glossary, which appears at the end of this text.

ACTIVITY ANALYSIS CHECKLIST

The **Activity Analysis Checklist,** shown in Figure 17-2, is a faster method of determining the particular components

1. *Name of activity:*

2. *Number of individuals involved:*

3. *Supplies and equipment:*
   List all tools, equipment, and materials needed to complete the activity. Optional items should be so designated.

4. *Procedure:*
   List all steps required to complete the activity.

5. *Cost:*
   List costs of all supplies and equipment. Large equipment, such as a kiln or jigsaw, is usually not included because it is only purchased once.

6. *Preparation:*
   List any processes that must be or could be completed before the treatment session. (This may be due to dangerous or complicated procedures, or because of limited treatment time.)

7. *Time:*
   List total amount of time necessary, including preparation and cleanup, if required.

8. *Space needs or setting required:*
   State requirements relative to where the activity will take place. (Activities performed in the clinic may not be appropriate for treatment in a patient's room.)

9. *Activity qualities:*
   Consider such factors as controllability, resistiveness, noise, cleanliness, practability, problem areas, and likely mistakes. List both positive and negative aspects.

10. *Amount of supervision:*
    Can the activity be completed independently, or must it be supervised? (To what degree?)

11. *Physical requirements:*
    Consider factors such as motions used (be specific), fine motor skills, gross motor skills, dexterity, eye-hand and bilateral coordination, posture/position (standing, sitting, leaning, bending, prone, supine, etc.), strength, endurance, and balance.

12. *Sensory requirements:*
    Consider visual, tactile, auditory, olfactory and gustatory factors.

13. *Cognitive factors:*
    Consider requirements for organization, concentration, problem solving, logical thinking, attention span, direction following (written, oral or demonstration), decision making and creativity.

14. *Emotional factors:*
    Consider aspects such as degree of structure, initiative, control, dependence, impulse control, frustration tolerance, opportunities to handle feelings, and role identification.

15. *Social factors:*
    Consider degree of communication, interaction, and competition required; opportunities for assuming responsibility and cooperating.

16. *Potential for adaption or modification:*
    Consider points 9 through 15.

17. *Precautions and contraindications:*

18. *Grading potential:*
    Consider how to change (simple, complex, rapid, or slow).

19. *Type of condition or problem for which activity is recommended:*

20. *Activity category:*
    (Functional, supportive, vocational, diversional)

21. *Expected primary therapeutic goals:*

22. *Other pertinent information:*
    Consider age appropriateness, gender identification, cultural considerations and vocational implications.

Figure 17-1. General activity analysis outline.[18]

of an activity, as it requires less writing than the general activity analysis outline (see Figure 17-1). Figure 17-3 shows the same form used to analyze the specific activity of constructing a leather coin purse. Although the form and the example emphasize psychosocial aspects, they easily could be modified to include criteria with a more definitive focus on physical performance deficts as well as other areas.

Example I: Play/Leisure Activity

1. *Name of activity:* Volleyball

2. *Number of individuals involved:* 8-15

3. *Supplies and equipment:* Volleyball, net, poles, score pad, and pen. Optional: Refreshments and prizes

4. *Procedure:* Stand in designated space. Reach to hit the ball over the net when it approaches you. Move side to side and front to back within your designated space to hit the ball. Rotate to the space on your left after score is made. Optional: Start a new game after the established score is reached.

5. *Cost:* None if equipment is available; otherwise about $60.00 (see item three).

6. *Preparation:* 5-10 minutes to obtain equipment and set up

7. *Time:* 1 hour and 5 minutes:
   5 minutes to set up equipment
   5 minutes to instruct group (process, rules, scoring)
   45 minutes for actual activity participation
   10 minutes to clean up, pack, and store equipment

8. *Space needs or setting required:* Outdoor area or large room free of obstacles and furnishings

9. *Activity qualities:* High potential for noise, due to excitement and competitve behavior. Participants may need assistance with procedures and scoring.

10. *Amount of supervision:* Direct to assure proper follow through

11. *Physical requirements:* Reaching, jumping, standing, turning, grasping, eye-hand coordination, balance, strength, and endurance

Activity: Check the appropriate box:	None	Min.	Mod.	Max.	Comments
1. Initiative					
2. Technical ability					
3. Manipulative ability					
4. Creative ability					
5. Concentrated effort					
6. Mechanical repetition					
7. Constant action					
8. Fine motor					
9. Gross motor					
10. Tactile					
11. Visual					
12. Auditory					
13. Olfactory					
14. Gustatory					
15. Time					
16. Modification of equipment					
17. Noise					
18. Degree of cleanliness					
19. Equipment and tool costs					
20. Materials costs					
21. Use of surplus or scrap materials					
22. Opportunity to express constructively:					
a. Affect or attitude					
b. Creativeness					
c. Originality					
d. Frustration					
e. Hostility					
f. Aggression					
g. Anger					
h. Obsessive-compulsive feature					
i. Need to excel					
j. Need to have supervision					
k. Narcissism					
l. Expiation of guilt					
m. Dependence					
n. Independence					
o. Masculine identification					
p. Feminine identification					
q. Regressive features					
23. Structure					
24. Controllability					
25. Pliability					
26. Resistiveness					
27. Predictability					
28. Concentration					
29. Problem solving					
30. Improve competence					
31. Improve efficacy					
32. Gradability					
33. Directions:					
a. Oral					
b. Written					
c. Demonstration					
34. Precautions					
35. Other					

Figure 17-2. Activity analysis checklist.

Activity: *Leather Coin Purse* Check the appropriate box:	None	Min.	Mod.	Max.	Comments
1. Initiative		✓			
2. Technical ability		✓			
3. Manipulative ability				✓	
4. Creative ability		✓			more if carving
5. Concentrated effort				✓	
6. Mechanical repetition				✓	
7. Constant action				✓	lacing
8. Fine motor				✓	lacing
9. Gross motor			✓		cutting
10. Tactile			✓		
11. Visual			✓		blind can lace
12. Auditory			✓		punching holes
13. Olfactory			✓		
14. Gustatory	✓				
15. Time		✓	✓		
16. Modification of equipment	✓				
17. Noise			✓		
18. Degree of cleanliness				✓	
19. Equipment and tool costs			✓		
20. Materials costs			✓		
21. Use of surplus or scrap materials			✓		
22. Opportunity to express constructively:					
a. Affect or attitude		✓			
b. Creativeness		✓			
c. Originality		✓			
d. Frustration		✓			
e. Hostility			✓		
f. Aggression		✓			stamping
g. Anger			✓		stamping
h. Obsessive-compulsive feature			✓		
i. Need to excel				✓	
j. Need to have supervision	✓				
k. Narcissism	✓				
l. Expiation of guilt		✓			
m. Dependence		✓			
n. Independence				✓	
o. Masculine identification		✓			
p. Feminine identification		✓			
q. Regressive features	✓				
23. Structure				✓	
24. Controlability				✓	
25. Pliability		✓			
26. Resistiveness		✓			
27. Predictability				✓	
28. Concentration		✓			
29. Problem solving				✓	
30. Improve competence				✓	
31. Improve efficacy				✓	
32. Gradability			✓		
33. Directions:					
a. Oral				✓	
b. Written				✓	
c. Demonstration				✓	
34. Precautions				✓	needle
35. Other					

Figure 17-3. Completed activity analysis checklist for constructing a leather coin purse.

12. *Sensory requirements:* Visual, tactile, kinesthetic; auditory helpful but loss can be accommodated

13. *Cognitive factors:* Attention span, concentration, problem solving, judgment, oral and demonstrated direction following, memory

14. *Emotional factors:* Initiative, frustration tolerance, activity tolerance

15. *Social factors:* Cooperative and competitive behavior; group interaction and potential for socialization. Nonparticipants can be encouraged to be "cheer leaders" or score keepers or to serve refreshments.

16. *Potential for adaptation or modification:* Good. May use a foam ball or a beach ball. May be played while seated. Playing for points and rotations may be omitted (also see gradation).

17. *Precautions and contraindications:* Participants with low tolerance may need frequent breaks; participants with short attention span or memory deficits may need frequent cueing. Avoid use with individuals with serious cardiopulmonary and respiratory problems. Thoroughly instruct in proper serving and other motions required to reduce potential for injury.

18. *Grading potential:* Rapid: Decrease time allocated and encourage increased participation. Slow: Decrease emphasis on time; allow game to proceed as tolerated; add breaks.

19. *Type of condition or problem for whom activity is recommended:* A wide variety. Not appropriate for the very young or those having pronounced perceptual and motor deficits.

20. *Activity category:* Functional and diversional

21. *Expected primary therapeutic goals:* Numerous; examples include those in items 9 to 13.

22. *Other pertinent information:* Prizes may be awarded for best serve, most points scored by a single person, good sportsmanship, etc.

Example II: Work Activity

This example illustrates a prevocational task used as one of the objective measurements of an individual's potential to work in a sheltered workshop environment.

1. *Name of activity:* Sorting and packaging screws

2. *Number of individuals involved:* 1 to 3 initially

3. *Supplies and equipment:* Chairs and table; 500 flat-head screws (250 1-inch and 250 1½-inch); 1 box of sandwich size plastic bags with ties; self-adhesive paper labels; one felt-tip marking pen for each person

4. *Procedure:* Sort screws according to size. Count and place 20 screws in a bag, seal the bag, mark the label with the correct size, and apply the label.

5. *Cost:* .03 to .05 cents per screw; .99 cents for 100 plastic bags; .50 cents per marker; .99 cents for box of 100 self-adhesive labels

6. *Preparation:* Minimal: 5 to 10 minutes to gather supplies and set up; determine monitoring methods

7. *Time:* 45 minutes, approximately:
   5 minutes to set up
   2 minutes to explain and demonstrate process
   25 minutes to perform task (task completion within allocated time is a requirement)
   5 to 10 minutes to clean up work area

8. *Space needs or setting required:* Quiet room to permit concentration and minimize distractions (no television, telephone, people entering and exiting, etc.)

9. *Activity qualities:* Structured, offers fairly immediate gratification, controllable, simple instructions, clean

10. *Amount of supervision:* Good potential for independence after initial learning. Monitor for fatigue, problems and observable behaviors

11. *Physical requirements:* Sitting or standing, reaching, bending, grasping, balance, eye-hand coordination; at least fair strength and endurance

12. *Sensory requirements:* Visual or tactile discrimination and integration or both; auditory loss can be accommodated

13. *Cognitive factors:* Concentration, attention span, direction following, memory, sequencing, decision making, time management, and organization

14. *Emotional factors:* Initiative, motivation, competition if working in group; frustration tolerance, and activity tolerance

15. *Social factors:* Independence; interaction not required unless set up as a task group; if so, still limited

16. *Potential for adaptation or modification:* Good. May be performed while sitting, standing or supine; can be adapted for a prosthesis. Easily adapted to a task group format (see gradation potential).

17. *Precautions and contraindications:* Observe for fatigue that may not be voiced. Confused people may ingest screws or ties.

18. *Grading potential:* Simple: Count screws of one size and shape; eliminate time requirement. Complex: Sort and count screws of varying sizes and shapes. May be accomplished slowly or rapidly.

19. *Type of condition or problem activity is recommended for:* Young adults, adults, and geriatric patients with a variety of performance deficits who need vocational preparation.

20. *Activity category:* Functional; vocational

21. *Expected primary therapeutic goals:* Improve independence, work tolerance, and work behaviors; identify needs for environmental modifications (table height, lighting, etc.).

22. *Other pertinent information:* Same process could be used for sorting and counting other materials such as mosaic tile for kits.

Example III: Self-Care Activity

1. *Name of activity:* Donning a shirt with front buttons
2. *Type of program:* Daily living task
3. *Type of patient indicated:* Variable
4. *Number of patients involved:* One or small group
5. *Materials and equipment needed:* Shirt or shirts with front buttons
6. *Cost:* Variable: Patients can have shirt brought from home if not available in setting
7. *Preparation required:* None
8. *Time involved:* Depends on patient; usually about 3 minutes
9. *Space needed or physical setting required:* May be completed at bedside or in clinic
10. *Qualities of activity:* Quiet, clean, practical; problems may occur in buttoning shirt incorrectly
11. *Amount of supervision required:* Minimal once demonstrated and learned; practice may be independent
12. *Directions required:* Oral and demonstration
13. *Procedure:*
    Unbutton shirt
    Position shirt
    Pick up shirt
    Put arm in shirt sleeve
    Pull shirt over shoulder
    Put other arm in shirt sleeve
    Pull shirt together
    Fasten buttons on shirt front
    Straighten shirt
14. *Physical functions or requirements:* May be performed sitting or standing, if patient has adequate balance; may also be performed in a supine position; dexterity and coordination are needed for buttoning. Motions involved include shoulder flexion and abduction when picking up shirt, elbow flexion and extension when pulling the shirt over the shoulder, forearm pronation and supination, wrist hyperextension, finger flexion, and neck flexion.
15. *Cognitive, sensory, perceptual motor functions:* Ability to comprehend simple verbal and demonstrated instructions; ability to cross the midline in bringing the shirt over the shoulder; vision and hearing not required
16. *Psychological functions:* Not frustrating; short-term; some judgment needed to avoid putting shirt on inside out or buttoning incorrectly; may be performed independently
17. *Potential therapeutic goals:*
    Increase daily living independence in area of dressing
    Aid in adjusting to residual abilities
    Improve tactile abilities (buttoning) and motor coordination
    Increase reality orientation (appropriate shirt for weather or season)
    Build self-esteem (success provides gratification)
    Aid in assuming responsibility (patient encouraged to dress daily)
18. *Gradation:* Learn to button first, then don shirt
19. *Potential for adaptation:* Use of a button aid or Velcro fasteners; pullover shirt can be used to eliminate buttons.
20. *Relationship to experience:* Necessary in life activities
21. *Precautions and contraindications:* Activity not limited to any particular diagnosis; maintain proper posture
22. *Comments:* Should be initiated early in the patient's treatment

Example IV: Homemaking Activity

An activity analysis of a cooking activity, which follows, is presented as a contrast to the dressing activity to emphasize the variety of ways an activity may be analyzed and also to contrast a simple activity with a complex one. Although detailed, this example tends to explore more general aspects of the activity in five rather than 22 categories. As experience and skill are gained, less detailed formats may be used.

Rosette Cooking

Materials Needed.
Rosette iron molds (80 different ones available)
Rosette iron handle
Deep fryer or heavy saucepan
Paper towels
Oil for frying
Metal tongs
$1/2$ cup evaporated milk
$1/2$ cup water
$1/4$ teaspoon salt
1 teaspoon sugar
1 egg, beaten
1 cup flour
garnishes: powdered sugar, cinnamon, whipped cream and/or fruit

Directions. Prepare batter in order listed; slowly stir in flour and beat until smooth.

Place approximately two inches of oil in deep fryer or heavy saucepan.

Heat oil to 365° F.

Attach rosette iron mold to mold handle.

Immerse iron mold in hot oil until thoroughly heated.

Lift out mold and blot excess oil with paper towel.

Dip mold into batter until it is $3/4$ covered. Do not cover the entire mold.

Hold the mold in the bowl for a few seconds; lift it out and shake off any excess batter.

Dip the batter-coated mold into the hot oil.

Once the rosette begins to brown slightly, lift the mold and let the rosette gently drop into the hot oil.

Using metal tongs, turn the rosette over and cook for a few more seconds.

Use the tongs to lift the finished rosette out of the oil and drain it on paper towels.

Sprinkle with powdered sugar, cinnamon, or other garnishes.

Type of Group or Individual Patient for Whom This Activity Is Appropriate. This activity is appropriate for a lower functioning patient group, due to its immediate gratification and success assured qualities. Close supervision and some assistance are required. Patient groups functioning at a higher level would also benefit from this type of activity. They would require minimal supervision and encouragement. It would provide a means of moving to higher level task skills required in many areas of daily living.

The activity can be structured to enhance group cohesiveness by delineating various tasks for small groups or individuals to perform. In this way, all members can make a contribution to the end product of the project group.

Precautions. The hot oil presents the main safety hazard and should be closely monitored at all times. Ingredients may need to be substituted to accommodate special diets.

Goals.
- Upgrade both basic and higher level daily living task skills
- Increase self-esteem
- Increase attention span and concentration
- Increase motivation to carry out a single project to completion
- Provide immediate, basic gratification and fulfillment
- Increase group cohesiveness through shared responsibility (may also be used with individuals)

SUMMARY

Activities are universal and historically have remained a primary foundation for the profession. Activity analysis is a deeply rooted concept, which has withstood the test of time and continues to be an important cornerstone for accurate assessment and effective intervention by occupational therapy personnel. The basic concepts and processes have been described to provide a fundamental understanding of the knowledge base and skills necessary for activities analysis. These skills include activity engagement principles, methods for developing skills, concepts of grading and adapting activities. Forms and examples of the analysis of specific activites were also presented.

Emphasis was placed on the need for the activity analysis process and the information that may be gained through exploration of activity properties and possibilities. Skill in activity analysis is essential to determine the validity of the activities used for assessment and treatment. A thorough and accurate activity analysis allows the practitioner to select the most appropriate activity, which is of interest to the patient, relates to his or her life tasks and roles, and provides opportunities for goal achievement.

Author's Note

Example III: Self-Care Activity and Example IV: Homemaking Activity were reprinted with the permission of the Occupational Therapy Assistant Program, Wayne County Community College, Detroit, Michigan.

Acknowledgment

The editor thanks Sr. Genevieve Cummings, CSJ, MA, OTR, FAOTA, for her editorial and content recommendations.

Related Learning Activities

1. Discuss some of the reasons occupatinoal therapy personnel use activity analysis.

2. Observe a person engaged in a work task. Identify the specific physical, cognitive and social skills required.

3. List the general categories of information that should be a part of an activity analysis.

4. Working with a peer and using the format for "Donning a Shirt with Front Buttons," complete an activity analysis for another dressing activity.

5. Using the format presented for "Rosette Cooking," complete an activity analysis for a different cooking activity and a craft activity.

References

1. Hopkins HL, Smith HD, Tiffany EC: Therapeutic application of activity. In Hopkins HL, Smith HD (Eds): *Willard and Spackman's Occupational Therapy,* 6th Edition. Philadelphia, JB Lippincott, 1983, p. 225.
2. United States Department of Labor, Employment, and Training Administration: *Dictionary of Occupational Titles,* 4th Edition. Washington, DC, U.S. Government Printing Office, 1981.
3. Tiffany EC: Psychiatry and mental health. In Hopkins HL, Smith HD (Eds): *Willard and Spackman's Occupational Therapy,* 6th Edition. Philadelphia, JB Lippincott, 1983.

4. Dunn W: Application of uniform terminology in practice. *Am J Occup Ther* 43:817-831, 1989.

5. American Occupational Therapy Association: *Reference Manual of Official Documents of the American Occupational Therapy Association.* Rockville, Maryland, AOTA, 1980.

6. Tuke S: *A Description of the Retreat: An Institution Near York for Insane Persons of The Society of Friends.* London, Dawson of Pall Mall, 1813.

7. Tracy SE: The place of invalid occupations in the general hospital. *Modern Hospital* 2(5):386, June, 1914.

8. Tracy SE: Twenty-five suggested mental tests derived from invalid occupations. *Maryland Psychiatric Quarterly* 8:15-16, 1918.

9. Slagle EC: Training aides for mental patients. *Arch Occup Ther* 1:13-14, 1922.

10. Dunton WR: The principles of occupational therapy. In *Proceedings of the National Society for the Promotion of Occupational Therapy, Second Annual Meeting.* Catonsville, Maryland, Spring Grove State Hospital Press, 1918, pp. 25-27.

11. Resolution Q: Definition of occupational therapy for liscensure. Minutes of the 1981 AOTA Representative Assembly. *Am J Occup Ther* 35:798-799, 1981.

12. Mosey AC: *Psychosocial Components of Occupational Therapy.* New York, Raven Press, 1986.

13. Hopkins HD, Smith HL (Eds): *Willard and Spackman's Occupational Therapy,* 6th Edition. Philadelphia, JB Lippincott, 1983.

14. Punwar AJ: *Occupational Therapy Principles and Practice.* Baltimore, Williams & Wilkins, 1988, Chapter 2.

15. Essentials and Guidelines for an Accredited Educational Program for the Occupational Therapy Assistant. *Am J Occup Ther* 45:1085-1092, 1991.

16. Early MB: *Mental Health Concepts and Techniques for the Occupational Therapy Assistant.* New York, Raven Press, 1987, pp. 274-275.

17. Trombly C, Scott AD: *Occupational Therapy for Physical Dysfunction,* 3rd Edition. Baltimore, Williams & Wilkins, 1989. Chapter 1.

18. Hopkins HL, Tiffany EG: Occupational therapy—base in activity. In Hopkins HL, Smith HD (Eds): *Willard and Spackman's Occupational Therapy,* 7th Edition. Philadelphia, JB Lippincott, 1988, pp. 93-101.

Appendices

Appendix A
SELECTED DEVELOPMENTAL SUMMARY

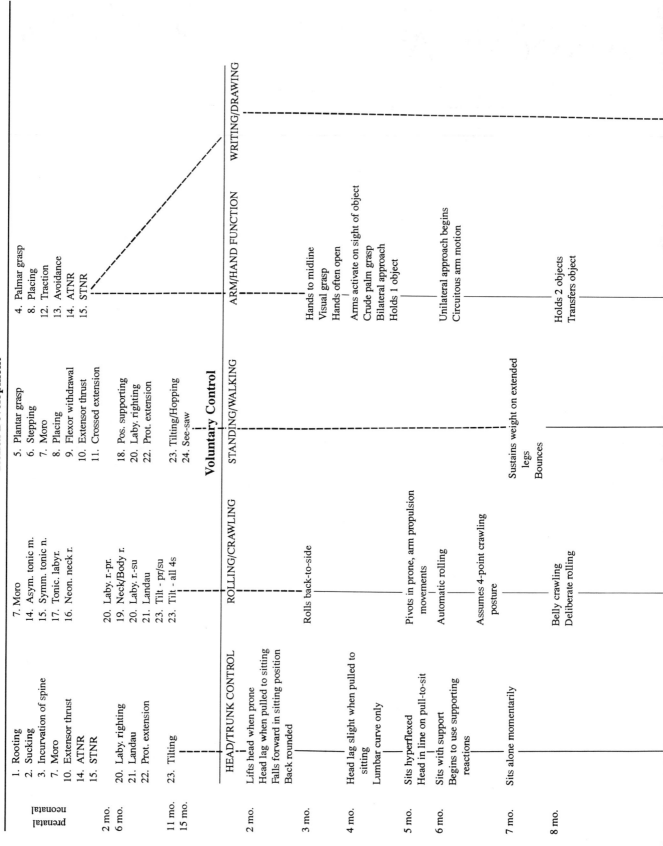

NEUROMOTOR DEVELOPMENT
Reflex Development

1. Rooting	5. Plantar grasp	4. Palmar grasp	
2. Sucking	6. Stepping	8. Placing	
3. Incurvation of spine	7. Moro	12. Traction	
7. Moro	8. Placing	13. Avoidance	
10. Extensor thrust	9. Flexor withdrawal	14. ATNR	
14. ATNR	10. Extensor thrust	15. STNR	
15. STNR	11. Crossed extension		
20. Laby. righting	18. Pos. supporting		
21. Landau	19. Neck/Body r.		
22. Prot. extension	20. Laby. righting		
	21. Landau		
	22. Prot. extension		
23. Tilting	23. Tilt - prf/su		
	23. Tilt - all 4s		

Voluntary Control

	HEAD/TRUNK CONTROL	ROLLING/CRAWLING	STANDING/WALKING	ARM/HAND FUNCTION	WRITING/DRAWING
2 mo.	Lifts head when prone Head lag when pulled to sitting Falls forward in sitting position Back rounded				
3 mo.		Rolls back-to-side		Hands to midline Visual grasp Hands often open	
4 mo.	Head lag slight when pulled to sitting Lumbar curve only			Arms activate on sight of object Crude palm grasp Bilateral approach Holds 1 object	
5 mo.	Sits hyperflexed Head in line on pull-to-sit	Pivots in prone, arm propulsion movements			
6 mo.	Sits with support Begins to use supporting reactions	Automatic rolling		Unilateral approach begins Circuitous arm motion	
		Assumes 4-point crawling posture			
7 mo.	Sits alone momentarily		Sustains weight on extended legs Bounces		
8 mo.		Belly crawling Deliberate rolling		Holds 2 objects Transfers object	

prenatal / neonatal
2 mo.
6 mo.
11 mo.
15 mo.

9 mo.
- No longer uses arms for support in sitting
- Assumes sitting independently
- Leans forward, re-erects
- Sitting to prone
- 4-point crawling
- Stands holding rail
- Release beginning

10 mo.
- Pulls up to rail and lowers
- Thumb and index tip prehension beginning

11 mo.
- Sits and pivots
- Lifts foot at rail
- Cruises

12 mo.
1 yr.
15 mo.
- Seats self in small chair
- Discards crawling
- Walks with one hand held
- Assumes standing on own
- Walks a few steps
- Falls by collapse
- Neat prehension
- Places cube on cube
- Casts object
- Marks by banging or brushing
- Marks rather than bangs

18 mo.
- Heel-toe progression in walking
- Walks sideways (17m)
- Walks backwards (17m)
- Crude release (on contact with surface)
- Holds crayon butt end
- Scribbles off page
- Whole arm movements
- One color

21 mo.
- Squats in play
- Down stairs hand held
- Tries to stand on 6cm walking board
- Kicks large ball
- Tower 5-6 blocks

24 mo.
2 yr.
- Runs well
- Walks with one foot on 6cm walking board (27cm)
- Less handedness shift
- Overhand grasp of crayon
- Wrist action
- Process rather than product

2 1/2 yrs.
- Jumps with both feet
- Tries standing on one foot
- Hops 1-3 steps on preferred foot
- Attempts to step on walking board (33m)
- Stands on 6cm walking board with both feet (38m)
- Throws ball with poor direction about 5-7 feet
- Throws bean bag into 12 in. hole from 3 feet
- Holds crayon in fingers
- Small marks
- Imitates vertical/horizontal stroke

3 yrs.
- Rides tricycle
- Alternates feet going up stairs
- Alternates feet part way on 6cm walking board (38m)
- Ascends small ladder alternating feet (38m)
- Towers 10 blocks
- 10 pellets into bottle, 30 sec.
- Catches large ball with stiff arms
- Throws ball without losing balance, 6-7 feet
- Handedness
- Copies circle
- Imitates cross
- Encloses space
- Simple figures
- Beginning designs
- Names drawing

3 1/2 yrs.
- Stands on 1 foot, 2 seconds
- Jumps from 8 in. elevation
- Leaps off floor with feet together
- Throws small ball 8-9 feet

Voluntary Control (continued)

	HEAD/TRUNK CONTROL	ROLLING/CRAWLING	STANDING/WALKING	ARM/HAND FUNCTION	WRITING/DRAWING
4 yrs.			Propels and manipulates wagon Skips on 1 foot only Down stairs foot-to-step Balance on 1 foot, 　4-8 seconds Walk 6cm board part way 　before stepping off Crouch for broad jump 　of 8-10in Hop on toes with both feet 　same time Carry cup of water without 　spilling Reciprocal arm motion in run- 　ning pattern Ascends large ladder, alternating 　feet (47m)	Throws ball overhand Beginning adult stance throwing Catches large ball, arms flexed 　but rigid	Pencil held like adult, wrist flexed Crude human figures "Suns" Copies cross
4 1/2 yrs.			Hops on 1 foot, 4 to 6 steps Alternates feet full length of 　6cm walking board (56m) Descends small ladder		More detailed human figures
5 yrs.			Roller skates, ice skates 　and rides small bicycle 　(5 or 6 yrs.) Skips alternating feet Stands indefinitely on 1 foot Hop a distance of 16 feet Walks long distance on tip toes Walks length of 6cm walking 　board in 6-9 sec. (60m) Running broad jump 28 　to 35in. Runs 11.5 feet per second Descends large ladder	Adult posture distance throwing 　Boys 24 feet 　Girls 15 feet Catches ball, hands more that 　arms, misses Bounces large ball	Buildings and houses Animals Idea before starting Copies triangle

Age	Gross motor	Strength / skills	Perceptual / drawing
6 yrs.	Stand on each foot alternately with eyes closed Walk a 4cm walking board in 9 seconds with one error Jump down from 12in landing on toes only Standing broad jump of 38in Running broad jump of 40 to 45in Hop 50 feet in 9 seconds	Reach, grasp, release and body movement smooth Catch ball, 1 hand *Grip strength Boys 11.3 lbs. Girls 3.2 lbs.	Finger and wrist movement Copies diamond
7 yrs.	Motor performance continues to become more refined (running, jumping, balancing, etc.) Strength increases Learns to inhibit motor activity	*Grip strength Boys 18.5 lbs. Girls 8.7 lbs.	
8 yrs.	Runs 5 yards per second Standing broad jump of 45in	*Grip strength Boys 26 lbs. Girls 14.4 lbs.	
9 yrs.		Distance throw Boys 60 feet Girls 35 feet	3-dimensional geometric figures Linear perspective
10 yrs.	Runs 6 yards per second Standing broad jump of 60in	*Grip strength Boys 45.2 lbs. Girls 33.8 lbs Distance throw Boys 95 feet Girls 60 feet	
11 yrs.			
14 yrs.	Boys standing broad jump 76in Girls standing broad jump 63in Boys run 6 yards, 8in per second Girls run 6 yards, 3in per second	*Grip strength Boys 71.2 lbs. Girls 46.2 lbs.	
17 yrs.	Boys run 7 yards per second Boys standing broad jump 90in.	Boys distance throw 150 feet	

*Dynamometer norms for dominant hand (average/mean) (unpublished) Scottish Rite Hospital for Crippled Children, Dallas, Texas.

SENSORIMOTOR DEVELOPMENT

Age	Vision	Other	Body Scheme	SOCIAL AND PLAY DEVELOPMENT	DAILY LIVING SKILLS
prenatal / neonatal	Rudimentary fixation / Reflexive tracking for brief periods	Sensorimotor Development (0-2 yrs.): •Tactile functions •Vestibular functions •Kinesthetic functions •Auditory functions •Olfactory functions •Gustatory functions		Individual—mothering person most important	
2 mo.	Sees light, dark, color and movement				
6 mo.					
11 mo.	Real convergence and coordination				
15 mo.					
2 mo.	Accommodation more flexible and eyes coordinate smoothly				
3 mo.					
4 mo.	Size and shape constancy				
5 mo.	Depth perception				
6 mo.	Visual tracking 90° V and H planes / Color perception / Acuity / Discriminates strangers				
7 mo.				Stranger anxiety	
8 mo.					
9 mo.					
10 mo.					Holds bottle / Finger feeds
11 mo.		Integration of body sides (1-4 yrs.): •Gross motor planning •Form and space perception •Equilibrium response •Postural flexibility		Immediate family group important	Drinks from cup (held) / Cooperates in dressing
12 mo.					
1 yr.					
15 mo.					Grasps spoon and into dish
18 mo.			"Tummy," legs, feet, arms, hand, face parts	Solitary or onlooker play	Feeds self, spills / Takes off hat, socks, mittens / Unzips zippers / Toilet trained daytime
21 mo.					Handles cup well

Age	Visual Perception	Tactile/Discrimination	Body Awareness	Play/Social	Self-Care
24 mo.		Strong tactile sense		Parallel play	Hold small glass 1 hand
2 yr.	Distinguishes vertical from horizontal lines			Imitation	Helps in getting dressed
					Pulls on socks
					Pulls up pants
					Removes shoes
2 1/2 yrs.					Strings beads, snips with scissors, opens jar lid, turns door knob
3 yrs.	Reacts to entire stimulus rather than separate parts		Planes of body related to objects	Associative play	Feeds self, no spilling
					Pours from pitcher
					Puts on shoes
					Removes pants
					Unbuttons
					Toilet training, independent
					Washes, dries face and hands
3 1/2 yrs.	Discrimination—notes similarities and differences (4 to 8 yrs.)	Discrimination in all functions (3 to 7 yrs.)			
4 yrs.	Needs more perceptual information (clues) than 10 yr. old		Thighs, elbows, shoulders, 1st and little fingers and thumb identified	Dramatic play	Brushes teeth
				Cooperative play	Dresses and undresses with supervision
					Laces shoes
					Distinguishes front and back of clothes
					Cuts line with scissors
4 1/2 yrs.	Distinguishes oblique, vertical and horizontal lines				
5 yrs.	May have difficulty with spatial orientation of objects (attending may resolve)		Learns 2 sides of body (left, right); can't locate		Dresses and undresses without assistance
6 yrs.			Identifies ring and middle finger		Ties shoe laces
			Locates left, right; details body parts		
7 yrs.	Errors for transformation in perspective, breaks and closures, transformation from line to curve, rotations and reversals resolved		Accurate left, right on self and in space	Competitive behaviors	Responsible for grooming

SENSORIMOTOR DEVELOPMENT

Vision   **Other**   **Body Scheme**

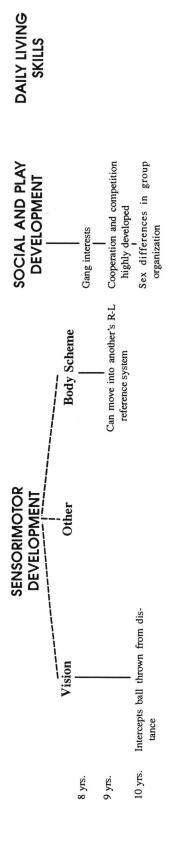

Can move into another's R-L reference system

8 yrs.

9 yrs.

10 yrs. Intercepts ball thrown from distance

SOCIAL AND PLAY DEVELOPMENT

Gang interests

Cooperation and competition highly developed

Sex differences in group organization

DAILY LIVING SKILLS

References

Ayres. (1962). Perceptual-motor training for children. *Approaches to the Treatment of Patients with Neuromuscular Dysfunction*. Third International Congress WFOT.

Barsch. (1967). *Achieving Perceptual-Motor Efficiency*.

Cratty. (1970). *Perceptual and Motor Development in Infancy and Early Childhood*.

Gesell. (1940). *The First Five Years*.

Espenschade and Eckert. (1967). *Motor Development*.

Llorens. (1970). Human development: The promise of occupational therapy. *Am J Occup Ther*. Rockville, MD: AOTA.

McGraw. (1945). *The Neuromuscular Maturation of the Human Infant*.

Mussen, Conger and Kagan. (1963). *Child Development and Personality*, 3rd ed.

Peiper. (1963). *Cerebral Function in Infancy and Childhood*.

Compiled by Mary K. Cowan, MA, OTR, FAOTA

Appendix B
RECREATIONAL ORGANIZATIONS
FOR PERSONS WITH DISABILITIES

American Alliance for Health, Physical Education and Recreation for the Handicapped Information and Research Utilization Center
1201 16th Street, NW
Washington, DC 20036
Phone: 202-833-5547

American National Red Cross
Program of Swimming for the Handicapped
17th and D Streets, NW
Washington, DC 20006
Phone: 202-857-3542

Handicapped Boaters
P.O. Box 1134
Ansonia Station
New York, NY 10023
Phone: 212-377-0310

National Association of Sports for Cerebral Palsy
United Cerebral Palsy Association of Connecticut
One State Street
New Haven, CT 06511
Phone: 203-772-2080

National Park Service
Department of the Interior
18th and C Streets, NW
Washington, DC 20240
Phone: 202-343-6843

National Wheelchair Athletic Association
Nassau Community College
Garden City, NY 11530
Phone: 212-222-1245

National Wheelchair Softball Association
P.O. Box 737
Sioux Falls, SD 57101

North American Riding Association
P.O. Box 100
Ashburn, VA 22011
Phone: 703-777-3540

American Athletic Association of the Deaf
3916 Lantern Drive
Silver Spring, MD 20902
Phone: 301-942-4042

American Blind Bowling Association
150 North Bellair Avenue
Louisville, KY 40206
Phone: 502-896-8039

American Wheelchair Bowling Association
2635 NE 19th Street
Pompano Beach, FL 33062
Phone: 305-941-1238

International Committee on the Silent Sports
Gallaudet College
Florida Avenue and 7th Street, NE
Washington, DC 20002
Phone: 202-331-1731 or 447-0360

National Association of the Physically Handicapped
76 Elm Street
London, OH 43140
Phone: 614-852-1664

National Inconvenienced Sportsmen's Association
3738 Walnut Avenue
Carmichael, CA 95608
Phone: 916-484-2153

National Therapeutic Recreation Society
1601 North Kent Street
Arlington, VA 22209
Phone: 703-525-0606

National Wheelchair Basketball Association
110 Seaton Center
University of Kentucky
Lexington, KY 40506
Phone: 703-777-3540

People-to-People Committee for the Handicapped
LaSalle Building, Suite 610
Connecticut Avenue and L Street
Washington, DC 20036
Phone: 202-785-0755

The President's Committee on Employment of the Handicapped
Subcommittee on Recreation and Leisure
Washington, DC 20210

Travel Information Center
Moss Rehabilitation Hospital
12th Street and Tabor Roads
Philadelphia, PA 19141
Phone: 215-456-9900

United Stated Deaf Skiers' Association
Two Sunset Hill Road
Simbury, CT 06070
Phone: 203-244-3341

National Handicapped Sports and Recreation Association
Capital Hill Station
P.O. Box 18664
Denver, CO 80218

National Spinal Cord Injury Foundation (Marathon Racing)
369 Elliot Street
Newton Upper Falls, MA 02164

Rehabilitation Education Center (Football)
University of Illinois
Oak Street at Stadium Drive
Champaign, IL 61820

Wheelchair Motorcycle Association
(All Terrain Vehicles)
101 Torrey Street
Brockton, MA 02410

Sports and Spokes
(W/C Sports Magazine)
5201 North 19th Avenue
Phoenix, AZ 85015

The Riding School, Inc.
275 South Avenue
Weston, MA 02193
Phone: 617-899-4555

S.I.R.E. (Self-Improvement Through Riding Education)
91 Old Bolton Road
Stow, MA 01775
Phone: 617-897-3396

Winslow Riding for the Handicapped
P.O. Box 100
Ashburn, VA 22011
Phone: 703-777-3540

Vinland National Center
3675 Ihduhapi Road
Loretto, MN 55357
Phone: 612-479-3555

National Foundation of Wheelchair Tennis
3855 Birch Street
Newport Beach, CA 92660

National Recreation and Park Association
1601 North Kent Street
Arlington, VA 22209

Disabled Sportsmen of America, Inc.
P.O. Box 26
Vinton, VA 24179

Wheelchair Pilots' Association
11018 102nd Avenue North
Largo, FL 33540

American W/C Pilots' Association
4419 North 27th Street, Apt. 3
Phoenix, AZ 85105

Winter Park Recreational Association (Skiing)
Handicapped Programs
Hal O'Leary, Director
Box 313
Winter Park, CO 80482

Appendix C
ASSESSMENT FORMS

Work Skill Assessment

	Yes	No
1. Willingness to start the task		
Agrees to start task without arguing	☐	☐
Shows enthusiasm about task	☐	☐
Starts immediately after directions have been given	☐	☐
2. Ability to follow directions		
Follows verbal directions correctly	☐	☐
Follows written directions correctly	☐	☐
3. Acceptance of supervision		
Accepts direction without showing resentment	☐	☐
Accepts criticism from supervisor without arguing or becoming defensive	☐	☐
4. Ability to sustain interest in the task		
Works continually without becoming distracted	☐	☐
Tolerates small frustrations without losing interest	☐	☐
Facial expression and posture indicate interest	☐	☐
5. Appropriate use of tools and material		
Uses familiar equipment for appropriate purposes	☐	☐
Handles equipment skillfully and safely	☐	☐
Uses material without wasting it	☐	☐
6. Appropriate rate of performance		
Accomplishes task successfully within the time limit	☐	☐
7. Acceptable level of neatness		
Keeps work area uncluttered	☐	☐
Maintains personal neatness	☐	☐
Cleans up when finished	☐	☐
8. Appropriate attention to detail		
Doesn't spend too much time or energy on unimportant details	☐	☐
Performs accurately when necessary	☐	☐
9. Ability to organize tasks in a logical manner		
Makes sure directions are clear before starting	☐	☐
Checks to see that all materials and supplies are ready before starting	☐	☐
Performs steps in logical sequence	☐	☐
10. Problem solving		
Recognizes when a problem exists	☐	☐
Attempts to solve problems without asking for help	☐	☐
Shows creativity in solving problems	☐	☐
Finds practical solutions to problems	☐	☐

Adapted from Mosey, AC: Activities Therapy. New York, Raven Press, 1973, pp. 112-120.

Social Skills Assessment

Dyadic Skills				
	Yes	**No**	**Skill Components**	**Comments**
1.			Expresses ideas clearly	
2.			Demonstrates appropriate affect	
3.			Initiates conversation	
4.			Maintains eye contact	
5.			Greets and calls people by name	
6.			Manners/habits are acceptable	
7.			Responds when spoken to	
8.			Responds beyond "yes" or "no"	
9.			Expresses feelings verbally	
10.			Shows consideration to others	
11.			Remains in contact throughout conversation	
12.			Speaks audibly and clearly	
Group Skills				
1.			Participates in group discussion	
2.			Asks for information	
3.			Contributes information	
4.			Asks for opinions	
5.			Contributes opinions	
6.			Encourages others	
7.			Assumes leadership role	
8.			Suggests operating procedures	
9.			Is willing to compromise	
10.			Accepts praise comfortably	
11.			Accepts criticism graciously	
12.			Supportive of others' contributions	

Used with permission from an unpublished manual by P. Babcock.

Appendix D

SAMPLE GROUP EXERCISE

The following patients have been working on craft activities in a parallel group. After discussion with the OTR supervisor, it was decided that the COTA should plan a *project* level activity that would meet the needs of the individuals in this group.

Patient	Observation	Plan
Ms. Wisenheimer	Is not interested in crafts. Identifies with staff. Is sarcastic and irritable.	Improve self-esteem. Allow some authority.
Ms. Gloomy Thoughts	Slowed down physically and mentally. Expresses feelings of inadequacy. Has difficulty making decisions.	Increase rate of performance. Provide activities that are easily recognized as useful and have a minimal number of steps.
Ms. Jitterbug	Capable and willing to work, but is tense, agitated and restless. Socializes well with others, but sometimes annoys others with interfering behavior. Needs immediate gratification.	Increase attention span. Provide tasks that are structured and short term. Provide for release of energy.
Ms. Detached	Offers minimal conversation. Appears sensitive to the needs to others. Usually chooses to sit by herself. Is unable to make decisions without help.	Develop personal identity and decision-making skills.
Ms. Picky	Is cooperative, conscientious and a perfectionist. Works slowly and is seldom satisfied with her work. Becomes irritated with the poor performance of others. Has trouble expressing her ideas.	Improve decision-making skills. Provide tasks that are easily corrected if mistakes are made. Develop behavior that is more tolerant of others.
Ms. Finagle	Undependable and manipulative. Appears friendly but talks about the other patients. Very bright and capable.	Develop dependable behavior. Provide activities that are intellectually stimulating and absorbing.

These patients are middle class young adults. All but one have completed high school and they all have had problems with chemical dependency. Using the information regarding project groups as a reference, respond to the following:

1. What activity could the COTA choose?
2. What steps are involved in the activity and how much time would each take?
3. What tools and materials would be required to complete the activity?
4. The supervisor has also asked the COTA to develop *task*-related behavioral goals for two of the patients—Ms. Gloomy Thoughts and Ms. Jitterbug. What goals might be appropriate for these patients? Is there a specific part of the activity that could be assigned to each of these patients in order to develop the desired behavior?
5. What goals might be appropriate for these patients? Is there a specific part of the selected activity that could be assigned to each of these patients in order to develop the desired behavior?
6. How might the activity be introduced to the group?
7. How would the group goal be explained to the members?

Prepared by Toné Blechert, COTA, ROH. From Fidler G: The task-oriented group as a context for treatment. Am J Occup Ther 1:43-48, 1969.

Appendix E
SOURCES FOR MICROSWITCHES

Supplies for Handmade Switches and Battery-Operated Devices

Chaney Electronics, Inc.
P.O. Box 27038
Denver, CO 80227

Digi-Key Corp.
P.O. Box 677
Thief River Falls, MN 56701

Microswitch
A Division of Honeywell
Freeport, IL 61032

Local Radio Shack stores

Commercial Microswitches, Controls and Interfaces

AbleNet
360 Hoover Street
Minneapolis, MN 55413

Adaptive Peripherals
4529 Begley Avenue North
Seattle, WA 98103

ComputAbility Corporation
101 Rt. 46
Pine Brook, NJ 07058

Don Johnston Developmental Equipment, Inc.
1000 N. Rand Road, Bldg. 115
P.O. Box 639
Wauconda, IL 60084

DU-IT Control Systems Group, Inc.
8765 Township Road #513
Shreve, OH 44676

Prentke Romich
1022 Heyl Road
Wooster, OH 44691

TASH, Inc.
(Technical Aids & Systems for the Handicapped)
70 Gibson Drive, Unit 12
Markham, ON L3R 4C2 Canada

Zygo Industries
P.O. Box 1008
Portland, OR 92707

Appendix F
SPLINTING RESOURCE GUIDE

Alimed, Inc.
297 High Street
Dedham, MA 02026
(800) 225-2610

Polymed Industries, Inc.
Splint Products Division
9004-H Yellow Brick Road
Baltimore, MD 21237
(800) 346-0895

Smith and Nephew/Rolyan, Inc.
N93 W14475 Whittaker Way
Menomonee Falls, WI 53051
(800) 558-8633

WFR-Aquaplast Corporation
68 Birch Street
P.O. Box 215
Ramsey, NJ 07446
(800) 526-5247

Fred Sammons, Inc.
Bissell Healthcare Corporation
Box 23
Brookfield, IL 60513-0032
(800) 323-5547
Distributors of the hand volumeter

J.A. Preston Corporation
60 Page Road
Clifton, NJ 07012
(800) 631-7277
Distributors of *Minnesota Rate of Manipulation Test*
(product of American Guidance Service, Inc.)

Johnson & Johnson Orthopedic Division
501 George Street
New Brunswick, NJ 08903
Distributors of Orthoplast®

Bibliography

CHAPTER 3

Breines E: Pragmatism as a foundation for occupational therapy curricula. *Am J Occup Ther* 41:522-525, 1987.

Cassidy JC: Access to health care: A clinician's opinion about an ethical issue. *Am J Occup Ther* 42:295-299, 1988.

Hasselkus B: Discussion of "patient" versus "client." *Am J Occup Ther* 39:605, 1985.

Serrett KD: Another look at occupational therapy's history: Paradigm or pair-of-hands? *Occup Ther Mental Health* 5:1-31, 1985.

Serrett KD et al: Adolph Meyer: Contributions to the conceptual foundation of occupational therapy. *Occup Ther Mental Health* 5:69-75, 1985.

Sharrott GW, Yerxa EJ: The issue is: Promises to keep: Implications of the referent "patient" versus "client" for those served by occupational therapy. *Am J Occup Ther* 39:401-405, 1985.

CHAPTER 4

Allen CK: *Occupational Therapy for Psychiatric Diseases: Measurement and Management of Cognitive Disabilities.* Boston: Litttle, Brown, 1985.

Bruce MA and Borg B: *Frames of Reference in Psychosocial Occupational Therapy.* Thorofare, NJ: Slack Incorporated, 1987.

Christiansen C: Occupational therapy: Intervention for life performance. In Christiansen C and Baum C (Eds.): *Occupational Therapy: Overcoming Human Performance Deficits.* Thorofare, NJ: Slack Incorporated, 1991.

Cynkin S: *Occupational Therapy: Toward Health Through Activities.* Boston: Little, Brown, 1979.

Kielhofner G: *A Model of Human Occupation: Theory and Application.* Baltimore: Williams & Wilkins, 1985.

CHAPTER 5

Llorens LA: Performance tasks and roles throughout the life span. In Christiansen C and Baum C (Eds.): *Occupational Therapy: Overcoming Human Performance Deficits.* Thorofare, NJ: Slack Incorporated, 1991.

CHAPTER 6

Clark FA et al: Occupational science: Academic innovation in the service of occupational therapy's future. *Am J Occup Ther* 45:300-310, 1991.

CHAPTER 7

American Occupational Therapy Association: *Entry-Level OTR and COTA Role Delineation.* Rockville, Maryland: AOTA, 1981.

Berger B: The sociology of leisure: Some suggestions. In Smigel, EO (Ed): *Work and Leisure: A Contemporary Social Problem.* New Haven, Connecticut: New Haven College and University Press, 1979.

Broderick T, Glazer B: Leisure participation and the retirement process. *Am J Occup Ther* 37:15-22, 1983.

Cheek N, Brunch W: *The Social Organization of Leisure in Human Society.* New York: Harper and Row, 1976.

Childs E, Childs J: Children and leisure. In Smith MA et al (Eds): *Leisure and Society in Britain.* London: Allen Lane, 1974.

Clayre A: *Work and Play, Ideas and Experience of Work and Leisure.* New York: Harper and Row, 1974.

Comfort A: Future Sex Mores: Sexuality in a Zero Growth Society. London: *Current* (February), 1973.

deGrazia S: *Of Time, Work, and Leisure.* New York: Doubleday, 1962.

DePoy E and Kolodner E: Psychological performance factors. In Christiansen C and Baum C (Eds.): *Occupational Therapy: Overcoming Human Performance Deficits.* Thorofare, NJ: Slack Incorporated, 1991.

Dumazedier J: *Toward a Society of Leisure.* New York: Free Press, 1967.

Friedman E, Havighurst R: *The Meaning of Work and Retirement.* Chicago, Illinois: Chicago Press, 1954.

Fuch VR: Women's earnings: Recent trends and long-run prospects. *Monthly Labor Review* 97(May):22-26, 1984.

Gilfoyle EM, Grady AP and Moore JC: *Children Adapt: A Theory of Sensorimotor-Sensory Development,* 2d ed. Thorofare, NJ: Slack Incorporated, 1990.

Havighurst R: The nature and values of meaningful free time. In Kleemier R (Ed): *Aging and Leisure: A Research Perspective into Meaningful Use of Time.* New York: Oxford University Press, 1961.

Hinojosa J, Sabari J, Rosenfield M: Purposeful activity guidelines and position paper. *Am J Occup Ther* 37:805, 1983.

Huizinger J: *Homoludens: A Study of Play Elements in Culture.* Boston: Beacon Press, 1951.

Kimmel D: *Adulthood and Aging.* New York: John Wiley and Sons, 1974.

Klinger J, Friedman F, Sullivand R: *Mealtime Manual for the Aged and Handicapped.* New York: Simon and Schuster, 1970.

Leonardelli CA: *The Milwaukee Evaluation of Daily Living Skills: Evaluation in Long-Term Psychiatric Care.* Thorofare, NJ: Slack Incorporated, 1988.

Llorens L: Changing balance: Environment and individual. *Am J Occup Ther* 38:29-31, 1984.

Mitchell E, Mason B: *The Theory of Play.* New York: AS Barnes, 1934.

Neulinger J: *The Psychology of Leisure: Research Approaches to the Study.* Springfield, Illinois: Charles C. Thomas, 1974.

Pebler D, Rubin K: *The Play of Children: Current Theory and Research Contributions to Human Development.* New York: Tanner and Basshardt, 1982.

Piepus J: *Leisure the Basis of Culture.* New York: Partheon Books, 1952.

Reilly M: *Play as Exploratory Learning.* Beverly Hills, California: Sage Publications, 1974.

Spencer JC: The physical environment and performance. In Christiansen C and Baum C: *Occupational Therapy: Overcoming Human Performance Deficits.* Thorofare, NJ: Slack Incorporated, 1991.

Thackery M, Skidmore R, Farley W: *Introduction to Mental Health Field and Practice.* New York: Prentice Hall, 1979.

Trombly CA, Scott AD: *Occupational Therapy for Physical Dysfunction.* Baltimore, Maryland: Williams & Wilkins, 1977.

Willard HS, Spackman CS (Eds): *Occupational Therapy,* 4th edition. Philadelphia: JB Lippincott, 1971.

CHAPTER 8

Cook EA, Luschen L, Sikes J: Dressing training for an elderly woman with cognitive and perceptual impairments. *Am J Occup Ther* 45:652-654, 1991.

CHAPTER 9

Babcock PH: *The Role of the OTA in Mental Health.* Unpublished manual. Minneapolis, Minnesota: St. Mary's Junior College, 1978.

Borg B and Bruce MA: *The Group System: The Therapeutic Activity Group in Occupational Therapy.* Thorofare, NJ: Slack Incorporated, 1990.

Davis CM: *Patient Practitioner Interaction.* Thorofare, New Jersey: Slack, Inc., 1989.

Kaplan K: *Directive Group Therapy: Innovative Mental Health Treatment.* Thorofare, NJ: Slack Incorporated, 1988.

Navarra T, Lipkowitz M and Navarra JG: *Therapeutic Communication: A Guide to Effective Interpersonal Skills for Health Care Professionals.* Thorofare, New Jersey: Slack, Inc., 1991.

Ross M: *Group Process: Using Therapeutic Activities in Chronic Care.* Thorofare, NJ: Slack Incorporated, 1987.

Ross M: *Integrative Group System: The Structured Five-Stage Approach,* 2d ed. Thorofare, NJ: Slack Incorporated, 1991.

CHAPTER 10

Barney KF: From Ellis Island to assisted living: Meeting the needs of older adults from diverse cultures. *Amer J Occup Ther* 45:586-593, 1991.

English O, Pearson G: *Emotional Problems of Living,* 3rd Edition. New York: WW Norton, 1963.

Evans J (Guest Ed.): Special issue on cross-cultural perspectives on occupational therapy. *Am J Occup Ther* 46(8):675-768, 1992.

Freeman J: *Crowding and Behavior.* New York: Viking Press, 1973.

Krefting LH and Krefting DV: Cultural influences on performance. In Christiansen C and Baum C (Eds.): *Occupational Therapy: Overcoming Human Performance Deficits.* Thorofare, New Jersey: Slack Incorporated, 1991.

Knutson A: *The Individual Society, and Behavior.* New York: Russel Sage Foundation, 1965.

Opler M: *Culture and Social Psychiatry,* Part II. New York: Atherton Press, 1967.

CHAPTER 11

Bessinger C: *The Video Guide.* Santa Barbara, California: Video Info Publishers, 1977.

Fuller J: *Prescription for Better Home Video Movies.* Los Angeles: HP Books, 1988.

Kerr RJ: *Video the Better Way: A New Art for a New Age.* Yokohama, Japan: Victor Company of Japan, 1980.

Lewis R: *Home Video Makers Handbook.* New York: Crown, 1987.

Quinn G: *The Camcorder Handbook.* Blue Ridge Summit, Pennsylvania: Tab Books, 1987.

CHAPTER 12

Closing the Gap. P.O. Box 68, Henderson, Minnesota 56044.

Control Battery Operated Toys: Instructions for Constructing a Large Area Flap Switch (LAFS) to Allow Disabled Children to Control Battery Operated Toys. G. Fraser Shein, Biofeedback Research Project, Rehabilitation Engineering Department, Ontario Crippled Children's Centre, 350 Ramsey Road, Toronto, Ontario, Canada M4G 1R8.

From Toys to Computers: Access for the Physically Disabled Child. Christine Wright and Mari Nomura, P.O. Box 700242, San Jose, California 95170.

Guide to Controls, Selection and Mounting Applications. Rehabilitation Engineering Center, Children's Hospital at Stanford, 520 Willow Road, Palo Alto, California 94304.

Homemade Battery Powered Toys and Educational Devices for Severely Handicapped Children, 2nd Edition. Linda J. Burkhart, R.D. 1, Millville, Pennsylvania 17846.

Information on Communication, Writing Systems, and Access to Computers for Severely Physically Handicapped Individuals. Trace Research and Development Center on Communication, Control and Computer Access for Handicapped Individuals, University of Wisconsin-Madison, 314 Waisman Center, 1500 Highland Avenue, Madison, Wisconsin 53706.

International Software/Hardware Registry. GC Vanderheiden, LM Walsted, Editors. Trace Research and Development Center for the Severely Communicatively Handicapped, University of Wisconsin-Madison, 314 Waisman Center, 1500 Highland Avenue, Madison, Wisconsin 53706.

More Homemade Battery Devices for Severely Handicapped Children with Suggested Activities. Linda J Burkhart, R.D. 1, Millville, Pennsylvania, 17846.

Wobble Switch Toy Control Switch: A Do It Yourself Guide. B Brown. Trace Research and Development Center for the Handicapped, University of Wisconsin-Madison, 314 Waisman Center, 1500 Highland Avenue, Madison, Wisconsin 53706.

CHAPTER 13

AOTA: *Technology Review '90, Perspectives on Occupational Therapy Practice.* Rockville, Maryland: American Occupational Therapy Association, 1990.

Brecher D: *The Women's Computer Literacy Handbook.* New York: New American Library, 1985.

Brewer BJ and McMahon P: Certified occupational therapy assistants and microcomputers. In Johnson JA (Ed.): *Certified Occupational Therapy Assistants: Opportunities and Challenges.* Binghamton, New York: Haworth Press, 1988.

Christensen WW, Stearns EJ: *Microcomputers in Health Care,* 2nd Edition. Frederick, Maryland: Aspen, 1990.

Clark EN (Ed): *Microcomputers: Clinical Applications.* Thorofare, New Jersey: Slack Inc, 1986.

Cromwell F (Ed): *Computer Applications in Occupational Therapy.* New York: Haworth Press, 1986.

Green P and Brightman AJ: *Independence Day: Designing Computer Solutions for Individuals with Disability.* Allen, Texas: DLM Learning Resources, 1990.

Naisbitt J, Aburdene P: *Megatrends 2,000.* New York: William Morrow, 1990.

Okoye RL: Computer technology in occupational therapy. In Hopkins HL, Smith HD (Eds): *Willard and Spackman's Occupational Therapy,* 7th Edition. Philadelphia: JB Lippincott, 1988.

O'Leary S, Mann C and Perkash I: Access to computers for older adults: Problems and solutions. *Am Jour Occup Ther* 45:636-642, 1991.

Smith RO: Technological approaches to performance enhancement. In Christiansen C and Baum C (Eds.): *Occupational Therapy: Overcoming Human Performance Deficits.* Thorofare, New Jersey: Slack Incorporated, 1991.

Thibodaux LR: Meeting the challenge of computer literacy in occupational therapy education. In *Target 2,000 Proceedings.* Rockville, Maryland: American Occupational Therapy Association, 1986.

Viseltear E (Ed): Special issue on technology. *Am J Occup Ther* 41:11, 1987.

Workman D, Geggie C, Creasey G: The microcomputer as an aid to written communication. *Br J Occup Ther* 51:188-190, 1988.

Zaks R: *Don't (Or How to Care for Your Computer).* Berkeley, California: Sybex, 1981.

CHAPTER 14

Cannon NM et al: *Manual on Hand Splinting.* New York: Churchill Livingstone, 1985.

Fess EE, Phillips C: *Hand Splinting Principles and Methods,* 2nd Edition. St. Louis, Missouri: CV Mosby, 1987.

Kiel JH: *Basic Handsplinting: A Pattern Designing Approach.* Boston: Little, Brown, 1983.

Malick M, Carr J: *Manual on Management of the Burn Patient, Including Splinting, Mold and Pressure Techniques.* Pittsburgh, Pennsylvania: Harmarville Rehabilitation Center, 1982.

Pedretti LW: *Occupational Therapy Practice Skills for Physical Dysfunction.* St. Louis, Missouri: CV Mosby, 1985.

Ryan SE (Ed.) *Practice Issues in Occupational Therapy: Intraprofessional Team Building.* Thorofare, New Jersey: Slack Inc., 1993.

Tenney CG, Lisak JM: *Atlas of Hand Splinting.* Boston: Little, Brown, 1986.

Ziegler EM: *Current Concepts in Orthotics—A Diagnosis-Related Approach to Splinting.* Menomonee Falls, Wisconsin: Rolyan Medical Products, 1984.

CHAPTER 15

Anderson L, Anderson J: A positioning seat for the neonate and infant with high tone. *Am J Occup Ther* 40:186-190, 1986.

Dahlin-Webb S: Brief or new: A weighted wrist cuff. *Am J Occup Ther* 40:363-364, 1986.

Gesior C, Mann D: Finger extension game. *Am J Occup Ther* 40:44-48, 1986.

Hopkins HL, Smith HD (Eds): *Willard and Spackman's Occupational Therapy,* 7th Edition. Philadelphia: JB Lippincott, 1988.

CHAPTER 16

Bissell J, Mailloux Z: The use of crafts in occupational therapy for the physically disabled. *Am J Occup Ther* 35:369-374, 1981.

Cynkin S, Robinson AM: *Occupational Therapy and Activities Health: Toward Health Through Activities.* Boston: Little, Brown, 1990.

Drake M: *Crafts in Therapy and Rehabilitation.* Thorofare, NJ: Slack Incorporated, 1992.

Fidler GS: From crafts to competence. *Am J Occup Ther* 35(9):567-573, 1981.

CHAPTER 17

Bing RK: Occupational therapy revisited: A paraphrastic journey. *Am J Occup Ther* 35:499-518, 1981.

Cynkin C, Robinson AM: *Occupational Therapy and Activities Health: Toward Health Through Activities.* Boston: Little, Brown, 1990.

Fidler GS: Psychological evaluation of occupational therapy activities. *Am J Occup Ther* 2:284-287, 1948.

Kircher MA: Motivation as a factor of perceived exertion in purposeful versus nonpurposeful activity. *Am J Occup Ther* 38:165-170, 1984.

Kremer ERH, Nelson DL, Duncombe LW: Effects of selected activities on affective meaning in psychiatric clients. *Am J Occup Ther* 38:522-528, 1984.

Lamport NK, Coffey MS and Hersch GI: *Activity Analysis Handbook.* Thorofare, NJ: Slack Incorporated, 1989.

Levine RE and Brayley CR: Occupation as a therapeutic medium: A contextual approach to performance intervention. In Christiansen C and Baum C: *Occupational Therapy: Overcoming Human Performance Deficits.* Thorofare, NJ: Slack Incorporated, 1991.

Reed K, Sanderson S: *Concepts of Occupational Therapy,* 2nd Edition. Baltimore: Williams & Wilkins, 1983.

Smith PA, Barrows HS, Whitney JN: Psychological attributes of occupational therapy crafts. *Am J Occup Ther* 13:16-21, 25-26, 1959.

West WL: Nationally speaking—perspectives on the past and future. *Am J Occup Ther* 44:9-10, 1990.

Glossary

This glossary is provided to assist the reader in learning new words and acronyms and their meanings. The index of the textbook should be used to locate specific terms so that they may be reviewed within context. In addition to the individual chapter definitions of terms, the following sources were used: *Uniform Terminology for Occupational Therapy*, 2nd Edition, 1989, (AOTA); *The Random House College Dictionary*, Revised Edition, 1990; *Roget's International Thesaurus*, 4th Edition; and the *Encyclopedia and Dictionary of Medicine, Nursing, and Allied Health*, 5th Edition, 1992.

Accommodation—Ability to modify or adjust in response to the environment. The changing of an existing schema as a result of new information.

Accuracy of response—Percentage of errors and the percentage of correct responses recorded during the tracking and selection time when using a switch or other device.

Action process— Purposeful action is a process of communicating feelings and thoughts as well as non-verbal messages (Fidler).

Active listening—Skills that allow a person to hear, understand and indicate that the message has been communicated.

Activities of daily living—An area of occupational performance that refers to grooming, oral hygiene, bathing, toilet hygiene, dressing, feeding and eating, medication routine, socialization, functional communication, functional mobility and sexual expression activities.

Activity analysis—The breaking down of an activity into detailed subparts and steps; an examination of the characteristics and values of an activity in relation to the patient's needs, interests and goals.

Activity analysis checklist—A form used to document activity analysis.

Activity categories—Groupings of activities frequently used for evaluation and treatment; categories include crafts, sensory awareness, movement awareness, fine arts, construction, games, etc.

Activity properties/characteristics—Factors that contribute to the therapeutic nature/potential of a particular activity, such as being goal directed, having significance to the individual, or requiring involvement, adaptability, or gradability, etc.

Activity tolerance—The ability to sustain engagement in a purposeful activity over a period of time.

Adaptation—The tendency to adjust to the environment; modification of an activity; changing of components required to complete the task.

Adaption—*see* Adaptation.

Adaptive equipment—Assistive devices or aids that allow a person with a handicap to participate in life activities.

Adaptive response—Active responses organized below the conscious level; a progressive movement from basic relations to adaptive responses to adaptive skills to adaptive patterns of behavior.

Adaptive skills—Abilities that enable the individual to satisfy basic needs and satisfactorily perform life tasks.

Affect—One's mood and related behaviors that reflect a mental attitude exhibited by emotions, temperament and feelings.

Affective skills—Abilities to interact appropriately in relation to inner feelings, emotional tone and mood; may be characterized by body language and gestures, as well as verbal content; relates to self-esteem, the ability to develop relationships and assume responsibility, etc. (*see* Affect.)

After-care houses—Halfway homes initially established by Ellis for people released from asylums.

Aggression—A primary instinct generally associated with emotional states that prompt carrying out actions in a forceful way; often manifested by exhibiting anger and destructiveness.

Alienist—An early term for psychiatrist.

ALS—Amyotrophic lateral sclerosis.

Ameliorate—Improve; to make or become better.

Analysis—*see* Activity analysis.

Anatomic arches (hand)—The longitudinal, distal transverse and proximal transverse arches that must be supported when making splints to assure comfort and to preserve the normal anatomic structure.

Approach—A method of treating or dealing with something.

Assimilation—The ability to absorb; to make information a part of one's thinking; a process by which experience is incorporated into existing knowledge. Incoming information is perceived and interpreted according to an existing schema that has already been established through previous experience.

Association—The ability to relate experiences from the past to present experience.

Asylums—Institutions often referred to as refuges for individuals who are unable to live independently in the community; historically, majority of residents were referred to as insane.

Attention span—The ability to focus on a task or tasks over a period of time.

Attitude—A pattern of mental views established through cumulative prior experiences; manner, disposition, feeling or position; may be consciously or subconsciously assumed.

Auditory—Of or relating to the reception, processing, and interpretation of sounds through the ears; includes the ability to localize and discriminate noises in the background.

Award of Excellence—The highest award bestowed on COTAs by the AOTA; recognizes the contributions of COTAs to the advancement of occupational therapy and provides incentive to contribute to the profession's growth and development.

Biopsychosocial—One of the component systems of occupation; model that illustrates how biologic, psychologic and social factors interact in an individual to affect occupational function or dysfunction.

Axiology—A branch of philosophy concerned with the study of values.

BASIC—Beginner's All-Purpose Symbolic Instruction Code; used for computer programming.

Behavior modification—A process of reinforcing desirable responses while ignoring undesirable ones; food, praise and redeemable tokens are some of the reinforcers used.

Bilateral integration—The coordination of the interaction of both sides of one's body when participating in an activity.

Biopsychosocial—One of the component systems of occupation; model that illustrates how biologic, psychologic and social factors interact in an individual to affect occupational function or dysfunction.

Body scheme—Awareness of the body and the relationship of body parts to each other.

Bolsters—Long, cylindrical, padded pieces of adaptive equipment used to assist in maintaining functional positions and to enhance activity management.

Bony prominences—Structures on the surface of the bones that have little tissue padding and must be accommodated in the construction and fitting of splints as well as in other situations.

Boot up—Turn on the computer and monitor.

Bulletin board—Computer program that is used to gain or exchange information, and send or receive messages (electronic mail).

Byte—In computer programming, a unit of information equal to one character.

Camcorder—An electronic device for making video recordings.

Career mobility—AOTA plan that allowed COTAs to become certified as OTRs after meeting specific criteria, including work experience, professional level fieldwork experiences and completion of the occupational therapist certification examination.

Categories of activity analysis (general)—Examples of components include, but are not limited to, motor, sensory, cognitive, intrapersonal and interpersonal skills, adaptions, supplies and equipment, cost, number of steps required, time involved, supervision required, space needed, precautions, and contraindications.

Categories of occupation—Occupation performance areas that include activities of daily living, work activities, or play or leisure activities.

Categorization—The ability to classify; to describe by naming or labeling; differentiating between differences and similarities.

Cephalocaudal development—Development that proceeds from the head to the lower extremities (tail).

Choice of occupation—The selection of an activity based on cultural exposure, individual values and interests, and special abilities.

Climate—Weather conditions that impact a person's external environment.

Cognition—A mental process involving thinking, judgment and perceptions to arrive at a level of knowing and understanding.

Cognitive disability—A series of functional units of behavior that cuts across diagnostic categories and interferes with task behavior.

Collaboration—Working with others in a shared, cooperative endeavor to achieve mutual goals.

Committee on OTAs—A group responsible for all developmental aspects related to the new occupational therapy assistant personnel designation in the profession.

Communication—The ability to receive and transmit messages verbally or nonverbally.

Community—Interaction among individuals; achieving a sense of union with others; interconnectedness; also refers to where an individual lives, such as a rural, urban or suburban area.

Competence—The ability to use dexterity and intelligence in the completion of tasks; (a sense of satisfaction is implied in completion); also a legal term referring to soundness of one's mind.

Components—Fundamental units or constituent parts; in relation to activities refers to processes, tools, materials, purposefulness, etc.

Concentration—The ability to focus on a specific portion of the total; to bring all efforts to bear on an activity.

Concept formation—The organization of information from a variety of sources is formulated into thoughts and ideas.

Conditioning—A learning process that alters behavior through providing reinforcements (instrumental or operant) or associating a reflex with a particular stimulus to trigger a desired response (classic—Pavlov).

Confidentiality—Maintaining secrecy regarding patient or other information; basic tenet of medical ethics.

Conflict—Opposition or competitive action relative to incompatible views.

Contraindication—A condition that deems a particular type of treatment undesirable or improper.

Control site—An anatomic site where the person can demonstrate purposeful movement.

Controversy—Dispute.

Cost-effective—Economical in terms of benefits gained in relation to money spent.

COTA Advisory Committee—Formed in 1986 by the AOTA Executive Board to replace the COTA Task Force; the group's goal is to identify COTA concerns and formulate suggestions for addressing them.

COTA Task Force—Group established by AOTA to make recommendations regarding COTA issues and concerns; later renamed the COTA Advisory Committee.

Cowan stabilizing pillow—A supportive pillow designed to assist children with balance problems to sit on the floor; an example of simply designed adaptive equipment.

CPU—Central processing unit of a computer.

Creativity—Originality of thought, process and expression.

Criteria of purposefulness—In activity, those standards by which an activity's therapeutic value is assessed; include being goal-directed, age-appropriate, and having relevance and purpose.

Crossing the midline—The ability to move the limbs and eyes across the midline (sagittal plane) of one's body.

CRT—Cathode ray tube.

Cultural environment—Characteristics common to a particular group that provide input to an individual's life; can include values, beliefs, rituals, food, apparel, etc.

Culturally sensitive—Showing awareness and appreciation of the significance of values, beliefs, rituals and traditions held by a particular group.

Custom—Pattern of behavior or practice that is common to members of a particular group.

Daily living skills—Those things performed each day that sustain and enhance life, such as dressing, grooming and eating.

Database manager—A computer software program that organizes and categorizes data.

DBM—Database manager.

Decision-making—The process of weighing options in order to reach the best conclusion.

Deformity prevention—The act of reducing or eliminating distortions or malformations of a part of the body by various means, such as the use of a splint; taking measures to avoid disfigurement orchange ina body part.

Dementia praecox—An early term for schizophrenia.

Depth perception—The ability to determine the relative distance between self and figures or objects observed.

Developmental level—Degree of achievement in an established progression; pattern of growth, development and maturation.

Developmental sequence—An established pattern of development and growth.

Differentiation—A process of altering behavior that requires the ability to discriminate which elements are necessary and those that are not in a given set of circumstances.

Difficulty level—Degree of complexity required to execute a particular activity or step.

DIP joint—Distal interphalangeal joint.

Discovery method—Involves teaching techniques such as emphasizing contrast, informed guessing, active participation and awareness; also referred to as the reflective method (Bruner).

Disruptions—Sudden changes in one's environment that require immediate attention and response.

Disk drive—Peripheral computer equipment that sends messages from a software program to the computer; also called the disk operating system (DOS).

Disorientation—Inability to make accurate judgments about people, places and time.

Disruption—A forced interruption in a person's life.

Disuse syndrome—Complications arising from inactivity; also referred to as hypokinetic diseases.

Documentation—Written records of the patient's health care that include information about current and future needs.

Doing—The act of performing or executing; a way of knowing (Meyer); a process of investigating, trying out and gaining evidence of one's capacities; potential becomes actual (Fidler).

DOS—Disk operating system of a computer.

Dualistic—A position that views humans as having mind/body separation.

Durability—Capacity of an object or piece of equipment to last for a length of time without significant deterioration.

Dyad—A relationship between two individuals in which interaction is significant.

Dyadic—Of or relating to the interaction of two individuals on a significant, one-to-one basis.

Dynamic splint—A splint that allows controlled movement at various joints; tension is applied to encourage particular movements.

Economic status—One's level of financial independence; also refers to social class, such as poor, middle class or rich.

ECU—Environmental control unit.

Effectiveness—Degree to which the desired result is produced.

Effects of occupation—Those factors influenced by engagement in various occupations; may be broadly categorized as biologic, psychologic and sociocultural; outome(s) of a purposeful, meaningful activity.

Efficacy—Power to produce intended results; effectiveness.

Efficiency—Producing the desired outcome in a timely, productive way.

Ego integrity—Acceptance of self, nature and one's life. The value of one's life is recognized and time is not spent grieving over what might have been.

Ego strength—An executive personality structure that effectively directs and controls a person's actions; requires effective evaluation of reality and impulse control and consideration of one's ethics and values.

Employment—Activity in which one is engaged; also refers to paid work.

Endurance—The ability to sustain exertion over time; involves musculoskeletal, cardiac and pulmonary systems.

Environment—All factors that provide input to the individual.

Environmental control unit—An electronic system with sensors that monitors and performs various tasks.

Epistemology—A dimension of philosophy that is concerned with the questions of truth.

Equilibration—Process whereby new knowledge attained is brought into balance with previous experience.

Ethics—Aspect of the axiology branch of philosophy that poses questions of value regarding the standards or rules for right conduct.

Evaluation tools—Tests, checklists, questionnaires, activities and other methods used to assess strengths and limitations.

Expiation of guilt—The making amends for wrong doings; may be expressed verbally or achieved through engagement in appropriate activities.

Extinction—The disappearance of a previously conditioned response due to a lack of reinforcement.

Facilitation—Techniques used to make the desired response easier.

Facilitator—An individual who assists in making a process easier; the individual who assists in helping one make progress in reaching a goal.

Feedback—Information individuals receive about their behavior and the consequences of their actions; guides future behavior.

Feeding and eating—The skills of chewing, sucking and swallowing, and the use of utensils.

Fidelity—The ability to maintain loyalties in spite of differences.

Figure ground—The ability to differentiate between background and foreground objects and forms.

Fine motor coordination/dexterity—The ability to perform controlled movements, particularly in the manipulation of objects, through the use of small muscle groups.

Firmware—Flat electronic cards that occupy slots inside the computer.

Form constancy—The ability to recognize various forms and objects in different environments, sizes and positions.

Frame of reference—A person's assumptions and attitudes based on beliefs and conceptual models.

Framework—A structure, plan or specified arrangement.

Functional communication—The ability to use communication devices and systems, such as telephone, computer and call lights.

Functional level—An individual's occupational ability based on his or her specific performance deficits and/or strengths.

Functional mobility—The ability to move from one position to another (eg, in bed or wheelchair) or transfer to tub, shower, toilet, etc.; driving and use of other forms of transportation.

Functional position—One in which the affected part or parts of the body will be able to function maximally in relation to performance requirements.

Functional requirements—Components of an activity that require motor performance and behaviors for adequate completion.

General systems theory—A method of organizing different levels and categories of information; components include open system, input, throughput, output and feedback; *see* individual headings for additional information.

Generalization of learning—The ability to apply previously learned concepts to similar, current situations.

Generativity—Concern for the establishment and guiding of the next generation; giving without expecting anything in return.

Genuineness—Characteristic evidenced by sincerity and honesty; authenticity.

Goal achievement—The completion of those tasks and objectives one has set out to accomplish.

Gradability— Refers to the process by which performance of an activity is viewed step-by-step on a continuum, moving from simple to complex, or slow to rapid.

Grandfather clause—An exemption from certain requirements based on previous experience and/or circumstance.

Gross motor coordination—The use of large muscle groups to make controlled movements.

Group—Three or more people who establish some form of interdependent relationship.

Group approach—Therapeutic intervention that focuses on meeting the needs of individuals through active participation with others (three or more).

Group-centered roles—Behavior patterns group members share and that are required for the group to function, maintain relationships and achieve group goals; example include encourager, gate-keeper, tension reliever, etc.

Group community—The desirable outcome of group member relationships; a union with others; group cohesion.

Group norms—Standards of behavior, stated or unspoken, that define what is accepted, expected and valued by the group.

Group process—The manner in which group members relate to and communicate with each other, and how they accomplish their tasks.

Guide for supervision—One collection of the teaching materials developed from the federally funded invitational workshops held between 1963 and 1968. Concepts from this document are included in the 1990 document, *Supervision Guidelines for Certified Occupational Therapy Assistants.*

Gustatory—Of or relating to the reception, processing and interpration of tastes.

Habit of attention—Tuke's key element in the use of occupations that required concentration, limited undesirable stimuli and expanded positive feelings.

Habituation—An individual's habits and internalized roles, that help to maintain activity and action.

Half-lapboard—Device that provides a table surface for people in wheelchairs.

Hand creases—Volar surface anatomical landmarks that must be considered when constructing and fitting splints; include distal and proximal palmar, thenar and wrist.

Hardware—The computer and all of its electronic parts.

Heterogeneous group—A group of people members vary in age, sex, values, interests, socioeconomic background or cultural background.

Holism—View of the human mind and body as being one entity.

Holistic view—*see* Holism.

Home health— Area of occupational therapy service delivery that focuses on therapeutic intervention in the home environment.

Homeostasis—The tendency of the system, especially the physiologic system, to maintain internal stability.

Homogeneous group—A group of people in which members share similarities such as age, sex values, interests, socioeconomic background or cultural background.

Hostility—An opposition in feeling or action; antagonistic attitude.

Human activity—Occupations including those necessary to satisfy basic needs such as survival, productivity, a sense of belonging, etc.

Human development—Levels of growth and maturation that occur at predictable intervals.

Human needs—Physiologic, psychologic and sociocultural requirements for one's well-being.

Hypokinetic disease—Complications arising from inactivity; also called disuse syndrome.

Immunity—The possession of biologic defenses against illness.

Individualized—Adapted to the particular needs and interests of a person.

Initial dependence—First stage of group development in which members are dependent on the leader and concerned about their respective places in the group.

Initiative—Ability for original conception and independent action.

Input—The ways a computer or video system can receive information; how it can be "put in"; also refers to the model of human occupation process of receiving information from the environment.

Inservice training—Educational opportunities such as seminars and workshops provided in the workplace.

Integration of learning—The ability to use previously learned behaviors and concepts by incorporating them into one's repertoire and using them in a variety of new situations.

Integrative school—Psychiatric position relative to the biopsychologic nature of individuals.

Interdependent—Relationship characterized by cohesion and a sense of community.

Interests—Activities that the individual finds pleasurable; those occupations that maintain one's attention.

Interfaces—Electrical circuits that connect switches to devices.

Interpersonal skills—Communications skills that help individuals interact effectively with a variety of people.

Intimacy—The ability to commit oneself to partnerships or concrete affiliations; to develop the ethical strength to abide by the commitment made, even if compromise or sacrifice is necessary.

Intrapersonal skills—Developing a clear and accurate sense of self.

Intrinsic—From within; innate, natural and true.

Intrinsic minus—Describes a position where the hand is in a functional position—15 to 30 degrees wrist extension, MPs moderately extended (as close to zero degrees as is comfortable), thumb in a gently (not maximally) abducted position from the palm.

Intrinsic plus—Describes a position counter to intrinsic minus (*see* Intrinsic minus).

Joint creases—Grooves in the skin related to joint movement.

Joystick—An input device that bypasses the computer keyboard and moves the cursor (position indicator) up, down, right and left and turns the machine on and off.

Kinesthesia—The ability to identify the sensation of movement, including the path and direction of movement.

Laterality—The use of a preferred body part, such as the right or left hand, for activities requiring a high skill level.

Learning—A relatively permanent change in behavior resulting from exposure to conditions in the environment.

Leisure—Nonwork or free time spent in adult play activities that have an influence on the quality of life.

Leisure patterns—Use of discretionary time (non-work) to engage in particular activities of personal interest.

Level of arousal—The degree to which one demonstrates alertness and responsiveness to stimulation from the environment.

Life roles—Refers to the variety of experiences that occupy one's time, including worker, student, caregiver, homemaker, mate, sibling, peer, etc.

Life space—The total activities or ways of spending time; everything that influences a person's behavior (eg, objects, people and values).

Life tasks—Those developmental tasks that must be accomplished by each person for successful living throughout the life span (Havighurst).

Lines of readiness—Foundation for treatment developed by OBrock involving construction of things, communicating things, finding out things, completing things, and excelling in things.

Mainframe—A large central computer with numerous terminals.

Manipulation—Ability to handle objects and use with some degree of skill in activity performance.

Mechanical assistance—Describes a situation where the patient is independent in carrying out activities with assistive or adaptive equipment.

Medication routine—A procedure of obtaining medication, operating containers, and take medication at the required times.

Memory—In splinting, the ability of the material being used to return to its original flat shape and size when reheated.

Mentally ill—Persons having diseases and disabilities that result in impaired mental function.

Metaphysics—A branch of philosophy concerned with questions about the ultimate nature of things, including the nature of humans.

Method of activation—Movement or means by which a control site will activate a switch.

Microswitch—A small electronic "on/off" switch.

Milieu—A social and physical environment; one's surroundings.

Mind/body relationship—Interdependence of mental and physical aspects of humans; holism.

Misuse syndrome—Conditions that arise from a change in structure or function of a body part due to improper use (eg, tennis elbow).

Mobility—The ability to move physically from one position or place to another.

Modem—Modulator/demodulator that allows computer signals to be sent over telephone wires.

Monitor—Peripheral equipment that displays computer information on a screen.

Motor development—Acquisition of control and movement skills in a sequence that is relatively unvaried and characterized by milestones (Gesell).

Mouse—An electronic device that provides input to the computer without use of the keyboard.

Muscle tone—A degree of tension or resistance present in a muscle or muscle group.

Narcissism—Egocentricity; dominant interest in one's self.

NDT—Neurodevelopmental treatment.

Needs—Lack of things required for the welfare of the individual.

Networking—Informal communication with others having common interests; a supportive system for sharing information and services.

Object manipulation—Skill in handling large and small objects, such as keys, doorknobs and calculator.

Obsessive-compulsive—Behavior marked by compulsion to perform repetitively certain acts or carry out certain rituals to excess, such as handwashing or counting.

Occupation—The full range of activities that occupy a person; goal-directed behavior fundamental to human existence focused on activities of daily living skills, work and play in occupational therapy; includes meeting survival needs as well as those that lead to a full and productive life; a dynamic changing process influenced by biologic, psychologic and sociocultural environments (Reed).

Occupational behavior—The result of one's ability to organize and take action based on skills, knowledge and attitudes, and to function in one's life roles; thorough mastery of the environment, with work and play being key elements; occupation is an integrating factor for improving patient behavior (Reilly).

Occupational nurse—Early designation given to specialized occupational work provided by nurses trained by Susan Tracy.

Occupational performance—Participation in activities of daily living, work activities, and play or leisure activities.

Occupational role—Endeavors that define the nature of the individual in terms of achieving his/her potential and social worth as a member of society (see Life roles).

Occupational science—The academic discipline being developed at the University of California based on the concept of occupation and the complexities of its components, including purposeful activities and role- and age-appropriate occupations.

Olfactory—Of or relating to the reception, processing and interpretion of odors.

Ontogenesis—Biologic term meaning there is repetition of evolutionary changes of a species during embryonic development of an individual organism.

Operation—(cognitive) A mental action that can be reversed.

Opportunity—Situation or condition favorable for goal-attainment; a therapeutic technique of structuring the environment; opposite of prescription.

Oral-motor control—The ability to exhibit controlled movements of the mouth, tongue and related structures.

Organization—The tendency of a person to develop a coherent system; to systematize.

Orientation—Refers to the degree to which one is able to correctly identify person, place, time and situation.

Orthostatic hypotension—Condition caused by a rapid fall in blood pressure when assuming an upright position after being recumbent for a period of time.

Osteoporosis—A metabolic condition in which bones become porous and brittle because of inactivity.

Output—Information that is sent or 'put out' from the computer; also refers to the model of human occupation process concerned with mental, physical and social aspects of occupation.

PA—Physical assistance.

Paddles—Electronic devices that bypass the computer keyboard or video system and provide information input via rotational movements.

Palmar grasp—A position in which all fingers and the palm are in contact with an object.

Paraphrasing—Restating in one's own words a message received.

Patient education—Materials and methods for providing specific instruction to recipients of occupational therapy services.

Perception—Ability to receive and interpret incoming sensory information.

Performance—Actions produced through skill acquisition; a subsystem of the model of human occupation concerned with neuromuscular, communication and process skills.

Phobia—An abnormal fear or dread.

PIP joint—Proximal interphalangeal joint.

Play—An intrinsic activity that involves enjoyment and leads to fun; spontaneous and voluntary activity engaged in by choice.

Pliability—Easily bent or changed; flexibility.

PNF—Proprioceptive neuromuscular facilitation.

Portability—Degree to which an object can be readily moved.

Position in space—The ability to determine the special relationship of objects and figures to self or to other objects and forms.

Postural control—The ability to assume a position and maintain it; proper alignment of body parts, orientation to midline, necessary shifting of weight, and righting reactions are important elements for accomplishment.

Practice settings—specific situational contexts in which health professionals work (ie, hospitals, nursing homes, psychiatric hospitals, etc.).

Praxis—The ability to do motor planning and to perform purposeful movement in response to demands from the environment.

Prescription—A directive or injunction; opposite of opportunity.

Prevention—Taking measures to keep something from happening.

Problem-solving—A process of studying a situation that presents uncertainty, doubt, or difficulty and arriving at a solution through definition, identification of alternative plans, selection of a likely plan, organizing the necessary steps in the plan, implementing it, and evaluating the results.

Problem-solving skills—Steps and techniques applied in problem-solving.

Processing the group—A time in group session when members openly discuss observations and feelings relative to a group activity in which they have participated.

Projective techniques—Methods and activities used to provide information about one's thoughts, feelings and needs.

Proprioception—An individual's awareness of position, balance and equilibrium changes based on stimuli from muscles, joints and other tissues; gives information about the position of one body part in relation to that of another.

Proximal-distal development—Development that begins in the parts closest to the midline and progresses to the extremities.

Psychodrama—Therapeutic technique in which patients enact or dramatize their daily life situations.

Psychomotor—Refers to activity that combines both physical and emotional elements.

Psychomotor skills—Movement abilities related to cerebral or psychic activity, such as gross motor skills, fine motor skills and coordination.

Purposeful activity—Those endeavors that are goal-directed and have meaning to the individual engaged in them; significant.

Quality of life—A combination of factors that contribute to one's degree of life satisfaction, such as enjoyable work, meaningful relationships, leisure fulfillment.

RAM—Random access memory of a computer.

Range of motion—Movement of body parts through an arc.

Rapport—The establishment of a harmonious relationship with another person or group.

Recapitulation—To review through a brief summary.

Reciprocal interweaving—Principle of motor development that states that the development of immature behavior and more mature behavior alternate in a constant spiral until matue behavior is firmly established

Recreation—A re-creating or renewal through participation in activities that satisfy, amuse or relax.

Recumbent—Pertains to lying down or reclining.

Reeducation—A process of relearning a task or behavior; also used to refer to retraining of specific muscles or muscle groups.

Reflection—The act of thinking about circumstances, events, activities and relationships; a summary of the affective meaning of a message, both verbally and nonverbally.

Reflective method—*see* Discovery method.

Reflex—An involuntary, immediate and unconscious response in reaction to sensory stimulation; may involve limbs and organs. Reflex movements are precursors to basic fundamental movements.

Reinforcement—The rewarding of desired behavior.

Repeatability—Ability to repeat performance over a specified length of time.

Response—Any item of behavior.

Right-left discrimination—The ability to discriminate one side of the body from the other side.

Roles—Pertains to the functions of the individual in society that may be assumed or acquired (homemaker, student, caregiver, etc.).

ROM—Range of motion; also refers to the Read only memory of a computer.

Safety—Taking measures to assure that risk, injury or loss will not occur; the application of measures necessary to prevent injury or loss of function.

SBA—Stand-by assistance.

Scanning—A technique that bypasses use of the keyboard and provides input directly to the cursor or arrow on the computer monitor.

Script—The written text followed when producing a film or a play.

Selection time—In electronics, the time needed to operate two switches or two functions of a switch.

Self-acceptance—Recognition and acceptance of one's strengths, limitations and related feelings.

Self-actualization—The highest level of need in Maslow's theory; refers to the desire to be fulfilled and achieve one's full potential.

Self-awareness—The ability to recognize one's own behavior patterns and emotional responses.

Self-centered roles—Individuals are primarily concerned with satisfying their own needs rather than those of the group; examples include withdrawing, blocking, dominating and seeking recognition.

Self-concept—Overall awareness or "picture" one has of oneself, both physically and emotionally, and including both positive and negative qualities.

Self-ideal—The way one would like to be seen by others.

Self-image—*see* Self-concept.

Self-management—The ability to use coping skills, exhibit self-control and manage time effectively.

Self-reinforcing—A process in which each success acts as a motivation for greater effort or a more complex challenge.

Sensory integration—The ability to develop and coordinate sensory input.

Sensory processing—The interpretation of sensory stimuli from visual, tactile, auditory, and other senses; information is received, a motor response is made, and sensory feedback is provided.

Sentient—Possessing sensory capabilities; the capacity to be highly sensitive and responsive to another person's feelings.

Sequencing—The placement of actions, concepts and information in a particular order.

Shaping—The use of prompts (and sometimes reinforcement) to promote desired behavior.

Skill acquisition—Learning or relearning to do something well based on knowledge, talent, training and practice.

Skill components—Distinctive attributes that lead to successful adaptation; include perceptual motor, cognitive, drive-object, dyadic interaction, primary group interaction, self-identity and sexual identity (Mosey).

Skill environments—Those settings that maximize the acquisition of skills through dynamic interaction.

Social conduct—Refers to one's ability to interact with others appropriately; includes the use of manners, gestures, self-expression, etc.

Social environment—Elements that comprise the relationships and places where one's social interactions occur.

Socialization—Process whereby skills in establishing interpersonal relationships with others are gained; implies community ties and societal involvement; development of the ability to interact with others appropriately with consideration to cultural and contextual factors.

Society of Friends—A religious group concerned with humane treatment of those in asylums; also known as Quakers.

Soft tissue integrity—Maintenance of skin and interstitial tissue condition, both anatomically and physiologically.

Software—Programs that send messages to the computer to perform certain functions.

Sold time—Time spent in meeting physiologic needs, such as sleeping, eating, bathing, eliminating and sexual activity.

Soldering—The process of fusing two pieces of metal together.

Specific needs—Those needs related to a definite goal or set of circumstances.

Splitting a wire—Process for dividing two portions of an electrical wire in order to make modifications for other uses.

Spreadsheet—A computer software program that manipulates numbers in a matrix of rows and columns.

Stability—Firmness in position; permanence; reliability.

Static splint—A splint used to prevent motion and to stabilize or immobilize a specific part in a functional position.

Stereognosis—Ability to use the sense of touch to identify objects.

Stimulus—Any input of energy that tends to affect behavior.

Strength—Muscle power and degree of movement is demonstrated in the presence of gravity or resistive weight.

Stress—Physical, mental or emotional strain or tension that interferes with the normal equilibrium of the individual.

Stripping a wire—A process of removing the plastic coating from a segment of wire.

Subcortical—Conscious attention is directed to objects or tasks rather than specific movements.

Superstition—Beliefs and practices that result from ignorance and fear of the unknown; irrational attitudes of the mind toward supernatural forces.

Supportive personnel—OT aides, technicians and COTAs who assist in the provision of services.

Synergy—Combined action; the correlated actions of several muscles working together or combined activities of organs of the body.

Synthesis of learning—A process whereby concepts that were previously learned are restructured into new patterns and ideas.

Tactile—The use of skin contact and related receptors to receive, process, and interpret touch, pressure, temperature, pain, vibration and two-point stimulation.

Task analysis—*see* Activity analysis.

Task group—Therapeutic activity where all members make a contribution to achieving the group goals through sharing in the completion of a task, such as planning and implementing a party.

Task roles—Functions necessary for a group to accomplish its objectives; examples include initiator/designer, information giver/seeker, opinion giver/seeker, challenger/comforter and summarizer.

Teacher's role—Primary function that helps the learner change behavior in specified directions.

Teaching process steps—Ten specific points that must be addressed to assure maximal teaching effectiveness related to objectives, content selection, modifications, units, materials, work space, preparation of student(s), presentation, tryout performance and evaluation.

Teaching/learning process—An interactive strategy involving the instructor and the learner in achieving desired goals.

Temporal adaptation—The way in which one occupies time and the appropriate balance of activities within specific and general time frames.

Terminal program—A communication program that allows a computer to link up with others via a modem to gain or exchange information.

Theoretical framework—An interrelated set of ideas that provides a way to conceptualize fundamental principles and applications.

Therapeutic potential—Degree of likelihood that therapeutic goals will be achieved.

Therapeutic value—The extent to which an activity or experience has potential for assisting in the achievement of particular goals.

Thermoplastic—Type of material that becomes soft and pliable when heated, without any change in basic properties.

Throughput—Refers to the model of human occupation; pertaining to one's internal organizational processes.

Topographic orientation—The ability to determine the route to a specified location; to identify the location of particular objects and settings.

Tracking time—The amount of time needed for the person to move from a resting position to activation of a switch.

Traditions—Inherited patterns of thought or action that can be handed down through generations or developed in a singular family unit.

Trial use—Utilizing a piece of equipment or an adaptive device for a specified length of time to determine its effectiveness and whether or not modifications are needed.

Values—Beliefs, feelings or ideas that are important and highly regarded and have value to the individual.

Vestibular—Receiving, processing and interpreting stimuli received by the inner ear relative to head position and movement.

Video feedback—Objective tool that provides information regarding the individual's performance, affect, interactions, and other factors; objective information received via the camera and tape.

Video lighting—Specific procedures that must be followed in using auxiliary illumination in videotaped productions.

Video maintenance—Procedures, such as cleaning, that must be performed periodically to assure that equipment will be operating maximally.

Visual—Of or relating to the reception, processing and interpretation of stimuli received by the eyes, such as acuity, color, figure ground and depth.

Visual closure—The ability to identify objects or forms from incomplete presentations.

Visual-motor integration—The coordination of body movements with visual information when engaging in activity.

Vocational exploration—A process of determining appropriate vocational pursuits through study of one's aptitudes, skills and interests.

Volition—Exercise of the will or will power; it guides choices of the individual and is influenced by values and interests.

Word processing—The use of a software computer program that composes, edits, moves, deletes and duplicates text.

Work—Skill in socially productive activities, including gainful employment, homemaking, child care/parenting, and work preparation activities.

Work-leisure continuum—Range of activities in which one engages throughout the life span, with varying amounts of time devoted to these pursuits.

Index

Practice Issues
in
Occupational Therapy

Intraprofessional Team Building

Practice Issues
in
Occupational Therapy

Intraprofessional Team Building

Editor

Sally E. Ryan, COTA, ROH

Faculty Assistant and Instructor
The College of St. Catherine
Department of Occupational Therapy
St. Paul, Minnesota

SLACK Incorporated, 6900 Grove Road, Thorofare, NJ 08086-9447

Dedicated to Shirley Holland Carr,
my teacher, mentor and treasured friend;
and to the advancement of the profession of occupational therapy.

Contents

Expanded Contents

About the Editor

A graduate of the first occupational therapy assistant program at Duluth, Minnesota, in 1964, Sally Ryan has entered her 29th year as a certified occupational therapy assistant and member of the profession. She has taken extensive coursework at the University of Minnesota as a James Wright Hunt Scholar, and at the College of St. Catherine, St. Paul. Her background includes experience in practice, clinical education supervision and management in long-term care; consultation; and teaching in the professional occupational therapy program at the College of St. Catherine. In the past, Ms. Ryan has served in a variety of leadership positions at the local, state, and national levels. She has served as representative to the American Occupational Therapy Association (AOTA) Representative Assembly from Minnesota; chair of the Representative Assembly Nominating Committee; a member-at-large of the AOTA Executive Board; member and on-site evaluator of the AOTA Accreditation Committee; and member and Secretary of the AOTA Standards and Ethics Commission. She

has also served as a member of the Philosophical Base Task Force, the 1981 Role Delineation Steering Committee, and as a consultant to the COTA Task Force. She is the immediate past Treasurer of the American Occupational Therapy Certification Board and continues to serve as a board member and member of the Disciplinary Action Committee. Ms. Ryan is the recipient of numerous state and national awards. She was the first COTA to receive the AOTA Award of Excellence, has been recognized as an Outstanding Young Woman of America and was among the first recipients of the AOTA Roster of Honor. The Minnesota Occupational Therapy Association has bestowed their Communication Award and Certificate of Appreciation Award on Ms. Ryan. She has been invited to present numerous keynote addresses, presentations, and workshops, both nationally and internationally. Frequently her topics focus on COTA roles and relationships and intraprofessional team building.

Contributing Authors

Harriet Backhaus received her certificate from the occupational therapy assistant program at Westminister College in Fulton, Missouri, an undergraduate degree in education from Harris College in St. Louis, and a master of arts degree in gerontology from Webster University also in St. Louis. She is currrently employed at the Program in Occupational Therapy at Washington University in St. Louis where she is involved in both clinical practice and undergraduate teaching. Ms. Backhaus is a member of the advisory committee for the occupational therapy assistant program at St. Louis Community College at Meramec, and recently completed a term as a member of the Certification Examination Development Committee of the American Occupational Therapy Certification Board. Her interest in therapeutic media and skill in selecting purposeful activities through activity analysis are widely recognized.

Patty L. Barnett is an Associate Instructor and Assistant Coordinator of Clinical Education in the Department of Occupational Therapy at the University of Alabama at Birmingham where she has the unique opportunity to teach both baccalaureate and technical students. She is also responsible for coordinating fieldwork education for occupational therapy assistant students. After joining the faculty in 1977, Ms. Barnett became involved in occupational therapy association activities at both the state and national level, serving on numerous committees, including coordinating the Southeast COTA Conference in 1980, the first in the nation. As a member of the American Occupational Therapy Association COTA Task Force and the COTA Advisory Committee, she was an advocate for COTA concerns and issues. In recognition of her commitment to advancing the role of the COTA, she was recognized by the Association as a member of the Roster of Honor and received the Alabama Occupational Therapy Association COTA Award of Excellence. She continues to be a strong COTA and student advocate.

Patricia K. Benham earned her undergraduate degree in occupational therapy from the College of St. Catherine in St.

Paul, Minnesota, and her master of public health degree from the University of Minnesota. Her practice has focused on pediatrics where she has held several positions in Texas and in Minnesota. She has been a faculty member in the department of occupational therapy at the College of St. Catherine and an instructor for the occupational therapy assistant program at the institution's St. Mary's campus. Ms. Benham is currently the representative from Minnesota to the American Occupational Therapy Association's Representative Assembly. She also is employed as a lobbyist for social reform and women's issues.

Teri Black has been a member of the faculty at the Madison Area Technical College Occupational Therapy Assistant Program for over 11 years. Before this appointment she was in clinical practice in the public school system in Madison, Wisconsin. In addition to her teaching responsibilities, Ms. Black is currently employed on an "on call" basis at the Salk County Health Center. She received her associate in arts degree as an occupational therapy assistant from Madison Area Technical College, and she is currently pursuing both an undergraduate and a master's degree in continuing and adult vocational education at the University of Wisconsin at Madison. A longtime advocate for the COTA role, she has served as the technical representative on several American Occupational Therapy Association Committees, including Directions for the Future. The association has recognized her many contributions through the Roster of Honor Award and the COTA/OTR Partnership Award. The latter was received jointly by Ms. Black and Carol Holmes, MA, OTR, FAOTA. After a three-year term as chair of the Wisconsin Occupational Therapy Regulatory Board, Ms. Black currently serves as the vice-chair. She is also a member of the Board of Directors of the American Occupational Therapy Certification Board.

Sheryl Kantor Blackman received her bachelor of science degree in occupational therapy from the University of Illinois at the Medical Center. She has been employed as a staff therapist, senior therapist and director of occupational therapy. As a senior therapist at the Rehabilitation Institute of Chicago for four years, she was recognized for her special expertise in developing programs and providing treatment for individuals with arthritis. Most recently, she served as the general manager of a seating and positioning company. Ms. Blackman's wide range of employment experiences confirms her versatility in many areas of professional practice. She has presented numerous papers and workshops on a variety of topics. Currently she is a full-time mother of two and works in home health care and provides consultation on a part-time basis.

Toné Blechert received a certificate as an occupational therapy assistant from St. Mary's Junior College and a baccalaureate degree in communications from Metropolitan State University in Minneapolis, Minnesota. She recently received a master's degree in organizational leadership from the College of St. Catherine in St. Paul. Throughout her career, she has held a number of leadership positions, including serving as chair of the American Occupational Therapy Association COTA Task Force and member of the steering committee and faculty member for the Professional and Technical Role Analysis (PATRA) project. She recently served as a member of the Board of Directors of the American Occupational Therapy Foundation. Ms. Blechert is a recipient of the Communication Award from Minnesota Occupational Therapy Association and has also received the Award of Excellence, the Roster of Honor and several Service Awards from the American Occupational Therapy Association in recognition of her leadership and many exemplary contributions to the profession.

Marcia A. Bowker is the owner and chief executive officer of Northern Restorative Services in Duluth, Minnesota, a private practice providing occupational therapy consultation and direct services to community businesses and health care facilities. She earned her bachelor of science degree in occupational therapy at Mount Mary College in Milwaukee, Wisconsin, and has since pursued coursework in varied practice areas including work injury, cumulative trauma, myofascial release and neurologic and orthopedic dysfunction and treatment. Ms. Bowker holds certification in neurodevelopmental treatment in adult hemiplegia (Bobath), and she is also certified in both the KEY and Isernhagen methods of functional capacity evaluation. She is currently the chair of the advisory committee for the occupational therapy assistant program at the Duluth Technical College in Duluth, Minnesota. A regular guest lecturer at the school, she is also a clinical supervisor for occupational therapy assistant students.

Terry D. Brittell received his associate of arts degree as an occupational therapy assistant from Mohawk Valley Community College in Utica, New York, and has completed

extensive coursework at Utica State College of Syracuse University. He was also an instructor and guest lecturer in the occupational therapy department at that institution as well as at Erie Community College and Regina Marie College. The co-author of *The Stress History Outline,* a standardized assessment, he has presented numerous papers and written articles for a variety of professional publications. Before his untimely death, he was the coordinator of the stress management program and the Mental Health Players group at the Mohawk Valley Psychiatric Center in Utica. Mr. Brittell served in a variety of leadership roles in the American Occupational Therapy Association, which included the Representative Assembly, the Executive Board and chair of the COTA Advisory Committee. He was an early recipient of the AOTA Award of Excellence and Roster of Honor, as well as the Service Award, in recognition of his many outstanding achievements. He was also a member of the Certification Examination Development Committee and the Board of Directors of the American Occupational Therapy Certification Board. Terry Brittell will long be remembered for his commitment and leadership and for his many professional contributions.

Ilenna (Leni) Brown is currently employed as the COTA Coordinator for Occupational Therapy Consultants, Inc., Bridgewater, New Jersey, and Assistant Director of Occupational Therapy at the New Jersey Veteran's Memorial Home at Paramus, where she is the clinical supervisor for technical level occupational therapy students. Ms. Brown holds an associate in applied science degree from Union County College in Scotch Plains, New Jersey, and has continued her studies at Sarah Lawrence College in New York. A recipient of the Roster of Honor and the COTA Award of Excellence from the American Occupational Therapy Association, she is also the first recipient of the COTA/OTR Partnership Award, along with Cynthia Epstein, MA, OTR, FAOTA. An active and dedicated participant in the voluntary sector, Ms. Brown has served on many boards and commissions, including Secretary of the American Occupational Therapy Certification Board.

Marianne F. Christiansen is an Assistant Professor and Director of the Occupational Therapy Assistant Program at the St. Mary's Campus of the College of St. Catherine in Minneapolis, Minnesota, where she has held a faculty appointment since 1981. She entered the profession as a COTA, earning her certificate from Houston Community College. Ms. Christiansen received her undergraduate degree in health science administration from Metropolitan State University in Minneapolis and a master of science degree in human and health services administration from the same institution. Professor Christiansen is a member of the Commission on Education of the American Occupational Therapy Association and an on-site evaluator for accreditation of occupational therapy assistant educational programs. An active advocate for COTA issues and concerns, she is currently a member of the committee responsible for writing the rules and regulations for statutory registration of occupational therapy practitioners in Minnesota.

Major Karen Cozean is presently the Chief of Occupational Therapy at Ireland Army Hospital in Fort Knox, Kentucky. She has served as an Army officer for over 11 years and has provided occupational therapy services at the Institute of Surgical Research Army Burn Unit, Brooke Army Medical Center at Fort Sam Houston, Texas. Major Cozean earned her undergraduate degree in occupational therapy from Eastern Michigan University at Ypsilanti, and she also holds a master of arts degree in management. Throughout her career, she has supervised many professional and technical students in occupational therapy and currently is a clinical preceptor for military occupational therapy assistant students.

Sister Genevieve Cummings is an Associate Professor and Chair of the Occupational Therapy Department at the College of St. Catherine in St. Paul, Minnesota, where she has held a faculty appointment since 1960. She received her undergraduate degree in occupational therapy from that institution and later earned a master of arts degree in child development from the University of Minnesota. Throughout her career, Professor Cummings has been recognized as an outstanding leader, and she has served in a number of capacities in the American Occupational Therapy Association, including a member of the Executive Board, Chair of the Standards and Ethics Commission and Representative from the state of Minnesota to the Representative Assembly. She is the recipient of many honors, including recognition by the Association as one of the first Fellows. She has also received the Occupational Therapist of the Year and the Communication Awards from the Minnesota Occupational Therapy Association.

Sherise Darlak is a certificate graduate of the occupational therapy assistant program at Houston Community College in Houston, Texas. While employed at the Texas Institute of Rehabilitation and Research, also in Houston, she was recognized for her expertise in treating patients with spinal injuries. She was also involved in providing occupational therapy services for the transitional living unit. Currently, Ms. Darlak is employed at Health South Rehabilitation Hospital in Humble, Texas, where she specializes in treatment of patients in pediatrics. She is also pursuing her interest in therapeutic recreational activities.

Margaret Drake is an Associate Professor of Occupational Therapy at the University of Alabama at Birmingham where she has held a faculty appointment since 1983. Professor

Drake earned her undergraduate degree in occupational therapy from the University of Puget Sound in Tacoma, Washington, a master of arts degree in art therapy and humanities at Goddard College, Plainfield, Vermont, and a doctoral degree in social science at the University of California at Irvine. Professor Drake's research has been used in comparative cultures in the field of art and in using art activities as an evaluative tool with homeless children. She recently spent a sabbatical year as a visiting professor of occupational therapy at the National Taiwan University School of Rehabilitation Medicine in Taipei.

Kathryn Melin Eberhardt is a graduate of South Suburban College (formerly Thornton Community College) in South Holland, Illinois, where she received an associate of applied science degree as an occupational therapy assistant. She received the Board of Governor's Bachelor of arts degree from Govenor's State University at University Park, Illinois. She is currently a full-time instructor in the occupational therapy assistant program at South Suburban College and also maintains a part-time practice in home health and acute rehabilitation. Ms. Eberhardt has served as the COTA liaison member of the Illinois Occupational Therapy Association (IOTA) board of directors and as a member of numerous local committees and task forces. The recipient of the COTA of the Year Award from IOTA in recognition of her many contributions, she currently is a member of the Illinois Department of Professional Regulation Occupational Therapy Licensure Board, representing certified occupational therapy assistants.

Jeffrey Engh holds an applied science degree as an occupational therapy assistant from St. Louis Community College at Meramec, St. Louis, Missouri, and is currently pursuing an undergraduate degree in business from Webster University in St. Louis. Mr. Engh is employed as an Industrial Rehabilitation Specialist at the SSM Rehabilitation Institute where his duties include coordinating rehabilitation services for industry and promoting industrial rehabilitation services. He is a frequent lecturer on this topic as well as the needs of older workers. In addition, he serves as chair of the advisory committee for the Occupational Therapy Assistant Program at St. Louis Community College at Meramec.

Cynthia Epstein is the President and Executive Director of Occupational Therapy Consultants, Inc., in Bridgewater, New Jersey. A nationally recognized master clinical therapist in geriatrics and a Fellow of the American Occupational Therapy Association, she has written and lectured extensively on the provision of restorative and consultative occupational therapy services in long-term care. Advocating a team approach, Ms. Epstein has designed and helped to implement specialized restorative programs that use the skills of the OTR/COTA team. As a consultant to facilities providing services to older persons, she has emphasized training and quality assurance as key aspects of team management. The new text, *Occupational Therapy Consultation: Theory, Principles and Practice*, which she co-authored with Evelyn Jaffee, enumerates these important consulting roles and functions. A graduate of the Boston School of Occupational Therapy at Tufts University, she also holds a master of arts degree in vocational rehabilitation from New York University. Ms. Epstein has been recognized for her outstanding contributions by many organizations. Most recently, she and Ilenna Brown were the first recipients of the COTA/OTR Partnership Award presented by the American Occupational Therapy Association in recognition of their productive partnership in gerontology.

M. Laurita (Lita) Fike is currently employed as the Assistant Dean, Department of Health Sciences and Associate Professor of Occupational Therapy at Texas Women's University in Houston. Ms. Fike earned her undergraduate degree in occupational therapy from the College of St. Catherine in St. Paul, Minnesota and later completed a master of arts degree in occupational therapy education from Texas Women's University. Throughout her career she has been recognized for developing model service delivery programs utilizing COTA/OTR teams. Ms. Fike has given numerous national presentations and has published in the *American Journal of Occupational Therapy* and the *Occupational Therapy Journal of Research*. She has also been a guest editor of the *American Journal of Occupational Therapy*.

Linda Florey earned her undergraduate degree in occupational therapy from the University of Iowa and her master of science degree in occupational therapy from the University of Southern California in Los Angeles, where she is currently pursuing a doctoral degree in occupational science. Ms. Florey is employed as the Chief of Occupational Therapy at the Neuropsychiatric Institute in Los Angeles. She has served in a variety of leadership positions at the state and national level, including Representative to the American Occupational Therapy Association's Representative Assembly, a member of the Accreditation Committee and the Communications Committee and a member of the Commission on Education Steering Committee. She has been recognized as a Fellow by the Association and is a member of the Certification Examination Development Committee of the American Occupational Therapy Certification Board.

Major Frank E. Gainer III is currently employed as the clinic supervisor of physical disabilities in the occupational therapy section at Walter Reed Army Medical Center in Washington, D.C. He entered occupational therapy practice as a COTA after graduation from Erie Community College in Buffalo, New York. He received his baccalaureate degree in occupational therapy from Western Michigan University at Kalamazoo and master of health science in occupational therapy degree, with a clinical specialty in adult psychiatry, from the University of Florida at Gainesville. The author of numerous publications, he has also presented papers at local, regional, national and international conferences. Major Gainer's professional experience includes drug and alcohol rehabilitation, mental health, adult physical disabilities and home health care, having served as a COTA supervisor in the majority of these settings. He holds certification in the neurodevelopmental treatment of adults with hemiplegia. A member of the Academy of Content Experts for the Certification Examination Committee of the American Occupational Therapy Certification Board, Major Gainer also serves on the executive board of the District of Columbia Occupational Therapy Association. His volunteer activities include work at an inner city clinic as a mobility instructor for those with visual impairments secondary to AIDS.

Elnora Gilfoyle is the Provost and Academic Vice President at Colorado State University in Fort Collins, Colorado. Before this appointment, she was the dean of the university's College of Applied Human Services. She is also a tenured full professor of occupational therapy at that institution, where she has held faculty appointments since 1981. Dr. Gilfoyle has served as the President of the American Occupational Therapy Association, as well as in numerous other leadership positions. The Association has honored her as the recipient of two of their highest awards—the Eleanor Clarke Slagle Lectureship for scholarly contributions and the Award of Merit for leadership. As a founding member of the Association's Fellow recognition (FAOTA), she has distinguished herself nationally through numerous presentations, workshops and publications including *Children Adapt*, 2nd Edition, published by SLACK Inc.

Dairlyn Gower has been an educator in the occupational therapy assistant program at Duluth Community College (formerly Duluth Area Vocational/Technical Institute) in Duluth, Minnesota, for the past 15 years. A graduate of that program, she has also earned a baccalaureate degree in vocational-technical education from the University of Minnesota at Duluth. Ms. Gower is currently the occupational therapy assistant vice chair, as well as a member of the Certification Examination Development Committee of the American Occupational Therapy Certification Board. She also was a member of the COTA Advisory Committee for the Professional and Technical Role Analysis (PATRA) study conducted by the American Occupational Therapy Association.

Madelaine Gray is the Executive Director of the American Occupational Therapy Certification Board (AOTCB) in Rockville, Maryland. Before assuming this position, she was the Associate Executive Director of the Department of Professional Services and the Deputy Executive Director of the American Occupational Therapy Association (AOTA). As a member of the AOTA staff, she directed several major credentialing activities, including role delineation studies to identify the expected competencies of entry-level COTAs and OTRs. She holds an undergraduate degree in occupational therapy from the University of New Hampshire and a master of arts degree in public administration from the University of Southern California. She is also a Certified Association Executive under the auspices of the American Society of Association Executives. Ms. Gray began her career in occupational therapy as a staff therapist in mental health and then became a fieldwork instructor in physical disabilities. She also served as an assistant professor in the Department of Occupational Therapy at the University of Southern California. She is a Fellow of the American Occupational Therapy Association in recognition of her many contributions to the profession.

Barbara (Bobbi) Hansvick is currently employed as a sales representative for a durable medical supply company in Minneapolis, Minnesota. She received her associate of arts degree from St. Mary's Junior College, also in Minneapolis. After graduation, she worked in long-term care settings where she was recognized for her innovative and holistic programing. Ms. Hansvick has also taught occupational therapy courses at the St. Mary's Campus of the College of St. Catherine. An active member of the American Occupational Therapy Association, she was a member of the Professional and Technical Role Analysis committee and chair of the Finance Committee for the Minnesota Occupational Therapy Association. She also served on the executive board in a variety of capacities.

Bonnie Hoffman holds a master of occupational therapy degree from Texas Women's University in Houston. As a Captain in the United States Army from 1980 to 1986, she was involved in occupational therapy assistant student training in various capacities, including instructor and clinical preceptor. While assigned as Chief, Occupational Therapy Branch at the Institute of Surgical Research at Brooke Army Medical Center, Fort Sam Houston, Texas, she was Program Coordinator and instructor for the Army occupational therapy and physical therapy burn management course. During her assignment at the burn unit, she became particularly interested in treatment alternatives for patients with facial disfigurement. This interest prompted her to leave the army to earn a master of arts degree at the University of Illinois at Chicago, where she specialized in maxillofacial prosthetics. Ms. Hoffman is currently in private practice in Fort Worth, Texas.

Dana Hutcherson is a staff occupational therapist at Sheltering Arms Hospital in Richmond, Virginia, where she is employed in the work hardening program. She earned her undergraduate degree in education from Longwood College, and later completed a master of science in Occupational Therapy at the Medical College of Virginia, Virginia Commonwealth University. Before her career in occupational therapy, Ms. Hutcherson taught art, health, physical education and driver education in Roanoke, Virginia. She developed and conducted a driver assessment program at Johnston-Willis Hospital in Richmond and provided consultation to driver trainers, educators and other therapists in the driver assessment and training of persons with disabilities. Ms. Hutcherson has also conducted and published research focusing on older adult drivers. She has served on the Advisory Council of Virginia Drivers with Disabilities and has also assisted occupational therapy students and therapists in career exploration in this specialized area.

Donna Jensen is the manager of occupational therapy and special programs at Riverside Medical Center in Minneapolis, Minnesota, where her duties include management of physical disabilities, cardiac rehabilitation, hand rehabilitation, work hardening, functional capacity assessments programs, and activities and recreation services in skilled nursing care facilities. She earned her bachelor of science degree in occupational therapy at Mount Mary College, Milwaukee, Wisconsin, and a graduate level certificate in business administration from the College of St. Thomas in St. Paul, Minnesota. Ms. Jensen was a contributing author to the book *Rehabilitation of the Multiple Sclerosis Patient for Health Care Professionals*. Her expertise as both a practitioner and a manager have been recognized widely. She was co-chair of the clinical education task force and is currently a member of the occupational therapy curriculum committees at the College of St. Catherine and the University of Minnesota. She is past chair of the Southwestern Minnesota Occupational Therapy Administrative Special Interest Group.

Robin A. Jones holds an associate of arts degree as an occupational therapy assistant from the Madison Area Technical College in Madison, Wisconsin, and a bachelor of science degree in public administration from Loyola University in Chicago. She is currently pursuing a master of arts degree in public service from DePaul University in Chicago. Her clinical expertise is primarily in the area of spinal cord injury, and she has published several chapters and articles on this topic. She has held a senior staff position at the Rehabilitation Institute of Chicago and served as an assistive technology specialist at the University of Illinois, Chicago. Ms. Jones pursued her interest in administration through employment as assistant to the director of the occupational therapy department at the

University of Illinois before becoming executive director of a community-based independent living center. She has also been Project Administrator for the Great Lakes Disability and Business Technical Assistance Center, providing consultation and education to the business community in six midwestern states about compliance with the Americans with Disabilities Act. Ms. Jones was the first COTA representative in the Representative Assembly of the American Occupational Therapy Association and is a recipient of the Award of Excellence and Roster of Honor from the Association.

Nancy Kari is an Associate Professor of Occupational Therapy at the College of St. Catherine in St. Paul, Minnesota, where she has been a faculty member since 1978. She received her baccalaureate degree in occupational therapy from the University of Wisconsin at Madison and a master's degree in public health from the University of Minnesota. Pursuing her interests in organizational governance and institutional change, she is also a member of the adjunct faculty with Project Public Life at the Humphrey Institute of Public Affairs at the University of Minnesota, a national initiative program to re-engage citizens in public life. Associated with this work, she co-directs the Lazarus Project, an action-research pilot program that investigates issues of empowerment within nursing homes. The goal of her pioneering work is to create a community model that is an alternative to the traditional medical and therapeutic models of governance. Professor Kari has published papers on team building and the politics of empowerment, and is a recent recipient of the Communication Award given by the Minnesota Occupational Therapy Association and the Cordelia Meyers Writer's Award given by AOTA.

Barbara A. Larson received her associate of arts degree as an occupational therapy assistant from St. Mary's Junior College in Minneapolis, Minnesota. She worked as a COTA in a variety of health care facilities and was also an instructor in the occupational therapy assistant program at St. Mary's Junior College. She received an undergraduate degree in occupational therapy from the University of Minnesota and is currently the director of the Work Center, Orthopedic Sports in Stillwater, Minnesota. Ms. Larson was President of the Minnesota Occupational Therapy Association and chair of the Legislative Committee where she was instrumental in directing numerous initiatives including landmark Medicare reimbursement changes. She was also co-chair of the American Occupational Therapy Association's annual conference and a board member of the organization's Political Action Committee. Recognized by the association as a recipient of the Roster of Honor, she has also received the Occupational Therapist of the Year Award from the Minnesota Occupational Therapy Association.

Ronna Linroth is employed as a Senior COTA at the Multiple Sclerosis Achievement Center in St. Paul, Minnesota and is the co-founder of the Multiple Sclerosis Allied Health Professionals group. She received her associate of arts degree from the North Dakota State College of Science at Wahpeton, and she is currently pursuing an undergraduate degree in occupational therapy at the College of St. Catherine in St. Paul, Minnesota. A strong advocate for advancing the role of the COTA, Ms. Linroth has written several articles and chapters in books and has held a variety of state and national leadership positions, including co-chair of the first COTA Consortium in Minnesota and a member of the COTA Task Force of the American Occupational Therapy Association. The Association has recognized her leadership and many contributions by awarding her the Roster of Honor. She is also the recipient of the Abigail Quigley McCarthy Award from the College of St. Catherine and the Certificate of Appreciation from the Minnesota Occupational Therapy Association. Ronna is dedicated to influencing public policy and has engaged in numerous legislative and bipartisan lobbying efforts on behalf of the profession, its members and recipients of services.

William Matthew Marcil began his occupational therapy career with an associate of applied science degree as an occupational therapy assistant from Maria College in Albany, New York. After working as a COTA for five years, he continued his occupational therapy education at the State University of New York at Buffalo where he received his undergraduate and master of science degrees. Mr. Marcil is currently employed in private practice in Virginia Beach, Virginia, where he specializes in home health care. In addition to his practice, he works as an AIDS educator and has published numerous journal articles and chapters in texts and has co-authored two books: *Terminal and Life-Threatening Illness* and *The Person with AIDS: A Personal and Professional Perspective*, both published by Slack, Inc. Mr. Marcil has also presented papers and workshops on these topics throughout the United States, Canada, Guam, Australia and New Zealand.

Susan McFadden has been the Director of Regulatory Affairs of the American Occupational Therapy Certification Board since January 1991. She also maintains a small private practice. Ms. McFadden received her undergraduate degree in occupational therapy from Virginia Commonwealth University and a master of arts degree in education with exceptional children from the Pennsylvania State University. She has actively contributed to the profession for over 25 years as a clinician, educator, author, public speaker and consultant. In acknowledgment of her efforts, her colleagues have elected her to the American Occupational Therapy Association's Roster of Fellows and have presented her with the Service Award. She is also the recipient of the Outstanding Occupational Therapist of the Year Award and Certificates of Appreciation from the Tennessee Occupational Therapy Association. Her national leadership activities have included serving as a member of the AOTA Accreditation Committee, chair of Certification Examination Development Committee and Secretary of the Board of Directors of the American Occupational Therapy Certification Board.

Adair M. Robinson is a staff therapist in the Occupational Therapy Section at Walter Reed Army Medical Center in Washington, DC. She earned her undergraduate degree in occupational therapy from Towson State University in Maryland and a master of arts degree in instructional systems development from the University of Maryland. Ms. Robinson is currently involved in a controlled efficacy study of in-patient rehabilitation services for military service members with traumatic brain injuries.

Denise A. Rotert is a member of the faculty in the Occupational Therapy Department at the University of South Dakota at Vermillion. She holds a baccalaureate degree in ocupational therapy from the University of Puget Sound and a master of arts degree in psychology, guidance and counseling from the University of Northern Colorado. While serving 20 years in the United States Army and achieving the rank of Lieutenant Colonel, she was director of the military occupational therapy specialist course for occupational therapy assistants. Ms. Rotert's clinical background is broad, with an emphasis in mental health practice, including fieldwork supervision of both technical and professional occupational therapy students. She has practiced and published in the area of substance abuse and is listed as a resource person for the American Occupational Therapy Association's *Guide on Alcoholism and Substance Abuse*. She has also presented lectures on stress management, executive stress and stress in organizations.

Marietta Cosky Saxon is an instructor and fieldwork coordinator in the occupational therapy assistant program at Anoka Technical College in Anoka, Minnesota, where she has been employed since 1981. Ms. Saxon received a baccalaureate degree in occupational therapy from Wayne State University in Detroit, Michigan. She has served as a master faculty member for the nationally recognized workshop, The Role of Occupational Therapy with the Elderly (ROTE), sponsored by the American Occupational Therapy Association and has produced videotapes on remotivation with the elderly and weaving techniques. As a staff therapist, consultant and educator, Ms. Saxon has worked closely with COTAs and values this role in the profession.

Major Melissa Wilde Sinnott has served in a variety of clinical assignments, including Director of Education and Research for the Occupational Therapy Section at Walter Reed Army Medical Center in Washington, DC. A member of the Army Medical Specialists Corps, she earned her undergraduate degree in occupational therapy from the University of New Hampshire, a master of arts degree in occupational therapy from San Jose State University in California, and a Doctorate of Philosophy in education administration from the University of Maryland at College Park. Major Sinnott is the liaison to the American Occupational Therapy Foundation and the research consultant for the Physical Disabilities Special Interest Section of the American Occupational Therapy Association. She has been involved in a variety of independent and collaborative research efforts and is particularly interested in qualitative design. Major Sinnot has recently became director of the occupational therapy assistant program at the Academy of Health Sciences, Fort Sam Houston, Texas.

Sallie Taylor is currently employed as the Projects Manager at Healthline Corporate Health Services in St. Louis, Missouri, where her primary responsibilities include obtaining and maintaining relevant agency certifications for evaluation and rehabilitation services, preparation of grants and proposals and facilitating professional development throughout the corporation. She received her undergraduate degree in occupational therapy from Richmond Professional Institute at Richmond, Virginia and a master of arts degree in education from the University of Florida at Gainesville. Her numerous publications include chapters on work-related topics and long-range planning in three editions of *Willard and Spackman's Occupational Therapy*. An active member of the American Occupational Therapy Association, Ms. Taylor has served as a member of the standing committee of the Work Special Interest Section and the association's Strategic Planning Committee. As a member of the Missouri Occupational Therapy Association, she has provided leadership in a number of areas which include serving as vice president and president.

Kent Nelson Tigges is an Associate Professor in the occupational therapy department at the State University of New York at Buffalo. He received his undergraduate degree in occupational therapy from the University of Kansas at Lawrence and a master of science degree in occupational therapy from the University of Southern California. The recipient of an international fellowship from the Republic of South Africa, Mr. Tigges developed the first undergraduate and master of science programs in occupational therapy in Africa at Pretoria College and Witwatersrand University, respectively. He is a member of the editorial board of the *American Journal of Hospice Care* and has published extensively internationally including co-authoring two texts: *Terminal and Life-Threatening Illness* and *The Person with AIDS: A Personal and Professional Perspective*, both published by SLACK Inc. The recipient of numerous state and national awards, he has been recognized by the American Occupational Therapy Association as a Fellow and by the World Health Organization as a Fellow in Health and Housing. Professor Tigges has assumed a number of leadership roles, including a five-year term as the chair of State Board for Occupational Therapy, New York State Education Department.

Javan E. Walker, Jr. is Director of the Division of Occupational Therapy and Associate Professor of Occupational Therapy at Florida Agricultural and Mechanical University in Tallahassee, Florida, where he developed the program. Before assuming this position, he was director of the occupational therapy assistant program at Illinois Central College in Peoria. Professor Walker began his occupational therapy career as a COTA in the United States Army. He earned his undergraduate degree in occupational therapy from Wayne State University in Detroit and a master of arts degree in education from Bradley University. He is currently a doctoral candidate at Illinois State University. After 15 years of active duty as an occupational therapist, Mr. Walker currently holds the rank of Lieutenant Colonel in the United States Army Reserves. In addition to his work as an educator and a clinician, he was recently elected as the Alternate Representative to the American Occupational Therapy Association Representative Assembly for the state of Florida. Professor Walker has provided consultation to long-term care facilities and mental health programs for the past 15 years, and he is actively involved with computer technology, both professionally and avocationally.

Toni Walski has served as the Occupational Therapy Program Director at Madison Area Technical College in Madison, Wisconsin, since 1971. Professor Walski received her undergraduate degree in occupational therapy from the University of Wisconsin at Madison and holds a master of science degree in adult education from Stout University in Menomonie, Wisconsin. She was recognized as a Fellow by the American Occupational Therapy Association for innovations in technical education and related professional activities at the state and national level. Professor Walski's career commitment to promoting COTA practitioners was kindled during her occupational therapy Level II fieldwork experiences, where she had the opportunity to learn from OTR/COTA teams in three different practice settings.

Patricia Watson entered practice as an occupational therapy assistant after graduation from St. Mary's Junior College in Minneapolis, Minnesota. She later received her bachelor of science degree in occupational therapy from the University of Minnesota. While working as a COTA at Sister Kenny Institute in Minneapolis, she was a clinical supervisor for occupational therapy assistant fieldwork students. Since completing her baccalaureate degree, Ms. Watson has worked in cardiac rehabilitation and general rehabilitation and in private practice in home health care. She has served on various committees and held several positions as a member of the executive board of the Minnesota Occupational Therapy Association. Currently, Ms. Watson is employed by Lifease in St. Paul, a company whose services focus on allowing the elderly to remain in their own homes through the use of environmental modifications, adaptive devices and services.

Melanie Wiener earned her bachelor of science degree in occupational therapy from the University of Florida at Gainesville. She has worked in a variety of occupational therapy settings and practices in Texas, Colorado and Alaska, including the Institute for Rehabilitation and Research in Houston and Craig Hospital and Hand Surgery Associates in Denver. Ms. Weiner has also worked in geriatric rehabilitation and home health, and she enjoys the diversity of experience provided by practicing in several different parts of the country.

Acknowledgments

I am indeed indebted to several persons who helped prepare this book. In the early stages of planning, many occupational therapy educational program directors, faculty members and practitioners responded to a lengthy survey. These OTRs and COTAs provided thoughtful critiques and comments, which were of great help in determining the focus of this second edition. Special thanks is offered to Dr. Louise Fawcett, who assisted with the interpretation of survey data, and to Phillip Shannon, who was a primary reviewer and consultant during the early planning stages of this edition. Appreciation is also offered to Shirley Holland Carr for constructive criticism of specific content areas.

The contributions of the highly skilled contributing authors are gratefully acknowledged. Their work, individually and collectively, is the great strength of this text. Forty-two occupational therapists and assistants have provided their extensive knowledge and expertise in preparing manuscripts. They come from diverse practice, education and research backgrounds; five OTR contributors are or were occupational therapy assistant program directors. Many of the authors, representing 16 states and the District of Columbia, have been actively involved in leadership roles in their state associations, as well as in the American Occupational Therapy Association (AOTA), the American Occupational Therapy Foundation, and The American Occupational Therapy Certification Board. Eighteen of the authors have been recognized by AOTA as Fellows or members of the Roster of Honor. In addition, 12 OTR/COTA authoring teams are featured in this edition. It has been a great privilege to work with these outstanding writers, and I convey my most sincere thanks to each of them.

I would also like to offer my thanks to the reviewers who provided critiques of the manuscript. Their objectivity and critical analysis of the content were most helpful in this developmental process.

Appreciation is also offered to Dr. M. Jeanne Madigan who assisted in writing a number of the related learning activities, which appear at the conclusion of each chapter.

Cheryl Willoughby, Editorial Director, and her staff at SLACK Inc., provided me with numerous resources, advice, critiques and overall editorial assistance. Their patience, coupled with expert problem-solving skills, helped me immeasurably in this enormous task. Publication of this text would not have been possible without their expertise and assistance.

I would like to acknowledge and express my personal gratitude to Sister Genevieve Cummings, chair, and all of the members of the faculty of the Department of Occupational Therapy at the College of St. Catherine for their support and encouragement during the many phases of this task. Their willingness to share resources and offer critiques and support was of great help.

To the many therapists, assistants, friends and family members who provided ideas, listened to my concerns and responded to my endless questions, I offer my most sincere appreciation. I regret that space does not allow me to list each of them individually.

Elena Malicova and Luba Nikolaeva assisted with a variety of office and household tasks for which I am most appreciative.

Thanking my husband Brian is most difficult. He filled many supportive roles including active listener, thoughtful responder, consultant, reviewer, typist, illustrator, errand runner, FAX sender, telephone monitor, and household manager. This project would never have been accomplished without his sense of humor, inspiration, insight, patience and remarkable ability to adapt. I am ever grateful.

Foreword

As health services reform measures seek efficient, economical and effective service delivery models and disciplines, our profession must constantly improve the utilization of the OTR/COTA team. Sally Ryan's *Practice Issues in Occupational Therapy: Intraprofessional Team Building* presents all of us in the profession with state-of-the-art strategies, attitudes and information critical for our success during this time of major adjustments to our industry.

Though the OTR/COTA team flourishes in many clinical and academic settings, it has been known to flounder or be non-existent in just as many. The speculation regarding the causes of our problems with the OTR/COTA team range from shortages, to role confusion, to inadequate numbers of new graduates, to antiquated regulations, to turf questions, to poor understanding of good management practices, to biases among us that go back many years. For most of us, if we have been part of a system where the OTR/COTA team is strong and well established, the basics of Ryan's message are familiar territory, yet her book offers us many refinements helpful in today's practice. If one really has not had the privilege of seeing a well balanced team in action, this book gives the reader the tools to initiate a dynamic OTR/COTA team as part of one's practice or curriculum.

The early days of my professional career in California and Minnesota were filled with the presence and the influence of great OTR/COTA teams at Rancho Los Amigos Hospital, Sharp Rehabilitation Center, in the Southern California OT Association and throughout my classes and fieldwork in Saint Paul. But I must admit that it was the mature, patient and skillful tutelage of those wonderful COTA's in my formative years that taught me the most about our professional team and about how to use my interpersonal skills therapeutically. These early impressions are extremely critical in setting up life-long professional expectations and attitudes.

Sally Ryan has created a very readable text that can be of invaluable assistance to students in any classroom or as a means of professional skills enhancement for the certified practitioner. It's the next best thing to personally being there. It will make a difference in how well the profession fares in future health, education and welfare service delivery systems.

Mary M. Evert, MBA, OTR, FAOTA
President, AOTA

Persons who share always get back more than they give. Sally Ryan has always shared her vision, her energy, and her knowledge for all of us to use as we build for the future. She is blessed with many colleagues and friends, and now she is blessed by knowing that she has produced a tool that thousands of clinicians will use to prepare for their professional roles. She will take great pleasure watching what happens as a result of her effort.

During the past two decades the roles and functions of therapists and assistants have grown. However, this growth will seem minuscule compared to that which will occur during the next two decades. The nation is facing a crisis. One of every seven Americans is impaired in their ability to carry out all of their daily tasks, which in turn impairs their ability to live independently. Occupational therapists and occupational therapy assistants will be called on more and more to help with this problem. As the nation plans strategies to address the needs of our people with chronic conditions, it will be necessary to build new systems of care that promote independence. Communities will need systems of care that promote health and prevent disabling conditions. Occupational therapists and occupational therapy assistants will play a critical role in this effort.

The reader of this book will find the knowledge and skills to work as an intraprofessional colleague and as a member of an interdisciplinary team to help persons overcome the deficits that impair performance. Use the knowledge well.

Carolyn Baum, PhD, OTR, FAOTA
Elias Michael Director and Assistant Professor
in Occupational Therapy and Neurology
Washington University School of Medicine
St. Louis, Missouri

Preface

The information age is very much upon us, with an explosion of new knowledge and skills and the availability of vast new sources of data and information never before so accessible. Rapid change is becoming the norm in our everyday lives and in our profession. Within this dynamic environment, it is important for an editor to carefully assess what information is essential, what is "nice" to know and what is not appropriate or necessary. At the culmination of this lengthy process, it was decided to change the format and expand the content of this text to two companion volumes. Originally published as the single title, the *Certified Occupational Therapy Assistant: Roles and Responsibilities*, this second edition has been divided and retitled to more accurately reflect the content and the intended audience. *The Certified Occupational Therapy Assistant: Principles, Concepts and Techniques* provides the reader with important foundations and fundamental information for entering practice. This companion volume, *Practice Issues in Occupational Therapy: Intraprofessional Team Building* builds on that material, providing greater development of key concepts through practical case study applications. Of equal importance, intraprofessional teamwork and team building strategies and discussion of key contemporary practice issues are major focuses. The text should provide both students and practitioners with valuable information which *integrates* the fundamental concepts, principles and techniques of the profession in the context of practice within multiple environments and systems, serving those with a wide variety of therapeutic intervention needs.

The following basic objectives used for the first edition have been readopted as a guide for developing, organizing and sequencing content: 1) provide an extensive and a realistic view of the roles and functions of occupational therapy practitioners, both in entry-level practice and beyond, 2) provide examples of how to successfully build intraprofessional relationships, and 3) be an important clinical reference and guide as well as a major classroom text.

Several documents published by the American Occupational Therapy Association (AOTA) were used as primary guides for content development: The *Entry-Level Role Delineation for Occupational Therapists, Registered (OTRs) and Certified Occupational Therapy Assistants (COTAs)*, the *Essentials and Guidelines for an Accredited Educational Program for the Occupational Therapy Assistant, Uniform Terminology for Reporting Occupational Therapy Services*, 2nd Edition and the *1990 AOTA Member Data Survey*. Data and information from the report *A National Study of the Profession of Occupational Therapy*, conducted by the American Occupational Therapy Certification Board, was also used. The 1992 document, *Standards of Practice in Occupational Therapy*, published by the AOTA, was another important source of information and is reprinted in the Appendix.

Sixteen new chapters have been added to this edition, as well as a glossary and related learning activities. Other chapters have been expanded and updated. The reader will also find more photographs, illustrations, charts and forms to enhance and emphasize important points. In addition, all chapters now open with a set of key concepts and a list of essential vocabulary terms. The key concepts are designed to assist the students in focusing their study on the fundamental subjects in each chapter. The essential vocabulary words are terms important to chapter content and occupational therapy practice, and appear in bold type at first mention. Every effort has been made to define each term clearly, both in context and in the glossary.

The book is divided into five major sections. The first section focuses on intervention principles, providing the reader with a basic understanding of some of the important concepts related to the process of therapeutic intervention, supervision guidelines and patterns and teamwork and team building.

Section Two focuses on the OTR and COTA team approach in therapeutic intervention. Case studies, organized developmentally, are used to illustrate how professional and technical personnel work together as a therapeutic intervention team in a variety of health care delivery systems. This major section might well be described as a definitive "map" for intraprofessional teamwork. Numerous examples of intervention strategies, both contemporary and traditional, are presented to provide the reader with dynamic examples of effective OTR and COTA partnerships in practice.

Contemporary models of practice are emphasized in Section Three. The reader is provided with both basic and advanced information related to work capacity assessment and work hardening. The role of the COTA as an activity director emphasizes the many skills required of an assistant who works in this capacity. The section concludes with a discussion of a head injury practice model.

The fourth section describes selected emerging models of practice. Although there are a variety of opportunities, stress management, hospice care and disabled driver education have been selected as examples of growing opporunities for OTR/COTA employment.

Section Five focuses on concepts related to documentation and components of management to carry out service operations. Fundamental principles are discussed and serve as a means for integrating some of the core concepts presented in preceding chapters. Strategies for building skill in this important aspect of clinical work are stressed.

Section Six, the final segment, presents contemporary practice issues and trends. The reader is given information on intraprofessional relationships and socialization as key elements of the professional socialization process. Principles of occupational therapy ethics and credentialing are also presented. The final chapter discusses the future of occupational therapy in terms of an environment of opportunity, offering new insights relative to the impact of current and future societal trends on health care in general and occupational therapy specifically.

When using this book, the reader should note the following:

1. In addition to the main chapter designations, all important chapter subheadings also appear in the Expanded Table of Contents. They are titled to reflect the major objectives of the writer(s) and the editor.

2. Every effort has been made to use gender-inclusive language throughout the book. In some instances, it was necessary to use "him or her," recognizing that this may be awkward for the reader. Exceptions to the use of gender-inclusive pronouns occur in the discussion of historical material, philosophical principles and in some quotations.

3. The term "patient" has been used frequently to describe the recipient of occupational therapy services. The authors and the editor recognize that this term is not always the most appropriate; however, it is believed to be preferable to other options currently being used. Exceptions have been made in some instances where terms such as "the individual," "the student" and "the child" have been used.

4. Related learning activities have been included at the conclusion of each chapter. Some of these were published previously in *The Certified Occupational Therapy Assistant: Roles and Responsibilities Workbook*.

5. Whenever a writing project of this magnitude is undertaken, inadvertent omissions and errors may occur. Although every attempt has been made to prevent such occurrences, the editor and authors hope that these errors, when found, will be called to their attention so that they may be corrected in the next printing.

In conclusion, I believe that this book and its companion volume will be a model and guidepost for occupational therapy teamwork in the delivery of patient services. It will serve as an incentive for the technically and professionally educated practitioners to discover the many ways in which their skills and roles complement each other. It will also be a catalyst for developing new skills and roles in response to the ever-changing needs of our society.

The former President of the American Occupational Therapy Association, Carolyn Manville Baum, summed it up best in her 1980 Eleanor Clarke Slagle Address when she stated:

"As a profession and as professionals, let us put our resources, intelligence, and emotional commitment together and work diligently toward the ascent of our profession. The health care system, the clients (patients) we serve and each of us individually will benefit from our commitment."

—Sally E. Ryan, COTA, Editor 1993

Occupational Therapy

A PROFILE

Occupational therapy is the art and science of directing participation in selected tasks to restore, reinforce and enhance performance; to facilitate learning of skills and functions essential for adaptation and productivity; to diminish or correct pathology; and to promote and maintain health. Its fundamental purpose is the development and maintenance of the capacity to perform those tasks and roles essential to productive living and to the mastery of self and the environment.

Because the primary focus of occupational therapy is the development of adaptive skills and performance capacity, its concern is with factors that serve as barriers or impediments to the individual's ability to function, as well as those factors that promote, influence or enhance performance.

Occupational therapy provides service to those individuals whose abilities to cope with tasks of living are threatened or impaired by developmental deficits, aging, poverty and cultural differences, physical injury or illness, or psychosocial and social disability.

The term *occupation* refers to a person's goal-directed use of time, energy, interest and attention. The practice of occupational therapy is based on concepts that acknowledge the following principles:

1. Activities are primary agents for learning and development, and they are an essential source of satisfaction.

2. In engaging in activities, the individual explores the nature of his or her interests, needs, capacities, and limitations; develops motor, perceptual and cognitive skills; and learns a range of interpersonal and social attitudes and behaviors sufficient for coping with life tasks and mastering elements of the environment.

3. Task occupation is an integral part of human development; it represents or reflects life-work situations, and is a vehicle for acquiring or redeveloping those skills essential to the fulfillment of life roles.

4. Activities matching or relating to the developmental needs and interests of the individual not only afford the necessary learning for development or restoration, but provide an intrinsic gratification that promotes and sustains health and evokes a strong investment in the restorative process.

5. The end product inherent in a task or an activity provides concrete evidence of the ability to be productive and to have an influence on one's environment.

6. Activities are "doing," and such a focus on productivity and participation teaches a sense of self as a contributing participant rather than as a recipient.

These principles are applied in practice through programs reflecting the profession's commitment to comprehensive health care.

*Adapted with permission from "Occupational Therapy: Its Definition and Function," Reference Manual of Official Documents of the American Occupational Therapy Association, 1980 (revised 1983), American Occupational Therapy Association, Inc.

Section I
PRINCIPLES OF PRACTICE

Therapeutic Intervention Process

COTA Supervision

Teamwork and Team Building

Building on the foundation established in the publication, *The Certified Occupational Therapy Assistant: Principles, Concepts and Techniques*, this section begins with the discussion of the basic principles that apply directly to therapeutic intervention. The components of the occupational therapy process are described, with examples of appropriate technical and professional roles noted.

Guiding principles and patterns of COTA supervision are also important themes. These are presented as they relate to various levels of personnel, service competency, patient condition, regulations and standards and general employment. Ryan has stated that ideally, supervision is a process of reciprocation and collaboration and should be viewed as a partnership between professional and technical personnel.

Career enhancement opportunities are also stressed, which emphasize options that will provide challenge, growth and advancement.

The final chapter in this section presents information about supervisory roles and responsibilities in the context of team work and team building both interdepartmentally and intraprofessionally. Specific stages of team development are presented together with characteristics, supervisor tasks, team member tasks, and communication issues associated with each stage. Emphasis is also placed on team member's needs in relation to ministration, mastery and maturation. The authors believe that intraprofessional team building is "critically important to the vitality and expansion of the profession."

Therapeutic Intervention Process

Sally E. Ryan, COTA, ROH

Introduction

The profession of occupational therapy has developed a specific plan for therapeutic intervention known as the occupational therapy process. It is made up of five distinct procedural categories that should be carried out in a particular order. (Exceptions are noted in the discussion of each category.) Service management is also considered as a sixth category. These sections are as follows:[1]

1. Referral
2. Assessment (including screening and evaluation)
3. Treatment planning
4. Treatment implementation (including periodic reevaluation)
5. Program discontinuation (including discharge planning and possibly follow-up)
6. Service management

The American Occupational Therapy Association (AOTA) has established general standards of practice for occupational therapy service programs and occupational therapy practitioners providing direct service. These standards were developed as guidelines to assist members of the profession. They have been reprinted in Appendix A because they detail important aspects of the occupational therapy process in which the certified occupational therapy assistant (COTA) serves an important role. In recent times, more specific standards of practice have been adopted in the areas of physical disabilities, developmental disabilities, mental health, home health, and school settings and other areas. They are published in the *Reference Manual of the Official Documents of the American Occupational Therapy Association*, which is available from AOTA.[2]

KEY CONCEPTS

Referral	Treatment implementation
Assessment	Program discontinuation
Treatment planning	Service management

ESSENTIAL VOCABULARY

Screening

Evaluation

Performance areas

Performance components

Problem solving

Activity analysis

Long-term objectives

Short-term objectives

Reevaluation

Follow-up

Referral

Requests for occupational therapy services may come from many sources including physicians, physical therapists, teachers, social workers and other health professionals, as well as parents and patients themselves. Referrals may be initiated and/or received by the occupational therapist either before or after the patient's initial screening. All referrals must be documented in writing and become a part of each patient's permanent record. The COTA may initiate patient referrals in the area of activities of daily living skills. When a COTA receives a referral, whether initiated or not, it must be given to the supervising registered occupational therapist (OTR) who is ultimately responsible for any action taken regarding the referral.[1]

The AOTA does not require that a referral be received before services can be provided. When there is no referral, the OTR must assume all responsibility for the delivery of services. In some instances, state laws or the requirements established by health care facilities mandate the receipt of a referral.[3] For example, the Commission on Accreditation of Rehabilitation Facilities (CARF), the Joint Commission on Accreditation of Healthcare Organizations (JCAHO), and Medicare regulations require that a physician's referral must be obtained if occupational therapy services are to be provided.[4] Figure 1-1 shows an example of a referral form used in a major hospital.

Assessment

The process of assessment includes both *screening* and *evaluation* and must take place before individual program planning. A thorough assessment provides a comprehensive "picture" of the patient based on a complete analysis of all of the screening and evaluation data. It is a predictor of the need for occupational therapy or other services and the estimated duration of treatment.

Screening

Screening of individuals who may benefit from occupational therapy services can be carried out by various health care providers. For example, a physical therapist may believe that a young man has stress management problems that are contributing to his diminished physical condition. A recreational therapist may note that a child has difficulty maintaining balance when participating in some play activities. Both of these individuals would be advised to seek an occupational therapy screening to determine the extent to which evaluation and treatment might alleviate or mediate the presenting problem.

The process of screening patients is necessary to determine whether a patient needs occupational therapy services.

Screening involves the collection and analysis of specific data and facts. Information is obtained by observing the patient while he or she is performing tasks or engaging in social interactions; through interviews with the patient, and family or significant others, such as a roommate or a close friend; or through a review of the patient's general history from sources that may include the medical chart, a psychologist's report or a teacher's appraisal. The COTA collaborates with the supervising OTR in the screening process by collecting and reporting selected information as requested. For example, he or she may use a structured interview form to gather information about the patient's educational background, employment history, hobbies and activities of daily living skills. If the occupational therapist's analysis of the screening information indicates that occupational therapy treatment would be beneficial, a comprehensive evaluation is performed.

Evaluation

The purpose of evaluation is to determine the patient's current level of functional performance and to identify performance deficits. The OTR is responsible for all aspects of the evaluation; however, the COTA may carry out some evaluative tasks under supervision. These tasks may include administering an interest checklist or an activity configuration and summarizing the information in a written report, or observing the patient in a specific situation and reporting on interpersonal skills, coordination, strength and endurance as they relate to activities of daily living skills and tasks.

The profession of occupational therapy is concerned with function and uses "specific procedures and activities to 1) develop, maintain, improve, and/or restore the performance of necessary functions; 2) compensate for dysfunction; 3) minimize or prevent debilitation; and 4) promote health and wellness.[3] The **occupational performance areas** and **performance components**, delineated in the document *Uniform Terminology for Occupational Therapy, Second Edition*, provide the framework for a comprehensive evaluation as follows:[5]

Occupational Therapy Performance Areas
1. Activities of Daily Living: grooming, oral hygiene, bathing, toilet hygiene, dressing, feeding and eating, medication routine, socialization, functional communication, functional mobility, and sexual expression
2. Work Activities: home management, care of others and educational and vocational activities
3. Play or Leisure Activities: exploration and performance

Performance Components
1. Sensory Motor Components: sensory integration, neuromuscular and motor
2. Cognitive Integration and Cognitive Components:

Patient _____
LAST   FIRST   M. INITIAL

Date Referral Received _____

Address _____ Zip _____

Address _____

Medicare # _____ Medicare #_____

_____

Contact Person _____ Phone # (_____) _____

Physician _____

Relationship: _____

Phone # _____

Primary Diagnosis: _____

Date of Onset: _____

Secondary Diagnosis: _____

Restrictions and Precautions: ☐ None ☐ Specify _____

Medical Prognosis: ☐ Excellent ☐ Good ☐ Fair ☐ Poor ☐ Guarded

☐ Patient ☐ Family is aware of Diagnosis and Prognosis

Physician's Plan of Treatment

☐ **Physical Therapy:** ☐ Evaluation and Treatment ☐ Other _____

Specify Rx/Modalities _____

Rehabilitation Goals: _____

Frequency _____ Duration _____ Wk/Mos Equipment: ☐ Yes ☐ No

☐ **Occupational Therapy:** ☐ Evaluation and Treatment ☐ Other _____

Specify Rx/Modalities _____

Rehabilitation Goals: _____

Frequency _____ Duration _____ Wk/Mos Equipment: ☐ Yes ☐ No

☐ **Speech Pathology:** ☐ Evaluation and Treatment ☐ Other _____

Specify Rx/Modalities _____

Rehabilitation Goals: _____

Frequency _____ Duration _____ Wk/Mos Equipment: ☐ Yes ☐ No

☐ **Social Work:** ☐ Evaluation and Treatment

Rehabilitation Goals _____

Physician Certification: I ☐ certify ☐ recertify that the above Skilled Rehabiliation Services are required and authorized by me.

_____
PHYSICIAN'S SIGNATURE   DATE

Figure 1-1. *Outpatient, Referral and Treatment Care Plan, adapted from Irene Walter Johnson Rehabilitation Institute, St. Louis, Mo.*

level of arousal, orientation, recognition, attention span, memory, etc

3. Psychosocial Skills and Psychological Components: psychological, social and self-management

Evaluation is necessary to determine the patient's strengths and weaknesses, needs and the degree of change possible through occupational therapy intervention. Occupational therapists and assistants use a variety of specific evaluations. Many are discussed in the individual case studies presented in Section II and the models of practice described in Section III.

The OTR analyzes and interprets screening and evaluation data to determine the total assessment results. Recommendations for continuance or dismissal from occupational therapy are made. Services other than occupational therapy that may assist the patient are identified and referral may be made.

Information obtained through a comprehensive evaluation also assists occupational therapy practitioners in determining the activities that will be most beneficial in assisting the patient in performance deficit areas.

Treatment Planning

According to Early, "treatment planning involves identifying the patient's problems and selecting goals that are reasonable to achieve and methods to achieve them."[6] Hopkins and Tiffany stress the need to use a **problem-solving** process in setting treatment objectives and carrying them out. This process is summarized as follows:[7]

1. Problem identification
2. Solution development
3. Development of a plan of action
4. Implementation of the plan
5. Assessment of results

In the treatment planning process, both long- and short-term objectives and time lines are established. Specific activities are analyzed, selected and sequenced to assist the patient in meeting the goals. Specific frames of reference, methods and approaches are also determined and adaptations are planned. The patient's goals, values, cultural identification, stage of biological and mental development, and interests and abilities are all carefully considered as an integral part of the process. The active involvement of the patient, as well as family members and significant others, in all phases of treatment planning is important and influences the overall effectiveness of the plan. Motivation and cooperation often increase when the patient has a thorough understanding of the treatment process and feels that he or she has had an integral part in the planning.

Failure to include the patient in planning may result in

ineffective or unnecessary intervention strategies. For example, if the patient is a woman who has had a stroke and needs to perform activities of daily living tasks with one hand, it is often a common practice in occupational therapy to include goals related to meal preparation. This may be stereotypical planning in some cases, as evidenced by the report of one COTA. The woman was placed in a cooking group and later told the occupational therapy assistant that her husband did all of the cooking and related tasks and she "never set foot in the kitchen nor did she plan to!" Another area where stereotypical planning might occur is housework. Setting goals related to tasks such as cleaning and doing the laundry would be inappropriate for a person who always hires outside help to do them and has the necessary financial resources to continue to do so. These brief examples illustrate the importance of including the patient in the treatment planning process. Outcomes of intervention must relate to the needs and priorities of the individual.

A strong background in a variety of different activities, together with knowledge and skill in **activity analysis**, is a critical factor in effective treatment planning. The therapeutic potential of age-appropriate activities and their various properties, components and potential for adaptation must be related to the specific treatment goals.

The COTA contributes to many aspects of the program plan; however, the OTR is responsible for the final plan that will best meet the patient's needs and objectives and is acceptable to the patient. The **long-term objectives** of such a plan are to develop, improve, restore or maintain the patient's abilities that allow for a more productive and meaningful life.[3] They may be quite broad in focus and are written to reflect the expected outcome of treatment.[4] The **short-term objectives** relate to the long-term objectives and contribute to their achievement. They must be stated in achievable, measurable outcomes and be met in a short enough time span to serve as a record of improvement. Short-term objectives address more immediate, specific goals. They may be viewed as "ministeps" that will lead to the desired result.[4]

Treatment planning is a critical component of the occupational therapy process. It involves "setting the problem" and identifying the steps necessary in "solving the problem."[8] The former is the role of the occupational therapist, and the latter is a collaborative OTR and COTA process, with the occupational therapist having the ultimate responsibility.

Treatment Implementation

All occupational therapy treatment is based on the treatment plan. Treatment implementation is putting the plan into action. Effective treatment requires the patient to participate in selected, purposeful activities designed to achieve the established goals. The COTA, working under close supervision, may implement a program for acutely ill individuals such as a patient who has had a recent stroke or someone who is depressed and suicidal.[1] Close supervision is essential because of the complex problems and degree of change frequently seen that may require a modified treatment approach or reevaluation by the OTR. If the patients are in a more stable, nonacute or controlled condition, the assistant may carry out treatment procedures with greater independence, as directed by the supervising OTR. The COTA may also be responsible for monitoring the patient's performance and providing a summary report. It is the COTA's responsibility to keep the supervising therapist informed of all changes in patient performance and any other pertinent facts. As treatment progresses and changes are noted, the assistant may contribute suggestions for program modifications and additions that will help the patient reach the established goals.[1]

In the event that the patient is not making satisfactory progress, the OTR will conduct a **reevaluation** to determine necessary changes in the program plan and the treatment procedures. Reevaluation refers to repeating certain assessments and analyzing the findings. Results may indicate that objectives have been set at too high a level or are unrealistic.[4] Perhaps methods, activities and/or time frames need to be modified. Specific aspects of the reevaluation may be delegated to the assistant. Reevaluation also takes place before discharge to determine discontinuation and discharge planning. Comparison of reevaluation data with that obtained in the initial evaluation provides an objective means of measuring change.

Program Discontinuation

Program discontinuation takes place when the patient has reached all of the established goals or it is determined that the patient can no longer benefit from occupational therapy services. Among other tasks, the COTA may assist in this process by providing specific information on progress or lack of progress to be included in a summary report. The COTA may also provide instructions for a home-based program, identify community resources and personnel, or recommend environmental adaptations that may assist the patient after discharge.

Although the standards of practice adopted by AOTA do not specify that patient **follow-up** must occur, it is desirable to gather such information to determine the effectiveness of treatment, general adjustment outcomes, and the degree to which the patient is able to resume social, family, work and leisure roles. This task could be performed collaboratively by an OTR and COTA, with the OTR determining the final conclusions. Follow-up also provides additional support to the patient in the transition from illness to wellness.

Service Management

Service management is a process that involves planning, structuring, developing, coordinating, documenting and evaluating the delivery of all occupational therapy services to ensure quality, efficiency and effectiveness. It is the organizational framework and system that supports the occupational therapy process in therapeutic intervention. Service management is essential in the delivery of occupational therapy services. Because this area has so many specific components, it will be discussed in depth in Chapter 28. Specific information relative to documentation may be found in Chapter 27.

Summary

Therapeutic intervention follows a specific plan called the occupational therapy process. This process includes sets of tasks that should be carried out in a particular order. Referral, assessment (including screening and evaluation), treatment planning, treatment implementation, (including reevaluation) and program discontinuation (including discharge planning and perhaps follow-up) are the major categories. Service management is a system that allows the occupational therapy process to be carried out. The COTA may participate in all aspects of the process as directed by the supervising OTR.

Related Learning Activities

1. Review the history and evaluation data for several patients of varying ages with both physical and mental problems. Work with a peer to develop potential treatment plans in the area of activities of daily living. Discuss your work with an OTR.

2. Use the treatment plans developed in item one as a basis for recommending specific treatment activities. Identify areas where additional information, if any, is needed. Discuss your work with an OTR.

3. Discuss specific roles the entry-level COTA can assume in the occupational therapy process.

4. What are some of the additional roles that may be assumed by experienced COTAs?

References

1. Entry-level OTR and COTA role delineation. *Am J Occup Ther* 37:802-809, 1981.
2. *Reference Manual of the Official Documents of the American Occupational Therapy Association*, Revised Edition. Rockville, Maryland, American Occupational Therapy Association, 1983, Chapter IV.
3. Commission on Practice Report. American Occupational Therapy Association, April, 1981.
4. Punwar AJ: *Occupational Therapy Principles and Practice*. Baltimore, Williams & Wilkins, 1988, p. 90.
5. Uniform terminology for occupational therapy—2nd edition. *Am J Occup Ther* 43:808-815, 1989.
6. Early MB: *Mental Health Concepts and Techniques for the Occupational Therapy Assistant*. New York, Raven Press, 1987, pp. 123-127.
7. Hopkins HL, Tiffany EG: Occupational therapy—a problem solving process. In Hopkins H, Smith H (Eds): *Willard and Spackman's Occupational Therapy*, Seventh Edition. Philadelphia, JB Lippincott, 1988.
8. Parham D: Toward professionalism: The reflective therapist. *Am J Occup Ther* 41:555-561, 1987.

COTA Supervision

Sally E. Ryan, COTA, ROH

Introduction

Throughout the history of the COTA, numerous questions have arisen regarding supervision issues. Questions continue about who supervises the COTA, under what circumstances, how frequently and whether the supervision is close or general. Other questions concern whom COTAs may supervise and the circumstances under which supervision may take place, as well as the experience necessary for assistants to provide supervision. This chapter discusses these issues and focuses on specific practice examples as well as guiding principles, patterns and responsibilities of supervision. Utilization issues and related concerns will also be discussed. The importance of career enhancement opportunities is also emphasized.

Supervision may be defined as the process of providing guidance and direction to employees and others. It involves assuming responsibility for the actions of workers, students, volunteers and others in carrying out the mission and goals of the unit, the department or the system within a given organization. It also involves overseeing, managing and providing leadership. Individuals who assume supervisory roles must possess strong interpersonal, intraprofessional and management skills. They must exhibit the ability to be role models, mentors, instructors, problem-solvers, arbitrators and evaluators. Successful supervisors are comfortable in their roles and are often characterized by their supervisees as effective, caring and involved. They are attuned to individual needs and are committed to helping individuals achieve their full potential, resulting in exemplary delivery of services and high job satisfaction. Moreover, they are effective team builders who have a keen understanding of the many ways that technical and professional staff members provide complementary skills, and they create an environment where collaboration is valued.

KEY CONCEPTS

Principles and patterns

Guidelines

Regulations and standards

Utilization of personnel

Career opportunities

ESSENTIAL VOCABULARY

Entry-level practice

Intermediate-level practice

Advanced-level practice

General supervision

Service competence

Occupational therapy aide

Volunteer

Cost-effective

Career enhancement

Close supervision

Terminology

For the reader to have a good understanding of the many facets of supervision, it is important to know the meaning of the following terms and designations:

Entry-Level Practice: The COTA or OTR who has less than one year of practice experience; the COTA is competent to deliver occupational therapy services, as stated in the current American Occupational Therapy Association (AOTA) entry-level role delineation, under the direction of an OTR.[1]

Intermediate Level Practice: The COTA or OTR who has one or more years of practice experience and is competent to carry out entry-level tasks; the COTA exhibits skills to carry out a variety of activities of daily living in treatment and may be developing additional, more advanced skills in a special interest area.[1]

Advanced Level Practice: The COTA or OTR who has three or more years of practice experience and has achieved the intermediate level; the COTA has demonstrated advanced level skills that may be clinical, educational or administrative.[1]

Close Supervision: "direct, on-site, daily contact."[2]

General Supervision: "frequent face-to-face meetings at the work site and regular interim communication between the OTR and the COTA by telephone, written report or conference."[2] According to Medicare guidelines, general supervision is "initial direction and periodic inspection of the actual activity; however, the supervisor need not always be physically present or on the premises when the assistant is performing services."[3] AOTA recommends that general supervision of the COTA should be used only "after service competencies have been determined by the supervising therapist."[4] These authors also emphasize that "contact by the supervising therapist may be less than daily, but should be a minimum of three to five direct contact hours per week for the full-time COTA."[4] In the case of the part-time COTA, supervision time is prorated.

Service Competence: "Implies that two people can perform the same or equivalent procedures and obtain the same results. This assurance is necessary whenever an OTR delegates tasks to a COTA."[2]

Occupational Therapy Aide: Designation given to individuals who perform routine tasks in the occupational therapy department. Through on-the-job training they learn skills in transporting patients, setting up treatment activities, maintaining supplies and equipment, and other related activities.

Volunteer: Unpaid worker who assists with varying tasks in the department such as typing, filing, preparing bulletin boards, serving refreshments, maintaining the library, and shopping for patients. (See Chapter 22 for additional information.)

Guiding Principles and Patterns

The AOTA has developed supervision guidelines for COTAs.[2] This document summarizes the requirements for supervision of COTAs in typical practice settings. It does not present information about assistants who practice as activities directors, educators, or in other nontraditional roles where they do not provide occupational therapy treatment services. Other principles of supervision are delineated in the *Executive Summary on Rules, Regulations, and Guidelines Governing Practice by and Supervision of Certified Occupational Therapy Assistants* available from AOTA.[3] A third resource is the AOTA Guide to Classification of Occupational Therapy Personnel.[1] In addition, the Entry-Level Role Delineation for Registered Occupational Therapists (OTRs) and Certified Occupational Therapy Assistants (COTAs) includes relevant supervisory information.[4] The following principles and patterns of supervision were drawn from these sources:

Related to Levels of Personnel:[1]

1. Entry-level COTAs require close supervision from an OTR or intermediate or advanced level COTA for delivery of patient services. General supervision by an experienced OTR or COTA is needed for management and administrative tasks. They do not have supervisory responsibilities.

2. Intermediate level COTAs require general clinical supervision from an intermediate or advanced level OTR. General supervision from an experienced OTR or advanced level COTA is needed for management and administration.

3. Intermediate level COTAs may provide "administrative supervision and clinical direction to entry-level COTAs" and occupational therapy assistant (OTA) level I and level II fieldwork students. They may supervise aides and volunteers.[1]

4. Advanced level COTAs require general clinical supervision from an intermediate or advanced level OTR; general management supervision is provided by an experienced OTR.

5. Advanced level COTAs provide "administrative supervision and clinical direction to entry-level COTAs" and OTA level I and level II fieldwork students. They supervise aides and volunteers.[1]

Related to Service Competency:[4]

1. It is the responsibility of the supervisor to establish the supervisee's level of service competency. A variety of methods, such as observation, videotaping, independent test-scoring, and co-treatment, can be used.

2. Service competency is more easily established for frequently used procedures. Infrequently used procedures may require closer supervision.

3. "It is recommended that the acceptable standard of percentage of agreement set by the OTR be met (by the supervisee) on three consecutive occasions before it is recorded that service competency has been established."[4]

Related to Patient Condition:

1. Regardless of the patient's condition, the COTA "may not evaluate independently or initiate the treatment process prior to the OTR's evaluation."[2] However, the COTA may contribute to the evaluation process.
2. More supervision is required for the COTA who is "working with a person whose condition is rapidly changing. . .because of the need for frequent evaluation, reevaluation, and treatment modifications."[2]
3. Treatment techniques that require "simultaneous reevaluation of the treatment response. . .are appropriately performed by an OTR."[3]
4. The COTA requires close supervision in implementing a treatment program for the acutely ill individual due to the complex problems and the degree of change frequently seen.[5]
5. The COTA may carry out treatment with a greater degree of independence for patients who are stable or nonacute or who have a controlled condition.[5]
6. It is the responsibility of the COTA to report all changes in patient performance and any other pertinent facts to the supervising therapist.

Related to Regulations and Standards:

1. It is the responsibility of every supervisor and supervisee to know and adhere to the supervisory and related regulations set forth by Medicare, Medicaid and other third party payers who provide reimbursement for occupational therapy services that the supervisor and supervisee carry out. For example, the Medicare guidelines for occupational therapy (Intermediary Manual, Part A, Section 3101.9) currently state that "while the skills of a qualified occupational therapist are required to evaluate the patient's level of function and develop a plan of treatment, the implementation of the plan may also be carried out by a qualified occupational therapy assistant functioning under the general supervision of the qualified occupational therapist."[3]
2. It is the reponsibility of every supervisor and supervisee to know and adhere to the supervisory and related regulations set forth by the Joint Commission on Accreditation of Healthcare Organizations (JCAHO) and the Commission for the Accreditation of Rehabilitation Facilities (CARF) when working for institutions that fall under their jurisdiction.
3. It is the responsibility of every supervisor and supervisee providing occupational therapy services in a state that has regulatory laws, such as licensure, registration or certification, to know and adhere to the supervisory and related regulations required by that state.
4. It is the responsibility of every supervisor and supervisee to know and adhere to the Standards of Practice (Appendix A) and the Principles of Occupational Therapy Ethics (see Appendix D) established by the American Occupational Therapy Association.

Related to General Employment:

Because supervision is a collaborative process between the supervisor and the supervisee, it is extremely important for each individual to have a clear understanding of his or her respective responsibilities.[6] Examples of these responsibilities are shown in Table 2-1.

Utilization of Personnel

Some occupational therapists serving as supervisors are recognizing the need to utilize COTAs more effectively due to increased demand for services, budget constraints, and limited availability of personnel. As Brooks has stated, "Role models and studies are needed to clearly demonstrate that OTRs working effectively with COTAs in a unified effort results in an expansion of occupational therapy services and is **cost-effective** as well."[7] The term "cost-effective" means producing the best results in relation to dollars spent. In a recent article on calculating cost-effectiveness of COTAs, Dennis presents convincing data that supports Brooks' assumption.[8] Linroth and Boulay also stress the need for employing more COTAs in terms of increased productivity and cost-containment. They state that, "Most occupational therapists intuitively know this but a good job of documenting and marketing this fact has yet to be done."[9] I agree. Over the past 20 years, concern has been voiced regarding the underutilization of assistants. The pattern of employment seen in many occupational therapy departments confirms the problem. For example, I have noted both personally and through informal surveys that in a geographic area with a more than adequate supply of highly qualified COTAs, it is not unusual to see major hospitals and other large facilities employing 20 or more OTRs and one or two COTAs. This fact is quite remarkable and indeed demonstrates an apparent inadequate utilization of personnel in some facilities. An interesting contrast is seen in the field of engineering where it is not unusual for one professional engineer to supervise six technicians. Despite great strides, the occupational therapy profession needs to increase its efforts to provide a better balance of

Table 2-1.
Examples of Supervisor and Supervisee Roles

Supervisor	Supervisee
Provide orientation to the facility and program	Participate in orientation activities
Assess periodically level of competency	Participate in competency assessment activities
Define and assign specific responsibilities	Carry out responsibilities effectively, seeking clarification if unsure
Establish criteria for performance evaluation and timelines	Discuss criteria and establish clear understanding of expectations
Schedule formal and informal meetings to identify problems, needs, and concerns and to solicit ideas	Participate regularly in meetings, openly and honestly discussing issues and providing feedback and ideas
Give feedback relative to areas of future growth and skill development, providing resources as needed	Seek new knowledge and skills and set professional goals
Develop and modify job descriptions	Recommend changes in job description

technical and professional personnel in the delivery of patient services.

The Army Medical Specialist Corps provides an example of effective utilization of assistants, as the ratio of COTAs to OTRs in the majority of their clinics in the United States is quite high. It is also significant to note that military workloads and levels of productivity are considerably higher than those found in the civilian sector.[10] More utilization models and related patterns of supervision such as these are needed to allow the occupational therapist to provide more services to more patients. Moreover, increased utilization of occupational therapy assistants can have an immediate impact on the growing personnel shortages the profession is experiencing in many areas.

Care must also be taken to ensure that COTAs are not overutilized. Failure to hire the proper level of personnel for the job requirements and to provide adequate supervision is unacceptable. Occupational therapy services *cannot* be provided by a COTA who is not receiving OTR supervision, and must be discontinued.[2] Evert, in her 1992 Presidential address, provides a scenario that typifies the supervisory dilemmas faced by many COTAs when an OTR is not available.[11] The COTA must often refuse to treat the patient, even in the face of administrative pressure to do so.

Career Opportunities

The supervisor must provide opportunities for challenge, growth and advancement for supervisees as vehicles for **career enhancement.** Strickland describes a career development planning model adopted by a large medical facility for employees in the occupational therapy department. Career ladders have been established that provide a variety of options for both OTRs and COTAs, including development of adaptive equipment and techniques, professional writing, educational presentations, and development of new programs and projects.[12] Opportunities such as these can be a shared collegial experience among OTRs and COTAs, which enhance day-to-day working relationships and, ultimately, job and career satisfaction.

Conclusion

Supervision is a complex and dynamic process that involves a variety of skills and abilities. Ideally, it is a process of collaboration and reciprocation between the supervisor and the supervisee. It should be viewed as a partnership between professional and technical personnel. Building on this concept, Chapter 3 presents detailed information on supervisory roles and responsibilities in the context of team building. Additional information on supervision may be found in Chapters 22, 28 and 29.

Summary

Supervision is a process of providing guidance and direction to others. It involves assuming responsibility for workers and others in carrying out the mission and goals of the unit, the department or the system within an organization. Knowledge of discipline-specific terminology and designations is necessary and provides a foundation for understanding occupational therapy supervision principles and patterns. These are delineated and discussed in terms of levels of personnel, service competency, patient conditions, regulations and standards, and general employment. Examples of supervisor and supervisee responsibilities are stressed. Models for increased utilization of technical personnel that demonstrate increased delivery of services in a cost-effective manner are needed. These models should also emphasize ways that technical and professional personnel can be challenged and achieve career growth through varied options. Career enhancement opportunities are necessary to build relationships with workers and increase job and career satisfaction.

Related Learning Activities

1. Conduct an informal interview with at least three supervisors and ask them to list their major responsibilities in terms of their supervisees.

2. Conduct an informal interview with at least three supervisees and ask them to list their major responsibilities to their supervisor.

3. Compare the information obtained in items 1 and 2 with the information shown in Figure 2-1, noting similarities and differences.

4. Role play the following scene with a peer: The OTR supervisor has asked you to administer a structured assessment that you have only performed once before. You are feeling very uncomfortable about this request. What actions will you take. After the role play, seek feedback and suggestions from your peer.

5. Interview a COTA who has at least one year of experience. Determine what career enhancement opportunities he or she is engaged in. Determine the role of the supervisor in this plan.

References

1. Schell BAB: Guide to classification of occupational therapy personnel. *Am J Occup Ther* 39:803-810, 1985.
2. American Occupational Therapy Association: Supervision Guidelines for Certified Occupational Therapy Assistants. *Am J Occup Ther* 44:1089-1090, 1990.
3. American Occupational Therapy Association: *Executive Summary on Rules, Regulations, and Guidelines Governing Practice by and Supervision of Certified Occupational Therapy Assistants.* Rockville, Maryland, American Occupational Therapy Association, 1990.
4. American Occupational Therapy Association: Entry-level role delineation for registered occupational therapists (OTRs) and certified occupational therapy assistants (COTAs). *Am J Occup Ther* 44:1091-1102, 1990.
5. American Occupational Therapy Association: Entry-level role delineation for OTRs and COTAs. *Reference Manual of Official Documents of The American Occupational Therapy Association, VII.1-VII.2.* Rockville, Maryland, American Occupational Therapy Association, 1981.
6. Early MB: *Mental Health Concepts and Techniques for the Occupational Therapy Assistant.* New York, Raven Press, 1987, Chapter 5.
7. Brooks B: COTA issues: Yesterday, today, and tomorrow. *Am J Occup Ther* 36:567-568, 1982.
8. Dennis M: Calculating cost effectiveness with the certified occupational therapy assistant. In Johnson JA (Ed): *Certified Occupational Therapy Assistants—Opportunities and Challenges.* New York, Haworth Press, 1988.
9. Linroth R, Boulay P: Certified occupational therapy assistants: Preparation for change. In Johnson JA (Ed): *Certified Occupational Therapy Assistants—Opportunities and Challenges.* New York, Haworth Press, 1988.
10. Personal correspondence, Roy Swift, EdD, OTR, FAOTA; Chief, Army Medical Specialist Corps, February, 1991.
11. Evert MM: New president's address: Daily practice dilemmas. *Am J Occup Ther* 43:7-9, 1993.
12. Strickland LR: Career ladder development for certified occupational therapy assistants. In Johnson JA (Ed): *Certified Occupational Therapy Assistants—Opportunities and Challenges.* New York, Haworth Press, 1988 .

Teamwork and Team Building

Toné F. Blechert, MA, COTA, ROH
Marianne F. Christiansen, MA, OTR
Nancy Kari, MPH, OTR

Introduction

Becoming a respected and accepted member of the team is an important goal. Effective teamwork can contribute to the welfare of one's patients, create high morale among staff members and foster a collaborative and an educational climate in the work setting.[1]

The term teamwork is often associated with **morale**. Morale refers to the attitudes of the employees in a department, whereas teamwork is the smoothly coordinated and synchronized action achieved by a closely knit group of employees.[1]

In an occupational therapy department, an effective team is built on the character and competencies of its members. Team efforts are strengthened as members improve their professional and personal abilities. For example, with practice and experience, an OTR or COTA team member may emerge as an expert in splinting techniques. Performance in this area may become so outstanding that no other team members could equal it. Another OTR or COTA may become an expert in the use of effective group skills. A dynamic strength of teamwork is that it frees each member to do some of the things he or she can do best in the occupational therapy process.

Occupational therapy personnel who are satisfied, contributing team members are helpful to patients and each other. These individuals demonstrate a basic personal security. They are most often those who are confident of their knowledge and abilities and comfortable and honest about their limitations. Once team membership skills are mastered, individuals can become involved in team building strategies.

KEY CONCEPTS

Teamwork qualities

Professional and personal abilities

Interdepartmental teaming

Intraprofessional team building

Basic needs and team behaviors

Organizational framework

Developmental team chart

ESSENTIAL VOCABULARY

Morale

Cooperation

Flexibility

Creativity

Job description

Ministration

Mastery

Maturation

Reciprocity

Causal map

Teamwork Qualities

Among the necessary qualities of a successful occupational therapy practitioner, several are worthy of discussion as they relate to effective teamwork.

Cooperation: Team members work together to achieve common goals. In this effort each individual must pay attention to details that make cooperation possible. The OTRs and COTAs on the team must be well informed about one another's activities. Cooperation allows the opportunity to teach and learn, to give and receive, and to increase the competence of all involved. A respectful attitude toward the other members of one's team is extremely important. As people work together more closely, they will learn a great deal of information about each other. Team members must be discrete and avoid petty gossip. Cooperation is more difficult if trust is broken.

Flexibility: A successful team member sees change as a positive element. Changing approaches and methods must be met with an open and accepting mind. This openness to change encourages all team members to think creatively and express ideas freely.

Creativity: Occupational therapy personnel pride themselves on their creative abilities. Certainly one would hope for an atmosphere that encourages creativity among staff members. Creativity implies individuality but should never be construed as unrestrained liberty.[2] Teamwork demands an environment that is permissive enough to allow new ideas to develop and yet structured enough to provide order and direction for all members.

In addition to cooperation, flexibility and creativity, one must also be aware of the purpose and philosophy of the work setting and understand his or her own duties and the duties of other departmental members. A **job description** is a list of the tasks that one is expected to perform. A written copy of one's job description as well as those of co-workers should be available to all members of the department so that no misunderstandings occur.

Interdepartmental Teamwork

The purpose of an interdepartmental treatment team is to provide the best possible service to the patient through the sharing of information and expertise and the coordination of services. The treatment team may be headed by a physician or other health professional depending on the setting. The members of the team may include anyone who works with the patient in any capacity. Other team members may be from physical therapy, therapeutic recreation, nursing, social service, vocational counseling or dietary departments. The following information describes roles of these team members in various settings.

Physician: A physician is a medical doctor who practices the science and art of preventing and curing disease and preserving health. Occupational therapy personnel work with physicians who have varying specialty backgrounds. A *physiatrist* is a medical doctor who specializes in physical medicine. A *psychiatrist* specializes in mental illness. These two specialists often direct treatment teams in the hospital setting.

Clinical Psychologist: The psychologist is not a medical doctor, although he or she may have a PhD degree. A clinical psychologist functions in three areas: diagnosis, psychotherapy and research. The psychologist administers diagnostic tests and conducts interviews. Psychological tests are made up of a kind of standard situation in which varying reactions of different patients may be observed. Many people are reluctant to reveal their thoughts in an interview, but may show a characteristic way of thinking in response to tests. Psychotherapy may be performed with individual patients or in patient groups, and families may be involved. Psychologists have a backgound in statistics and research methods and are prepared to assist staff members who wish to do research by helping construct experimental procedures and interpret results.

Nurse: The role of the nurse is to be aware of the total nursing needs of patients. The nurse is responsible for seeing that these needs are met through preparing, administering and supervising a patient care plan for each patient. This responsibility involves evaluating the patient's physical, spiritual and emotional needs. The scientific basis for applying scientific principles in performing nursing procedures and techniques must be known. The nurse must be able to perform therapeutic measures prescribed and delegated by the physician and must be able to observe and evaluate patient symptoms, reactions and progress.

Social Worker: The role of the social worker is to provide contact between the patient and the community, enabling one to make the best use of the resources available. Social workers may work in public or private hospitals, community settings such as welfare agencies, centers for emotionally disturbed children, corrections institutions and schools. In a private hospital, patients are referred by physicians to discuss problems such as lack of funds, placement of patients in nursing homes and similar community-related needs. The patient is helped by referral to an appropriate agency.

Physical Therapist: A physical therapist provides treatment for patients with disabilities resulting from disease or injury. Various modalities are used in physical therapy, including light therapy, which involves ultraviolet and infrared light; electrotherapy, which may involve diathermy and electrical stimulation; hydrotherapy, which includes equipment such as the Hubbard tank, whirlpool and contrast baths; mechanical therapy, which involves massage, traction and therapeutic exercise of various kinds; and thermotherapy, which involves heat such as paraffin baths and whirl-pool. The purpose of the treatment may be to relieve pain, to increase function of a body part by improving muscle strength and joint range of motion, or to teach patients to ambulate with the help of crutches, canes and other aides.

Therapeutic Recreation Specialist: A therapeutic recreation specialist uses free play, exercise and other activity to meet treatment needs. Group recreation may encourage more positive relationships with others, improve body image, allow an outlet for emotional release, aid circulation and other body functions, and provide enjoyment and relaxation. Some activities used in therapeutic recreation are swimming, music, games and contests, dancing, dramatics, special events, and outings. Leisure counseling is also provided.

Vocational Counselor: The vocational counselor may be employed by a federal rehabilitation organization such as Vocational Rehabilitation or by the institution itself to test patients' vocational abilities. A patient may have to change occupations depending on the extent of illness or injury. For instance, a truck driver who has had a heart attack may need to find a less demanding job. The vocational counselor administers aptitude tests and does predischarge planning for special training and job placement. The OTR and COTA may work with the vocational counselor in evaluating the patient's work readiness, tolerance, coordination, and special skills. The vocational counselor is concerned with the patient's postdischarge plans.

Dietitian: The function of the dietitian is to manage the preparation and serving of food for patients. This job includes planning and preparing many special diets. The occupational therapy assistant may be asked to be present at mealtime to help the patient with physical disabilities such as a stroke to learn to eat independently again. The occupational therapy department must work with the dietary department in scheduling needs for various activities.

In summary, one must understand the functions of other departments and personnel to achieve the following objectives:

1. Establish a climate of mutual respect and sound working relationships
2. Develop appreciation of the importance of the other treatment procedures and intervention services
3. Communicate scheduling needs and changes
4. Cooperate to provide the best possible treatment
5. Avoid unnecessary duplication of services

Information about the roles of other health care providers and departments may be found in the Case Studies and Models of Practice sections of this text.

Intraprofessional Team Building

Although the information on effective team building presented in this section can be applied to all members of the health care team, the focus is on the intraprofessional relationship between occupational therapists and occupational therapy assistants. "The relationship of teamwork to the effectiveness of service delivery within the profession of occupational therapy" is a major theme.[3]

Napier and Gershenfeld[4] define team building as a process that facilitates the development of a group of people with respect to their unique needs, their degree of readiness and their past experience with team building activities. They also point out the importance of team members having opportunities "to experience each other in a wide variety of situations" as well as through activities that "provide permission for a group to look at its own behavior and also to explore new ways of approaching problems in order to be more effective."[4]

The term *effectiveness* is one of the "buzz words" of the 1990s. Increased health care costs, productivity demands and personnel shortages, coupled with maldistribution and attrition patterns, have produced problems in the effective delivery of occupational therapy services.[5] In geographic areas where there is an ample supply of both therapists and assistants, often only therapists are hired or when assistants are hired they are underutilized. The latter situation "results in a loss of job satisfaction, decreased commitment and attrition for assistants."[3] With increased demands for cost-effective services, every effort must be made to reduce this attrition. Intraprofessional team building is one solution. It is "critically important to the vitality and expansion of the profession."[3]

Basic Needs

Effective team building is founded on the principle that team members' needs must be met or team dysfunction will occur. Needs may be categorized as follows:[6,7]

Ministration: Ministration refers to one's need to feel a sense of closeness with co-workers; to feel safe, guided and supported; and to experience acceptance, trust and respect. An example is the occupational therapy assistant student who is beginning the first level II fieldwork experience. Team members who provide extra orientation, anticipate questions, and indicate a willingness to listen to the student's fears and uncertainties help meet the individual's ministration needs. When a team member states that it is okay to make a mistake and demonstrates an understanding that errors are an inherent part of the learning process, the student feels a certain level of safety and support.

Mastery: Mastery involves role exploration, influencing others and performance review. This need can be met in a variety of ways such as developing a high level of expertise and an enhanced role in a particular area of therapeutic intervention. Stress management, wheelchair positioning and construction of adaptive devices are a few examples. Opportunities are sought to provide leadership to others

TABLE 3-1.
Developmental Team Chart

Stage of Team Development	Characteristics	Supervisor's Tasks	Team Member's Tasks	Communication Issues
I. INITIATION STAGE Exploration and definition of member roles and responsibilities within the context of team and work settings.	Before and in the beginning phase of team formation, individuals may experience self-doubt, lack of trust, tole amibiguity, and a degree of powerlessness in the work setting.	Promote atmosphere of acceptance and trust: • State expectations openly • Encourage discussion of members' expectations • Encourage commitment to team building by helping members to: • Identify skills, areas of strength and interest • Provide opportunities to increase self-esteem Provide general definition and direction for newly formed team • Define the situation and resources available • Define roles and responsibilities for team members	Learn and explore role expectations. Begin to share resources, identify own areas of expertise and interests.	Express anxieties and insecurities of new relationships. Verbalize support for team efforts. Demonstrate acceptance and begin to develop trust.
II. TRANSITION STAGE Adjustment and rearrangement of roles to create a team.	Team members experience increased anxieties, defensiveness and struggles for control. Reclarification and adjustments of roles are evident. Group norms are forming. Relationship issues are important at this stage.	Provide encouragement. Manage conflict openly. Provide structures for team to make decisions, solve problems, and set priorities. Effectuate intervention strategies if needed. Reclarify roles, team goals.	Develop skills, gain confidence. Learn about the organizational structure. Commit self to teamwork. Begin to identify and deal with conflicts openly.	Begin to identify and deal with conflicts openly. Verbalize group norms and values. Encourage team affiliation by engaging in community building activities.
III. WORKING STAGE Tasks are identified and achieved.	Team members experience cohesion and productivity. Conflicts are dealt with openly and are effectively managed.	Refine leadership skills. Allow team members more autonomy and support development of their professional skills. Provide liaison functions for team with the external organization. Help team members find solutions to difficult problems; provide resources and support services. Assess and evaluate work relative to the team's overall performance.	Participate fully as a team member in the planning, decision-making, and execution of tasks. Clarify personal goals. Ask for needed direction/ support from supervisor. Participate in evaluation of task completion. Develop sense of mastery.	Communicate support, and challenge members through feedback. Discuss how methods of problem solving, decision-making, and conflict management occur in the team.

through assuming supervisory and educational roles. Review of performance is actively sought from one's supervisor or other knowledgable person.

Maturation: Maturation is characterized by personal and professional goal renewal, risk taking for goal achievement and the empowerment of others. This need is illustrated by the COTA who seeks activities and programs that maintain as well as expand professional roles. Seeking new responsi-

TABLE 3-1. (continued)
Developmental Team Chart

Stage of Team Development	Characteristics	Supervisor's Tasks	Team Member's Tasks	Communication Issues
IV. INTERDEPENDENCE STAGE Team members are effective in their work and achieve interdependence in their working relationships.	Team members are mutually supportive, take pride in the team, value each other, and experience the team as interlocking roles.	Model collegial relationships. Become a mentor; empower others. Continue to develop personal and professional skills.	Reflect on self as a professional, reassess goals, offer peer evaluations. Learn to think about issues from multiple points of view. Take risks; achieve greater competency.	Express valuing of team members and demonstrate support for each others' achievements.
V. SEPARATION Team separation may occur at any stage; however, characteristics and tasks will be different depending on the maturity of the team.	Team members experience anxiety as they anticipate separation. There is an awareness of the successes and failures of the team.	Ensure opportunity for and assist members in summarizing, integrating, and interpreting the team experience. Provide a framework that will help members evaluate the team effort and individual roles. Allow time for members to resolve unfinished business and express feelings about the separation.	Summarize the team experience and the attainment of personal and professional goals. Evaluate personal and team performance. Define tasks for new members.	Express feelings about separation. Avoid withdrawal or distancing of members. Give and receive feedback; discuss the application of current experiences to future teams.

bilities involving risks, such as developing a new program, and becoming a mentor to another person are other ways that this need can be achieved.

These three needs, as they relate to the intraprofessional socialization process, are discussed in greater depth in Chapter 28.

Team Building Behaviors

In the early 1960s, Levinson[6] and his colleagues studied a group of workers at a new company. Their studies revealed that the employees were engaged in a process of fulfilling mutual needs and expectations. A climate of successful **reciprocity** was built (reciprocity refers to a mutual giving and receiving or exchange) and the following contributing behaviors were observed:[3,6]

1. Others are treated as individuals.
2. Individual differences are appreciated.
3. Relationships are established with those who are different.
4. Flexibility is shown in stressful situations.
5. Satisfaction is derived from a wide variety of sources.
6. Strengths as well as limitations are accepted.
7. Realistic self-concepts are exhibited.
8. Activity and productivity are evident.

These behaviors and others are important to the success of teamwork and team building efforts.

Organizational Framework

A **causal map** representing the profession as a whole is shown in Figure 3-1. It illustrates the relationships between the health of the profession and practitioner's need satisfaction.[3] Relationships that demonstrate cause and effect between personal and professional subsystems are described in relation to the total system.[8] An important theme shown is that teamwork leads to personal growth, productivity, and quality care and increased the status of both the department providing services and the entire profession.[3]

Developmental Team Building

The developmental team chart shown in Table 3-1 presents a team building process organized according to stages of team development, characteristics of the particular stage, supervisor tasks, team member tasks and communication issues. The levels of ministration, mastery and maturation are also delineated. When using this chart it is important for the reader to consider the following factors:[3]

1. Information may be used to assess current team functioning.

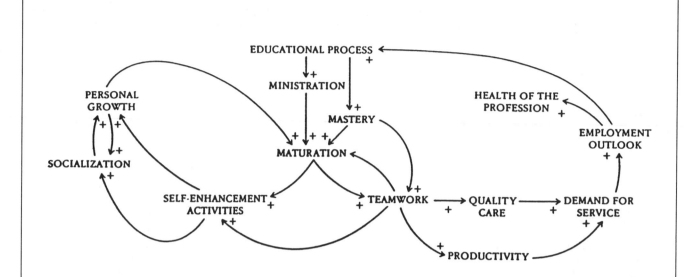

Overview
The driving force in the system is the educational process. If it is successful, the student will graduate and enter the field with a basic understanding of meeting ministration and mastery needs. When an individual's ministration and mastery needs are met, maturation can occur. The quality of teamwork is enhanced and continuously reinforced by the satisfaction of these three needs.

Personal Subsystem
As a person matures, there is an increased interest and ability to participate in self-enhancement activities. Such participation enables further socialization within the profession. Increased socialization in one's career as well as involvement in self-enhancement activities leads to personal growth. As maturation is reinforced, a climate is created that facilitates appreciation and support for continued involvement in self-enhancement activities.

Professional Subsystem
Effective teamwork evolves when people's ministration, mastery, and maturation needs are met and people are able to interact in a manner that will help them grow. As this occurs in a work setting, productivity will increase. This kind of teamwork provides quality care. Both productivity and quality care will have an effect on the demand for service as other health professionals, administrators, patients, and the public gain respect for occupational therapy services. The demand for service has implications for the employment outlook. As jobs increase, more people will be interested in entering the field and will enroll in educational programs. The increased demand for occupational therapy personnel contributes to the health and stability of the profession as a whole.

Whole System
Both the professional and personal subsystems interconnect and loops are formed. All of the loops in the diagram are reinforcing loops. If the relationships are positive as described, then the health of the system can grow at an exponential rate. However, if there is a decrease or problem at any point in the system, it will have a negative effect on the organization. For example, negative effects may be manifested as increased attrition, loss of professional identity, and an eroded financial base.

Figure 3-1. *Causal Map*

2. Factors that may enhance group functioning are listed.
3. The stages listed are not absolute and may overlap.
4. Teams are unique and their experiences may not always parallel the chart.
5. Teams evolve according to their experiences in preceding stages.[9-11]

Summary

Effective teamwork and team building are essential processes in the profession of occupational therapy. They contribute to quality service delivery and morale, and they can also have a significant influence on reducing COTA attrition. Teamwork qualities include cooperation, flexibility and creativity. Occupational therapy practitioners work with a variety of interdepartmental personnel to share information, coordinate schedules, and provide the most effective overall treatment, avoiding overlap and duplication. Intraprofessional teamwork and team building are equally important. A causal map illustrates an organizational framework that identifies the relationship between the health of the profession and need satisfaction of its practitioners. The basic needs of ministration, mastery and maturation provide a theme that carries over into the developmental team chart, which presents a team building process organized according to specific developmental stages of teams. The identification of team characteristics, supervisor and member tasks and communication issues provides a matrix that can serve as an important tool for improved intraprofessional team building.

Related Learning Activities

1. Observe various teamwork activities in a health care setting. List the characteristics that appear to contribute to effective teamwork.

2. Participate in a self-assessment exercise with a peer. Identify the characteristics that each of you possess that would contribute to teamwork and team building relationships.

3. Review the material on professional team members and identify the areas of their services that may overlap with those provided by occupational therapy personnel.

4. Study the chart found in Table 3-1 and list additional team member and supervisor tasks for each of the levels as they relate to a particular team problem you have experienced.

5. List and discuss additional communication issues for the stages of team development in terms of a specific personal team situation.

References

1. Beggs D (Ed): *Team Teaching: Bold New Venture*. Indianapolis, United College Press, 1962, pp. 44-47, 131, 456-465.
2. Terry G: *Principles of Management*. Homewood, Illinois, Richard Irwin, Inc., 1977.
3. Blechert TF, Christiansen MF, Kari N: Intraprofessional team building. *Am J Occup Ther* 41:576-582, 1987.
4. Napier RW, Gershenfeld MK: *Making Groups Work*. Boston, Houghton Mifflin Company, 1983.
5. American Occupational Therapy Association: Member data survey: Executive summary. *OT Week* June 6, 1991.
6. Levinson H: *Men, Management and Mental Health*. Cambridge, Harvard University Press, 1962.
7. Blechert TF, Christiansen MF: Intraprofessional relationships and socialization: The maturation process. In Ryan SE (Ed): *The Certified Occupational Therapy Assistant: Roles and Responsibilities*. Thorofare, New Jersey, Slack, Inc., 1986.
8. Roberts N, Anderson D: *Introduction to Computer Simulation: A Systems dynamics modeling approach*. Reading, Massachusetts, Addison-Wesley, 1983.
9. Brill N: *Teamwork: Working together in the Human Services*. New York, JB Lippincott, 1976.
10. Corey G: *Theory and Practice of Group Counseling*. Monteray, California, Brooks/Cole, 1981.
11. Hagberg J: *Real Power: Stages of Personal Power in Organizations*. Minneapolis, Winston Press, 1984.

Section II
INTERVENTION STRATEGIES—THE TEAM APPROACH

Part A: Childhood

Part B: Adolescence

Part C: Young Adulthood

Part D: Adulthood

Part E: The Elderly

This section provides the reader with specific, illustrative examples of the many ways in which the OTR and the COTA work together effectively as a team. Seventeen chapter-length case studies are presented representing a wide variety of age groups, problems, intervention strategies and treatment settings. Basic medical information is also reviewed in relation to each case scenario.

Many of the case studies are based on actual events and situations whereas others are composites. Names, personal information and other pertinent data have been changed to protect the identity of actual occupational

therapy patients.

It is very important for the reader to note that the case studies are examples, *not recommended standards*, for the intraprofessional team approach in the delivery of occupational therapy services. The authors have expressed their professional opinions based on actual experiences as well as hypothetical and ideal situations. The overall goals of the authors and the editor are to promote the profession of occupational therapy through the intraprofessional team approach and to provide quality health care services efficiently and effectively.

Part A
CHILDHOOD

The Child With Visual Deficits

Patricia K. Benham, MPH, OTR

Introduction

In 1986, Congress passed the Education of the Handicapped Amendments (PL 99-457), which mandated early intervention services for children aged birth to two years old and their families. This chapter reviews current federal legislation affecting services for children and presents a case study of a toddler with a visual handicap. The occupational therapy early intervention plan is discussed in the context of the requirements of PL 99-457. Both the occupational therapist and the certified occupational therapy assistant (COTA) described in this case study are practicing at the advanced level as defined by the American Occupational Therapy Association (AOTA) document *Guide to Classification of Occupational Therapy Personnel*.[1]

Family Centered Approach to Early Intervention

AOTA supports a family-focused approach to early intervention. This position is clearly articulated in the Occupational Therapy Services in Early Intervention Position Paper published by the AOTA and included in the manual *Guidelines for Occupational Therapy Services in Early Intervention and Preschool Services*.[2]

This family-centered philosophy recognizes the parents as consumers and enables them to collaborate with professionals in the planning and implementation of a treatment program for their child. Using this framework, occupational therapy personnel view the child as a member within a family and deliver services in ways that strengthen and support the family. The

---

KEY CONCEPTS

Family-centered approach	Treatment goals
Legislative mandates	Play and feeding activities
Medical and family history	Transition planning
Cultural implications	Follow-up
Developmental assessment	

ESSENTIAL VOCABULARY

Individualized education plan

Developmental delay

Individualized family service plan

Retrolental fibroplasia

Apnea

Sepsis

Takata's play history

Segmentation

Moro reflex

Hypotonic

infant or toddler who is at risk benefits from a prevention model that recognizes the needs and strengths of the primary caregivers and empowers them to interact proactively with their child.

Legislative Mandates

The Education of All Handicapped Children Act (PL 94-142) was enacted in 1975. This federal legislation mandated that states provide free and appropriate educational services to all school-aged children, regardless of their handicapping conditions. The Act specified that related services, which include occupational therapy, be provided when deemed a necessary component to the child's special education program. Each child must have an **Individualized Educational plan** (IEP), which documents the services to be received and the goals of the child's program. It ensured the right to due process and the provision of the educational program in the least restrictive environment.[3]

This legislation authorized grant programs, research, dissemination of information, model projects and specialized training and assistance to state and local programs in order to support the implementation of the law. It also established Child Find, a service to identify at-risk and handicapped children beginning at birth. Additional information about this legislation may be found in Chapter 6.

Although PL 94-142 encouraged the expansion of services to preschool-aged children who were handicapped by offering incentive dollars to states (Section 619, The Preschool Incentive Grant), services were not mandated until 1986 when Congress passed the Education of the Handicapped Amendments (PL 99-457).[4] This law is significant for several reasons. It amended PL 94-142, Part B, to include three- to five-year-old preschoolers with handicaps, and it supported the establishment of early intervention programs for infants and toddlers (Part H). Under Part H, states receive financial assistance to plan and implement statewide comprehensive, coordinated, multidisciplinary, interagency programs that offer early intervention services for infants, toddlers and their families.[4]

The regulations affect children from birth through age two years who need early intervention services because they are either experiencing developmental delays or have a diagnosed physical or mental condition that has a high probability of resulting in developmental delay. The state may include those at risk for developmental delays if early intervention services are not provided. Each state determines the parameters and criteria for eligibility, so the occupational therapist and assistant must be aware of the guidelines in the state where they are practicing.[4]

Developmental delays may occur in any one or more of the following areas: physical development, cognitive development, language and speech development, psychosocial development, or self-help skills. Each statewide system of early intervention must have its own definition of "developmental delay" and describe the procedures to be used to determine the existence of a developmental delay.[4]

The law defines occupational therapy as a service that addresses the functional needs of a child related to the performance of self-help skills; adaptive behavior and play; and sensory, motor and postural development. These services are designed to improve the child's functional ability to perform tasks at home, at school and in community settings. Occupational therapy is an early intervention service for children from birth through age two years and their families. This differs from Public Law 94-142 in that occupational therapy is defined as a related service and provided only when occupational therapy is necessary to meet the educational needs of the child.[4]

This legislation attempts to make families the focal point of service. To assure a family-centered approach, the regulations state that a voluntary family assessment/interview must be designed to include the strengths and needs of the family as they relate to enhancing the child's development. Occupational therapy practitioners would be likely to participate in family assessments in the areas of self-care, play and positioning.

The assessment of the child and the family is necessary to formulate the **Individualized family service plan** (IFSP). Although similar to the IEP required by PL 94-142, the IFSP places more emphasis on the collaboration of the family and professional services.

The IFSP must include information about the child's status; family; projected outcomes of intervention; and the methods, criteria and timelines that will be used to determine progress. A case manager must be identified, as well as the early intervention services or other services necessary to meet the needs of the child and family. The ISFP must include the steps to be taken at age three years, which will support the child's transition, if applicable, into an appropriate preschool program.

In summary, PL 99-457 states that infants and toddlers aged birth to two years and their families may receive occupational therapy services. Occupational therapy is considered a primary early intervention service and can be provided along with or separate from other health or educational services. Under PL 94-142 and the amendments of PL 99-457, preschool- and school-aged children may receive occupational therapy services when defined as a related service necessary to allow the child to benefit from the special education program.

Case Study Background

The focus of the following case study is a child with a visual impairment as a result of **retrolental fibroplasia** (RLF). This bilateral condition may occur as the result of a child being placed in an incubator that has an excessive amount of oxygen. The elevated oxygen levels destroy the rapidly growing blood vessels in an infant's retina. When the child is returned to normal room air, the blood vessels grow back haphazardly, and scar tissue forms. As the scar tissue contracts, it pulls the retina away from the choroid, causing the retina to detach. It is difficult to determine the degree of functional damage for an infant affected by RLF; however, blindness usually develops within several weeks. Once blindness occurs, there is no effective treatment. Other factors that contribute to the origin and development of the disease include **apnea** (temporary cessation of breathing), asphyxia, **sepsis** (presence of pathogenic microorganisms or their toxins in the blood or other tissues), nutritional deficiencies, and a large number of blood transfusions given during a short period of time.[5]

Referral Information

Alejandro was 15 months old when he was referred to the Early Intervention Program at the state Department of Health and Human Services by his pediatrician after an initial examination that revealed delays in several areas of development on the Denver Developmental Screening Test.[6] Alejandro was diagnosed as developmentally delayed and visually impaired as a result of RLF.

A case manager was assigned and the early intervention team members began their assessments. Team members included a teacher of the visually handicapped, an orientation and mobility specialist, a psychologist, an ophthalmologist, an occupational therapist and an occupational therapy assistant.

Assessment Information

Family History

An initial meeting was scheduled with the early intervention team and the parents. The Family Needs Survey was administered, revealing the parent's primary needs for services and information.[7] The survey data and a subsequent interview with both parents indicated the following information.

Alejandro's family included his mother, father, and two older female siblings, aged three years and five years. The family had recently moved to the United States from Honduras as a result of the father's employment opportunities. The parents met while attending college in the United States. The father, who is Hispanic, and the mother, who is

Anglo, are professionals and employed outside of the home. The relationship between the parents is supportive and caring, with equal sharing of family responsibilities. The father expressed acceptance of his son, but disappointment that his child would not be "the son of his dreams."

The survey identified the parent's need for more information about their child's development and specific ideas regarding how to teach and play with their son despite his handicap. The parents also requested more information about RLF, hoping to understand better the condition themselves and explain it to others, especially the grandmother.

The extended family is an integral part of this family system. Family members share personal confidences, occasions of sadness and happy celebrations. They understand that their lives are intertwined by their family history, their faith in God and the future of their children. The paternal grandmother lives with the family and cares for the children while the parents work. Although the mother and the grandmother love and respect one another, friction has arisen between them as a result of differences in cultural expectations.

The mother-in-law apparently believes that Alejandro's condition is a result of *mal-puesto* (bad luck). She believes that the blindness was caused by a "hex" that was put on Alejandro's mother while she was pregnant. The grandmother and the mother differ in their expectations for Alejandro. Because of volunteer work in the local high school with retarded children, the mother has seen that children with handicaps are capable of leading independent lives, and she hopes Alejandro will be able to lead an independent life as well. The grandmother believes that a child with a handicap should be accepted "as he is." To "push" Alejandro to do things that upset him is wrong in her view. The grandmother is resistive to the parent's attempts to broaden their son's experiences, such as encouraging him to try new foods. The parents are opposed to the grandmother's "old-fashioned" belief in home remedies and the use of folk healers, referred to as *curanderos*. They refuse to allow her to perform rituals for healing Alejandro's ailments.

The family expressed a desire to have only one or two professionals involved in their son's care, and preferably those who speak Spanish, because the grandmother, who is one of the primary caregivers, does not understand English. Because the COTA speaks Spanish and English, she will work closely with the occupational therapist in the assessment and programing aspects of this case.

Medical History

Alejandro was 15 months at the time of referral. Born prematurely at 32 weeks' gestation, he weighed 3 pounds. He suffered severe respiratory distress and required oxygen, which resulted in a visual impairment diagnosed as RLF.

When he was discharged from the hospital at age 3 months, no motor impairments were noted, and the extent of his visual impairment was unknown. The parents were told that he was blind and to expect his development to be slower than normal. The family received no follow-up care other than that routinely provided for a newborn. Because financial resources were limited, no specialized services were sought. Although the parents were concerned about Alejandro's delay in development, they assumed it was an inherent part of his blindness.

Developmental Assessment

Based on the referral information and the parent interview, the OTR and the COTA determined that the following areas would be included in the occupational therapy assessment:

1. Fine and gross motor development
2. Reflex maturation
3. Self-care activities
4. Sensory-motor development
5. Play development

The Developmental Programming for Infants and Young Children was used for the assessment.[8] The OTR administered the perceptual-fine motor, gross motor and self-care sections of developmental evaluation. The Milani-Comparetti Motor Development Screening Test was also used by the OTR to evaluate the emergence and disappearance of primitive and postural reactions.[9] The COTA used **Takata's Play History** (An assessment used to assist in measuring a child's play and family interactions in the home.) as a tool to assist her in making observations of the child's play and family interactions in the home.[10] The OTR and the COTA used the Sensory History developed by Ayres to interview the parents and grandmother concerning Alejandro's reponses to tactile, vestibular, visual, gustatory-olfactory and proprioceptive input.[11] The COTA also observed the child's response to tactile and vestibular stimulation during play interactions.

Assessment Results

The results of testing and observations indicated that Alejandro's gross motor, fine motor, self-help and play development were delayed. His gross motor development was typical of blind children; that is, the milestones achieved are those that do not require self-initiated mobility. He is able to sit alone briefly, but usually uses his arms for support. No trunk rotation was noted and he is not able to achieve a sitting position independently. In a prone position, he uses reciprocal crawling with his trunk still on the ground. He moves by using lateral flexion to weight shift. Occasionally, he will attempt to support himself on his hands and knees and rock back and forth. He raises his head when in a prone position on extended arms but has weak neck extensors and a lack of visual motivation to maintain

the position. Rolling is achieved accidentally. If he hears his mother's voice, he will try to follow the sound, resulting in spontaneous rolling.

Beginning **segmentation** (movement characterized by differentiating the head from the trunk) is noted. Because he cannot deliberately control the rotation, he is often frightened by the movement. When pulled to standing and held in a supported standing position, he is beginning to bounce up and down. He does not pull himself to a standing position independently, nor does he attempt supported walking. He appears to be fearful in this antigravity position.

Primitive reflexes appear integrated, although he still responds with a slightly exaggerated **Moro reflex** (flexion of thighs and knees; fanning and then clenching of fingers, with arms first thrust outward then brought together as if embracing something)[12] when startled by unexpected noises or a change in position. Righting reactions are emerging in prone, supine and sitting. Muscle tone is slightly **hypotonic** (abnormally reduced tonicity or tension).

His fine motor development has been compromised by his resistance to tactile exploration and his visual impairment. He is performing skills in the eight-month to nine-month range. He can easily transfer objects from hand to hand and uses a neat pincer grasp to hold a small piece of dry cereal. He voluntarily releases objects. Index finger poking has not emerged, but he is beginning to isolate the finger during play. He does not reach for objects by using sound location. This critical skill is necessary for reaching objects in his environment.

In self-care activities he is performing at the 9- to 11-month age range. He is able to chew, take food off a spoon and hold his bottle. He will not hold a spoon or finger feed himself. He refuses to try new foods and mealtime is often unpleasant.

Play skills are limited primarily to solitary play. He is social and enjoys hearing his siblings nearby, but he does not actively seek participation in their play activities. The COTA observed that the grandmother was extremely protective of Alejandro and chided the other children if they bumped him or tried to engage him in play. His play experience is limited, and he frequently engages in self-stimulating behaviors such as eye poking, waving his hands in front of his face, and rocking. Because he still uses his hands to support himself in sitting, his hands are not free to manipulate objects.

The sensory history revealed that he does not enjoy "rough-housing" and cries when moved unexpectedly. He enjoys being rocked, but he does not like being held firmly or cuddled. Alejandro is orally defensive and does not readily mouth objects. He is resistive to tactilely exploring his parents' faces. He does not enjoy putting his hands in soft or "messy" textures.

The teacher of the visually handicapped assessed Alejandro's functional vision using the Functional Vision Inventory for the Multiple and Severely Handicapped.[13] Based on this assessment and the ophthalmologist's medical assessment of the child's eyes, Alejandro was thought to have remaining vision that he was not using optimally. The vision teacher made recommendations that were to be incorporated into the IFSP regarding optimal lighting conditions, distance of objects, object size and visual field presentation.

Treatment Planning

The OTR and the COTA, in collaboration with the other early intervention team members and the family, developed a holistic plan to address the needs and strengths of the family and child. This plan would be carried out in the home twice a week. Because the primary caregiver would be the Spanish-speaking grandmother, it was determined that the bilingual COTA would provide a home program in the areas of feeding and play under the OTR's supervision. The COTA would document and maintain a record of the child's progress in relation to specific feeding and play skill development goals. The OTR would make a home visit once a week in the evening when both parents would be present. Treatment sessions would be videotaped to document progress and to ensure the accuracy of the home program instruction.

The family identified the following areas of needs:
1. To have the child participate in play with siblings
2. To understand the child's condition and to have realistic expectations
3. To have the child become independent in feeding
4. To decrease the child's self-stimulation behaviors
5. To have the child walk independently
6. To have the parents and grandmother appreciate each other's point of view regarding treatment

The following areas of child and family strengths were identified:
1. Alejandro's desire to participate in family interaction
2. The parents' desire to encourage independence
3. Grandmother's interest in child's well-being

The following treatment goals were incorporated into the IFSP:
1. Decrease blindisms or mannerisms
2. Stimulate remaining vision
3. Decrease tactile defensiveness
4. Increase independence in feeding
5. Encourage normal play development and interaction with siblings
6. Increase tolerance for vestibular stimulation
7. Develop adequate righting and equilibrium reactions sitting, kneeling and standing
8. Enhance age-appropriate gross and fine motor development

It was agreed that the COTA would focus on the goals related to play and feeding. These goals will be further developed to illustrate the format used for each treatment goal in the IFSP developed by the Federal IFSP Task Force and the National Education Expert Team in 1988.[14]

Feeding Long-Term Goal—6 months: Alejandro will feed himself using a spoon or fingers as appropriate with minimal assistance and compliant behavior.

Short-Term Objectives—1 month:
1. Alejandro will consistently tolerate his hand on the spoon using a hand-over-hand backward chaining technique as his grandmother directs food toward his mouth at mealtimes.
2. The grandmother will introduce one new food each week, using a positive but firm approach with Alejandro.

Activities:
1. During play time, place Alejandro's hand on a spoon and move him through the motions of banging the spoon on various surfaces. Talk about the different sounds and whether the noises were loud or soft. To direct his visual attention to the spoon or object, wrap it with fluorescent tape. Initially, place him in a supported sitting position, as he is not able to maintain unsupported sitting. This will free his hands. As sitting balance improves, encourage him to sit with one arm support and gradually move to independent sitting with hands engaged in play at midline. Gradually decrease the pressure of the "helping hand" on his hand until he is holding the spoon independently.
2. During snack time put peanut butter or honey on the spoon and encourage him to bring the spoon to his mouth. Initially, the spoon may need to be redirected 100% of the way, but the distance for which assistance is required should be gradually decreased. Visually impaired children need to have experiences that will enhance body perception, so telling him about his hand and where it is in relation to his mouth is important. Because Alejandro is also orally defensive, thus decreasing the amount of oral play in which he engages, he needs assistance in developing proprioceptive awareness of the hand-to-mouth pattern.
3. Encourage fingerfeeding by having him fingerpaint with whipping cream. Allow him to put his fingers in the mouth of his grandmother to give her a taste, and encourage him to lick his fingers. He will benefit from variety in his sensory experiences, so add puffed rice cereal and fruit-flavored gelatin cubes to the whipped cream to add tactile and oral texture.
4. Make arrangements for the grandmother to visit a preschool classroom for visually impaired children during lunchtime to observe independent self-feeding. Also arrange to have a Spanish-speaking mother of

one of the children talk to the grandmother about the progress her child has made with self-feeding.

Play Long-Term Goal—6 months: Alejandro will initiate a play activity by reaching for a toy given a sound or light cue, with minimal prompting.

Short-Term Objectives—1 month:

1. Alejandro will visually attend to toys for 45 seconds when a light is shined on them.

2. Alejandro will demonstrate a preference for social interaction by belly crawling toward a sibling playing nearby to increase proximity to them.

Activities:

1. In a darkened room, shine a flashlight on a toy and direct Alejandro's face in the proper direction. Gradually increase the length of time he looks at the toy. Direct his hand toward the toy. Present toys such as Lite Brite® while he is in a prone position, thereby also encouraging him to maintain neck extension for a prolonged period. This enhances visual attention and encourages use of remaining vision and to reach toward sound cues.

2. Encourage sibling interaction by playing games such as "So Big" and "Patty Cake." Start out engaging him in play with one sister initially to facilitate one-to-one interaction. Be sure that his sister is in close enough physical contact so that Alejandro can feel her presence. Gradually, increase the distance so that he will have to reach arm's length to pass a ball or tickle his sister. Be sure interactions are fun for both children.

3. As Alejandro improves in his tolerance of vestibular stimulation, increase the use of activities that have physical and tactile components, such as rolling up in a blanket with his sister or riding "horsey back."

4. The grandmother and the parents will need to be reminded to let the siblings comfort each other if there is an accident or hurt feelings during their play. This can be encouraged by having them hug or kiss the hurt or rub it to make it feel better as an additional tactile activity. Alejandro has been overprotected from the normal day-to-day bumps, bruises and disagreements that occur among siblings. Efforts need to be made to allow the children to solve their own problems to empower the children and solidify Alejandro's family position.

Several examples of additional specific treatment activities are shown in Figures 4-1, 4-2, 4-3, 4-4 and 4-5.

Treatment Implementation

The COTA met with Alejandro and his family twice weekly in their home. The OTR made weekly visits in the

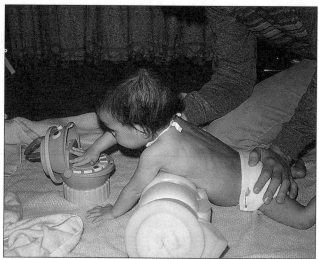

Figure 4-1. *A bolster provides trunk support allowing arms to extend to play with the Big Mouth Singer®.*

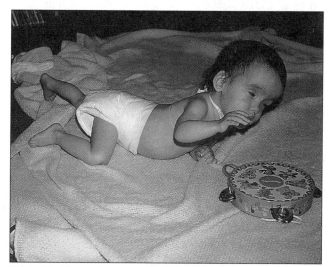

Figure 4-2. *Eliciting location and reaching through the use of a tamborine.*

evening to maintain contact with the family and to modify the treatment activities as needed.

Although the grandmother was initially resistive to the interfering *metida* (busy body or nosy person), she now looked forward to the COTA's visits. The COTA valued and respected the grandmother's religious and cultural beliefs and incorporated them into the treatment activities as appropriate. It was agreed to postpone the visit to the classroom for the visually impaired until the grandmother had a greater comfort level about speaking English in public.

After a month of therapy, an informal conference was held to reassess the plan. This conference was initiated by the COTA who had noted the grandmother's comments that the mother was critical of her progress with Alejandro. It was discovered that Alejandro's mother was envious of the closeness that had developed between the grandmother and

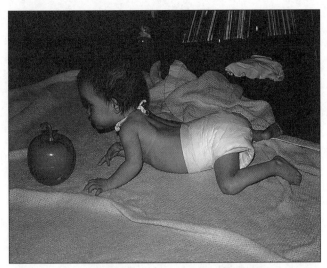

Figure 4-3. *The Happy Apple® provides sound as stimulus for self-initiated belly crawling.*

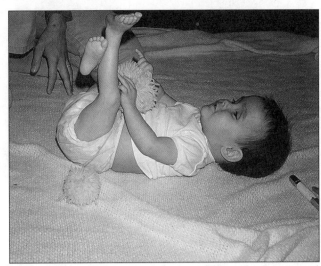

Figure 4-5. *A handmade yarn pom-pom is used for tactile awareness and body stimulation.*

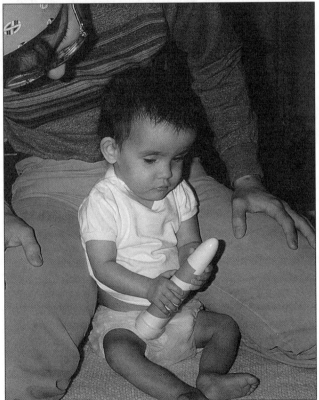

Figure 4-4. *A supported sitting position allows both hands to be engaged in activity using a battery-powered vibrator wrapped with fluorescent tape.*

her grandson because of the increased interaction while they were engaged in purposeful activities.

The mother longed for physical contact with her son, but contact was limited by Alejandro's negative reaction to touch. The treatment plan was modified to include specific treatment activities that the mother could do with her son during their evening routine. For example, at bath time bubbles were used to make a hat or a beard, and a nozzle was used to gently spray water on his arms. Textured towels and varied drying pressure were used to wipe him dry. Alejandro's love of music was used as an inducement to allow his mother to hold him gently and rock him before bedtime.

Alejandro achieved the short-term goals of tolerating his hand on the spoon, with assistance from his grandmother in directing the food to his mouth and accepting one new food each week. He was able to feed himself finger food independently with few prompts. Graham crackers, refried beans and lemon yogurt proved to be three of his new favorites. He also was able to attend visually to toys, particularly his talking teddy bear and large plastic keys, for 45 seconds or more when a light was shined on them. He initiated belly crawling toward his siblings when they were nearby and often entered into their social interaction by "Patty Cake" clapping and laughing with them, and attempting to join in their singing of Spanish and English folk songs. Although bumps, bruises and normal sibling disagreements continued to occur, the grandmother was able to exercise more restraint in letting the children settle these minor episodes, rather than rushing to protect and comfort Alejandro as in the past.

Treatments were continued at two visits per week by the COTA and one visit by the OTR for the next five months until the long-term goals were achieved. Since Alejandro was making rapid progress, the occupational therapist had to make frequent modification in the treatment objectives. Throughout treatment, periodic videotaping was a useful tool in documenting progress.

Transition Planning

The OTR scheduled a meeting with the family in their home two weeks before the anticipated date of discharge from the occupational therapy program. Segments of the videotape were reviewed, demonstrating the many goals that Alejandro had achieved. The parents and the grandmother indicated their appreciation and thought that the entire family had benefited from the intervention program. The case manager would continue to follow Alejandro and his family, assisting them in identifying appropriate community resources and groups as necessary. He would also receive services from the teacher of the visually impaired, primarily for premobility training. Preschool services that Alejandro would be eligible for were also discussed.

Follow-Up

During the family's semiannual follow-up visit to the center, one month before Alejandro's third birthday, transition plans were made. The ISTP defines the steps necessary to facilitate the transition of toddlers to preschool services if such services are required. Although Alejandro had made outstanding progress in the program described in the preceding sections, it was agreed that he would continue to require assistance to maximize his independence. Review of his records indicated that he is age-appropriate in self-care activities and play interactions. His gross motor skills are age-appropriate but he lacks fluidity in his movements because of inadequate postural responses and an intolerance for novel movement patterns. He no longer demonstrates tactilely defensive behaviors and shows age-appropriate hand development. Alejandro and his family were referred to the occupational therapy preschool program where goals were established that related directly to his educational goals. His occupational therapy program will focus on increasing postural security, spatial orientation and body awareness. Achieving these goals will enable him to develop the skills necessary for independent orientation and mobility. Goals in the tactile areas will now focus on fine discrimination to facilitate pre-Braille activities.

Related Learning Activities

1. Compare and contrast PL 94-142 and PL 99-457.

2. Choose a treatment goal from those listed and identify additional activities that would facilitate Alejandro's development in that area.

3. Work with a peer and develop a list of other activities that could be used for treatment with a visually handicapped child.

4. Visit a preschool program that provides services to visually impaired children. Observe the roles of at least three different professionals and describe some of the services they offer.

5. Write to the American Foundation for the Blind, 15 West 16th Street, New York, NY 10011, and request information about the services they offer.

6. Describe the differences between the role of the therapist in a family-centered intervention program and a traditional intervention model.

References

1. Schell BAB: Guide to classification of occupational therapy personnel. *Am J Occup Ther* 39:803-810, 1985.
2. American Occupational Therapy Association: Guidelines for occupational therapy services in early intervention and preschool services. Position Paper, 1989.
3. Education for All Handicapped Children Act of 1975. PL 94-142. *Fed Regist* 20 United States Congress:1401, 1975.
4. Education of the Handicapped Act Amendments of 1986. PL 99-457. *Fed Regist* 20 United States Congress:1400, 1986.
5. Thomas CL (Ed): *Taber's Cyclopedic Medical Dictionary*, Sixteenth Edition. Philadelphia, FA Davis, 1989.
6. Frankenberg WK, Dodds JB, Fandel AW: *Denver Developmental Screening Test Manual*, 2nd Edition. Denver, Ladoca Project and Publishing Foundation, 1970.
7. Baily D, Simeonsson R: *Family Needs Survey*. Chapel Hill, North Carolina, Frank Porter Graham Child Development Center, 1985.
8. Rogers SJ, D'Eugenio DB: *Developmental Programming for Infants and Young Children*. Ann Arbor, University of Michigan Press, 1977.
9. Milani-Comparetti A: Routine development examination in normal and retarded children. *Dev Med Child Neurol* 9:631,766, 1967.
10. Takata N: Play as prescription. In Reilly M (Ed): *Play as Exploratory Learning: Studies in Curiosity Behavior*. Beverly Hills, California, Sage, 1974.
11. Ayres AJ: *Sensory History*. Torrance, California, Ayers, 1977.
12. Miller BF, Keane CB (Eds): *Encyclopedia and Dictionary of Medicine, Nursing, and Allied Health*, Fifth Edition. Philadelphia, WB Saunders, 1992.
13. Langley BM: *Functional Vision Inventory for the Multiple and Severely Handicapped*. Chicago, Stoelting Co., 1980.
14. Dunst A, Trivette M, Deal S: *Family Support Scale, Enabling and Empowering Families: Principles and Guidelines for Practice*. Cambridge, Massachusetts, Brookline Books, 1988.

The Child With Mental Retardation

Susan M. McFadden, MA, OTR, FAOTA

Introduction

This chapter presents a case study of a mentally retarded child enrolled in a Head Start Program who received occupational therapy services through a private practice. The case study illustrates a hypothetical example of one model of a collaborative relationship between a certified occupational therapy assistant (COTA) and a registered occupational therapist (OTR). To better visualize the child's situation, a brief description of the private practice and the Head Start Program follows.

Mental Retardation

The American Association on Mental Deficiency (AAMD) defines mental retardation as "significant subaverage general intellectual functioning existing concurrently with deficits in adaptive behavior and manifested during the developmental period."[1] An overall slowness in development is characteristic of children with **mental retardation** and this slowness makes them seem younger than they actually are. During the preschoool years, mentally retarded children consistently fall behind other preschoolers in their ability to learn, to remember what they have learned, and to solve problems. In the preschool years, **adaptive behavior**, referred to in the AAMD definition, means a child's ability to use language, play with others and do things independently.

Experts generally agree on four levels of mental retardation: mild, moderate, severe and profound. These levels refer to different levels of IQ (intelligence quotient) and adaptive behavior and to different abilities to learn. Mildly mentally retarded children are sometimes called **educable mentally retarded**. They should be able to learn most activities in the classroom, but will probably need more help and practice than other children. Moderately mentally retarded children are sometimes

KEY CONCEPTS

Cultural/ethnic differences	Referral
Private practice	Feeding and dressing activities
Project Head Start	Assessment checklist
Developmental delay	Program discontinuation

called **trainable mentally retarded**. These children tend to behave like children about half their age. They benefit from the use of simpler language to explain things, and from breaking activities down into small parts that can be taught and practiced one at a time. **Severely and profoundly mentally retarded** children, like infants, need help with most of their daily needs. Some severely and profoundly mentally retarded children never develop speech and may have severe handicaps, such as those found in cerebral palsy (see Chapter 6).

Cultural or ethnic differences have sometimes been confused with mental retardation, and cultural differences can sometimes lead to mislabeling a child as mentally retarded. Because a child may not have seen or been taught the same kind of social behavior that children from middle-class families have learned as "normal" or because the family speaks a language other than English or a nonstandard English dialect, children from minority and low-income families can appear mentally retarded when their test scores are compared to those from middle-class families. The problem may not be with the children, but with the tests.

The child in the case study that follows was diagnosed as being moderately mentally retarded. Children who are moderately mentally retarded develop at about half the rate of nonretarded children the same age. Therefore, moderately mentally retarded three- to five-year-old children are more developmentally similar to nonretarded children who are one and one-half to two and one-half years old. As will be described in the case study, Jason, in addition to being moderately mentally retarded, experienced other developmental delays. In other words, his developmental skills are not commensurate with his mental age.

Private Practice

In selecting a COTA for a private practice position, several factors must be considered. As with an OTR, private practice is not recommended for a new graduate. Since a private practice is a unique model for a collaborative COTA and OTR relationship, the COTA should have several years of experience, demonstrate maturity and independence, and be self-directed before entering into such a model. Supervision of a COTA by an OTR in a private practice situation is often minimal. Circumstances generally do not allow for much direct observation of the assistant, and supervision cannot be conducted on a daily basis. Because of the indirect nature of supervision, good verbal and written communication skills are necessary for all involved in such a collaborative relationship.

I established a private practice several years ago and have contracts with a nursing home, a long-term care state psychiatric facility, a state institution for the retarded and a private institution for the adult retarded. The occupational therapy services provided to these facilities included direct patient services of screening, evaluation and program planning, as well as indirect services that include teaching aides or technicians, general in-service training and program planning. As the private practice grew, more and more facilities, including a Head Start program, requested services from the occupational therapist, and it became necessary to subcontract with other occupational therapy personnel on a part-time basis.

Project Head Start

Project Head Start was launched in 1965 as a federally funded preschool summer program, part of the antipoverty campaign of the Johnson administration. The program is now administered by the Head Start Bureau, Office of Human Development Services, US Department of Health and Human Services, and has expanded to a year-round service. Head Start was conceived as a child development program to provide comprehensive educational, social and health services to preschool children of low-income families. As a matter of policy, children with handicaps have always been included in the program. Head Start began as an entirely center-based program, with children transported to a particular center to receive services. **Home-based programming**, with home visitation and some services provided in the home, was introduced in 1972. One reason for adding home-based programming may have been that home-based services were more easily accepted by culturally divergent families than were "traditional" medical or educational services.

Since 1975, the provisions of P.L. 94-142 have formed the basis for Head Start services to its handicapped enrollees and their families. Although all Head Start programs must follow certain federal guidelines, individual programs vary widely regarding the services provided, staff utilized, and screening tools administered. Because Head Start programs cannot assume total responsibility for the hiring of full-time staff for the many services needed, they contract with other agencies to provide some services, such as occupational therapy. The child described in this case study was enrolled in a resource center program one day a week and received home-based programming one day a week.

Case Study Background

At the time of enrollment in the Head Start Program, Jason was three years old, the only boy and the second child in a family of three children. His sisters were six years and one year; the mother was a housewife with an eighth grade education. The father was unemployed, doing "fix-it" type work for individuals when possible; he also had an eighth grade education. Jason's family lived in a rural area, approximately 100 miles from a major city. The family income was estimated at $4,200 per year. Jason's parents reported that he had no major health problems, but they sensed that something was different about Jason when compared to his sisters.

Referral

As a part of its services, Head Start identifies families in need so that problems can be detected at an early age and services provided to help the children and families overcome these adversities. Jason's sister came to the attention of Head Start when she was three years old, and the family was then enrolled in the Head Start Program. Since the family had already been identified by the program, a screening process was initiated with Jason when he was three years old. The results of this screening indicated that Jason was significantly delayed in the areas of fine motor development, cognitive-verbal development, and gross motor development. The activities that Jason was not able to do when screened included building a tower of seven blocks, buttoning one button, stringing four beads in two minutes, naming 8 of 11 pictures, repeating two-digit sequences of numbers, balancing on one foot for two seconds, walking on tiptoes when shown, and walking up stairs using alternating feet. The screening test used with Jason at 36 months indicated that he was functioning below 30 months of age, the lowest level of the screening tool. Because of the delay in fine motor, cognitive-verbal, and gross motor areas, a psychological evaluation was recommended for Jason, and he was enrolled in a home-based Head Start program. The psychological evaluation revealed that Jason was moderately mentally retarded. The psychological examiner believed that an occupational therapy evaluation was necessary because Jason was not performing self-help skills appropriate to his mental age.

Assessment

Jason was evaluated by the OTR at the Head Start resource center. At the time of scheduling, Jason had just turned four. The occupational therapist's evaluation indicated that his reflex maturation was appropriate for his age, with no primitive reflexes present; his range of motion, strength and muscle tone were normal. Jason's sensory awareness appeared to be normal, as he responded to pinprick and rough and soft surfaces on his extremities.

As part of the occupational therapy assessment, the Developmental Test of Visual Motor Integration by Berry and Buketnica was administered to Jason. On this design copying test, the child received a score of 2 years, 11 months. This score was within the range for a four-year-old moderately retarded person. In explaining expectations to the parents as well as the COTA, they were reminded that moderately retarded children develop at about half the rate of nonhandicapped children the same age. Therefore, Jason, a moderately mentally retarded child of four years of age was more developmentally similar to children without handicaps who were two years old.

Using the Gesell Developmental Scales as a guide, The OTR determined that Jason was able to perform most fine motor tasks for two-year-olds; however, the mother indicated that Jason was having difficulty undressing, dressing and feeding himself. Because the home is a more natural environment, the COTA was assigned to visit the home and to assess Jason in these areas. The COTA gathered data on the activities of daily living skills of undressing, dressing and eating by observing Jason perform these activities. Results were recorded on two different forms shown in Figures 5-1 and 5-2. The combined use of these recommended forms included an approximate age level, as shown in the first, and a more detailed task analysis through use of the second.

A developmental type checklist with age levels was not available for feeding; however, using the information available in Copeland, Ford and Solon,[2] and the previously mentioned forms as a model, it was possible to gather similar information on eating skills.

To ensure that sufficient data were collected, the COTA made two home visits to observe Jason's performance of dressing, undressing and feeding skills. The checklists previously described were used to record information observed on each visit. The assistant also noted the physical features of the home environment and assessed the parents' knowledge of Jason's developmental needs and their ability to manage his behavior.

Partial results of the COTA's assessment of Jason's dressing, undressing and feeding skills are summarized in Figure 5-3.

An important aspect of the occupational therapy evaluation was determining Jason's need for occupational therapy services. Based on the self-help skills one would expect from a moderately mentally retarded child, it was evident that Jason was not able to execute many of the skills appropriate for his mental age. The COTA's results showing that Jason was in fact functioning more like a one-year-old in dressing, undressing and feeding were a key factor in determining the child's need for occupational therapy services. Also contributing to the recommendation for services was the COTA's impression that the parents did not understand that Jason should have been performing the dressing, undressing and feeding skills equiva-

Name:	Date:

Approximate Age	Skill	Achieved Independently	Achieved with Help	Not Achieved
One year	Cooperates in dressing			
	Holds arm out for sleeve			
	Holds foot up for shoe			
	Puts hat on head and takes it off			
	Likes to pull shoes off			
	Pushes arms through sleeves and legs through pants			
	Removes socks			
Two years	Removes unfastened garment (coat)			
	Purposely removes shoes if laces are untied			
	Helps push down garment			
	Finds armholes in T-shirt			
Two and one-half years	Removes pull-down garment with elastic waist			
	Tries to put on socks			
	Puts on front-button type of coat, shirt or sweater			
	Unbuttons one large button			
Three years	Puts on T-shirt with some assistance			
	Puts on shoes without fasteners (may be wrong foot)			
	Puts on socks with some difficulty turning heel			
	Independent with pull-down garment			

Figure 5-1. *Development Predressing Checklist from Dunn, M.L.: Skill Starters for Self-Help Development. Tuscon, Communication Skill Builders, 1983.*

Child's name: Date: Pretest of dressing skills	Independent	Verbal assistance	Physical assistance	Description of method child uses to complete the task
Undressing trousers, skirt 1. Pushes garment from waist to ankles 2. Pushes garment off one leg 3. Pushes garment off other leg				
Dressing trousers, skirt 1. Lays trousers in front of self with front side up 2. Inserts one foot into waist opening 3. Inserts other foot into waist opening 4. Pulls garment up to waist				
Undressing socks 1. Pushes sock down off heel 2. Pulls toe of sock, pulling sock off foot				
Dressing socks 1. Positions sock correctly with heel side down 2. Holds sock open at top 3. Inserts toe into sock 4. Pulls sock over heel 5. Pulls sock up				
Undressing cardigan 1. Takes dominant arm out of sleeve 2. Gets coat off back 3. Pulls other arm from sleeve				
Dressing cardigan flip-over method 1. Lays garment on table or floor in front of self 2. Gets dominant arm into sleeve 3. Other arm into sleeve 4. Positions coat on back				
Undressing polo shirt 1. Takes dominant arm out of sleeve 2. Pulls garment over head 3. Pulls other arm from sleeve				
Dressing polo shirt 1. Lays garment in front of self 2. Opens bottom of garment and puts arms into sleeves 3. Pulls garment over head 4. Pulls garment down to waist				
Undressing shoes 1. Loosens laces 2. Pulls shoe off heel 3. Pulls front of shoe to pull shoe off toes				
Dressing shoes 1. Prepares shoe by loosening laces and pulling tongue of shoe out of the way 2. Inserts toes into shoe 3. Pushes shoe on over heel				

Figure 5-2. *Pretest of Dressing Skills Data Sheet from Copeland, M., Ford, L., and Soloes, N.: Occupational Therapy for Mentally Retarded Children. Baltimore, University Park Press, 1976.*

Skills	Normal Developmental Age (Years)	Moderately Retarded Child (Years)	Jason
Removes socks	1	2	Yes
Likes to pull off shoes	1	2	Yes
Pushes arms through sleeves	1	2	Yes
Removes unfastened garment	1	4	No
Purposely removes shoes	2	4	No
Helps push down garment	2	4	No
Finds arm holes in T-shirt	2	4	No
Buttons large front buttons	3	6	No
Puts on shoes without fasteners	3	6	No
Independent with pull-down garment	3	6	No
Drinks well from cup	1.5	3	Yes
Handles glass with one hand	2	4	No
Moderate spillage from spoon	2	4	No
Likes to spear food with fork	3	6	No

Figure 5-3. *Dressing and Feeding Skills*

lent to a two-year-old and performing other skills compatible with his mental age.

Program Planning

In collaboration with the OTR, the COTA developed a program to treat Jason in the home once a week. The therapist and the assistant agreed that approximately nine visits would be necessary for Jason to accomplish the following occupational therapy treatment objectives:

1. Remove an open front garment independently
2. Put on an open front type garment independently
3. Feed himself independently using a spoon with moderate spillage from the spoon

An additional goal was to provide the Head Start resource teacher with information to assist Jason in meeting these objectives. After several home visits had been made, the COTA agreed to arrange for Jason's parents to visit the resource center. Involving the parents and the resource teacher in the program added to the day-to-day consistency and provided more opportunity for Jason to practice the skills in the occupational therapy program.

Treatment

Five of the nine occupational therapy treatments were directed toward attaining the undressing and dressing objectives. The COTA selected an initial dressing activity of playing "dress up" using a variety of hats and shirts. The assistant had noticed Jason's interest in police officers and firefighters and obtained their hats and shirts for Jason to use in practicing skills. Figure 5-4 shows one technique for teaching a child to remove a front-button shirt.

As an initial feeding activity, the COTA selected playing in the sand with a spoon to learn a scooping technique. The assistant noted that Jason was able to grasp the spoon while scooping and had adequate eye-hand coordination. The OTR concurred with the COTA's recommendation that a session of manual guidance in an actual meal setting was the next step in teaching Jason to feed himself. The COTA then requested that the mother prepare a meal for the next treatment session that would require Jason to use a spoon. During the meal, the COTA noticed that Jason had a good hand-to-mouth pattern as he attempted to eat using his fingers. The assistant provided **manual guidance** by placing her hand over Jason's hand as he filled the spoon and brought it toward his mouth. Whenever Jason attempted to use his fingers to feed himself, the COTA instructed him to use the spoon and followed this directive by guiding his hand toward the spoon. The assistant also pointed out to Jason's mother that she should tell Jason what to do instead of what not to do.

A detailed **task analysis** of the objective "student will feed himself with a spoon on command after attaining five consecutive, positive responses on each step" can be seen in Figure 5-5. This task analysis combines the use of manual guidance as indicated in the odd-numbered steps and the use of **gestures**[2] (body movements used to express ideas, opinions or emotions).

Jason's mother was present during all occupational therapy treatment sessions, and care was taken to ensure that her

Skill: Remove a Front-Button Shirt

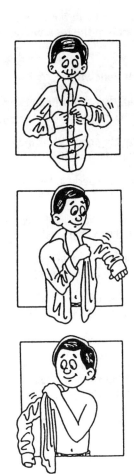

Objective:	Student will remove a front-button shirt.
Approximate Developmental Age:	Two years
Materials:	Use a front-button shirt, jacket, sweater, or pajama top that is too large or that fits loosely.
Note:	Start by unbuttoning or unzipping garment for student. Take same arm out first to help establish a routine.
Position:	Sitting or standing
Task Analysis:	Backward chaining. Trainer prompts student through entire process, leaving last part or parts for student to complete.

1. Student removes garment with one arm half in.
2. Student removes garment with one arm in.
3. Student removes garment with one arm in and one half in.
4. Student removes garment when pulled off shoulders.
5. Student removes garment.

Figure 5-4. *Pre-Dressing Skills: Skill Starters for Self-Help Development. Dunn, M.L.: Tuscon, Communication Skill Builders, 1983.*

questions were answered. The COTA concluded each session by asking the mother to continue modeling the demonstrated techniques during the next week.

The COTA documented each weekly treatment session by noting the date, length of session, time of day, activities presented and Jason's response to the activities. The assistant then discussed the results of each occupational therapy treatment session with the OTR and described the activities planned for the next week.

Program Discontinuation

Jason's progress toward meeting his occupational therapy objectives proceeded as anticipated. After nine sessions in the home and one visit to the resource center, Jason had achieved all of the occupational therapy objectives. The OTR and the COTA discussed Jason's achievements and agreed that the occupational therapy program should be discontinued. In a final home visit, the assistant reviewed Jason's progress during the treatments with both parents. She explained **developmental expectations** (age-appropriate goals) in undressing, dressing and feeding for Jason and enumerated activities that the parents should continue to ensure that Jason maintained his newly learned skills.

Final notes were made regarding Jason's treatments, and all progress notes were signed and turned over to the OTR. The therapist then informed the Head Start Program of Jason's progress, skill achievement and discontinuation of occupational therapy services. The OTR also

Feeding Task Analysis

The student will feed himself with a spoon on command after attaining five consecutive positive responses on each step of the task analysis below.

TASK ANALYSIS STEPS

The student will:

1. Let you use his hand to hold the spoon, scoop the spoon into the dish, lift the spoon to his mouth, and put the spoon in his mouth.

2. Put the spoon in his mouth from lip level after you have picked up the spoon using his hand, scooped it into the dish, lifted it to mouth level, and gestured for him to put it in his mouth.

3. Put the spoon in his mouth from lip level after you have picked up the spoon using his hand, scooped it into the dish, and lifted it to mouth level.

4. Put the spoon in his mouth from chin level after you have picked up the spoon using his hand, scooped it into the dish, lifted it to chin level, and gestured for him to put it in his mouth.

5. Put the spoon in his mouth from chin level after you have picked up the spoon with his hand, scooped it into the dish, and lifted it to chin level.

6. Put the spoon in his mouth from shoulder level after you have picked up the spoon using his hand, scooped it into the dish, lifted it to shoulder level, and gestured for him to put it in his mouth.

7. Put the spoon in his mouth from shoulder level after you have picked up the spoon using his hand, scooped it into the dish, and lifted it to shoulder level.

8. Put the spoon in his mouth after you have picked up the spoon using his hand, scooped it into the dish, lifted it above the dish, and gestured for him to put it in his mouth.

9. Put the spoon in his mouth after you have picked up the spoon using his hand, scooped it into the dish, and lifted it above the dish.

10. Put the spoon in his mouth after you have picked up the spoon using his hand, scooped it into the dish, and gestured for him to put it in his mouth.

11. Put the spoon in his mouth after you have picked up the spoon using his hand and scooped it into the dish.

12. Scoop into the dish and lift the spoon to his mouth after you have gestured for him to do so and after you have used his hand to pick up the spoon and put it into the bowl.

13. Scoop into the dish and lift the spoon to his mouth after you have used his hand to pick up the spoon and put it into the bowl.

14. Scoop into the dish and lift the spoon to his mouth after you have gestured for him to do so and after you have used his hand to pick up the spoon and take it to the dish.

15. Scoop into the dish and lift the spoon to his mouth after you have used his hand to pick up the spoon and take it to the dish.

16. Scoop into the dish after you have gestured for him to do so, and lift the spoon to his mouth after you have handed him the spoon.

17. Scoop into the dish and lift the spoon to his mouth after you have handed him the spoon.

18. Eat independently on command.

Figure 5-5. *Feeding Task Analysis. From Popovitch, D.: A Prescriptive Behavioral Checklist for the Severely and Profoundly Retarded. Austin, Texas, PRO-ED, Inc., 1981, Vol. II.*

forwarded the necessary documentation to the Head Start resource center.

Although the role of the COTA in this case presentation was hypothetical, the case itself was based on an actual experience and represents one example of how an experienced assistant can work in an advanced level of practice in a collaborative relationship with an OTR. It should be noted in at least one state (as this text is being written), state law prohibits COTAs from practicing in a home setting without on-site supervision from a OTR. It is understood that efforts are being made to change this supervisory regulation.

Related Learning Activities

1. Administer an activites of daily living checklist to a child between the ages two and four years of age and prepare a report of the findings. Compare the results with the norms for the Gesell Developmental Appraisal.

2. The COTA used the activity of scooping sand with a spoon to prepare Jason to eat with a spoon. Identify two other activities that could also be used.

3. Dressing and eating were analyzed in this chapter. Analyze another activity such as walking up stairs. Determine the skills involved and the developmental progression.

4. Discuss with peers why it is important to assess Jason's parents' knowledge of his needs and ability to manage his behavior.

References

1. Grossman HG (Ed): *Manual on Terminology and Classification in Mental Retardation*. Baltimore, Garamond/Pridemark, 1973.
2. Copeland M, Ford L, Solon N: *Occupational Therapy for Mentally Retarded Children*. Baltimore, University Park Press, 1976.

The Child With Cerebral Palsy

Teri Black, COTA, ROH
Toni Walski, MS, OTR, FAOTA

History of School System Practice

Public education of children with handicapping conditions has evolved in the 20th century. By 1918, all states had established compulsory attendance laws for school-aged children, which indirectly prompted development of "special education" facilities for retarded children. In 1911, New Jersey became a pioneer in legislating educational programs for the retarded, and by 1955 most states had passed similar requirements.

The decades of the 1930s and 1940s witnessed organization of separate regional or city-wide schools specializing in serving children with physical handicaps, thereby allowing them to remain at home rather than being institutionalized. Occupational therapists were first employed in these orthopedic schools.

In 1961, President Kennedy established the President's Panel on Mental Retardation, and in 1966 the Bureau of Education of the Handicapped (BEH) was established as part of the US Office of Education. During the 1960s, occupational therapy broadened its scope to serve students with developmental problems.

During the 1970s, federal legislation revolutionized special education and greatly increased the need for school system therapists. Related education services such as occupational therapy were required by law to enable students with handicaps to function more effectively in their school programs. Occupational therapists extended services to the learning disabled during this decade, and increased understanding of neurophysiology dramatically changed approaches for treating movement disorders. Whereas earlier interventions had focused on developing compensatory movement patterns, the emerging emphasis was on neuromuscular techniques that facilitate sensorimotor integration to provide normalization of movement and function and to promote learning.

ESSENTIAL VOCABULARY

Educable mentally retarded

Trainable mentally retarded

Cerebral palsy

Choreoathetoid

Diplegia

Hemiplegia

Quadriplegia

Hypertonicity

Atonic

Reinforcers

Parental priorities

KEY CONCEPTS

Historical perspectives

School system practice

Public Law 94-142

Initial screening

Evaluation findings

Recommendations

Intervention

OTR/COTA collaboration

Occupational therapy has continued to evolve and diversify its school services. Practitioners collaborate with school team members in the mainstreaming of youngsters with handicaps in regular education classrooms and in many specialized programs such as infant stimulation, preschool early intervention/prevention, elementary and secondary special education and prevocational assessment.

The roles of other school-based Related Services personnel and their relationship to occupational therapy providers are summarized in Table 6-1.[1]

Public Law 94-142: Education of All Handicapped Children Act

Major court cases from 1950 to the early 1970s, which dealt with racial segregation or exclusion of retarded and physically disabled individuals from public schools, supported a constitutional right to free and appropriate education. Beyond the courts, federal laws, which included The Education of the Handicapped Act of 1970, Section 504 of The Rehabilitation Act of 1973, and The Right to Education Amendments Act of 1974, also paved the way for Public Law 94-142, The Education Of All Handicapped Children Act of 1975. This law sought to: "...assure that all handicapped children have available to them a free appropriate public education which emphasizes special education and related services designed to meet their unique needs, to assure that the rights of handicapped children and their parents or guardians are protected, to assist states and localities to provide for the education of all handicapped children, and to assess and assure the effectiveness of efforts to educate handicapped children."[2]

Children with handicaps were defined as: "...children who are mentally retarded, hard of hearing, deaf, orthopedically impaired, other health impairments, speech impaired, visually handicapped, or seriously mentally disturbed children with specific learning disabilities who by reason thereof require special education and related services."[2]

Public Law 94-142 outlined six requirements for providing education services:[2]

1. *Zero reject*: All handicapped youngsters must be given a free, appropriate public education. As of 1980, states were required to provide education services for 3- to 21-year-olds.
2. *Nondiscriminatory evaluation*: Unbiased or culture-free assessment instruments for evaluating all areas of suspected disability must be provided through a multidisciplinary team of teachers and other specialists.
3. *Individualized education plan*: For each student whose evaluation indicates special needs, an individualized education plan (IEP) must be written and

updated yearly. Figure 6-1 illustrates the multidisciplinary team process in developing the IEP.

4. *Least restrictive environment*: Handicapped children must be mainstreamed to the fullest extent possible; therefore, placement in a regular classroom is preferred over special education, and the latter is preferred to an institutional setting. (Note: Previously, Section 504 of The Rehabilitation Act of 1973 had made it illegal for any public or private organization receiving federal money to discriminate against a person with a handicap. Such agencies must take steps to make buildings and programs accessible, so persons with handicaps can learn and work on an equal basis. As a civil rights act, a grievance procedure was provided and noncompliance could result in a cutoff of federal funds).
5. *Due process*: Procedures must safeguard the appropriateness of the educational plan. If needed, parents, guardians, or surrogates appointed by public agencies can institute an impartial hearing process on behalf of the child.
6. *Parental involvement*: Parents or guardians must participate in developing each student's IEP, and parents should participate in public hearings and advisory boards that influence state educational plans for children with handicaps.

States have also enacted laws that detail education of individuals with handicaps within their jurisdiction. Rules governing Related Services are available through the State Department of Education. Professional guidelines for COTAs relative to supervision, roles and functions are available from the American Occupational Therapy Association. In addition, state regulatory bodies and state occupational therapy associations should be consulted about COTA practice within a given state.

School Setting Background

Garfield Elementary School serves 315 neighborhood students. Special needs children are transported to Garfield from other sections of the district. There are five self-contained special education classrooms: one for Learning Disabled (LD); two for mildly retarded referred to as **educable mentally retarded** or EMR (approximate IQ 55 to 70); and two for moderately retarded, referred to as **trainable** mentally retarded or TMR (approximate IQ 40 to 55). Each of these classrooms is staffed by a special education teacher and an aide. Several students with physical disabilities also attend regular classes.

Related Services includes one half-time occupational therapist, a half-time physical therapist, and a full-time COTA. A health aide provides transportation and personal

Table 6-1.
Overview of Similarities and Differences Between Occupational Therapy and Other Related Services

Discipline	Role and Function in the School System	Relationship to Occupational Therapy
Adaptive physical education	Concerned with sports activities and fitness of disabled children	Common concern with physical activity and fitness of disabled children. Adaptive physical education teachers use more generalized strategies and group activities. Occupational therapists can prescribe individual treatment program geared to ameliorating specific dysfunction.
Perceptual motor training and optometry	Concerned with visual-perception and visual-motor function	Perceptual motor trainers and optometrists are concerned with visual-motor integration primarily related to gross motor activity. Occupational therapists are concerned with visual motor integration as related to gross and fine motor as well as sensory processing.
Physical education	Concerned with sports activities and fitness	Common concern with student's engagement in physical activity and fitness. Occupational therapists are concerned with student's other limitations that may interfere with physical education.
Physical therapy	Concerned with assessing, remediating, and habilitating physical and motor dysfunction	Common concern with motor function. Occupational therapists are concerned with motor function in relationship to engagement in occupation or activity.
Psychology	Concerned with child's psychological and intellectual processing	Occupational therapists are concerned with sensory-motor processing as a substratum of intelligence, and sensory-motor processing as a substratum of the child's social/emotional/psychological state.
Speech pathology	Assesses, remediates, and habilitates speech/language and communication disorders	Common concern with oral-motor function. Occupational therapy intervention focused more on oral development as related to eating, reduction of drooling, or on motor skill to utilize adaptive communication device.
Vocational education	Preparation for and training in vocational skills leading to employability	Both concerned with engagement in vocational activities. Occupational therapists more involved in sensory, motor, and technologic adaptation necessary to allow the individual to function most effectively.

From Royeen, C., Promoting occupational therapy in the schools, American Journal of Occupational Therapy, 42, pp 715, 1988. Reprinted with permission

Some of the information in this table is from the paper "Neuroanatomical and Neuropathological Aspects of Apraxia in Adults and Children," presented by S. Cermak and L. Cermak in April 1979 at the 59th Annual Conference of the American Occupational Therapy Association in Detroit. Adapted by the authors' permission.

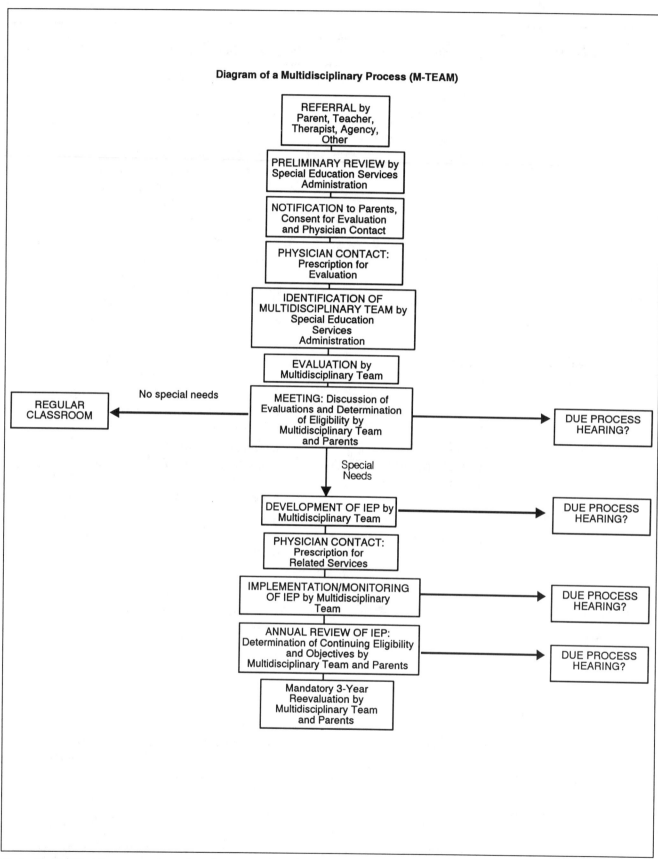

Figure 6-1. *Multidisciplinary team process for evaluating an individualized education plan.*

care assistance to students. The speech and language therapist provides services to Garfield, as well as three other schools. In addition, a social worker, a psychologist and special education consultants are available as needed. The part-time school nurse occasionally consults with Related Services regarding students' self-management of catheters, ileostomies, injections etc.

Case Study Background

Jennifer, a 5-year-old girl with cerebral palsy (CP), has also been diagnosed as being educably mentally retarded. **Cerebral palsy** is a diagnostic category applied to a number of nonprogressive movement and posture disorders resulting from damage to a child's immature brain. Several other disorders—mental retardation, seizures, visual and auditory deficits, speech and language disabilities, and behavior problems—may also challenge the affected child. Because brain maturity occurs at approximately 16 years of age, a variety of events that occur before then, such as chromosomal abnormalities, intrauterine conditions, prematurity, birth complications and childhood injury or illness, can produce the brain injury associated with cerebral palsy. Causes are generally but not always identifiable.[3]

There are many classifications of cerebral palsy; however, three groups predominate: spastic (pyramidal), **choreoathetoid** (extrapyramidal), and mixed. Furthermore, labels such as **diplegia**, **hemiplegia**, and **quadriplegia** indicate whether two extremities, one side of the body, or all four extremities, respectively, are primarily involved.[3]

Children with spastic cerebral palsy sustain damage to the motor cortex or to the pyramidal tract of the brain. In such cases, **hypertonicity** (abnormally increased tone or strength) of affected muscle groups prevents smooth initiation of movement and threatens stability of the body. Muscle contractures and weakness, hyperactive reflexes, and underdevelopment of limbs are also associated with the spastic diagnosis.

Choreoathetoid cerebral palsy (Jennifer's diagnosis) involves damage to pathways outside the pyramidal tract and particularly to the basal ganglia. There are involuntary movements of arms and legs, which increase with stress and seem to disappear with sleep. Typically, there is difficulty controlling movement and posture. Muscle tone decreases or increases variably and can particularly affect oral-motor control, producing difficulties with drooling, sucking, swallowing, and speaking. Besides choreoathetosis, other forms of extrapyramidal involvement include "lead pipe" rigid and "floppy" **atonic** (absence of tone) cerebral palsies.

Brain damage is often extensive in mixed-type cerebral palsy, and children can show signs of both pyramidal or extrapyramidal involvement and other developmental disabilities.

Referral

Jennifer was referred by her classroom teacher, who noted motor problems that limited her performance in academic and self-care activities. She was five years, seven months when she was first seen by occupational therapy personnel.

The referral was initially forwarded to an administrative office that coordinates services city-wide. This office sent a notification of referral to the parents and included a request for parental permission to evaluate the child and communicate with the physician. When the parents' consent form was received and the physician's prescription for an evaluation had been secured, appropriate school team members were contacted to evaluate the child, a process that required three weeks. This procedure launched the multidisciplinary team (M-team) process, which must be concluded within 90 days.

While the supervising OTR communicated with the doctor regarding specific aspects of the medical history, the COTA began compiling Jennifer's occupational therapy file, including copies of the referral, parental consent, physician's prescription for evaluation and any previous medical or therapy records. The COTA was responsible for maintaining necessary records and communications throughout the student's involvement in occupational therapy.

Assessment

Initial Screening

An initial screening was performed to judge Jennifer's potential need for occupational therapy services and to determine further evaluations that would be necessary. Using an outline form developed by the OTR supervisor, the COTA reviewed the child's file and summarized pertinent details of her educational background, clinical condition and present level of functioning.

The COTA also prepared a mailing to Jennifer's parents, which included a cover letter, Related Services information pamphlet and a questionnaire. The questionnaire solicited information regarding home **reinforcers** (preferences in food and activities), **parental priorities** (functioning problems that concerned parents), emotional adjustment, play patterns and preferences and any behavior problems that bothered the parents, such as tantrums, head banging, biting and screaming during the night.[4]

Another aspect of the screening process involved gathering information from Jennifer's teachers. The COTA used a a structured interview/behavioral checklist to gather data that might indicate the child's potential problems in educational, gross motor, fine motor, tactile sensation, vestibular sensation, auditory language, visual perception and psychosocial adjustment areas.[4]

These findings were then reported to the OTR who, after analysis and synthesis of the screening information, determined that Jennifer could benefit from a more in-depth occupational therapy evaluation.

Evaluation

Jennifer's evaluation was largely performed by the occupational therapist, as the complexity of the child's clinical condition and the particular evaluation instruments required knowledge of sensorimotor development to make necessary observations and judgments. Several of the performance component evaluations were standardized, yielding normative comparisons of age equivalency.

Occasionally, the COTA assisted with the evaluation by positioning Jennifer appropriately for goniometric range of motion and standing by for added safety during the assessment of gross motor and locomotor functions such as balancing and jumping, thereby freeing the therapist to observe movement more closely. The COTA also contributed observations of Jennifer's performance in the classroom, playground and lunchroom, which helped to confirm the functional effects of performance component problems detected in the formal evaluation.

The COTA evaluated dressing skills using a developmental checklist and contributed greatly to the evaluation of Jennifer's functioning in the areas of grooming and hygiene, object manipulation, psychosocial adjustment and play, integrating observations with relevant feedback from Jennifer's parents and teachers. Because of Jennifer's neuromuscular disability, her ability to eat was evaluated by the OTR. Specific tests administered by the occupational therapist included the Milanni-Comparetti, Goodenough-Harris Drawing Test, Beery-Buktenica Developmental Test of Visual-Motor Integration (VMI) and an early childhood fine motor checklist.

Jennifer was cooperative, though distractible during evaluation activities. Her attention span was improved in a low-stimulus environment. Muscular tone and body posturing increased as she attempted motor tasks.

After the three-week evaluation period, the OTR and the COTA met formally to review their respective assessments and observations, and the OTR prepared the report shown in Figure 6-2 and the following sections.

Referral/Background

A brief narrative summary of the referral, Jennifer's background and the evaluation process, including dates and

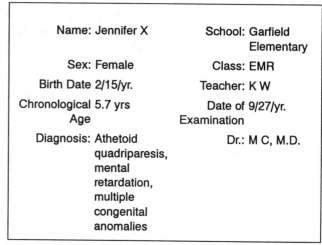

Name: Jennifer X   School: Garfield Elementary

Sex: Female   Class: EMR

Birth Date 2/15/yr.   Teacher: K W

Chronological 5.7 yrs Age   Date of 9/27/yr. Examination

Diagnosis: Athetoid quadriparesis, mental retardation, multiple congenital anomalies   Dr.: M C, M.D.

Figure 6-2. *Report of Jennifer X based on evaluation by OTR and COTA.*

specific instruments and procedures used, appeared in this section and was followed by these findings.

Sensorimotor Components: Sensory Integration

Sensory Awareness/Processing:
1. Visual: Visual acuity and field appear within normal limits. Jennifer has difficulty isolating eye from head movements for smooth visual tracking and scanning.
2. Tactile: There is some tactile hypersensitivity if touched unexpectedly or when agitated. Jennifer shows difficulty locating light touch or two-point stimuli applied to her face and hands. She seems unaware when her chin is wet from drooling.

Sensory Motor Components:Neuromuscular

1. *Reflex*: Jennifer uses many postural fixations to compensate for instability in the trunk, shoulders and hips. Her arms make writhing motions distally. Righting reactions and equilibrium responses are delayed and unreliable.
2. *Range of motion*: Joint range of motion is generally within normal limits. She exhibits slight tightness in right shoulder external rotation. Mild scapulohumeral fixation at the left shoulder can be disassociated with facilitation. Hyperextension at the metacarpophalangeal (MP) and interphalangeal (IP) joints is present bilaterally. Jennifer may be at risk for spinal curves due to low muscle tone and unusual posturing. In addition, she tends to "W" sit to stabilize herself.
3. *Muscle tone*: Jennifer's overall tone is variable, but generally hypotonic. She often appears "floppy," but will stiffen her arms, legs and mouth musculature when she becomes excited or performs motor activities. Bilateral upper extremity tone fluctuates between normal and mild spasticity, with slight resistance felt in shoulder adduction, internal rotation and elbow

flexion.

4. *Strength and endurance*: Jennifer shows limited strength and endurance in trunk, shoulders and hips. Bilateral hand weakness interferes with classroom activities, and weak lateral grasp limits dressing. She shows poor endurance in most repetitive exercises or multistep tasks, although distractibility and increasing tone also interfere.

5. *Postural control*: Jennifer's hypotonic trunk and lack of co-contraction at the shoulders and hips contribute to poor sitting balance. Her balance is also jeopardized by increased muscle tone triggered by excitement, verbalization or hand use; typically, Jennifer's knees extend and elbows flex with athetoid movements distally.

Sensory Motor Components: Motor

1. *Gross motor coordination*: Jennifer functions at approximately the three-year-old level of gross motor skills on the Milanni-Comparetti test. She shows lack of proximal co-contraction and stability, and she is unable to perform any gross motor activities that require hip stability. When asked to stand from a squat position, Jennifer exhibits tongue thrust and arm posturing. Generally, she does not perform gross motor tasks in a smooth, coordinated manner; for instance, when pulling herself forward on a scooter board, her shoulders elevate to her ears.

2. *Laterality*: Jennifer is right dominant and tends to neglect using her left hand assistively.

3. *Bilateral integration*: Jennifer is hesitant in using her left arm in bilateral activities such as catching a bouncing ball or stabilizing her paper when drawing. Jennifer experiences difficulty isolating movements so that one arm can be used separately from the other in cutting with a scissors or holding clothing while dressing. Again, postural instability, muscle tone increases and weaknesses interfere with smooth use of two hands.

4. *Fine motor coordination/dexterity*: Jennifer performs at a three-year-old level on an early childhood fine motor checklist. She has difficulty with quick release of objects and can isolate her index finger more easily on her right hand. She reverts to a primitive squeeze/raking pattern when her posture is stressed because of poor positioning in her chair. Repetitive hand movement results in a building of muscle tone and extraneous posturing. On the Goodenough-Harris Drawing Test, Jennifer's production of a man was unrecognizable.

5. *Visual-motor integration*: The Beery-Buktenica Developmental Test of Visual Motor Integration (VMI) score is three years, two months. Because motor performance influences results, this score may not reflect her perceptual ability.

6. *Oral-motor control*: The palate is slightly high but stays clear of food while Jennifer is eating. Musculature is hypotonic overall; however, abnormal increased tone patterns of lip retraction and purse-string puckering are seen as associated movements in speaking and eating, especially when Jennifer is excited or distracted. Chewing action of the jaw is mostly vertical, with slight rotary motion to the right and left. Lip closure is loose, but with increasing tone, lip retraction or purse-string action is seen, indicating emergence of a less controlled pattern. Jennifer compensates for weakened lip closure by keeping her fingers to her lips. Tongue movements can be lateralized to the right, but are decreased toward the left. Drooling increases as tone rises.

Cognitive Integration Components

Attention span: Jennifer is able to attend to tasks for 10-minute intervals in a low stimulus room. She is highly distracted by environmental stimulation such as noise and touch, usually requiring verbal cues to bring her back to a task.

Psychosocial Skills/Components

Psychological, social and self-management: Jennifer is reinforced by verbal praising of her accomplishments or interacting with her favorite toys. She adapts fairly well to new situations, but seems to prefer the same routine. Fast changes or stimulating environments trigger increased muscle tone and distractibility. Jennifer communicates more readily on a one-to-one basis than in a classroom group. She tends to play with girls from her class, and she has a few other acquaintances, who assume helper rather than playmate roles.

Occupational Performance Areas: Activities of Daily Living Skills

1. *Grooming, oral hygiene, bathing and toilet hygiene*: Jennifer requires moderate assistance in most tasks. She can brush her teeth after the toothpaste has been applied to the brush, but needs supervision for thoroughness. She manages her hair using a round bristle brush and washes herself independently with a mitt-type washcloth. Jennifer has good bowel and bladder control, but needs help pulling up her pants and handling fasteners.

2. *Dressing*: Jennifer needed assistance of varying degrees throughout the evaluation process. She was able to take clothes off with minor assistance in handling fasteners. After initial assistance, she can pull on T-shirts. Given extra time she can pull on socks.

3. *Feeding and eating*: Jennifer shows suckling and sucking patterns in drinking and consuming an ice

lollipop. At times she doesn't swallow the last bit of liquid as promptly or completely as she did when in a suck-swallow sequence. A munching/tongue thrust pattern is seen in eating, and biting through hard or sticky foods is difficult.

During lunch, Jennifer sits on a picnic bench with classmates. A foot rest would allow her to plant her feet to compensate for trunk instability. Her elbows rest on the table with shoulders in internal rotation. Presently, she shows free forearm rotation on the right, holding a spoon loosely in a dagger or shovel grasp. She picks up and positions her spoon using her right hand only. Jennifer tends to bite off pieces of food versus cutting them to size, and shows inconsistent use of her left hand to assist in cutting food or stabilizing dishes. Trunk instability affects her performance of a smooth, controlled hand-to-mouth movement.

4. *Functional communication*: Jennifer has great difficulty articulating speech. Overall body tone, lip retraction and drooling increase as she tries to speak.

5. *Functional mobility*: Jennifer walks with a shuffling gait and wide base of support. She can roll and crawl reciprocally but cannot hop, skip, balance on one foot or climb stairs. In two-foot jumping, she is barely able to clear the floor.

Occupational Performance Areas: Work Activities

1. *Educational activities*: Using her right hand, Jennifer holds a pencil in a loose lateral grasp and writes using gross arm versus finer wrist and hand motions. Repetitive hand activity results in increased muscle tone, and Jennifer reverts to increasing shoulder movement and a more gross grasp of the pencil. Bilateral hand and finger weakness interferes with classroom activities such as cutting with a scissors, squeezing a glue bottle, opening jars, manipulating door knobs and operating faucets. Generally, objects should be larger or built-up for adequate handling.

Occupational Performance Areas: Play or Leisure Activities

Play performance: Jennifer tends to observe others on the playground. She will occasionally climb on lower equipment, but avoids swings and slides. During unstructured classroom time, she chooses eight- to ten-piece wooden puzzles and shape sorting toys. Jennifer's mother has expressed concern with her tendency to watch television. She has asked whether a microcomputer might provide her with a more constructive outlet.

Assessment Summary and Recommendations

Jennifer is functioning at approximately the three-year

level in gross, fine and visual motor components of performance and activities of daily living. Many motor delays prevent maximal participation in her school program. Major interfering factors are as follows:

1. Lack of proximal stability, co-contraction, and strength of the trunk, shoulders and hips, which limit her ability to steady her body for sitting or arm use during classroom tasks.

2. Variable, but generally hypotonic or "floppy" muscle tone, resulting in poorly graded movements; increasing tone and associated stiffening of mouth, arm and leg musculature when stressed or performing motor tasks.

3. Lack of disassociated or isolated movements, so that using one arm separately from the other makes daily tasks difficult.

4. Generalized poor strength and endurance due to aforementioned factors and some unwillingness or inability to attend to tasks for a prolonged period.

5. Oral motor problems affecting eating, drinking and speaking, which increase when the student is excited or involved in motor activities.

Occupational therapy recommends direct services and environmental adaptations to promote proximal stability, normalize muscle tone, promote more coordinated and isolated movement patterns, improve arm and hand strength and endurance, develop better oral-motor function, and build independence in activities of daily living. Consultative services with teachers are also advised to provide techniques for adapting classroom activities.

Program Planning

Using the assessment data, the OTR and the COTA collaborated in formulating a hierarchy of occupational therapy goals and corresponding measurable objectives for the occupational therapy portion of the IEP. A specific intervention plan was developed that detailed techniques, media choices and sequence of particular activities. The COTA made numerous suggestions and provided specific recommendations about environmental modifications and adaptive equipment that would improve Jennifer's level of functioning. The initial IEP established is shown in Table 6-2.

The OTR contacted the parents to discuss the rationale for treatment and the need for mutual coordination, particularly in the area of activities of occupational performance intervention. Plans for future communication were also established.

The COTA forwarded a copy of the occupational therapy evaluation to the physician and requested a prescription authorizing treatment. After the prescription was received,

Table 6-2.
Occupational Therapy IEP

Annual Objectives	Programming and Assessment Procedures	Time Line	Progress to Date
Jennifer will be able to: 1. Exhibit increased proximal stability at the hips, shoulders, and trunk across settings.	Provide weight bearing in a variety of positions—4-point, prone over the bolster. Promote weight bearing and inhibition through joint compression. Consult with classroom teacher to have her encourage weight bearing when possible.	School Year 19yr	There is evidence that weight bearing is effective in decreasing extraneous movements; arm and hand flapping decreases after weight bearing on palms.
2. Demonstrate reliable righting and equilibrium reactions when balance is challenged.	Change positions from 4-point to kneel to side sit with facilitation at key points—shoulder girdle, hips. Use tilt board to challenge reactions. Have Jennifer straddle bolster or lie prone lengthwise on bolster while tipping it. Have Jennifer sit on therapist's lap, leaning side to side.		She rolls in an uncoordinated way. When balance is challenged, Jennifer's arms reach to the side and front. She is able to maintain a pivot prone position for several seconds.
3. Demonstrate more coordinated, controlled fine motor skills, including the following: a. Maintain good sitting position. b. Demonstrate a finer prehension grasp on utensils (as opposed to lateral or shovel grasp). c. Perform bilateral activities. d. Practice voluntary release of objects.	Have Jennifer participate in a fine motor group session once weekly, co-planned by OTR and classroom teacher. Complete a fine motor checklist to obtain baseline of functional ability. a. See goal 6 and approaches. b. Provide functional activities, eg, grooming tasks, hair/teeth brushing, dressing. c. Promote manual functioning—using ruler, writing, cutting paper with easy-grip scissors, stringing large beads, opening wide-mouth jars, operating computer and other classroom manipulatives. d. Practice release through bean bags, balls, cubes, peg board activities.	Fall 19yr and Spring 19yr	Checklist completed; will keep on practicing skills that Jennifer has difficulty completing in a smooth, coordinated manner. Still uses a more lateral, shovel-type grasp, which is weak; has difficulty staying on task for multistep tasks. Will continue fine motor group one time weekly, and individual therapy two times/week.

the assistant was responsible for monitoring the prescription anniversary date so that a renewal could be secured if necessary. The COTA also made sure that copies of all current and subsequent evaluations and plans were forwarded to the central special education office, the parents and the physician.

Intervention

The OTR and the COTA collaborated in providing direct services. Because of the complexity of this child's clinical condition and the need to use certain neurodevelopmental modalities, the OTR assumed a primary treatment role. The OTR/COTA team assumed the following responsibilities with regard to Jennifer's specific objectives.

Objective 1—Stability of trunk, shoulders and hips: The OTR performed treatment in this area, with the COTA assisting as needed. The COTA reinforced this treatment goal by monitoring Jennifer's positioning during school activities and advising her teachers and parents on appropriate positioning.

Objective 2—Righting and equilibrium reactions: The OTR provided neurodevelopmental treatment (NDT) on a one-to-one basis. The COTA assisted when two people were needed to perform a particular technique. The assistant also reported relevant observations of Jennifer's daily functioning in school and reinforced neurodevelopmental treatment principles in classroom positioning.

Objective 3—Fine motor skills: A weekly fine motor group was planned collaboratively with the classroom teacher and conducted by the OTR or the COTA. The COTA also worked with Jennifer individually twice a week, emphasizing academic-related activities such as manipulating buttons, crayons and scissors.

Table 6-2. (continued)
Occupational Therapy IEP

Annual Objectives	Programming and Assessment Procedures	Time Line	Progress to Date
4. Demonstrate lip closure and decrease drooling.	Provide oral facilitation 15 minutes before lunch every day. Use following techniques: inhibitory pressure—repeat 4-5 times; tongue pressure—broad handle of spoon—repeat 6 times; stretch pressure—quick stretch—3 times, upper and lower lip stretch from cheek to corner of mouth 3 times; sucking—suck on ice or popsickle—stretch pressure; straw drinking—tight fitting lid hole for straw.	School Year 19yr	Jennifer's active lip movements have increased slightly, but she still shows lack of active strong lip and cheek muscles in eating and drinking. Protrusion of tongue decreased slightly; not seeing good controlled sideward movements. Still exhibits some lip retraction when she is excited, but is able to close lips around spoon more consistently since facilitation techniques have been used.
5. Maintain a clean mouth at meals.	Provide verbal and sensory cues to remind when food is on mouth, so she will use napkin.	School Year 19yr	With verbal cues, Jennifer will reach out, pick up napkin, and wipe face, but is not always consistent with this.
6. Assume an erect sitting posture with head up, chin tucked, and feet stabilized, for self-feeding and fine motor skills.	Consult with classroom teacher to choose chairs which will allow Jennifer to maintain both feet on the ground or supply foot rest. Construct a portable foot rest to attach to lunchroom bench where Jennifer eats, promoting more stability in sitting.	School Year 19yr	Jennifer can assume correct position 75% of time during eating, with verbal reminders.
7. Demonstrate independent dressing skills. a. Practice a finer prehension grasp. b. Decrease the amount of assistance needed with fasteners.	Provide predressing activities: buttons through plastic lids, peg board activities and such, to practice skills necessary for fasteners—eg, zippers, unzipping, buttons, snaps, untying shoes, practice taking on or off pull-over shirts, putting on shoes and socks.	School Year 19yr	Jennifer has progressed in speed of putting on shirt and jacket and most other undressing skills; still needs minimal assistance with fasteners.

Objective 4—Lip closure and drooling: Increase lip closure and decrease drooling during eating (see objective 5).

Objective 5—Clean mouth at meals: The OTR designed a feeding facilitation program, and she and the COTA alternated in performing neuromuscular facilitation of oral musculature before Jennifer's lunch. The COTA supervised Jennifer and other children with similar problems for positioning and self-feeding in the lunchroom.

Objective 6—Correct posture to enable improved arm and hand use: Jennifer was instructed in the use of abdominal muscles and correct positioning by the OTR. The COTA monitored Jennifer's posture in different school situations, giving her verbal reminders as necessary. The assistant also constructed two foot rests of appropriate heights so that she could sit more securely on regular classroom and lunchroom furniture.

Objective 7—Dressing independence: The COTA practiced dressing-related skills with Jennifer in therapy sessions twice weekly and provided adaptive equipment and clothing modifications as needed. The assistant periodically reassessed Jennifer's level of function using a dressing skills checklist. The COTA was also responsible for coaching classroom aides about the type and amount of assistance to offer Jennifer in dressing and self-care related to bathroom use and physical education activities.

The COTA coordinated Jennifer's home reinforcement program with the family. This process involved teaching proper positioning, adaptive procedures and adaptive equipment use.

The OTR shared the occupational therapy plan with Jennifer's classroom teacher, and they exchanged ideas about how OT goals might be mutually reinforced through the academic part of the IEP. For instance, having Jennifer crawl on her palms in moving about the classroom could provide

---

Table 6-3.
OTR/COTA Working Relationship[5,6]

I. *Responsibilities of OTR Supervisor*:
The OTR supervisor is responsible for the development and utilization of staff in assuring quality and cost efficiency of OT services. The OTR supervises receipt of referrals, exercises professional judgment in delegating tasks to appropriate OT personnel, and oversees task performance in accord with accepted standards of professional practice.

II. *Style of Supervision*:
To foster staff member growth and motivation, a collaborative style of supervision is developed, which involves technical personnel in sharing responsibility and decision making regarding tasks they have been delegated.

III. *Roles of OTR/COTA Team Members*:
  A. Occupational Performance Intervention
    1. Activities of daily living—grooming, oral hygiene, bathing, toilet hygiene, dressing, feeding and eating, medication routine, socialization, functional communication, functional mobility and sexual expression.
    2. Work activities—home management, care of others, educational activities and vocational activities.
    3. Play or leisure activities—exploration and performance.
  B. Performance Component Intervention
    1. Sensory motor components—sensory integration, neuromuscular and motor.
    2. Cognitive integration and cognitive components—level of arousal, orientation, recognition, attention span, memory, sequencing, categorization, concept formation, intellectual operations in space, problem solving, and generalization, integration and synthesis of learning.
    3. Psychosocial skills and psychological components—Psychological, social and self-management.

OTR or COTA with General Supervision

COTA ROLE: OTRs and COTAs may work similarly in assessment, planning and implementation of such interventions.

OTR or COTA with General or Close Supervision

COTA ROLE: COTAs may perform assigned assessment, planning and intervention tasks depending on OTR's consideration of the following factors:
  1. Condition of patient/client
  2. Proficiencies of the COTA supervisee
  3. Complexity of evaluation or therapy modality
  4. Standards of government and regulatory agencies
  5. Practice standards and guidelines of OT profession
  6. Requirements of third-party reimbursers

---

additional exercise to promote proximal stability. It was also noted that several children in Jennifer's class shared a common fine motor goal, so activities were coordinated with the special education teacher to establish a fine motor group within the classroom.

The COTA frequently advised regular classroom teachers who may have little background in working with students with handicaps. For instance, Jennifer's physical education teacher tended to have her "sit out" during most class activities. After consulting with the OTR, the COTA met with the teacher to clarify Jennifer's performance abilities and realistic precautions and then made recommendations regarding ways the student could be included in regular gym activities.

Throughout the treatment program, the COTA shared observations, questions and suggestions with the supervising therapist. The assistant maintained anecdotal notes on students receiving treatment and discussed them with the OTR in preparation for the spring IEP updates.

Conclusion

The COTA makes many valued contributions to Related Services and the delivery of occupational therapy services in a school setting. Employment of a COTA provides the additional manpower to extend occupational therapy services, thereby offering the benefits of more therapy time per child. A full-time, on-site assistant can greatly aid the therapist by maintaining communication with Related Services, teachers and families, thus promoting continuity of occupational therapy services and facilitating mainstreaming. The COTA assures that Related Services and occupational therapy approaches are reinforced throughout the school day, so that functional gains made in therapy are better integrated into students' daily academic routines. Other areas of responsibility include maintaining the therapy room, ordering supplies and equipment and supervising occupational therapy assistant students on fieldwork assignment.

Table 6-3 outlines the general roles and areas of mutual collaboration of the occupational therapy intraprofessional team members.[5,6]

Related Learning Activities

1. Practice administering a developmental skills checklist to a normal child. After you feel comfortable with it, obtain permission to administer it to a child with a handicap.

2. Plan a gross motor group activity for four children who are trainable, mentally retarded and are clumsy in their movements.

3. Identify activities that could be used in a home program for school-aged children with normal intelligence who have fine motor problems.

4. Dicuss ways parents can become involved in the education of their child with a handicap.

References

1. Royeen CB, Marsh D: Promoting occupational therapy in the schools. *Am J Occup Ther* 42:713-117, 1988.
2. Education for All Handicapped Children Act, 1975, P.L. 94-142. *Fed Regist*, August 23, 1977, sec. 601.
3. Miller BF, Keane CB: *Encylopedia and Dictionary of Medicine, Nursing, and Allied Health*, Fifth Edition. Philadelphia, WB Saunders, 1988.
4. Gilfoyle EM: *Training: Occupational Therapy Educational Management in Schools*, Volume 2. Rockville, Maryland, American Occupational Therapy Association, 1980.
5. Practice Statement: COTA Supervision. Wisconsin Occupational Therapy Association, 1985.
6. Commission on Practice: *Uniform Terminology*, Second Edition. Rockville, Maryland, American Occupational Therapy Association, 1989.

The Child With a Conduct Disorder

Linda Florey, MA, OTR, FAOTA

Introduction

Conduct disorders are the most common behavior disorders in children.[1] The key feature of this condition is a persistent pattern of behavior in which the basic rights of others and the major age-appropriate social roles or expectations are violated. Physical and verbal **aggression** (angry and destructive behaviors aimed at dominance) are common. Children with this disorder often initiate aggression, and they may be physically cruel to people or animals. They may steal and the stealing may involve confrontation with the victim, such as in the case of a mugging. Cheating and lying are common, and often children with this disorder are truant from school and have episodes of running away from home. Typically, children with a conduct disorder have low self-esteem, which they hide by portraying themselves as uncaring.[2]

Conduct disorder is more common in boys than girls by a ratio of 3:1. Children with severe conduct disorder often develop antisocial personality disorders as adults; however, many achieve reasonable social and occupational adjustment.

Case Study Background

Randy is an 11-year-old boy who was admitted to the child inpatient unit with a diagnosis of conduct disorder. Randy currently lives with his mother, 16-year-old brother, and his mother's boyfriend. His parents were divorced when he was two years old, and Randy sees his biological father on weekends.

KEY CONCEPTS

Family background	Goal setting
Initial evaluation	Intervention groups
Assets and deficits	Cub Scouts

ESSENTIAL VOCABULARY

Conduct disorders

Aggression

Oppositional behavior

Findings

Peer interactions

Multidisciplinary team

Behavioral control

Task skills group

Workshop task group

Play group

Randy has a long history of **oppositional behavior**. In preschool, his teacher reported that he pushed and shoved other children and was more impulsive than other children of the same age. In elementary school, his first and second grade teachers reported incidents of physical and verbal aggression toward other children. This behavior included making insulting remarks to peers if things didn't go his way and biting and punching other children during recess and after school. In the fourth grade, Randy was placed in a class for the seriously emotionally disturbed (SED) for part of the day and in the fifth grade he was in the class for the SED for the entire day. Randy was admitted to the inpatient unit because of increasing aggression at home and in school, including tantrums in which he threw furniture.

Initial Evaluation and Findings

The OTR and COTA worked together to obtain an assessment of Randy's prior and current pattern of play and socialization, task performance, play interests and visual motor skills. The specific evaluaion, its format, purpose, the responsible OT personnel and findings follow:

Evaluation: "Typical Day Interview"
Format: Semistructured interview
Purpose: To determine patterns of daily living, school, play activities, chores and time management
Staff: OTR
Findings: Randy reported that during the week he went to school, watched TV after school, and on the weekend, he "hung out." When asked about friends he said he didn't need any and that kids in his class were "babies" and "stupid." He was unable to name any games, sports or hobbies in which he engaged on a regular basis. He said that he sometimes went to movies with his dad and brother and had played catch a few times with his mother's boyfriend.

When asked, Randy said that he was responsible for cleaning his room and for stacking the dishes in the dishwasher after the evening meal. Throughout the interview he challanged the authority of the occupational therapist, asking why she needed to know something and telling her that she asked too many questions.

Evaluation: Task performance using Westphal Decision Inventory
Format: Structured checklist
Purpose: To determine decision making, problem solving ability, attention span
Staff: COTA
Findings: Randy was given a simple three-step project to complete. At first he was resistant to engaging in the project asking "Why do I have to do this anyway?" and

saying that it was "stupid." The COTA explained that all the children on the unit learned activities as part of their program. He then listened to directions and completed the first two steps. He made a minor mistake during the third step, attempted to correct it himself and could not. He then pushed it across the table, telling the COTA that he didn't want to do the "dumb" project anyway. The COTA corrected the mistake and Randy was able to successfully complete the last step. He attended to the project for the full 45-minute period with encouragement to continue when he became discouraged.

Evaluation: Observation of socialization in occupational therapy workshop and on the unit using observation guide
Format: Semistructured guide
Purpose: To determine frequency and content of interactions with peers and adults
Staff: OTR and COTA
Findings: Randy was seen in occupational therapy participating with another peer in a structured table game. He understood the rules of the game, but became easily frustrated when the game did not go his way. He tried to manipulate the rules to his advantage and to cheat. He tended to be controlling in his **peer interactions** (verbal and nonverbal interchanges with individuals of a similar age), such as making choices for his peer and deciding who would go first.

Randy was also observed during free time on the inpatient unit. He selected games characterisic of a younger child, which required little interaction with others, and consistently cheated so that he would win. He bragged and was bossy and critical of his peers. He attempted to align himself with adults, saying that the other kids were "babies" and he couldn't play with them.

Evaluation: Developmental test of visual motor integration
Format: Structured test that uses form copying
Purpose: To determine developmental or age equivalent status of visual motor skills
Staff: OTR
Findings: Randy received a raw score of 32, which corresponds to an age equivalent of 11 years 2 months, and a percentile rank of 53. This indicates that Randy had adequate visual motor skills.

Summary of Assets and Deficits

With the findings of the initial evaluation, the OTR summarized Randy's assets and deficits as follows:
Assets:
- Adequate task performance skills
- Adequate attending behavior
- Adequate visual motor skills
Deficits:
- Lack of identified play interests

- Lack of reported peer friendships
- Poor social interaction skills
- Poor impulse control

Program Planning

The program planning process on the children's inpatient unit is the same as that on the adolescent unit (see Chapter 8). Basically, the goals for the individual patients are implemented within programs broadly designed to meet the needs of most children. Specific activities and tasks are selected and paced to encourage increasing levels of skill, responsibility, interpersonal control and responsiveness.

Program planning is completed within the context of the **multidisciplinary team**, which includes representatives from psychiatry, psychology, social work, nursing, the school, and recreation therapy. Pertinent findings from the other disciplines were that Randy obtained a high average IQ measure of 118 and that he tested above grade level in all school subjects except reading comprehension and spelling. He was also noted to be controlling and dominating with peers. Interviews with the mother and biological father conducted by the social worker revealed that both parents had difficulty controlling Randy. The interviews also corroborated the findings of the occupational therapist with regard to peer friendships. The mother reported that Randy had bullied most of his playmates and that he currently had no friends.

Randy's anticipated length of stay was two months. He was expected to return to live with his mother and to attend classes for the SED at school.

In collaboration with the COTA, the OTR set the following measurable short-term and long-term goals:

Short-Term Goals

1. Randy will play simple games without cheating.
   Time Frame: Two weeks
2. Randy will ask for help when he encounters a problem.
   Time Frame: Two weeks
3. Randy will share materials with others
   Time Frame: Two weeks

Long-Term Goals

1. Randy will tolerate a one-hour group without incident of overt frustration leading to aggression.
   Time Frame: Four weeks and throughout hospitalization
2. Randy will independently solve problems that arise in task performance.
   Time Frame: Five weeks and throughout hospitalization

3. Randy will work with another peer to complete a cooperative project.
   Time Frame: Four weeks
4. Randy will identify three or more play interests.
   Time Frame: Four weeks and throughout hospitalization
5. Randy will state his needs in a positive manner.
   Time Frame: Four weeks and throughout hospitalization

Intervention

Randy was scheduled for the following occupational therapy groups:
- Cooperative Task Group
- Workshop Task Group
- Play Group
- Social Skills Group
- Cub Scouts

The COTA and OTR, working as a team, used the treatment groups to focus on the short-term and long-term goals. Together they determined Randy's progress and made revisions in the program. When short-term goals were met, long-term goals were then implemented. Randy was encouraged throughout all assigned treatment groups to deal with his frustration in an assertive, not an aggressive manner, to independently problem solve and to interact positively with his peers. Positive role modeling, emotional support, discussion and feedback on behaviors were the specific means of intervention used. Randy was also on a total unit system of **behavioral control** in which he was given warnings and "time outs" for unacceptable behavior such as verbal or physical aggression toward another peer. This behavioral program was implemented by all team members so that Randy would have consistent expectations of his behavior.

Treatment Implementation

Throughout his hospitalization Randy was involved in the task skills group and the play group. He participated in the social skills group at the beginning of his hospitalization. After learning to adhere to the basic skills of listening to others, waiting his turn and expressing his views in a positive manner, he was placed in the more complex social group of Cub Scouts. The COTA led the task groups, and the OTR led the play and social skills groups. Both the OTR and the COTA conducted the Cub Scout group. Randy's progress in the task and play groups and the Cub Scouts is reviewed.

Task Groups

The **task skills groups** were held five times weekly. There were four patients in each group. In the cooperative task group, patients are required to work with a peer on an assigned project to promote and encourage those skills required to get along with others (sharing, respecting others opinions and compromising). Initially, Randy attempted to take control of the project, deciding on color selection and assigning parts of the project to his peers. When the COTA intervened, restating the cooperative goals of the group, Randy refused to participate, saying the group project was "babyish." The COTA then assigned each child a specific task and with prompting, Randy completed his share. Randy had difficulty compromising and had to be prompted to consider the wishes of others. By the fourth week of hospitalization, he was able to listen to the suggestions of others, obey majority decisions on the project and work to task completion.

The **workshop task group** consisted of offering several choices of projects for patients to work on independently. The process of choice promotes the first steps in problem solving. A selection of choices, provided by the COTA, was geared toward success, but also allowed for creativity and problem solving. Randy initially chose a clay project which allowed him several choices (such as shape and color), as well as a certain amount of frustration to overcome (breakage and uncertainty about how well it would "fire"). He decided on a small pinch pot. When one he constructed collapsed because it was too thin, he said he didn't want to do it anymore. Pointing at the clay, he said, "This is for babies" and "I hate it." The OTR and the COTA noted that Randy seemed to label incidents as "babyish" when he perceived himself as being unsuccessful. They decided to structure his choices to include short-term projects in which they felt he would succeed and to provide him with additional instruction on the projects outside of group time. After individual attention and instruction, Randy was able to complete projects and seemed better able to share the materials and the attention of the COTA with other children. He did well with small craft activities in which he gained immediate tangible results. He also responded well to clear expectations for behavior.

Play Group

The **play group** was comprised of three to four children. The objective of the group was to play games according to rules, using the correct sequence of turn taking, in which they would accept winning and losing as "good sports." The competitive aspects of the game were deemphasized. Table games and gross motor games were used. This group was particularly difficult for Randy because of his tendency to dominate and boss his peers and his desire to be a winner at all costs. Simple games that focused on taking turns were used in the beginning, and progression was made to games requiring more skill and strategy. Randy wanted to be in control and often blamed his peers for cheating and making him miss targets or plays. On several occasions he had to be briefly excluded from the games because of verbal aggression toward his peers. After these "time outs" he was able to respond to redirection and reengage in the game.

Cub Scouts

The Cub Scout troop at the psychiatric hospital is a legitimate pack chartered with the Boy Scouts of America. The pack includes both Cub Scouts and Webelos. Weekly den meetings are conducted by the OTR and the COTA who serve as den leader and assistant den leader, respectively. Approximately six to eight children are included in the pack.

Within the meeting structure, the patients participate in the business meeting, which includes learning and reciting the Cub Scout promise, working toward achievement pins in areas such as artistry and forestry, and partcipating in scouting events, which include the "Genius Kit Competition" and the "Pinewood Derby Races." Scout shirts, scarves and neckslides are loaned to the children during their stay. The objective of having a chartered troop within the hospital is to promote socialization, cooperation and leadership within the context of a bona fide community group. Children who have been scouts can continue to participate in these activities, and the organization itself provides an age-appropriate after-school resource in which children can be engaged after discharge.

During the fourth week of hospitalization, the OTR talked with Randy about promoting him from the social skills group to the Scouts, as he was now listening to others, waiting his turn and beginning to express his views in a positive manner. Randy was excited about being a Cub Scout. Both the staff and the patients on the unit held the Scouts in high regard, and the troop served as a symbol of status and belonging. From the beginning, Randy's participation in Scouts was a positive, successful experience. He adapted to the structure of the meetings and was able to share materials and attention and to talk to his peers without becoming bossy and negative. He needed a few prompts and reminders to wait his turn but responded positively to the clearly stated expectations. The COTA asked Randy to work with a new scout member on the unit to help him learn the promise. Randy complied with this request and volunteered to help all new members learn the oath. In the sixth week of hospitalization, Randy was elected "Denner of the Pack." He called the meetings to order, led the business meeting, and served as a role model for the other scouts. He was in a position of control with his peers, but he had been elected by them and had to obey the general rules of fair play, which also applied to him. Randy now legitimately belonged to something and he had earned a position of esteem among his peers.

Program Discontinuation

One week before discharge, the OTR scheduled a meeting with Randy's mother. The OTR and the COTA determined that Randy did well under conditions in which clear expectations for behavior and for performance were broken down to focus on short-term, tangible results. The OTR telephoned the district executive for the Boy Scouts of America to determine the troop or den closest to Randy's home and school. In the meeting with Randy's mother, the OTR and the COTA reviewed her child's progress and strongly recommended that he join the scout troop and other structured after-school activities as a means of promoting and enhancing social interaction with peers and productive achievement. Randy had done well in the hospital scout troop, and he was interested in continuing this activity. The troop provided him with a tangible sign of belonging to a peer group and had taught him social rules for successful interaction and achievement.

Acknowledgment

The author wishes to extend appreciation to Ellen Castillo, COTA, for contributing ideas that were most useful in developing this case study.

Related Learning Activities

1. Discuss behaviors commonly exhibited by children with a conduct disorder with your peers.

2. Develop a list of games that could be used with children such as Randy.

3. What specific three-step projects could have been used as a part of Randy's evaluation?

4. Obtain a copy of a Cub Scout Handbook and become familiar with the basic objectives and activities of the organization.

References

1. Strauss C, Lakey B: Behavior disorders in children. In Adams H, Suther P (Eds): *Comprehensive Handbook of Psychopathology*. New York, Plenium Press, 1984.
2. American Psychiatric Association: *Diagnostic and Statistical Manual of Mental Disorders*, Third Edition-Revised. Washington, DC, American Psychiatric Association, 1982.
3. Westphal M: A Study of Decision Making. Unpublished master's thesis, University of Southern California, 1967.

Part B
ADOLESCENCE

The Adolescent With Depression

The Adolescent With Chemical Dependency

The Adolescent With Burns

The Adolescent With Depression

Linda Florey, MA, OTR, FAOTA

Introduction

Depression is a disorder of mood in which there is a loss of interest or pleasure in almost all activities. Feelings of unhappiness or misery dominate. Associated symptoms include disturbance in appetite, disturbance in sleep, psychomotor **agitation** (irregular action, unrest or disquiet) or retardation, decreased energy and recurrent thoughts of death, or suicidal ideation or attempts. Although the essential features of depression are similar throughout the life cycle, specific hallmarks are associated with different ages. In adolescence, negative or antisocial behavior may be dominant. Other common signs include irritable mood, restlessness, grouchiness, sulkiness, aggression, feelings of wanting to leave home, or not being approved of or understood. Additionally, the adolescent may withdraw from social activities, may experience difficulties in school and may be inattentive to personal appearance. The onset and duration of a major depressive episode are variable. The most serious complication of this disorder is **suicide** (taking one's own life).[1]

Case Study Background

Ann, a short, attractive 15-year-old adolescent was admitted to the adolescent inpatient service with the diagnosis of **post-traumatic** (after injury produced by violence or other outside agent) stress disorder with depressed and anxious affect. Ann was born in Oklahoma, and shortly after her birth her mother and father separated. Her mother moved to Los Angeles and left Ann and her two older siblings, ages three years and five years, in the care of her father. Ann's father

---

KEY CONCEPTS

Post-traumatic stress disorder

Assessment roles and methods

Interdisciplinary planning

Craft workshop

Cooking group

Discharge planning

died when she was four years old, and from age four years to seven years, she and her older brothers were cared for by her paternal aunt and uncle. During this period, Ann's mother kept in contact with her family and brought Ann to live with her and her new husband and stepson when friends suspected that Ann had been **sexually abused** (experienced forced sexual contact) by her uncle.

At 10 years of age, Ann began to be sexually abused by her 14-year-old stepbrother. She became pregnant by him when she was 13 years old. Her mother assumed that Ann was "getting fat" and did not learn of her pregnancy until she took her to a doctor for a respiratory infection. Ann was afraid to tell her mother how she became pregnant, as she feared her stepbrother might hurt her.

When Ann was seven months pregnant, police were called by neighbors to stop a family argument. The police questioned Ann about her pregnancy and she admitted to them that her stepbrother had abused her for several years. The stepbrother was arrested and convicted and began serving his sentence in jail. The Department of Public Social Services recommended that Ann attend a support group for victims of **incest** at a psychiatric facility. Incest refers to sexual relationships between family members or very close relatives.

Ann's baby was put up for adoption, and she continued to live with her mother and stepfather. Tension in the home became unbearable for Ann. Her stepfather continually blamed her for causing his son to be in jail, which led to several fights with Ann's mother. During a support group session, Ann said she was planning to kill herself and was then referred to the adolescent psychiatric inpatient service.

Assessment

As part of the interdisciplinary treatment plan, Ann was scheduled for an occupational therapy assessment. A screening process to determine the need for occupational therapy services was not performed. It is an expectation of the facility that all patients receive an assessment to determine the focus and frequency of occupational therapy intervention. The assessment is documented in the chart within the first ten days of admission. This assessment is referred to as the initial occupational therapy assessment. An additional evaluation may be performed at a later time to probe **deficit** areas identified in the initial assessment. The term deficit means inadequate behavior or task performance.

The COTA reviewed the medical chart and reported the history to the occupational therapist as described in the case study background section. The first step in the assessment process was for both the COTA and OTR to meet briefly with Ann to explain occupational therapy services, prepare her for the evaluation process, and to gain an impression of her willingness and ability to participate in the evaluation process. Because of Ann's ability to maintain eye contact, listen to information and ask questions, the occupational therapy team determined that although the patient was shy, she was receptive to the evaluation process.

Initial Evaluation and Findings

The initial evaluation served as an indicator of her level of function with respect to interests, time management, task performance, socialization and vocational interests. Ann participated in five evaluations. The specific evaluation, its format, purpose, the responsible occupational therapy personnel and **findings** (results) follow.

Evaluation: "Typical day interview"
Format: Semistructured interview
Purpose: To determine patterns of daily living, school, leisure activities, chores, and time management
Staff: OTR
Findings: Ann spent most of her prehospital days in school. She devoted other time to self-care activities, chores and homework. She was responsible for assisting with meal preparation and clean up and household chores in addition to caring for her room. She spent a little time in the evenings reading or watching television. She reported that she had no close friends, but occasionally she would walk to and from school with a classmate. She did not engage in any hobbies or special interests. Ann said that she had never had any hobbies as she was "too busy with homework."

Evaluation: NPI Interest Checklist[2]
Format: Structured checklist
Purpose: To determine ability to discriminate interests, to identify clusters of interest
Staff: COTA
Findings: Ann was able to discriminate strength of interests. Her strong **interests** were in the category of activities of daily living (eg, sewing, housekeeping, cooking). Her secondary interests were in the category of social recreation. Her least preferred interests were in the area of culture and education.

Evaluation: Task performance using Westphal Decision Making Inventory[3]
Format: Structured checklist
Purpose: To determine decision making, problem solving ability, attention span
Staff: COTA
Findings: Initially, Ann was unable to decide on a project and was given several suggestions. She then selected a simple structured task that required minimal problem solving. She required one-step verbal instructions with demonstration. She was able to recognize problems but initially required assistance to implement problem solving. She

attended to her project for the full 50-minute session, completed it, and verbalized enjoyment and satisfaction with the quality of her completed work. She stated that she wanted to learn how to do more 'things' in future sessions.

Evaluation: Observation of socialization on unit, in OT workshop and in OT cooking group using observation guide

Format: Semistructured guide

Purpose: To determine frequency and content of interactions with peers and adults

Staff: OTR and COTA

Findings: In the occupational therapy workshop and on the unit, Ann sat with the group and watched what occurred, but did not initiate conversation with peers. She approached staff when she had a question, eg, "When do I have school?" When approached by peers and staff, she responded with short sentences.

Ann was observed with two peers in a cooking group that was conducted in a small kitchen adjacent to the workshop area. Ann listened to the conversation of her peers, occasionally laughed, responded to questions, but did not initiate any comments. When she was asked to measure some ingredient, she approached the COTA, asking, "What is one third of a cup?" She said that she had never used a measuring cup, and she didn't know how to use one.

Evaluation: Adolescent Role Assessment[4]

Format: Semistructured interview

Purpose: To determine strengths and deficiencies in occupational choice process

Staff: OTR

Findings: The majority of Ann's scores indicated marginal behavior but no obvious student **role dysfunction** (inability to carry out responsibilities). She reported that she liked school but that her grades had dropped from Bs to Ds because she hadn't been able to concentrate for the past several months. She was enrolled in the tenth grade. Her favorite subject was typing. Ann said that she wished to finish high school and thought she might be a typist. She stated, "That's what my mom wants me to be." She also said she had once thought that she wanted to be a policewoman or a model but now thought these ideas were "silly" because she wasn't strong enough to become a policewoman or pretty enough to be a model. Ann indicated that she had done some baby sitting but had never had any other work experience outside the home environment.

Summary of Assets and Deficits

Based on the findings of the initial evaluation, the OTR summarized Ann's assets and deficits as follows:

Assets:
- Pleasant and cooperative
- Good attention span
- Eager to learn
- Learns quickly from verbal and demonstrated instructions
- Discriminates interests

Deficits:
- Difficulty initiating interaction with peers
- No reported friendships
- No diversified interests or hobbies
- Difficulty with measurement concepts in cooking
- Delayed occupational choice process

Program Planning

Program planning for individual patients is completed within the context of the existing occupational therapy program. The program is broadly designed to promote goals for most adolescent patients while addressing individual patient needs. The setting of treatment goals and the analysis, selection and sequencing of activities to meet the goals are guided by two main dynamics: simple to complex and dependence to independence. Goals and activities are thought of as a continuum in which tasks and situations are paced to encourage increasing levels of difficulty and responsibility. Initial goals guide treatment intervention. They are usually broad in scope and become more focused in reaction to the patient's response to treatment.

Program planning is also accomplished within the context of the interdisciplinary team. The members of different disciplines discuss the findings of their evaluations and goals of intervention and determine overall patient goals, anticipated length of hospitalization, and anticipated plans for discharge.

Ann's anticipated length of stay was three months. Depending on her family's response to family therapy, Ann would either return to her home or be placed outside the home.

The OTR formulated short-term and long-term goals, as well as time frames, for Ann. The OTR and the COTA formulated the following methods of intervention:

Short-Term Goals
1. Initiate peer interaction in structured groups
   Time Frame Three weeks
2. Increase repertoire of interests
   Time Frame Two weeks
3. Select projects independently
   Time Frame Four weeks
4. Increase complexity of task skills
   Time Frame Two weeks
5. Increase measurement skills
   Time Frame Three weeks

Intervention

Ann was scheduled for the occupational therapy craft workshop with five peers three times weekly to increase interest and task skills and independent selection of projects. The COTA was responsible for working with Ann to increase the complexity of task skills within her selected projects (eg, moving from simple one-step projects to long-term projects requiring multiple steps. If Ann did not select a project independently, the COTA would provide her with choices. The COTA would also engage Ann in simple conversation.

Ann was scheduled to attend the adolescent cooking group with three peers once weekly to increase her peer interaction, measurement skills and skills in meal preparation. Once Ann initiated conversation with her peers, she would be placed in a social skills group with an increased focus on social interaction.

Long-Term Goals

1. Initiate peer interaction spontaneously
   Time Frame: By the end of hospitalization
2. Increase awareness of interests and capacities and relate them to occupational choice
   Time Frame: Six weeks and throughout hospitalization
3. Incorporate interest areas into leisure time on ward
   Time Frame: One month and throughout hospitalization

After Ann had begun to independently select and execute projects based on her interests, she would be placed in an occupational exploration group to discuss the occupational choice process and to learn job-related skills such as filling out an application for employment. After Ann had demonstrated ability to work independently at various levels of task complexity, she would be encouraged to bring projects to the ward to work on in her spare time.

Treatment Implementation

Throughout her hospitalization, Ann was involved in the occupational therapy craft workshop and an adolescent cooking group. She was also part of a social skills group and an occupational exploration group for limited time periods. The occupational exploration group was conducted by the occupational therapist. The cooking group was led by the assistant, and the craft workshop and the social skill group were conducted by the OTR and the COTA. Ann's progress in the craft workshop and the cooking group is reviewed, as these groups reflect the working relationship between the therapist and the assistant.

Craft Workshop

Ann was involved in the craft workshop three times a week with five other peers. In the first session, the COTA gave Ann an introduction to the workshop, explaining the type of projects that could be selected. Initially, Ann was unable to select a project. She seemed overwhelmed with the choices available and uncertain of her capacities. She said "too many things" and "I've never done this." The COTA assured Ann that she would teach her and help her with whatever project she selected. She then presented Ann with three projects based on her strong interests.

Ann selected a simple three-step sewing project and learned quickly. In other sessions, the COTA suggested more complex projects, each of which built upon skills Ann had just acquired. Ann continued to learn quickly and began to work independently. Throughout the initial sessions, Ann was encouraged to sit next to her peers, and both the OTR and the COTA would initiate conversations about the projects, different individual interests and ward activities. When Ann encountered a problem, she was encouraged to ask for suggestions from her peers if they were familiar with the steps.

In subsequent sessions, Ann exhibited an increased interest in her peers and in the various projects on which they were working. She began to spontaneously initiate contact and conversation and to select projects independently. She continued to learn quickly and work carefully. Ann also asked to bring projects to the unit. This overall pattern continued throughout her hospitalization. Ann's interests, complexity of skills, independence and social spontaneity increased. She seemed aware of her own capacities and was able to take risks in new learning situations. Her "I've never done this" set was replaced by an "I'll try it" set.

The occupational therapist was responsible for developing and monitoring the treatment plans for all of the patients in the group and was primarily responsible for implementing the plan with two patients in the group, one of whom was Ann. In this group the COTA and the OTR worked side by side to validate one another's observations of patients' response to treatment.

Cooking Group

Ann was involved in a lunch-time cooking group with three to four peers throughout her hospitalization. All members within the group were responsible for planning the menu and participating in meal preparation. On a rotating basis, one member of the group was responsible for the overall coordination of tasks.

Cooking was another of Ann's strong interest areas and one in which she had engaged at home. This combination of interest and skill in a smaller group may have made Ann more confident in this situation. In the third session, she began initiating conversation and joking with her peers while engaging in a goal-oriented activity. Ann's initial problems in using measuring cups decreased with specific teaching and practice. No problems with other measurements, such as using a ruler, were noted in other areas.

During the third month of hospitalization, Ann became "bossy" with her peers and angry with them if something wasn't done the way she wanted. For example, Ann told one group member to "cut the onions smaller." Her peer responded by grating the onion onto miniscule pieces. Ann responded angrily, "you never do anything right." After such an interaction, The COTA arranged time later in the day to talk to Ann to explore reasons for her behavior. In most instances, Ann was usually angry at another peer for something that had happened outside of the cooking group. The COTA encouraged Ann to express her feelings in the context in which they occurred.

The cooking group was a positive experience for Ann. She enjoyed the group and continued to socialize spontaneously with peers and staff members invited to the group. She also began to assume a leadership role on the unit in the area of cooking. Ann took responsibility for organizing and implementing baking of birthday cakes and making evening snacks. Her skills and confidence in this area generalized to her daily ward routine.

The COTA was responsible for conducting the cooking group. The format of this group is more structured than the craft group because it is focused on meal planning and preparation. The OTR and the COTA in consultation with the other members of the treatment team selected the patients for the group based on their need to socialize, work cooperatively, increase independence and skill level, or a combination of these skills. After each session, the COTA discussed the performance of the patients with the OTR. During these meetings, strategies were developed to deal with Ann's anger.

Program Discontinuation

Ann was hospitalized for four months and was discharged to a group home for adolescent girls. One month prior to discharge, the OTR and the COTA began meeting with Ann to help her formulate plans for entering the home. Before scheduling her visit to the home, they helped Ann formulate questions to ask about life in the home so that she could enter the situation with as much information as possible. They involved Ann in a role play meeting with the housemother in which she asked questions about general living arrangements, proximity to public transportation, school and community resources, as well as the daily routine, responsibilities and leisure activities in the home.

They also role played approaches for entering a new peer group.

Ann was excited when she returned from her visit. She said that the housemother and the six girls who lived at the home were "nice" and "friendly." She would have some chores to do, one of which was to help in meal preparation for dinner. She said, "It will be almost like the cooking group and I love cooking." She also stated that her mother could visit her whenever she wished. The housemother had told her that all of the girls had privileges at the YWCA, which was located five blocks from the home. Ann noted that the YWCA had a swimming pool but no craft workshop. She felt, however, that she could buy some supplies for projects if she saved money from the allowance she would be getting.

All staff members who had worked with Ann were encouraged by her positive reaction to her new living situation. It was felt that she had benefited from the hospitalization. Ann and her mother had developed a good relationship and Ann's perception of herself had changed markedly. She no longer felt she was at the "mercy" of the wishes and desires of others with no option on life but that she now had skills, abilities and choices ahead of her.

Related Learning Activities

1. Practice role playing behaviors that would help an adolescent patient enter a new peer group. Ask a peer to provide feedback.

2. Obtain a copy of the interest checklist (see reference listing). Use this tool with at least three individuals of varying ages. Determine other interests that might be added to the checklist to reflect contemporary trends.

3. Working with a peer, plan a specific cooking activity for an adolescent group in a psychosocial inpatient setting. Indicate basic equipment and supplies necessary, general precautions to be observed and goals that could be met.

References

1. American Psychiatric Association: *Diagnostic and Statistical Manual of Mental Disorders*. Washington, DC, American Psychiatric Association, 1982.
2. Matsutsuyu J: The interest checklist. *Am J Occup Ther* 23:323-328, 1969.
3. Westphal M: A Study of Decision Making. Unpublished master's thesis, University of Southern California, 1967.
4. Black M: Adolescent role assessment. *Am J Occup Ther* 30:73-79, 1976.

The Adolescent With Chemical Dependency

LTC Denise A. Rotert, MA, OTR, Retired
MAJ Frank E. Gainer III, MHS, OTR

Introduction

Dependence on chemicals/substances to relieve pain, get "high" or reduce the effects of stress has been in existence for as long as human beings. The medical profession identifies **alcohol dependence** (alcoholism), drug dependence and **cross addiction** (addiction to a variety of chemical substances) as a disease. The disease is chronic, progressive and fatal, but can be halted through abstinence from abused substances.

The third edition of *The Diagnostic and Statistical Manual of Mental Disorders-Revised*, also referred to as DSM III-R, distinguishes between psychoactive **substance abuse** and **substance dependence**, whether the substances are alcohol, narcotics or marijuana. The essential feature of psychoactive substance dependence is a cluster of cognitive, behavioral and physiologic symptoms that indicate the person has impaired control of psychoactive substance use and continues use of the substance despite adverse consequences. The symptoms of the dependence syndrome include, but are not limited to, the physiologic symptoms of tolerance and withdrawal. In most instances, withdrawal is associated with a rising level of symptoms from restlessness and shaking to hallucinations and **delirium tremens** (the DTs).[1] The latter may be the result of acute substance withdrawal and can lead to convulsions. Psychoactive substance abuse is continued use despite knowledge of having a persistent or recurrent social, occupational, physiologic or physical problem that is caused or exacerbated by the use of the psychoactive substance. Some symptoms of the disturbance have persisted for at least one month or occurred repeatedly over a longer period of time. In addition, the individual has never met the criteria for psychoactive substance dependence for this substance.[1]

KEY CONCEPTS

Adolescent developmental tasks

Occupational therapy questionnaire

Time utilization history

Art and craft activities

Life skills development group

Time management group

Communication skills group

Recreational activities group

ESSENTIAL VOCABULARY

Alchohol dependence

Cross addiction

Substance abuse

Substance dependence

Delirium tremens

Adolescence

Problem solving

Antabuse

Communication worksheet

Alanon

No other disease generates such an intensity of emotions and is so misunderstood as substance abuse. Biases toward the substance abuser include viewing the individual as one who lacks willpower, one who enjoys the situation and does not want to change, or who is antisocial and cannot be treated.

Adolescence is a time of change and turmoil. The adolescent undergoes a significant change in physical development. Rapid growth, poor posture and physical and social awkwardness occur. The two primary developmental tasks of the age are achievement of independence and establishment of identity. Achievement of independence is characterized by conflicts with authority figures, which develop as the adolescent struggles with emancipation from parents. Establishment of identity is characterized by a search for definition of one's own values. Peers become a primary support system as well as a basis for identity; dress, actions and behaviors are all associated with the peer group. Peer pressure becomes a more significant force than family relationships. The adolescent has feelings of ambivalence and frequently will test both limits and capabilities.

Drugs or alcohol can be used by adolescents to help overcome inadequate feelings, to feel a part of the peer group and to get good feelings when "high." Typically, the adolescent withdraws from age appropriate activities because the heavy substance use interferes with the acquisition of skills and task achievement related to performance in general. When adolescents attempt to abstain, they often find themselves lagging behind peers in social, academic and athletic skills. Difficulty concentrating, recalling information and interacting with others is made worse by the anxiety related to falling behind peers in achievement levels. Adolescents choose a "negative identity" because it is so difficult to fit in with their contemporaries who have developed competence in age-related skills.

It is not possible to separate drug and alcohol problems among adolescents. Evaluation of substance abusers illustrates the ease with which one drug may be substituted for another when the drug of choice is not available. Generally, once a problem with alcohol or another drug arises, there is an increased vulnerability to substance dependence problems of all kinds.

Case Study Background

Tom, a 16-year-old male, was admitted to the adolescent unit of a drug and alcohol recovery program. The precipitating events that led to his admission were his repetitive tardiness from school, being suspended twice for fighting and smoking marijuana, and decreased academic performance. In addition, he had been charged with driving while intoxicated (DWI) approximately four months before ad-

mission. When the school authorities confronted him with these incidents, Tom admitted to drinking and smoking marijuana heavily and feeling out of control. He requested help in dealing with his problems.

During an intake assessment for the program, Tom and his parents were interviewed and the following information was gathered. Tom was the oldest of three children and had a younger brother and sister. He lived in a small city and his family was middle class. His parents separated one year ago but had not divorced. The children lived with their mother but saw their father regularly. Tom's mother was a licensed practical nurse who worked full time on rotating shifts in a local hospital. His father was an alcoholic but had been abstinent for the past nine months. Tom reported that his mother was the disciplinarian in the family, and that "they got along fine." In addition, he stated that he and his father got along but had difficulties in the past when his father had been drinking. The mother expressed some concern over Tom's legal and academic problems, deteriorating interactions with the family and changing behavior. She stated that Tom used to be a good student, dependable and helpful around the house. Currently, he was staying out all night, involved with a "bad bunch" and wanting to sleep all day.

Tom started drinking at the age of 13 years with heavy use over the past two years. His substance of choice was beer, although he would drink anything available, and he smoked marijuana. He had tried some other drugs but did not continue them because of unavailability, expense or dislike. He drank three nights per week, primarily weekends, and drank more when on vacation. He had one arrest for driving while intoxicated at which time his blood alcohol content was 0.12, which is over the legal limit in most states. Tom had experienced the following: loss of control, increased tolerance, increased preoccupation, sneaking drinks, gulping drinks and three blackouts. His withdrawal symptoms included restlessness, loss of appetite, difficulty sleeping and agitation. He had not attempted suicide, although he reported having thoughts of suicide at the time his parents separated.

Evaluation

In conjunction with group therapy, individual counseling, family therapy and educational sessions, Tom was referred to occupational therapy for evaluation as part of his treatment program on the unit. This decision was made at a multidisciplinary treatment planning meeting.

Appointments were arranged by the certified occupational therapy assistant (COTA) for all new referrals to the department. At the time appointments were scheduled for Tom, the COTA provided him with a brief introduction to occupational therapy services.

Before the evaluation, Tom's medical record was reviewed to gather any pertinent data. The occupational therapy evaluation consisted of a questionnaire requesting demographic information; an educational, work, leisure and social history; and time clock figures representing an average school day and nonschool day before his admission to the program. An example of this form is shown in Figure 9-1. After Tom completed the questionnaire, he was interviewed by the occupational therapist. The interview focused on the information contained on the questionnaire. In addition to conducting the interview with Tom, the OTR made preliminary observations and assessed the data.

Interview results included the following information:

- *Educational history*: Tom was a junior in high school; therefore, his occupational role was as a student. His grade average was "C," which had consistently decreased over the past year. He was failing two courses.
- *Work history*: He had a part-time job at a department store loading and unloading merchandise and had worked there for a year. There had been no noticeable change in his work performance, and no one at work had spoken to him about his drinking or marijuana use.
- *Leisure history*: Tom's leisure activities consisted of partying, chasing girls, auto repair and going to movies. At school, he had been involved in the history and language clubs, the debate team and varsity football but had dropped all extracurricular activities except football.
- *Social history*: Tom was fairly popular and had a number of school friends; however, he had fewer friends than the previous year. Five or six of Toms's friends also used alcohol and drugs. Tom stated that he had liked how he looked and was pleased with his potential and accomplishments before becoming heavily involved with alcohol and marijuana. He thought other people saw him as "nice and fun to be with." He disliked his shyness, difficulty talking with girls and his loss of self-confidence. Tom indicated he would like to be more responsible, to resume some of his former activities, and to cut back on his alcohol and marijuana use.
- *Time utilization history*: Tom's time clocks demonstrated a lack of balance between school, work, leisure, self-care, rest and sleep activities. After he dropped some of his extracurricular activities, and began to stay out all night, the time for sleep and constructive leisure were identified as primary problem areas.

The interview also included behavioral observations of Tom's social skills, his reactions to questions asked, his insight into the ways that substance dependence had interrupted his life-style, his ability to make decisions and his self-concept.

Tom appeared somewhat unsure of himself because he had difficulty answering some questions and maintaining eye contact. His social skills were appropriate during the interview, although Tom expressed that this was a problem for him in other social situations. His insight into how substance dependence had caused him problems in his daily living functioning demonstrated that he lacked the initiative to follow through with plans. Tom understood that his substance dependence had caused problems, but he had not made a commitment to totally stop substance use. He was cooperative during the interview and agreed to full participation in the occupational therapy program.

Treatment Planning

When the evaluation was completed, the OTR met with the COTA to discuss the results. Together they developed the following treatment plan based on contributing input and observations that both had gathered during the evaluation.

Goal Achievement

Tom was unclear about what he wanted but knew that he had potential to succeed. He was easily influenced by his peers. In addition, he had difficulty making a commitment and directing his attention and behavior to long-term goals.

The following treatment outcomes were identified:

1. Complete a task utilizing the problem-solving approach.
2. Establish a set of personal goals and an action plan for achievement of those goals.
3. Develop a life plan for use after discharge which does not include drugs or alcohol.

Time Management

Tom became easily distracted when he was involved with school and extracurricular activities. He stated that he got bored, but on further questioning, he indicated that he was feeling overwhelmed. This feeling was related to his inability to recall facts and to follow directions.

The following treatment outcome was identified: Develop a time management plan that includes a balance of school, work, leisure, self-care, rest, and sleep activities and provides for need satisfaction.

Self-Concept

Tom expressed some discontentment about himself because he was not able to stand up for his beliefs, because he was shy when talking to girls, and because he had lost confidence in himself.

The following treatment outcomes were identified:

1. Identify realistic, personal strengths and weaknesses.
2. Demonstrate increased assertiveness, communication and socialization skills.

Emphasis on age-appropriate skills was the basis of the treatment outcomes. These skills were required to facilitate accomplishment of developmental tasks.

Before implementing treatment, the COTA discussed the plan with Tom. The discussion centered on the problems identified from the evaluation, treatment outcomes for resolution, and the occupational therapy media and methods that would be used to reach the treatment outcomes.

Treatment Implementation

Based on treatment outcomes identified with Tom and an analysis of activities, the following occupational therapy media and sequence of activities were outlined.

Art and Craft Activity

A variety of activities were identified that would meet the specific outcomes for treatment. The activities had to require goal setting, organization, and time management and provide a success experience to help bolster Tom's self-concept. He was allowed to choose an activity from the identified list. This choice afforded him an opportunity for active participation in the treatment process and would motivate and commit him to the task. Tom ultimately chose a woodworking project; however, he did have difficulty making the choice. To complete the project, he was required to utilize the **problem-solving** method with guidance from the occupational therapy staff. The problem solving method had the following components: establishing a goal, step-by-step planning and goal completion.

Tom's goal was to complete a wooden cassette tape holder for his personal use. He was required to draw plans for the holder, sequence the steps, select the materials, have the plans approved and learn about tools and materials before beginning work on his project. Actual work on the tape holder included cutting out pieces of wood, sanding them, constructing the holder, staining and finishing it.

Three 50-minute treatment sessions were conducted weekly in the occupational therapy clinic. In addition, Tom was evaluated during each session for the following factors:
1. Attention span
2. Frustration tolerance
3. Motivation
4. Decision/choice making
5. Ability to make commitment and follow through
6. Ability to follow written and verbal instructions
7. Ability to handle constructive criticism and act accordingly
8. Ability to delay gratification

The COTA was responsible for monitoring safety and supervising Tom while he completed his project in the clinic. The assistant also ensured that Tom used the steps in the problem solving method. Tom was given assistance as needed, and the COTA provided him with feedback on the progress of his project.

Life Skills Development Group

Life skills development groups, geared to specific problem areas, were scheduled on the unit. Each patient was specifically placed in a group on the basis of identified treatment outcomes. When patients were scheduled for a group, they were required to make a commitment to attend sessions, participate in the tasks and activities for that group, and provide input to other group members. The life skills development groups were task-oriented, structured learning groups designed for skill acquisition through hands-on experience.

The OTR and the COTA co-facilitated the life skills development groups. Both were responsible for ensuring that the patients remained task oriented, and they elicited feedback from the patients about the topic of discussion.

Tom was scheduled for three of the life skills groups and attended the one-hour sessions on alternate days from clinical activities. In the goal setting group, Tom identified short-term and long-term education, work, leisure and social goals for himself. He initially wrote out his goals, shared them with the group, and received feedback from other group members. Once the goals were finalized, he established priorities, developed a plan of action, and shared his plan with the group. The final portion of the goal setting process addressed barriers to goal achievement and solutions to those barriers.

The final phase of this life skills development group was to develop a life plan for use after discharge. The primary purpose was to help Tom formally identify how he would manage a substance-free life-style to include goals and a plan of action as well as a support system. His support system included an Alcoholics Anonymous (AA) sponsor, AA involvement, Narcotics Anonymous (NA) involvement, **Antabuse** (a drug used in alcoholism treatment), if needed, and a plan for time utilization. Alateen involvement was also recommended in order for Tom to understand how his father's alcoholism had affected him. His plan would coincide with the aftercare plan, which he developed as part of his treatment regimen.

Time Management Group

The second group in which Tom participated focused on time management. Tom brought his time clocks (see Figure 9-2.) to the group and shared them with the other members. He described problem areas and received feedback. After the problem areas had been identified, Tom indicated those over which he had control, such as leisure time, and those over which he did not have control, such as school time. He evaluated his clocks to see if there was an imbalance between school, work, leisure, self-care, rest and sleep

NAME : _____

AGE: _____   SEX: male / female

HOME ADDRESS: _____

EDUCATIONAL BACKGROUND:

Current School Grade: _____

Average Grades in School: _____

Are you failing any subjects: _____

If yes, what? _____

Favorite Subjects: _____

Least Favorite Subjects: _____

Do you get along with others at school? _____

Explain: _____

WORK BACKGROUND:

Current Paid Job(s): _____

What other jobs have you had in the past? _____

Have you ever been fired from a job? _____

If yes, why? _____

What do/did you like about these jobs? _____
_____

What do/did you dislike about these jobs? _____
_____

Do you get along with others at work? _____
_____

Explain: _____
_____

What are your responsibilities at home? _____
_____

Do you get along with others at home? _____
_____

Explain: _____
_____

Figure 9-1. *Occupational Therapy Questionnaire.*

LEISURE INTERESTS

What do you do to have fun? _____

_____

List the activities that you usually do by yourself: _____

_____

List the activities you usually do with others: _____

_____

What clubs, organizations, and/or teams do you participate in? _____

_____

What do you usually do while you are drinking/drugging? _____

_____

How would you describe your skills or talents? _____

_____

List those activities you used to participate in but no longer do: _____

_____

SOCIAL HISTORY

Do you find it easy to do the following:

Socialize with others? _____ Why or why not? _____

_____

Start conversations? _____ Why or why not? _____

_____

Share feelings and emotions? _____ Why or why not? _____

_____

Describe your strongest points: _____

_____

Describe your weakest points: _____

_____

What are your goals for the future? _____

_____

What effects have your drinking/drugging had on your life? _____

_____

Do you want to get and stay sober? _____

_____

What would you like to change about yourself or your life to help you be sober? _____

_____

Figure 9-1. *(Continued)*

Fill in time clocks for a typical day by blocking (pie shapes) activities.

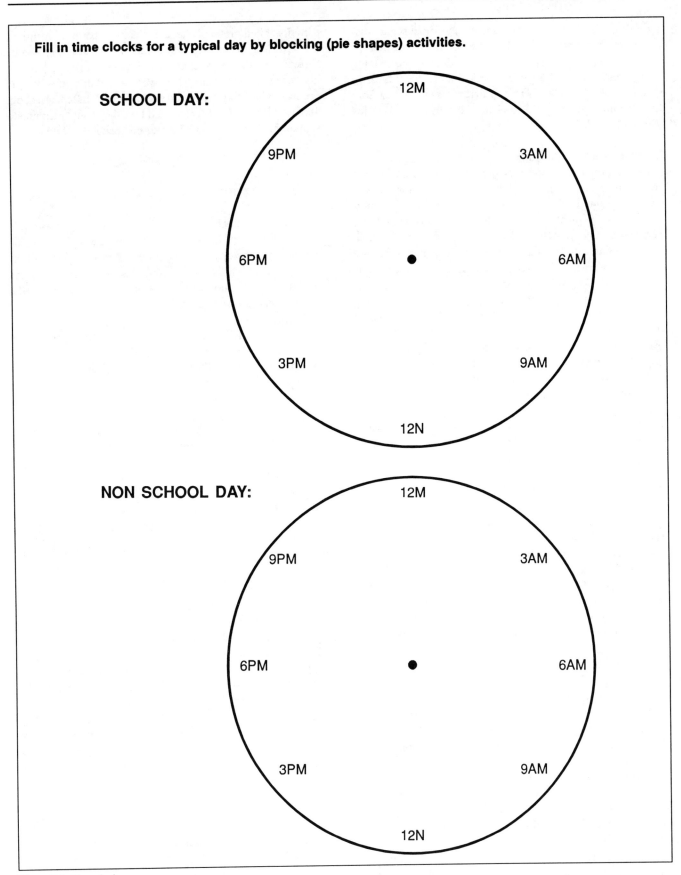

Figure 9-2. *Time clocks.*

activities. He then developed ideal time clocks and discussed the barriers that were keeping him from reaching his ideal clocks, such as peer pressure. Methods for taking charge and overcoming those barriers were identified. In addition, occupational therapy provided assistance to Tom for planning unstructured time on the unit as well as his weekend passes.

Communication Skills

In the communication skills group, Tom completed a **communication worksheet,** which included his own definition of communication, identifying what types of communication were the most difficult or easiest and why, identifying personal barriers to communication, such as no eye contact, and communication enhancers, such as maintaining eye contact. He practiced assertiveness and socialization skills through role playing situations with peers in areas such as initiating and ending conversations, and he received group feedback. After these exercises, Tom identified his personal strengths and weaknesses in writing and shared them with the group. Ways to capitalize on his strengths and to improve his weaknesses were also established.

Tom maintained a "feelings" journal throughout his treatment program. The journal included feelings that Tom experienced throughout the day and identification of the situations that were associated with those feelings. By using the journal, Tom had a cumulative source of information to share with staff and other patients.

Recreational Activities

Tom participated in structured, physical activities, which included volleyball, bowling, and softball, twice a week. The intent of these activities was to promote physical fitness, to encourage involvement in team sports and games, to provide socialization and to explore alternative leisure activities. The COTA was responsible for supervising the physical activities and was also an active participant. Observations related to leadership qualities, competitiveness, cooperativeness and sportsmanship were reported to the occupational therapist during their daily meetings.

Recreational outings were scheduled twice a month and Tom participated regularly. These outings were designed to help patients learn how to have fun without the use of substances. The outings also provided the opportunity for patients to identify community resources to use as alternatives to substance dependence and allowed for appropriate socialization. Examples of these outings included picnics at local parks, attending concerts and sports events and visiting museums. Supervision of the recreational outings was rotated among the unit staff members. The occupational therapy assistant arranged for the logistical support, which included general scheduling, transportation and lunches.

Family involvement was an integral part of this drug and alcohol rehabilitation program. Tom's family was invited to participate in a group picnic and a familiy sports competition, and Tom was pleased that they agreed to come to these events. Efforts were also made to include his parents in other facets of his treatment program. They were scheduled to visit the occupational therapy clinic on several occasions to learn about Tom's treatment, his progress and how they could continue to support his life plan when he returned home.

Documentation and Reporting

Throughout treatment, the COTA and OTR were role models for Tom in terms of appropriate behavior. The occupational therapy assistant made behavioral observations of Tom's work skills, motivation, frustration tolerance, and level of socialization and reported these findings to the occupational therapist at their daily meetings.

Occupational therapy services were documented in Tom's treatment record. The OTR was responsible for recording the results of the evaluation and treatment plan in Tom's medical record. In addition, these findings were discussed at the multidisciplinary treatment planning conferences, which both the COTA and the OTR attended. Continued observations were made and regular reevaluations were completed and noted as they occurred. Program changes were based on Tom's participation and progress in treatment. Progress was discussed with Tom and his family, documented in the record by the OTR and the COTA, and shared with the multidisciplinary team. Treatment outcomes formulated by occupational therapy and the other disciplines were integrated into an overall treatment program for Tom that was a part of his treatment record.

Program Discontinuation

The drug and alcohol recovery program that provided Tom's treatment was a six-week, closed-ended program. Approximately two weeks before discharge, the COTA scheduled a meeting with Tom and his parents. The occupational therapist conducted this meeting and discussed the family's role in supporting Tom in his life plan. One of the specific ways they could help in carrying out his aftercare was to become involved in **Alanon,** a support group for family members and significant others involved with alcoholics.

Acknowledgments

The authors wish to thank the following individuals and groups for their invaluable assistance in providing information, content and editorial suggestions: Elaine Diepenbrock,

MEd, CCMHC, at Second Mile House; the Occupational Therapy Section staff members at Walter Reed Army Medical Center; and the Tri-Service Alcoholism Recovery Department at the Bethesda Naval Hospital.

Editor's Note

The authors have prepared this chapter in their private capacity. No official support or endorsement by the US Army or the Department of Defense is intended or should be inferred.

Related Learning Activities

1. Using a medical dictionary or encyclopedia, look up the following terms and describe their characteristics: hallucinations, delirium tremens, convulsions and delusions.

2. Describe some of the stereotypes about a substance abuser's character.

3. Visit a high school in your area and find out what programs are used to teach students about substance abuse and dependence.

4. Attend an Alcoholics Anonymous, Alanon or Narcotics Anonymous group meeting; summarize their goals and methods of treatment.

5. Discuss two problems present in substance dependence that are not present in substance abuse.

References

1. American Psychiatric Association: *Diagnostic and Statistical Mannual of Mental Disorders*, Third Edition-Revised. Washington, DC, American Psychiatric Association, 1987.

The Adolescent With Burns

Bonnie E. Hoffman, MOT, OTR
MAJ Karen Cozean, OTR

Introduction

Each year approximately 1% of the population sustains a burn in the United States.[11] Of this percentage, over 1 million people need medical care for their burns.[2] Patients with severe burns require lengthy hospital stays. Their life is abruptly changed and learning to live with pain, disfigurement and loss requires tremendous personal strength, as well as support from the patient's family. Sixty-six percent of burn injuries occur in home accidents.[3] Careless cigarette smoking, electrical problems and cooking equipment account for most sources of fires.[4]

Burns can occur by electrical, chemical, or thermal (steam, flame, hot liquids or metals) contact.[5] The depth and size of the burn determines the outcome for wound care, risk of infection, need for grafting, occurrence of hypertrophic scarring and functional performance of the patient.[6]

The size of the burn must be calculated to determine medical care. A patient's fluid needs for resuscitation, risk for infection, and chances for survival depend on calculations of total body surface area (TBSA) and depth of the burn. The percentage of the body surface area is usually estimated by the *Rule of Nines*. The body is divided into surface areas of 9%. For example, each arm is 9%; each leg is 18%; the anterior trunk and the posterior trunk are each 18%; the head and neck are 9%; and the perineum and genitalia are 1%. For children younger than 15 years, the percentages differ. Their legs represent less surface area and the head and neck more; however, proportions change as children grow.[6]

KEY CONCEPTS

Types and characteristics of burns	Edema control
Assessment tools and activities	Analysis and adaptation of activity
Goal development	Splinting
Therapeutic positioning	Skin grafting

ESSENTIAL VOCABULARY

First-degree burn

Second-degree burn

Exudate

Esthetic

Third-degree burn

Debridement

Triage

Diuresis

Conformers

Hypertrophic

Venous stasis

Maceration

Burn depth is measured by degrees or skin thickness. A **first-degree burn** involves only the epidermis or superficial layer of the skin. Healing time is usually three to six days. The skin surface is bright red, painful and sensitive. Sunburn is an example of a first-degree burn.[7]

A **second-degree burn** or partial-thickness burn involves the epidermis and part of the dermis. It may be superficial or deep depending on the damage. The skin of a superficial second-degree burn is moist, red and very painful and has blisters with copious **exudate** (a fluid that has escaped from the blood vessels).[8] The healing time is usually three weeks. A deep, partial thickness burn is not as sensitive, but is still **esthetic** (has sensation) and is darker red, pale or colorless and less pliable. Skin grafting may be necessary because healing is slow, often accompanied by hypertrophic scarring. This type of burn can convert to a full-thickness burn if it becomes infected. Some causes of partial-thickness burns are flash, such as electrical or flammable substance, brief exposure to flames or scalds.[7]

A full-thickness or **third-degree burn** destroys the epidermis and dermis layers of the skin. Deeper tissue and bone can be destroyed as well. The skin is dry and "leathery" in texture, and it may be charred black, yellow-brown or translucent. Superficial veins may be thrombosed just beneath the skin surface. The skin is not painful because the superficial cutaneous nerves are destroyed. The cause of injury can be flame, immersion scalds, chemicals or electricity. Skin grafting is necessary to gain wound closure.[7]

Case Study Background

Bill, a 17-year-old high school student, was burned when he lit a cigarette after filling a lawn mower with gasoline in the garage. He was able to put out the flames by rolling against the wall. Bill sustained a 26% TBSA burn with 21% being second-degree to the head, chest, forearms, hands, thighs and legs. Five percent were third-degree burns involving the neck, right forearm and the dorsum of both hands. He was taken by ambulance to the hospital emergency room and admitted to the burn unit.

During the next two months, the patient underwent three surgical procedures for split-thickness autografting: 1) 14 days after injury for both arms and hands, 2) two and one-half weeks later for thighs and right arm, and 3) three weeks later for spots on left thigh and right arm.

Occupational therapy personnel began following the patient immediately after admission for prevention of contractures and deformity, preservation/restoration of functional abilities and assistance with psychological adjustment. When the patient was discharged from the hospital two and one-half months after injury, the supervising occupational therapist referred him to another outpatient

clinic where he was treated for one additional year until he had returned to full functional independence and the burn scar had matured. Throughout treatment in this clinic, the occupational therapist and the entry-level COTA collaborated closely because of the possible complications that can occur with a patient who has major burns.

Because the long-range effects of the burn injury can delay recovery and result in loss of function, it was the policy of the burn unit to refer the patient to each service of the burn team for screening and evaluation. This referral was automatic by the physician in charge. As a result, Bill's treatment was initiated within three hours after arrival.

Assessment

Screening

Before the patient arrived on the unit, initial screening was accomplished by reviewing the emergency room referral information. This review indicated that the upper extremities were involved. While the patient was undergoing initial **debridement** (removal of all foreign material and contaminated or devitalized tissue),[8] the admission note was reviewed for historical data such as respiratory tract injury, fractures, and preexisting disease that might affect edema or infection. The "Rule of Nines" figures and Lund-Browder tables were reviewed as soon as they were available for location, percentage and degree of burn.

The injury was sustained from a flash burn. Because he was wearing only cut-off shorts, Bill had burns to most of the exposed anterior areas except his face, which he had protected with his hands. No complications were noted. The fact that both hands had areas of third-degree burns placed Bill in the critical burn category, and was an indication for occupational therapy intervention to preserve/restore his functional ability. Figure 10-1 shows the extent of the burns.

Evaluation

Evaluation was more detailed with each stage of recovery. Initial evaluation was performed at the patient's bedside after **triage**, a procedure used to determine priority of medical needs and proper place of treatment.[8] While he was appropriate in his response to questions, his medication was "wearing off" and the pain made concentration difficult. Hence, interaction was informal and brief, and data gathering was mostly observational. Although initial information gathering was structured by the occupational therapy interview form, it was accomplished in short segments scheduled between medical, nursing and therapy procedures and was further limited by the patient's pain at the time.

The patient had an intravenous line in his left arm for resuscitation fluids. There were also two heat lamps in use to help him maintain body temperature. He did not have a

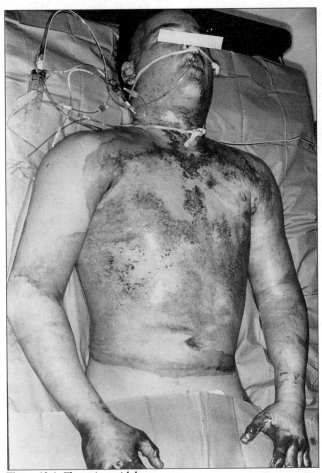

Figure 10-1. *The patient with burns.*

catheter. His hips and knees were flexed while arms were adducted and elbows flexed. Edema was noted, particularly in the upper extremities. Third-degree burns were present on the anterior neck and chest (1.5% TBSA), posterior right forearm (1.5%), dorsum of both wrists and hands (1% each); and there was questionable third-degree injury of the right index and long fingers. While shoulder and elbow joints had been spared, his chest burn extended close to the right axillary region, and the right forearm burn wrapped radially to within 0.5 inch of the antecubital fossa. Other burn wounds were second degree over muscle belly areas and were clear of joints. This visual assessment was the basis for determining the occupational therapy intervention to reduce edema in the upper extremities and to maintain therapeutic positioning of the upper extremities and neck.

Later, Bill was able to demonstrate to the COTA that he had adequate bed mobility for nursing care and functional grasp for feeding. The physical therapy (PT) evaluation revealed full active range of motion (AROM) of upper and lower extremities except for the right hand, which lacked one finger's breadth of full flexion due to edema. This assessment indicated that the patient had the capacity to

perform other self-care activities such as dressing. However, since this burn unit used the open method of burn treatment, he was not specifically evaluated in this area until his wounds were closed. The open method of treatment involves exposure of the burned area to air, with minimum clothing worn.

From the time of admission, Bill was also observed for psychological adjustment by all staff for effects on his self-concept, his interaction with others (especially family), and his situational coping skills (to treatment in early stages and to resuming former activity/interaction later). Nonverbal signs such as change in affect, decreased activity level and decreased appetite were also monitored and reported to appropriate staff members.

With completion of fluid resuscitation and beginning of **diuresis** (excretion of urine), about 72 hours after admission, Bill passed the critical period and was assessed for the second stage of treatment. During this wound healing period, the OTR and COTA monitored edema and positioning, psychological status, orientation and comprehension on a daily basis. An additional area of emphasis at this stage was the monitoring of AROM and normal movement patterns. Since the physical therapist had reported that Bill was unable to demonstrate full AROM at the beginning of exercise sessions and took some time to stretch out, Bill was evaluated for pregraft splinting to maintain range of motion and normal alignment patterns. As the time for grafting approached, postgrafting splints were discussed with the physician. Because burns on both hands and the right forearm were over or near joints, splints were indicated for immobilization.

The COTA evaluated sensation in noninjured areas using 2-point discrimination and temperature testing, five days after admission and 30 minutes after medication. Because the palms were not involved, responses were within normal limits. As the burn wounds healed, the upper extremities were evaluated for protective sensation using sharp/dull discrimination, temperature and light touch. Bill was found to be hypersensitive. The sensorimotor components of coordination, strength and endurance were evaluated through combined efforts of the OTR, the COTA and the physical therapist. Each morning the occupational and physical therapists met to review the patient's performance of the previous day. Initially, occupational therapy staff observed feeding skills and involvement in self-care to assess coordination, and the physical therapy department worked with the patient in active and active assistance range of motion exercise, observing the motion achieved to avoid infection through reopening of wounds. As endurance increased and wounds closed, the physical therapist could then use a goniometer and dynamometer for objective measurement. It was possible for the COTA to measure hand function objectively using tools such as the Minnesota Rate of Manipulation Tests, the Purdue Pegboard Test and the Bennett Hand Tool Assessment.

Other areas of skill, such as self-care and communication, were also assessed. His ability to perform hygiene and dressing tasks was observed. The COTA gave Bill writing and typing tests to establish a baseline before treatment. Results indicated decrease of fine dexterity and strength of the right upper extremity, which also affected speed on bilateral activities.

Program Planning

Goal Development

The OTR and COTA collaborated in developing treatment goals based on the information gathered through ongoing assessment. The long-range goals of acute care were as follows:

1. Through splinting, positioning and therapeutic activity, contractures and deformity will be prevented to all involved joints by daily occupational therapy intervention. Upon discharge, Bill will have no functional limitations.
2. Through weekly participation in the patient support group, which provides a supportive, accepting treatment environment utilizing puposeful daily activity, Bill will regain self-confidence and return to school.

The short-term goals established for Bill were as follows:

1. The pitting edema in both upper extremities will be eliminated within four days by continuous upper extremity (UE) elevation in slings, AROM, and self-care skills, such as eating. Upper extremity positioning in the slings will be monitored every hour by the staff and Bill will perform AROM exercises two times daily with the therapist and four times daily independently.
2. Bill will be assessed on daily rounds for any signs of skin/joint contracture development and for signs of breakdown. Should a contracture develop, the contracture will be corrected through night splinting. If beginning signs of skin breakdown are observed, a positioning device will be fabricated to eliminate pressure.
3. The occupational therapy staff will provide patient education on occupational therapy procedures and reassure and support Bill's performance in therapy daily. Computer games, board games and role playing with other patients and the COTA will provide psychological support and increase self-esteem upon discharge. Bill will demonstrate functional independence in self-care skills two weeks before discharge.
4. Splints immobilizing the newly grafted right upper extremity will be assessed three times a day by occupational therapy staff to monitor position,

prevent loose dressings and to check with the patient for any signs of skin/joint discomfort. Grafted areas will not move so that healing can occur. Splints will be worn continuously for five days. The first dressing change will occur five days postoperatively.
5. Through daily functional activities, strengthening exercises, splinting and positioning, maintenance of AROM will be maintained or increased.

Techniques and Media

The OTR and COTA again collaborated in selecting techniques and media to achieve treatment goals and in sequencing the activities. Priority during resuscitation was edema reduction, which was accomplished through elevation using slings on intervenous (IV) poles for height adjustment and/or foam wedges to place the extremities higher that the level of the heart as shown in Figures 10-2 and 10-3.

Prevention of tissue trauma was accomplished through daily skin checks of pressure points. Since the patient had good bed mobility and was aware, no problems were noted.

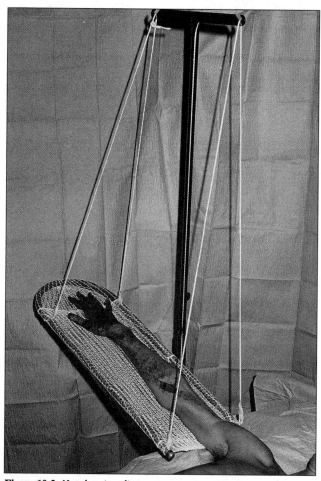

Figure 10-2. *Net elevation sling.*

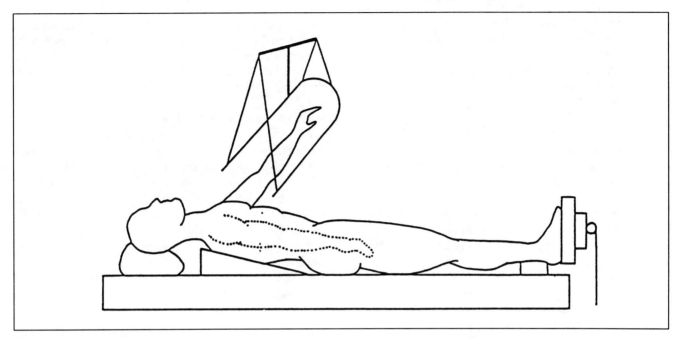

Figure 10-3. *Supine positioning.*

Soft tissue contracture and deformities were prevented or managed through therapeutic positioning opposite the expected deformity, using a foam back wedge to extend the neck, and slings to extend the elbows and abduct the shoulder. The following list details these and other commonly used antideformity positioning techniques and assistive devices.

1. *Head*:
   Position of comfort: rotated to one side.
   Optimum position: neutral.
   Devices: foam head donut; ear donut if side lying.

2. *Anterior Neck*:
   Position of comfort: flexed when burn is symmetric; add a rotational component when burn is asymmetric.
   Optimum position: extension with head in midline and head of bed elevated.
   Devices: foam back wedge, shoulder roll, folded towels, thermoplastic or foam collar with/without conformer inserts.

3. *Shoulder*:
   Position of comfort: adduction often with a slight internal rotation.
   Optimum position: 90-degree abduction and 15- to 20-degree flexion.
   Devices: net arm slings on IV poles, arm troughs, foam axillary wedges, breakfast tables with foam wedges or pillows, and airplane splints.

4. *Elbow*:
   Position of comfort: flexion and pronation
   Optimum position: anterior burn—extension and supination; posterior burn—consider resting in about 10 to 20 degrees of flexion.
   Devices: arm slings on IV poles, thermoplastic extension splints, Tubigrip, conformers/inserts.

5. *Wrist*:
   Position of comfort: flexion often with component deviation.
   Optimum position: 30 to 40 degrees extension (exception is dorsal burns requiring a neutral wrist position).
   Devices: soft rolls, hard cones, thermoplastic cock-up splints.

6. *Hand*:
   Position of comfort: Metacarpophalangeal (MPs) joints flexed to 30 to 40 degrees; proximal interphalangeal joints (PIPs) flexed to 45 degrees; distal interphalangeal joints (DIPs) flexed to 10 degrees.
   Optimum position: MPs in 90 degrees flexion; PIPs and DIPs in full extension.
   Devices: thermoplastic splint in antideformity position (position of advantage) as shown in Figure 10-4, nail traction, web spacers (foam, elastomer), and pressure garments.

7. *Thorax*:
   Position of comfort: flexion.
   Optimum position: prone with healed anterior burns but flat in supine position while still open.
   Devices: Prone—chest foam with diaphragm cut out, head donut, knee donuts; supine—flat or back wedge.

8. *Hip*:

Position of comfort: flexion, abduction and external rotation.

Optimal position: supine, completely flat with neutral rotation and slight abduction.

Devices: foam separators as needed.

9. *Knee*:

Position of comfort: flexion.

Optimum position: extension.

Devices: thermoplastic knee tabs, metal long leg splints; foam heel wedges.

10. *Ankle and Heel*:

Position of comfort: inversion and plantar flexion.

Optimum position: neutral in all planes.

Devices: foot board, foot drop splint, heel wedges, pillows.

During the wound closure phase, the same techniques were used as during resuscitation/critical care but with several additions. Edema reduction was still a concern. The patient was allowed to be out of bed and encouraged to exercise. However, elevation was still used whenever the activity would permit and always when the patient was at rest. The same adjustable IV pole slings were used during the pregrafting phase of care. Foam wedges were used in the postgrafting stage.

Tissue trauma was of concern particularly for splinted areas. Skin was checked every time the splint was removed.

Soft tissue contracture was managed through positioning and static night splinting during this phase. Hands were splinted with maximum flexion of the MPs and full interphalangeal (IP) extension as shown in Figure 10-4. Elbows were extended in slings at night.

Grafts were protected through custom-fitted static splints shown in Figure 10-5. The type of splint was determined by the OTR in collaboration with the physician. They were used continuously until grafts adhered (about five to eight days) and were used as night splints until full hand motion was regained.

Strength and range of motion were maintained through combined occupational and physical therapy efforts. While the physical therapist provided ranging and exercise twice a day, the OTR and the COTA primarily used self-care and leisure activities to achieve range of motion. Particular media for such activities was chosen for ease of cleaning and freedom from irritating materials.

As healing occurred, hypersensitivity was reduced and skin was toughened through patient application of pressure and texture, beginning with lotion massage in the early stage and progressing to having Bill rub various fabrics and the use of desensitization boxes containing different types of substances.

Independence in physical daily living skills was pursued through simulated work situations that included skills necessary for school, such as writing drills, typing drills,

computer use, calculator use and drafting problems, engaged in over gradually increasing periods of time. Psychological support was provided primarily through role playing, discussion and stress management techniques to assist with situational coping.

Analysis and Adaptation of Activity

Bill was a high school senior planning on majoring in engineering at a local college. He was active on the debate team and enjoyed playing the guitar in his spare time. Whenever possible, activities were chosen by the OTR to involve these interests while meeting treatment goals. The COTA was instrumental in modifying and monitoring the use of the activity. Range of motion and strengthening activities included oversized games positioned to require maximum stretch of the upper extremities. Hi-Q, checkers and chess were among Bill's favorites. Pieces were graded from large to small to improve grasp. Strengthening was accomplished by adding Velcro to the board and game pieces, using wrist weights or both. A typewriter, calculator and mazes were used for dexterity; and Bill was encouraged to practice his guitar when on pass. Just before discharge, when the wounds were well healed, he was given macramé and leather lacing, which had been modified with instructions for maximum stretch of shoulder abduction and graded with wrist weights.

Hand and elbow splints as shown in Figure 10-5 were monitored daily for fit and were revised with decreased edema and increased motion until the optimal antideformity position was achieved. Foam positioning devices and neck collars were modified to achieve desired antideformity position. **Conformers** (silastic elastomer inserts, custom molded to provide total contact with scar tissue) were worn under the collars to provide even pressure as **hypertrophic** (increased volume of tissue) scar began to form toward the end of Bill's stay in the hospital.

Discussion of Goals and Methods

While Bill had some difficulty with concentration due to pain during the resuscitation period, he was able to comprehend most of the interaction with the occupational therapy staff. As he improved, both the OTR and COTA reviewed the goals of treatment, the procedures and media to be used and potential complications (eg, edema, graft loss, soft tissue contracture, hypertrophic scarring and deformity). The family was unavailable during the day, so the COTA interacted with them in the evenings to ensure their understanding and support during the treatment program.

The burn team made rounds every morning, and changes in Bill's program plan were discussed for each stage of recovery. The OTR entered the initial evaluation, assessment and program plan in the chart. Progress notes and changes in the plan were documented by either the OTR or COTA after they discussed observations.

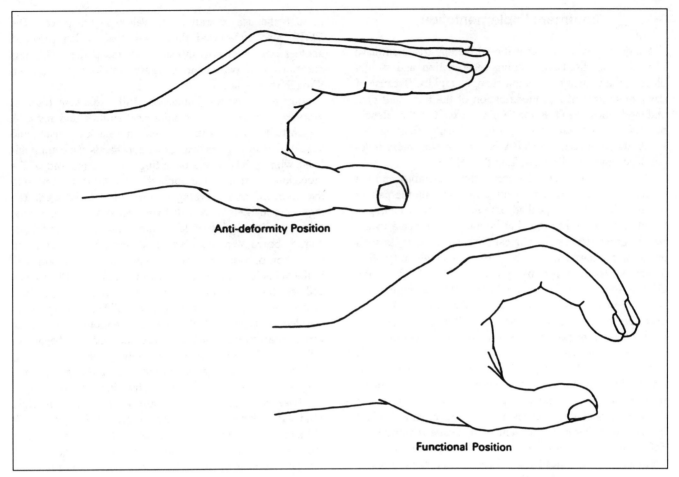

Anti-deformity Position

Functional Position

Figure 10-4. *Hand positions.*

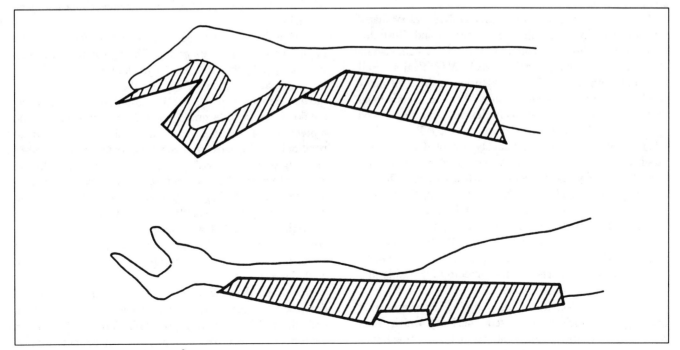

Figure 10-5. *Antideformity splints.*

Treatment Implementation

Many aspects of the occupational therapy treatment have already been discussed. During resuscitation and wound closure, the patient's condition changed rapidly. Because of daily reassessment and modification of the treatment plan and modalities, the OTR and COTA worked together closely to ensure continuity and quality of care. (During the rehabilitative phase, the COTA performed with more independence and less direction from the OTR.)

Throughout treatment the occupational therapist and the assistant both sought to maintain a rapport with the patient to help with psychological adjustment. Bill was encouraged to interact with other individuals and to participate in the patient group, led by the clinical psychiatric nurse, as soon as he was allowed out of bed. He was taught relaxation techniques to aid in controlling pain. Both the OTR and the COTA always explained procedures before beginning and provided verbal reinforcement during the patient's performance. Treatment was timed for about 30 minutes after pain medication, when possible, so as to decrease discomfort and increase compliance.

For the first three days after admission, treatment consisted of patient education to ensure follow through, elevation of his upper extremities to reduce edema, and therapeutic positioning of his arms in abduction and slight horizontal flexion to prevent soft tissue contraction/deformity. Net slings on adjustable IV poles were used. A shoulder roll was placed just below the base of the neck to facilitate neck extension. No pillow was allowed. Bill was checked at least three times a day to ensure proper elevation and positioning.

After diuresis began on the third day, Bill was evaluated for antideformity hand splints as discussed and illustrated previously. On his right hand, he was able to demonstrate about 60% of metacarpophalangeal (MP) flexion. Full proximal interphalangeal (PIP) extension of the right index and long fingers was achieved only when the occupational therapist blocked the MP joints in flexion, indicating a need for night splinting to protect and position the PIP joints. The other splint was worn continuously except during supervised occupational therapy activities and when being exercised by the physical therapist or when bathing. The left hand required only night splinting since it was stiff but still had full AROM. To allow maximum functional use and exercises, the COTA did not apply the splint until bedtime each night. The OTR removed both of Bill's splints each morning before rounds to check for pressure areas and the need for adjustments. Therapeutic antideformity positioning of neck and arms was continued.

Bill was supervised 30 minutes morning and afternoon at board games, such as oversized checkers, which were positioned vertically to achieve stretch of the upper extremities and to discourage neck flexion. Resistance was provided

through the use of weights or Velcro in the pieces. The COTA also supervised these activities, which provided another opportunity to interact with the patient. Bill was encouraged to participate in these activities on his own throughout the day.

Fourteen days after admission, Bill underwent his first grafting procedure on his upper extremities and neck. A 1-inch foam ring was used to maintain neck extension and keep his head aligned. His arms and hands were immobilized with splints in the operating room at the end of the procedure, fabricated and applied by the OTR. On return to the ward, his arms were again elevated and abducted. The legs were also elevated with foam blocks placed under the calves to allow drying of donor sites on the posterior thighs. A foot board was provided for comfort and to assist in prevention of **venous stasis,** a condition where blood flow in the veins is stopped or significantly reduced. Bill was on bed rest for five days until the drying was accomplished. When the patient's arms were immobilized and legs were elevated, occupational therapy intervention consisted of verbal interaction. When daily dressing changes began, an OTR or COTA was on hand to reapply splints.

About eight days after surgery, when the grafts were judged adherent by the physician, all splints were changed to nightwear and the regular program was resumed. The right hand was lacking enough flexion to grasp a fork, so a built up handle was provided. As soon as motor function improved, the handle was discontinued, even though this change made use of the fork less comfortable. Feeding was used to encourage increased active motion through functional activity. Pegs were used for game pieces to encourage making a fist and positioned to require reaching and neck extension.

During the second surgery, 32 days after the injury, the thighs and right arm were grafted. The right elbow was again immobilized by the OTR. Although Bill was on bed rest, his left arm and hand were free, and the COTA was able to provide treatment at the bedside. Since his left hand was nondominant, a plate guard was provided until he became more skilled at feeding. Space was not available for vertical positioning of games, so major emphasis was on forward reaching and strengthening. Pieces were either attached to Velcro or weighted. No weight was used on the arm because the skin was still fragile. A foam neck collar was worn during activity to prevent flexion. Eight days after surgery, the right elbow splint was changed to nightwear. Bill was allowed to walk short distances and be up in a wheelchair. At that point the regular occupational therapy treatment could be resumed.

About 45 days after injury, Bill's neck rotation had decreased, and the grafted area blanched with slight motion, both the result of scarring. The OTR fabricated a silastic conformer and incorporated it into the neck collar to provide even pressure to the scar. This collar was worn continuously except for exercise sessions and bathing. Either the OTR or COTA performed skin checks twice a day to prevent **maceration,** a softening of tissue. An elasticized stockinette was applied to both forearms, and web spacers were applied to the right hand to manage hypertrophic scars, which were beginning to form.

Fifty-three days after injury, Bill underwent his last surgical procedure for spots on his left thigh and right arm. No splints were needed for immobilization. Bed rest lasted four days. Occupational therapy treatment was similar to that provided after the second surgery, but with some additional media since the wounds were now essentially closed. Graded activities included macramé, leather lacing and woodworking for range of motion, strengthening and endurance. Typing and writing drills were given to establish a database and provide treatment in preparation for his return to school. A right hand-based index and ring finger PIP extension splint was fabricated by the COTA and checked by the OTR. It was worn during the day. At night, static finger extension splints were worn. Self-desensitization of healed areas was continued under close supervision by the OTR. The therapist also measured the patient for pressure garments, even though he would be discharged to the outpatient occupational therapy facility by the time the garments arrived.

As discharge approached, the patient expressed more anxiety and concern about his appearance and the reaction of others. Bill was encouraged to verbalize his fears, and the OTR and COTA worked with him in role-playing situations. Before discharge, the COTA assisted the OTR in completing a sensorimotor evaluation and reviewed proper care of the skin and the need to continue a therapeutic home program with Bill and his family.

Program Discontinuation

Inpatient treatment was discontinued with wound closure. Although Bill had done well with treatment goals, rehabilitation was just beginning. Hypertrophic scarring was beginning to form and would not be mature for 12 to 18 months. He was referred to the outpatient clinic with an appointment in one week and a home program for range of motion, sensory reeducation and scar control until he could be assessed by the outpatient facility. The OTR provided the facility with a summary of inpatient treatment to ensure continuity of care.

Conclusion

This case study emphasizes the role of the OTR and COTA in the acute care of patients with major burns.

Primary emphasis is on prevention of deformity, with differences in rehabilitation techniques and media depending on the status of wound healing.

The OTR is responsible for initial screening, evaluation, program coordination and discharge planning. The entry-level COTA will need close supervision until he or she is thoroughly familiar with the antideformity positioning and splinting so essential to functional recovery. Once the COTA has attained a level of expertise with which both the OTR and the COTA feel comfortable, the COTA may function more independently. The COTA is also primarily responsible for patient involvement in therapeutic activity for range of motion and situational coping. Because of the many physiological and psychologic complications that the acutely burned patient experiences during this period, the roles of the OTR and the COTA may not always be clearly differentiated and may frequently overlap and complement each other. It is essential that the COTA and the OTR work closely as a team to achieve maximum results in treating acutely burned patients.

Editor's Note

The authors have written this chapter in their private capacity. No official support or endorsement by the US Department of the Army or the Department of Defense is intended or should be inferred.

Related Learning Activities

1. Use a medical text to gain additional information about the following: 1) split-thickness autografting, including indications for its use, complications and precautions; 2) Rule of Nines and Lund-Browder Tables; and 3) the causes and importance of controlling edema.

2. Using additional readings, outline the appropriate occupational therapy goals for a burn patient at each of the following stages: initial, before grafting, after grafting, healing and convalescent-rehabilitative.

3. Make a chart of 20 different craft activities and indicate the following: 1) the equipment and supplies needed for each; 2) the suitability for patients in bed; 3) those that thorough cleaning after each use is not possible; and 4) those that involve or do not involve irritating substances.

4. Outline how you would adapt and grade leather lacing to promote increasing range of motion and strength.

5. Discuss with peers why OTR and COTA roles are not always clearly defined and differentiated when working with the acutely burned patient.

References

1. Maley MP: Burn education and prevention. In Hummel RP (Ed): *Clinical Burn Therapy.* Boston, John Wright PPSG, Inc, 1982, p. 509.

2. National Center for Health Statisitics: *Persons Injured and Disability by Detailing Type and Class of Accident, United States 1971-1972.* Rockville, Maryland, US Department of Health, Education, and Welfare, 1976.

3. O'Shaughnessy EJ: Burns. In Stolov WC, Clowers MR (Eds): *Handbook of Severe Disability.* Washington, DC, US Department of Education and Rehabilitation Services, 1981, pp. 409-418.

4. Clarke F, Ottoson P: Fire death scenarios and fire safety planning. *NFPA Fire Journal* May, 1976, p 22.

5. Dyer C: Burn care in the emergent period. *J Emerg Nurs* 6:9, 1980.

6. Pruitt BA: The burn patient: Initial care. *Curr Probl Surg* 16(4):11-12, 1979.

7. Pruitt BA, Goodwin CW: *Early Care of the Injured Patient*, 4th Edition. New York, American College of Surgeons, 1990, pp. 288-290.

8. Miller BF, Keane CB: *Encylopedia and Dictionary of Medicine, Nursing, and Allied Health*, 5th Edition. Philadelphia, WB Saunders, 1992.

Part C
YOUNG ADULTHOOD

The Young Adult With a Spinal Injury

The Young Adult With Schizophrenia

The Young Adult With Rheumatoid Arthritis

The Young Adult With a Spinal Injury

M. Laurita Fike, MA, OTR
Melanie Wiener, OTR
Sherise Darlak, COTA

Introduction

Spinal cord injury (SCI) is a devastating and usually permanent condition, which results in paralysis and loss of sensation below the site of the **lesion** (a pathologic or traumatic interruption in tissue or loss of function). Approximately 8,000 people receive spinal cord injuries each year, and it is estimated that 500,000 people with SCI now live in the United States.

The most common cause of spinal cord injuries is trauma, frequently as a result of motor vehicle accidents, but also from diving and other sports injuries, industrial accidents, falls and gunshot or knife wounds. Other causes include hemorrage or thrombosis of the spinal cord arteries and diseases such as multiple sclerosis, amyotrophic lateral sclerosis and tumors. Some children born with **meningomyelocele**, a condition in which the spinal cord fails to close and connect properly, will have the same problems as those associated with traumatic spinal cord injury.

Immediately after SCI, there is a period of shock, in which all reflex activity below the level of the lesion is obliterated; the patient is completely flaccid, with loss of bowel and bladder control. This period lasts from a few hours to as long as three months. This period is followed by a period of hyperactive spinal reflexes, which result in spasticity, usually in the legs, but sometimes in the arms and hands as well. If the spinal cord injury was fully transected, the injury is considered complete, and the person will remain fully paralyzed and insensate below the level of injury. In many cases, however, the spinal cord is only partially damaged and the injury is incomplete; thus, some degree of motor or sensory return may be expected.

ESSENTIAL VOCABULARY

Lesion

Meningomyelocele

Orthostatic hypotension

Blood pressure monitoring

Autonomic dysreflexia

Decubitus ulcers

Heterotopic ossification

Bradycardia

Tenodesis

Quad pegs

Self-catheterization

KEY CONCEPTS

Characteristics of spinal cord injury

Sitting program

Assessment components/activities

Patient and therapist goals

Adaptive equipment

Intervention activities

Community reintegration

In addition to loss of movement and sensation, people with spinal cord injuries may also have other complications. The most common injury occurs at C5-C6, and slightly more than 50% of SCI results in quadriplegia. Sixteen percent of injuries are very high, at the C-1 to C-6 level. Quadriplegics and some high paraplegics have a decreased vital capacity because of decreased lung expansion; they have decreased ability to cough and are susceptible to upper respiratory infections. Their endurance and energy levels are low. People with spinal cord injury may also experience **orthostatic hypotension** (rapid fall in blood pressure when assuming an upright position), resulting in fainting or blackouts because of pooling of blood in the abdomen. The most dangerous problem associated with spinal cord injuries of T-4 and above is **autonomic dysreflexia**. This condition is a high increase in blood pressure, usually due to distension or infection of the bladder and is considered a medical emergency which can be fatal if not treated promptly.[1]

A major problem associated with the long-term effects of SCI is skin breakdown, or **decubitus ulcers** (bed sores or pressure sores, often over a bony prominence). Pressure on the skin of the buttocks, thighs, knees and/or heels may be unrelieved because the person with a spinal cord injury is insensate and sometimes unable to shift weight in bed or in a wheelchair. Healing of decubitus ulcers may take months and sometimes requires surgery. If the ulcers become infected, the condition can be life-threatening. Other long-term problems include osteoporosis of disuse, in which calcium is lost from the long bones of the legs, making them fragile and susceptible to pathologic fractures, and **heterotopic ossification**, in which osseous material is deposited at the knee, hip, elbow or shoulder, leading to bony contractures and decreased range of motion.

The major goal for all rehabilitation specialists is to educate people with spinal cord injuries about their condition, related problems and therapeutic options, so that they may resume control of their lives. In occupational therapy, people with SCI participate in learning new ways to perform or direct their self-care, choose and acquire adapted equipment, explore vocational and recreational options, and begin reintegrating into the community.

Case Study Background

Nancy was 25 years old when she sustained a C-6 fracture (incomplete) of the spinal cord after a 20-foot fall from a balcony. She was originally admitted to an acute care trauma center where she was placed in Gardner Wells tongs with traction for 27 days. Surgery was not indicated. Following traction, she was placed in a SOMI brace (Figure 11-1) during the day and a Philadelphia collar at night (Figure 11-2). The patient's hospitalization at the acute care center was uncomplicated except for one instance of **bradycardia** (slowness of the heartbeat) five days after admission, which resolved spontaneously. Her bladder was managed with intermittent catheterization every four hours. Oral laxatives and suppositories were used for bowel management. Nancy received occupational and physical therapy daily, consisting of range of motion and strengthening exercises for her arms and limited training in activities of daily living. Two months after her accident, she was transferred from the acute care hospital to a rehabilitation facility that specializes in the treatment of the spinal injured

On the day of Nancy's admission to the rehabilitation facility, the occupational therapy department received the standard referral from the physician requesting occupational therapy evaluation and treatment; referral to occupational therapy is a routine order for all patients. The physician stated on the referral that the patient's neck was stable enough for the patient to sit, using only a soft collar as a brace for her neck and head. The occupational therapy (OT) unit supervisor assigned the patient to two staff members who worked as partners, one of whom was a registered occupational therapist (OTR) and the other a certified occupational therapy assistant (COTA). After the OTR and the COTA jointly reviewed the referral and decided which partner would conduct specified portions of the initial assessment to determine the patient's needs in occupational therapy.

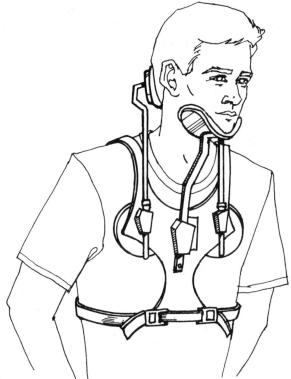

Figure 11-1. *SOMI brace. Adapted from Arthritis: Rational Therapy and Rehabilitation by R.L. Swezey, p. 89, with permission of W.B. Saunders Co., Philadelphia, PA, 1978.*

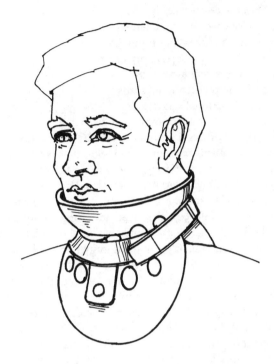

Figure 11-2. *Philadelphia collar. Adapted from Arthritis: Rational Therapy and Rehabilitation by R.L. Swezey, p.88, with permission of W.B. Saunders Co., Philadelphia, PA, 1978.*

Before meeting the patient for the first time, both partners read the medical chart to obtain pertinent background information. The OTR and the COTA were able to coordinate their time so that they could introduce themselves to the patient together. They explained that they were from the OT department and briefly described their respective roles as partners. They informed Nancy that the COTA would begin the screening process later that day.

First, however, as is customary at the facility, the partners needed to start the patient on a "sitting program," so that she could come to the OT clinic for assessment in a wheelchair. Arrangements for the sitting program were made during this first visit to the patient's room.

In order for the patient to sit, the OTR had to complete a skin assessment to determine if there were any contraindications to sitting, such as red skin areas, skin breakdown, abrasions, bruises or a rash. The OTR examined Nancy's skin on her lower back and buttocks, paying particular attention to the seating surface and bony prominences. The OTR then filled out the skin assessment form, noting any scars, pressure areas or potential problem areas. Copies of the form were filed in both the medical chart and the occupational therapy chart. The patient was noted to have a mild rash due to incontinence, but this was not severe enough to prevent limited sitting.

The COTA then measured the patient's hip width to determine the size of the wheelchair and seat cushion that the patient needed. She consulted with her partner to choose the type of wheelchair and seat cushion most appropriate for Nancy. Because the patient had reported dizziness and light-headedness when sitting at the acute care hospital, the partners decided that a full reclining back wheelchair was indicated and that the patient should initially sit at a 60-degree angle.

The patient also reported minimum sensation in the buttocks area, and a special seat cushion was recommended. This foam cushion had been tested during research at the facility, and was thought to provide adequate pressure distribution for most spinal injured patients.

The COTA obtained an appropriate wheelchair and cushion and arranged for the nursing staff to dress and help transfer the patient to the chair. Before transferring the patient to the wheelchair for the first time, the COTA took Nancy's blood pressure while she lay supine in bed, again immediately after the transfer, and then every five minutes until the pressure readings were stable. Significant drops in blood pressure can indicate **orthostatic hypotension,** a common problem for people with new spinal injuries, and the patient can suffer light-headedness or even loss of consciousness. The patient's blood pressure was 120/80, a normal baseline. During the initial sitting session, pressure dropped to 105/70, but stabilized at 110/75. The COTA continued to monitor Nancy's blood pressure every 10 minutes during the first session.

Assessment

Initial Screening

The occupational therapy initial assessment at the rehabilitation facility routinely consists of six parts:

1. Database
2. Areas of occupational performance affected
3. Occupational performance components affected
4. History/comments
5. Patient's initial goals
6. Occupational therapy intervention

According to departmental policy, the COTA could be responsible for completing parts 1, 2, 4, and 5; the OTR was required to complete parts 3 and 6.

Part 1, the database, included the patient's name, age, sex, date of referral, date of onset, type of admission, hospital room number, diagnosis and/or medical involvement, and a description of life roles and occupations before onset. A separate section was used to record initial grip and prehension strength readings. The COTA obtained some of the information from the medical record and interviewed the patient to gather other pertinent facts. Nancy was noted to have a cervical spinal injury at the sixth vertebra, which resulted in involvement of all four extremities, and loss of bowel and bladder control. Her life roles and occupations before her injury had included being a daughter and sister and an employee of a geophysical company, for whom she did computer-related work. She had no grip or prehension in her right (dominant) hand; in her left hand she had one pound of gross grip strength and approximately one pound of prehension strength in lateral prehension, three-point prehension, and single-point prehension.

For Nancy, the areas of her occupational performance affected by her injury included self-care, work, education and leisure. Through interview and observation, the COTA noted that the patient was unable to perform the following specific activities independently: eating, dressing, personal hygiene, functional mobility, homemaking, vocational and avocational.

Pertinent history obtained through an interview noted that Nancy had attended college in New York and had graduated with a degree in mathematics. Her parents lived near New York City. Nancy had three brothers, one of whom was a hemophiliac, while another had Down syndrome. She enjoyed traveling and skiing, and had also participated in team sports. Nancy had recently planned to return to work in New York; her accident occurred at her going-away party.

The COTA also discussed Nancy's initial goals with her, as these would suggest Nancy's level of understanding and acceptance of her condition as well as provide the COTA with direction to encourage the patient's active participation in rehabilitation. Nancy stated that her goals were "to walk out of the hospital" and to get back the use of her hands.

After these areas of the initial assessment were completed, the COTA showed Nancy a document entitled "Patient and Therapist Goals." These goals are based on the facility's many years of experience in working with spinal injured persons and are considered "generic" goals; more individualized goals are developed as each patient proceeds through the rehabilitation process. By discussing these "generic" goals with Nancy, the COTA was helping Nancy understand the role of occupational therapy as well as helping her explore a broader range of goals. Columns are provided for both the staff member and the patient so that each may place a check by those goals that, for example, the COTA felt applied to Nancy and those that Nancy would like to accomplish. The COTA and Nancy jointly identified the following goals:

- Increase sitting time
- Increase upper extremity muscle strength
- Increase upper extremity joint range of motion
- Improve trunk balance
- Increase endurance
- Improve independent living skills
- Evaluate and train in use of orthotic equipment if needed
- Improve coordination and dexterity

- Order necessary equipment
- Explore avocational interests
- Pursue homemaking training
- Participate in adaptive driver's training
- Improve safety awareness
- Evaluate prevocational skills
- Take functional out-trips
- Follow a home program upon discharge

At the end of the first session, the COTA's portion of the initial assessment was completed. She then explained the "sitting program" to Nancy, emphasizing the need to build up general sitting tolerance, but also skin tolerance, by gradually increasing the amount of time spent sitting. The COTA also reinforced the need to change position frequently, by doing weight shifts which the patient would learn in physical therapy, and the importance of checking the skin for pressure areas. After returning Nancy to her room, the COTA waited 20 minutes and then checked Nancy's skin. She appeared to tolerate the session well.

The next day the OTR transported Nancy to the clinic for parts 3 and 4 of the initial assessment. The occupational performance components affected by her spinal injury included muscle strength, range of motion, muscle tone, coordination, pain, sensation, body image, self-esteem, family relationships, and ability or need for adaptive techniques and equipment. While interviewing and observing the patient, the OTR used the session to advance the sitting angle of the chair to 70 degrees, which the patient tolerated well.

Program Planning

After the patient was returned to her room, the OTR completed part 6 of the initial assessment, occupational therapy intervention, which consists of writing the formal plan for Nancy's occupational therapy (OT) program. The OTR reviewed the "Patient and Therapist Goals" completed by the patient and the COTA, as well as the information recorded by the COTA on the other parts of the assessment form. The OTR also discussed with the COTA her impressions and concerns about Nancy.

Although Nancy was always to be treated as a unique individual, based on the occupational therapy initial assessment of her rehabilitation needs, she appeared able to benefit from a typical OT spinal injury program at this facility.

Short-Term Goals

The OTR specified the following short-term goals, which were to be completed within one week:

- Complete manual muscle test (MMT).
- Complete sensory evaluation.
- Complete evaluation of personal independence (EPI).

- Begin hand skills assessment.
- Increase progressive sitting to 1.5 hours three times per day at a 90-degree angle.

Each week new short-term goals would be established, based on Nancy's progress.

Long-Term Goals

The OTR listed the following long-term goals, which were expected to be completed by discharge:

- Patient will be independent in feeding, dressing and personal hygiene.
- Patient will sit eight to ten hours daily with no problems.
- Patient will acquire basic homemaking skills.
- Patient will acquire necessary equipment.
- Patient will explore vocational and leisure interests.
- Patient will receive home program before discharge.

These long-term goals are also typical for persons with spinal injuries at the facility, and experience over time has demonstrated that most patients like Nancy will be able to meet these goals during their hospitalization. The OTR and COTA discussed the goals and how they would be individualized for Nancy. Then both staff members signed and dated the initial assessment form.

Continued Evaluation

For the rest of the week, while beginning treatment to achieve her goals, Nancy also continued to receive specific tests of her functions. These evaluations provided the baseline information from which her progress could be measured. These same evaluations would be repeated periodically throughout her hospital stay and immediately before discharge and the results compared with these initial findings.

First, the OTR completed the MMT and the sensory evaluation, and found that the patient differed from the picture of a "complete" C-6 spinal injured person because she retained voluntary bilateral elbow extension, wrist flexion and left wrist and finger motion. Her left arm was significantly stronger than her right arm. Nancy's sensation was tested to the T-12 dermatome level for pain, light touch, pressure, temperature and proprioception. In general, Nancy had intact sensation to the C-6 level, impaired sensation to the T-12 level, and no sensation below that level. Proprioception was intact throughout, except for her fingers on the right hand, which appeared to have no sensation. The OTR felt that sensation appeared better on the left side than on the right, as Nancy responded more quickly when touched on the left.

That same day the COTA completed the EPI, (Evaluation of Personal Independence), a test of physical daily living skills standardized at the facility. The COTA observed while Nancy performed a variety of tasks that included communication, eating, hygiene and dressing. Then she graded Nancy's performance from "1" to "4" with "4" being the most independent, on specific activities within each daily living skill area. In general, Nancy was independent in most areas of communication, required minimum to moderate assistance in eating and sink hygiene, and required maximum assistance for all other areas. Her total score on the EPI was 520 of a possible 748.

The next day the COTA completed a hand skills assessment, which had also been standardized at the facility. Nancy was unable to perform any bilateral hand skills subtests and scored below 65% of the score for able-bodied persons on unilateral skills. The COTA also noted that on the unilateral tests Nancy stabilized herself by using one arm to hold onto the arm rest of the wheelchair, which suggested that poor trunk balance might be interfering with Nancy's ability to use both hands together.

This completed the evaluation process for the patient. Baseline data had been obtained in the areas of personal independence, muscle strength, hand skills, coordination and sensation. Goals had been established jointly with Nancy, and long-range goals for occupational therapy had been decided. Short-term goals would be updated weekly.

The partners decided that the COTA would take primary responsibility for Nancy's day-to-day occupational therapy program, with the OTR monitoring treatment by discussing the patient's progress with the COTA on a weekly basis, giving feedback and suggestions when appropriate, reading the COTA's progress notes before weekly interdisciplinary team rounds, and by treating Nancy on the COTA's days off.

Treatment Implementation

Week One

Although evaluation was the primary focus during Nancy's first week at the facility, treatment had also been in progress. The COTA ensured that the patient could continue the level of self-care she had attained in the acute care hospital by providing a universal cuff for different utensils. This cuff holds items to the palm of the hand and is useful when people have little or no grasping strength. Nancy used the cuff on her left hand initially, inserting her toothbrush, comb and eating utensils. The COTA then made arrangements with other staff for these items to remain within Nancy's reach so that she could maintain the highest possible level of independence. The universal cuff is shown in Figure 11-3.

The COTA also began passive range of motion to prevent joint stiffness in the right (nonmoving) hand and fingers. Although some facilities use resting or static orthoses to prevent joint deformity and to facilitate development of functional hand positions, at this facility range of motion exercises and training with dynamic orthoses are used,

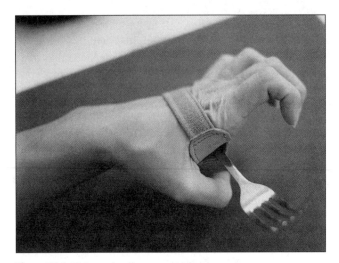

Figure 11-3. *Universal cuff.*

unless the patient exhibits spasticity, which was not a problem for Nancy. The COTA instructed Nancy in the performance of short, upper extremity exercises to prevent deconditioning, including the use of one-half and one pound wrist weights during simple active range of motion exercises.

In general, the patient tolerated her first week of treatment well, although she became light-headed on several occasions when first transferred into her wheelchair. This problem was easily corrected by tilting the chair back for one minute at the beginning of each sitting session.

Week Two

By week two, the COTA felt that Nancy was ready to begin a more active therapy program. She asked her if she would like to try a ceramic project to improve her strength, endurance, and coordination. Nancy agreed and selected a small decorative ceramic box that had been previously poured using a mold. Nancy used a cleaning tool with a 1.5 inch foam built-up handle to help increase the grip strength in her left hand. Moving the tool in a variety of planes to clean the seams of the box facilitated coordination. In addition, the COTA placed a one-pound wrist weight on Nancy's right arm and a 2-pound weight on the left. Lifting her left arm to clean the seams and using her right to stabilize the ceramic project helped promote bilateral strength and endurance. She was able to work on this project for 20 minutes, but required several rest periods.

The COTA taught Nancy to perform self-range of motion by using her more functional left hand to move her right wrist and fingers. She also cautioned her against hyperextension of her fingers while her wrist was also extended, as this could excessively stretch the flexor tendons and prevent an effective **tenodesis** (wrist extension and finger flexion) grasp.

Although her left hand was more functional, Nancy

elected first to attempt writing using her dominant right hand. Because Nancy had no functional pinch in her right hand, the COTA applied a wrist-driven flexor hinge (reciprocal) orthosis from the department's supply of training equipment as shown in Figure 11-5. Follow-up studies at this facility indicate that early introduction to and training with such devices result in greater retention and use after discharge. The greatest long-term use of reciprocal orthoses is by patients whose activities involve fine motor coordination, such as extensive writing and drawing. If a reciprocal orthoses proved practical for Nancy, a customized device could be made for her by the Orthotics Department. Because such devices are quite expensive, the need for them must be carefully evaluated. By extending her wrist, Nancy could bring her fingers and thumb together to form a tripod pinch to hold a pencil. The COTA used simple connect-the-dot and tracing exercises to promote coordination, but Nancy had great difficulty with these, often overshooting the dots and drawing extremely crooked lines. Her attempt to write her name was barely legible. Aluminum tooling using a mold and a built-up tool handle was introduced to assist in developing writing skills (Figure 11-4).

The COTA worked with Nancy to establish adequate telephone skills since she received and made many calls. No special equipment was needed because the COTA was able to suggest adaptive ways of lifting and holding the phone using both hands in place of a single handed palmar grasp. In self-feeding, Nancy continued to use her left, nondominant hand, but she progressed from a universal cuff to utensils with 1.5-inch built-up handles. This change gave her more control and she spilled less food. She was also pleased that she was eating more "normally." The COTA also worked with her on using a knife and Nancy was able to cut soft foods, but still needed assistance with tougher items. Nancy began using the built-up handles for her personal hygiene as well.

Since Nancy was tolerating sitting at 90 degrees, the

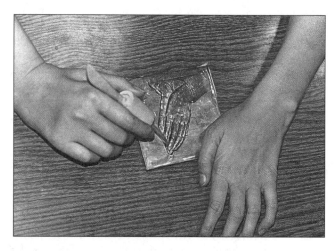

Figure 11-4. *Aluminum tooling mold and built-up tool.*

COTA decided to procure an upright wheelchair with **quad pegs** (projections from the metal push-rim) on the wheels, so that Nancy could begin moving herself around the building. This modification would give her more independence, and the pushing would also increase her upper extremity strength and overall endurance. During this second week, however, Nancy was able to push only 10 to 12 feet before tiring. At the same time her sitting time was advanced to 2.5 hours, three times a day, with no skin problems.

Week Three

At the beginning of week three, the COTA used the dynamometer to re-evaluate Nancy's grip strength on the left. She found it had increased from 1 to 2.5 pounds. There was still no measurable grip in the right hand. The patient continued to clean her ceramic piece and work on metal tooling, but the COTA cut the diameter of the built-up handles from 1.5 inches to .5 inch. Wrist weight cuffs were continued, and the COTA used positioning of the ceramic project to force Nancy to reach higher and farther. Nancy was also able to increase the length of time she could work to 25 minutes.

Since the patient enjoyed playing cards and board games, the COTA suggested that these would be good activities to help promote right-hand dexterity and coordination. She demonstrated tenodesis grasp for Nancy, and had her use this technique to pick up game pieces and cards with her right hand. Nancy would alternate use of her hands as the right hand was not as functional as the left and tended to fatigue easily.

Nancy practiced propelling her wheelchair each day and was able to push herself approximately 20 feet. Her sitting time was advanced to 3.5 hours, twice a day, with the additional option of 2 evening hours, which brought her total sitting time to an average of 8 hours a day. She continued to have no skin problems, and she took the responsibility for asking her nurse or therapist to assist her in performing weight shifts to reduce skin pressure.

Nancy expressed the desire to attempt writing with her left hand. With a .5 inch foam handle on a pencil, she was able to write more quickly and legibly than with the reciprocal orthosis on her right hand (Figure 11-5). She decided she would like to practice with her left hand before deciding which hand she preferred to use for writing.

During this week, as she did every week, the COTA spent time discussing the physical and psychological value of each activity used in therapy with Nancy. This approach appeared to help Nancy continue to be motivated and to actively participate in her rehabilitation program.

As she did each week of the patient's stay, the COTA wrote a narrative progress note for the medical record. The OTR reviewed this note and discussed the patient's progress with the COTA. The OTR then reported on Nancy's progress at interdisciplinary rounds.

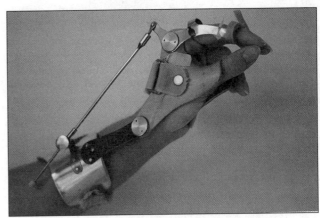

Figure 11-5. *Wrist-driven flexor hinge (reciprocal) orthosis.*

Week Four

At the end of the first month of her hospitalization, Nancy appeared to have gained significant upper body strength and endurance. On the left, her lateral pinch had increased to two pounds and her grip strength to three pounds. The COTA and Nancy decided to remove the foam handles from her self-care equipment and her ceramic brush and metal tool. Nancy expressed pleasure that she no longer required such equipment.

The patient continued to paint her ceramic project, with wrist weights increased by one pound each, and positioning of her project was also increased. She was independent in moving her wheelchair around the clinic to get her ceramic materials and to set up her work area, as well as putting her supplies away at the end of therapy. Her handwriting improved gradually. Although awkward, she could write legibly within the lines of standard notebook paper using her left hand. She decided that she preferred to use her left hand to write, because she did not like how the orthosis looked on her right hand. At this point Nancy was using her left hand for most activities of daily living skills, and in effect had switched dominance. This adjustment was supported by both the COTA and the OTR, as Nancy continued to have functional gains in her left hand, with very slow progress on the right.

Because Nancy's coordination and her endurance had improved, the COTA suggested that she try typing with a typing stick in a universal cuff on her right hand. Nancy was able to use isolated finger movements to type with her left hand. She was familiar with the keyboard and typed 45 words per minute (wpm) before her injury. On her initial typing trial she typed 9 wpm with two to three errors per line. By the end of the week she was able to type 12 wpm with very few errors.

The COTA provided Nancy with minimally resistive therapy putty and reviewed a hand exercise program with her. Because Nancy was very motivated, the COTA granted her request to do the exercises in her room during her free time. At the same time, the COTA cautioned the patient to exercise for only ten minutes twice a day initially, to avoid overtiring the muscles.

Because Nancy's trunk balance had improved and she was maneuvering her wheelchair safely and with greater endurance, the COTA suggested that she try out a lightweight model, as many patients with spinal injury, and younger people in particular, tend to prefer the sport-type wheelchairs for their permanent use. The chair selected did not have pegs on the wheel rims, so Nancy used push mitts to create friction and give her a stronger push. Using the lighter chair, she was able to push herself 60 feet with only two rest intervals.

Nancy's sitting time was increased to four hours twice daily, with an optional two hours in the evening. This sitting schedule continued for the duration of her hospitalization, and she continued to tolerate the schedule well, with no skin problems.

Week Five

It is customary at this facility for the interdisciplinary team to hold a discharge planning meeting with the patient and family members if possible. Nancy's mother came from New York to participate in the meeting and she remained for one week to become familiar with her daughter's rehabilitation program. The COTA met with the OTR before the meeting to discuss the occupational therapy goals that should be accomplished before discharge. The COTA attended the meeting and reported that in addition to the activities Nancy had been doing, she could become independent in dressing, simple meal preparation and in operating a personal computer. The COTA also said that Nancy would need to order a wheelchair, as she was currently using one from the OT equipment pool. Nursing staff felt the patient should be independent in **self-catheterization** (independent management of bladder drainage system) and turning and positioning in bed, and the physical therapist stated Nancy should become independent in all transfers to and from her wheelchair.

Nancy agreed with all the goals except ordering the wheelchair. Although the physician had been explicit with her regarding her prognosis (there had been no motor return in the legs), Nancy still believed she might walk, and did not want to buy a permanent wheelchair. She also said that although friends had invited her to live with them upon discharge, she would prefer to get her own apartment. The team felt that her daily activities would take more time and energy than they had before her injury and recommended that she consider having a roommate who could provide some assistance. The social worker planned to help Nancy work out suitable living arrangements before discharge.

Nancy's mother attended occupational therapy sessions with her daughter for the remainder of the week and participated in educational experiences, such as learning to assist her daughter with transfers in physical therapy and getting items set up for Nancy's self-care.

During this week, the COTA had to change Nancy's therapy time so that Nancy could work on self-catheterization on a regular basis. The COTA was aware that at some facilities occupational therapy personnel also work with the patient on self-catheterization and bowel programs, particularly in the development of the necessary hand skills and acquisition of adaptive equipment. At this facility, however, the "Cath Team," a group of specially trained technicians supervised by the nursing department, was responsible for assisting Nancy in meeting this goal. Other team members, such as the COTA, primarily provided support, reinforcement and schedule changes as needed.

The patient noticed movement in her right hand and discussed this with the COTA, who reported it to the OTR. The OTR re-evaluated Nancy's active range of motion and muscle strength on her right, and found that she had gained approximately 10 degrees of active range in metacarpophalangeal (MCP) flexion and extension. Nancy was extremely anxious to work toward strengthening the muscles of her right hand and had to be cautioned not to overwork her muscles. The OTR agreed to re-evaluate her range every day until discharge to detect any improvement.

Because Nancy's previous and future vocational interests had involved computers, she was interested in learning to operate the microcomputer in the OT department and began the first of the three training tapes. She was able to insert and remove the disk from the disk drive and to operate the tape recorder independently.

With the COTA's help, Nancy began working on upper body dressing and learned to put on a pullover shirt. She needed minimum assistance getting a front-buttoned shirt around her back while in her wheelchair, but could button it independently.

During this week the COTA obtained permission for Nancy to have a day pass to begin community reintegration. She arranged for Nancy to go to the zoo and to a restaurant with her mother. Nancy reported that it was "very therapeutic" for her to be away from the hospital setting for the first time in three months. She pushed her wheelchair for a short period around the zoo and became very tired, but she was proud that she was able to feed herself at the restaurant, needing only to have her steak cut. She also said this day pass helped her to realize how tired she would become if she did everything for herself when she was discharged. Nancy and the COTA discussed other out-trips she could take, either with an OT group, or with Therapeutic Recreation, and Nancy signed up for an outside activity the following week.

Week Six

Nancy continued to make steady gains. Her left hand grip increased to six pounds. She had nearly 20 degrees of active range at the MCPs of her right hand. Her handwriting was more legible, and she was typing 16 wpm. She was independent in wheelchair mobility throughout the day. In addition to the computer, she worked on a calculator and an adding machine. These were machines she had used on the job in the past and anticipated using them in the future, so the COTA recommended working on hand function and vocational goals at the same time. Nancy finished her ceramic project and gave it to her mother as a going-away present. The COTA suggested copper tooling for a new activity, advising Nancy that it would be more difficult because of the resistance of the copper, but that it would help Nancy work toward greater strength and coordination. Nancy chose a mold of a skier, one of her favorite sports, and worked with a three-pound weight on her right wrist and a four-pound weight on her left.

With the COTA's help, Nancy practiced putting on her pants, using the elevating head of her bed to assist her to a sitting position and to maintain trunk stability. However, she was unable to roll side to side to pull the trousers over her hips. Although rolling could be worked on in OT, it was being worked on as a major exercise in physical therapy, so the COTA and Nancy agreed to address other occupational therapy goals and to continue to work on dressing the next week.

Week Seven

This week Nancy was able to roll side to side and learned to pull her pants over her hips. It took her 45 minutes to dress herself.

Nancy had finished the copper tooling and was ready to sand the mounting board. The COTA set up the table so that sanding could be performed on an inclined plane to work for increased strength and endurance. Because of the increased difficulty of this task, the wrist weights were removed.

During this week, Nancy worked on meal preparation and was able to complete a simple meal of a salad and grilled cheese sandwich. She needed no special equipment, but did use adaptive techniques for holding and stabilizing cooking utensils. The COTA reviewed energy-saving techniques, such as placing frequently used items within easy reach. Modifying a regular kitchen to make it wheelchair accessible was discussed in detail. The COTA also talked with Nancy about safety precautions, especially the possibility of burns and cuts on the hands and arms due to diminished sensation.

Nancy's right hand active range had increased significantly, and she was now able to use utensils with a 2-inch foam handle. She was able to alternate hands for eating and for other self-care activities, which seemed to reduce her fatigue as well as provide additional exercise to the right hand.

Nancy was still not psychologically ready to order a permanent wheelchair. In view of her impending discharge, the COTA arranged to order a rental wheelchair for Nancy.

Week Eight

During the final week of Nancy's hospitalization, the focus was on refining her skills, completing discharge evaluations, and providing a home program.

Nancy was able to dress herself in 30 minutes, except for her shoes and socks, which she was still not strong enough to put on. The COTA completed a final EPI, and a discharge hand skills assessment. Nancy had a score of 690 out of a possible 748 on the EPI, as compared with 520 at admission. Her hand skills scores increased by 20% in both hands.

The OTR completed a discharge evaluation of muscle strength and sensation. Nancy had gained an average of one half of a muscle grade in her upper extremities in all but the thumb and interphalangeal movements of her right hand. Her sensation appeared to be intact to the C-7 level. All of the discharge evaluations indicated that Nancy had made significant progress during her admission.

Nancy completed her copper tooling project and the last of the computer training tapes. In addition, she had completed the goals set for her by nursing and physical therapy: She could transfer independently, turn in bed and perform self-catheterization.

Program Discontinuation

After discussing Nancy's progress and discharge status with the OTR, the COTA completed a written home program for Nancy. On Nancy's last day of treatment, the COTA reviewed the home program with her. The program included recommendations for progressive activities that Nancy could perform independently in her apartment to improve her strength, endurance and coordination.

The COTA recommended that Nancy increase her sitting time of four hours by one-half hour per week. Since she only needed to return to bed for a few minutes to perform self-catheterization, she could increase her tolerance to eight to ten hours at a time if she wished. The COTA stressed to Nancy the importance of monitoring her skin for red areas each day and for decreasing her sitting time if red areas appeared. If actual skin breakdown occurred, Nancy was instructed to call her physician without delay.

The COTA also made sure that the rental wheelchair fit well and was adequate for Nancy's needs. The COTA reviewed wheelchair and cushion care, instructing Nancy to contact the rental agent if any problems occurred.

Realizing that Nancy had a very high level of motivation, with the potential for overexertion, the COTA again cautioned her to rest adequately and to exercise only as prescribed on the home programs from physical and occupational therapy. She also discussed with her the ways to ask for help when needed.

Finally, the COTA and Nancy discussed occupational

therapy goals for her readmission in two to three months. Nancy wished to continue working on the "Patient and Therapist Goals," which had been discussed at admission. In particular she wanted to complete the adaptive driving program and learn to drive with hand controls, for which she would need more upper extremity strength (Chapter 26). The COTA also suggested to Nancy that the second admission would be a good time to look at the need for a permanent chair, as the rental was a standard and not a lightweight, and Nancy agreed to discuss it at that time. In addition, Nancy wanted to explore heavier homemaking skills, such as ironing, vacuuming and additional meal preparation. Through her home program she could continue to work on building her strength and endurance as she had done during her hospitalization, and this would help her to be ready for more advanced work on the next admission.

Nancy was discharged to an apartment, with a roommate, two months after her admission to the rehabilitation center.

Related Learning Activities

1. Use a reference text to gather more information about the following items: Gardner Wells tongs, SOMI brace, and Philadelphia collar.

2. Obtain a catalog and learn more about the purpose and cost of the following assistive devices and adaptive equipment: universal cuff, dynamic orthosis, quad pegs, reciprocal orthosis and push mitts.

3. Working with a peer, determine what other craft activities could be used with patients with spinal cord injuries similar to those described in this case.

4. Obtain information about independent living facilities in your community for individuals with handicaps. Determine whether they are suitable for a quadriplegic.

5. Study your home or apartment and list all of the changes that would be necessary to make it wheelchair accessible.

Reference

1. Trombly CA (Ed): *Occupational Therapy for Physical Dysfunction*, 3rd Edition. Baltimore, Williams & Wilkins, 1989.

The Young Adult With Schizophrenia

Patty L. Barnett, COTA/L, ROH
Margaret Drake, PhD, OTR/L ATR

Introduction

Schizophrenia refers to a group of mental disorders characterized by mental deterioration resulting in **delusions** (false beliefs based on incorrect interpretation of reality), **hallucinations** (sensory impressions that have no basis in external stimulation), inappropriate affect, and impairment in social and occupational functioning.[1] There is a deterioration of the person's ability to function at work and in social situations and to perform self-care. Individuals tend to withdraw from the external world because of inability to "cope with reality and the demands of everyday living."[1] Newer findings show that many people with schizophrenia have disturbances of brain circuitry and some measurable physical differences in brain structures, as well as chemical imbalances in the brain.

Case Study Introduction

Owing to legislative reassignment of mental health funds, a state mental hospital was scheduled to close. Five hundred patients had to be relocated. The legislature had reappropriated funds from the hospital budget to be given to the home counties of each of the patients to set up a program for these relocations.

Jefferson County was the home of about 70 of those needing placement, so the county mental health association designed a program requiring the services of occupational therapists (OTRs), occupational therapy assistants (COTAs), social workers and a recreational coordinator. The program was located in a community-based center with an existing sheltered workshop. Adequate space was provided for additional offices and an occupational

---

KEY CONCEPTS

Characteristics of schizophrenia

Community-based programming

Scorable Self-Care Evaluation

Assessment activities

Treatment activities

Vocational rehabilitation

therapy clinic. Occupational therapy treatment took place in the center, where patients were brought by van for a six-hour program, five days a week. Occupational therapy practitioners also provided treatment in the individual group homes whenever necessary (PRN basis).

Case Study Background

Gordon was a resident of one of the new group homes established in Jefferson county when he was referred to the occupational therapy department at the center. A review of his history indicated that he was 27 years old and had resided in an upper middle class suburban community. He was the middle child of three. His mother's career as a concert violinist was stifled for a number of reasons, and she had started to mold Gordon into the musician she had always wanted to be. He had been considered a child protegé. Gordon had willingly participated in this unstated plan by taking lessons and giving recitals until his first schizophrenic episode at age 16. Before his five-year stay in the state hospital, he had numerous admissions at the local acute psychiatric unit of a major hospital and a private psychiatric hospital. At the time of the latter inpatient stay, the psychiatrist recommended that Gordon receive ongoing long-term care. It was thought that this action would also improve the entire family's mental health. Gordon had been diagnosed as schizophrenic from the onset, but the refined diagnosis for admission to the state hospital was schizophrenia, undifferentiated type.

Gordon's childhood had been unremarkable, with the exception of a lack of peer interaction due to his mother's insistence on his violin practice. Teachers reported Gordon was a good student, but expressed concern about his social isolation. No other unusual behaviors were noted until Gordon was in the eleventh grade. At this point, he became very strongly infatuated with his social studies teacher, who gently rebuffed his adolescent advances. His response to this apparent rejection ranged from abusive statements to auditory hallucinations. His "voices" had seemingly been telling him that the teacher was attracted to him and desired more than a student-teacher relationship. His increasingly disturbed behavior after this episode resulted in Gordon's first hospitalization. Subsequent **exacerbations** (increase in severity of the disease or its symptoms)[1] and rehospitalizations were related to hallucinations about a variety of slightly older women.

Gordon's older sister had provided a nurturing, protective and controlling influence. His relationship to her had been similar to the one he had with his mother. His younger brother, an athlete and popular school leader, had maintained a close affiliation with his father, but almost no brotherly relationship with Gordon. Gordon indicated his closest family kinship was with his mother.

The father was a highly respected manager of a local television station. This job frequently required elaborate social gatherings at their home. Gordon's increasingly bizarre behavior had been an embarrassment at these events. The state hospital admission had removed him from his home and community, where his presence had been extremely disruptive to the family's life; however, the family remained supportive and genuinely interested in his receiving appropriate care.

Medication had controlled Gordon's worst symptoms but caused mild **tardive dyskinesia**, an impairment of voluntary movement,[1] which had been controlled by a change to a different type of medication. Over the course of five years in the state hospital, a variety of antipsychotic (neuroleptic) medications were tried before an effective combination of antipsychotic and **anticholinergic drugs** was found. Anticholinergic drugs are used to control the side effects of antipsychotic medications. These side effects may include Parkinsonian symptoms such as rigidity and an immobile face.

Gordon's return to his home community was expected to cause adjustment problems for the family, because his parents, who were approaching retirement, remained in their home but were considering buying a condominium.

A discharge summary from the state hospital that preceded his placement in a group home indicated dysfunction in socialization and self-care skills and absence of work and some prevocational skills. Gordon had his violin in the hospital but was unable to use it often because of the medication's side effects and also because the violin was locked up most of the time.

Assessment

One COTA and one OTR were assigned to work together as a team with a group of the recently relocated patients. The occupational therapy staff at the center established a plan to evaluate each patient on arrival. A multidisciplinary team screened patients before choosing them for treatment at the center. Because of Gordon's past treatment and diagnosis, the following assessments were chosen: the Scoreable Self-Care Evaluation (SSCE)[2] and the Schroeder Block Campbell Adult Psychiatric Sensory Integration Evaluation (SBC).[3] Socialization skills were evaluated informally by the occupational therapy team. The outcomes of these evaluations were the basis of an individual program plan for the sheltered workshop as well as the occupational therapy treatment plan.

The OTR/COTA team's goal was to complete the battery of evaluations within a week after Gordon's first attendance at the center. They both met with the patient the first day to introduce themselves, briefly explain the purposes of the program and to verify their choice of assessments. Both team members had read the discharge summary and family history provided by the state hospital before their first meeting with Gordon.

The most crucial aspect of reentry into the community is self-care; therefore, the Scorable SSCE was initiated first. This structured test was administered by the COTA under the supervision of the OTR. The SSCE scoring record form used to gather this data is shown in Figure 12-1. The results indicated the following information:

Initial Appearance

The first area evaluated was initial appearance. Gordon's clothing was mismatched. His dress slacks did not fit his 6'1" frame. It was obvious he had been wearing his clothes for some time, as they were speckled with spots and stains. His appearance was unkempt with a day's growth of whiskers and recently cut but uncombed hair. His fingernails were dirty, untrimmed and tobaccco-stained. Gordon had the typical schizophrenic "S" posture with slumped shoulders and **lordosis** (forward curvature of the lumbar spine).[1] His arms hung limp at their sides, confirming the occupational therapist's decision to also administer the SBC.[3]

Orientation

Gordon's orientation was appropriate. He knew where he was and he could sign his name and give his birth date. He was unable to accurately give his home address, although he attempted to remember. Gordon's concept of time appeared to be almost absent. He did not wear a watch and stated he hadn't worn one since admission to the state hospital. Gordon reported this had caused him considerable problems since he often had been late for or missed scheduled appointments. He also stated that when his parents had seen him the previous Friday they had promised to buy him a new watch and some new clothes.

Hygiene

On the section of the SSCE addressing hygiene, Gordon was unable to say how often a person should shower, wash one's face and hair, shave, brush teeth or comb hair. He said he had been told when to do these activities in the hospital but indicated he didn't know how often they were required for adequate hygiene.

Communication

When Gordon was given the telephone book and asked to look up emergency numbers, he exhibited unfamiliarity with the process of using the book.

First Aid

He could recall having had a first aid class in high school but could not remember any life-saving and first-aid procedures.

Food Selection

Gordon was presented with a blank menu sheet and asked to plan a balanced meal. He was unable to take the first step by naming a main dish he was accustomed to eating; however, he said he "loved barbequed pork rinds" and noted "they almost never have them" in the snack machine at the hospital.

Household Chores

In organizing household chores such as dishwashing and laundry, Gordon was given cards on which were printed specific tasks to place in the proper sequence. He laid the cards in a row on the table and began to read them aloud, suddenly turning his head to the side to say, "No this is women's work. I'm not going to do this because she just wants me to do it with her so she can be my girlfriend. She is just like my social studies teacher in high school." He then turned to the COTA and said, "You want me to do this so you can touch me!" When the COTA asked who he had just been speaking to, he said the voice had told him not to do women's work and to be beware of women trying to seduce him. Because the patient did not appear excessively agitated, the COTA, speaking in a calm voice, assured Gordon that she did not wish to be his girlfriend and that her goal was to help him. Gordon's facial expression demonstrated that he accepted her statement. In a pleading tone of voice he said, "I really want help. Please help me." The evaluation continued without disruptions.

Safety

In analyzing picture cards for dangerous situations, the patient seemed to be unaware of basic safety practices.

Leisure Pursuits

When asked about leisure pursuits, Gordon was unable to name any except playing the violin and smoking. He continued to discuss his desire to do more with his violin.

Transportation

Gordon was handed a city map and asked to find the street where his parent's home was located. He acted confused and overwhelmed with the task.

Financial Management

Gordon appeared to have no problem with simple monetary transactions; however, he was unfamiliar with the basic check writing procedure, paying bills and budgeting. Gordon knew that the group home operator would manage his money and provide him with an allowance for items such as cigarettes, snacks and grooming supplies.

The next day the OTR and COTA discussed the results of this evaluation. They continued with their planned administration of the SBC. The COTA administered two parts of the assessment: body image and self-reported childhood

	Score		Maximum Possible Points
Personal care	_____	1. Initial appearance	8
	_____	2. Orientation	7
	_____	3. Hygiene	6
	_____	4. Communications	6
	_____	5. First aid	24
	_____	SUBTOTAL	51
Housekeeping	_____	1. Foods selection	26
	_____	2. House chores	10
	_____	3. Safety	6
	_____	4. Laundry	15
	_____	SUBTOTAL	57
Work and leisure	_____	1. Leisure activity	4
	_____	2. Transportation	4
	_____	3. Job seeking	4
	_____	SUBTOTAL	12
Financial management	_____	1. Making correct change	4
	_____	2. Checking	11
	_____	3. Paying personal bills	5
	_____	4. Budgeting	10
	_____	5. Procurement of supplemental income	1
	_____	6. Source of income	6
	_____	SUBTOTAL	37
Total score			157

Patient: _____

Date tested: _____

Figure 12-1. *Scorable Self-Care Evaluation scoring record form. From Clark EN and Peters M. (1984). The Scorable Self-Care Evaluation. Thorofare, NJ: SLACK, Inc.*

history. The OTR interpreted the results of these two sections. Figure 12-2 shows the SBC summary sheet.

Body Image

In the body image section, Gordon was directed to draw a person. He took more than half an hour to draw the minute details of the female figure's clothing and hair. He appeared to be hallucinating during the drawing, turning his head to the side and "talking to the air." The COTA recognized that

the picture was of her.

Childhood History

On the self-reported childhood history, Gordon discussed his family environment. He felt he could never achieve the perfection in music that his mother desired. When asked about other family members who might have had mental illness, Gordon recalled that his mother's brother had been in a mental hospital in the West. He appeared to remember

Client _____

Primary diagnosis _____

Secondary diagnosis _____

Physical diagnosis _____

Medication _____ # ____ ____ ,

Medication _____ # ____ ____ ,

Medication _____ # ____ ____ ,

Age _____ Sex _____ Subject No. _____

DSM III ___ ___ ___ • ___ ___ 1st Test Date ___ / ___ / ___

DSM III ___ ___ ___ • ___ ___ 2st Test Date ___ / ___ / ___

DSM III ___ ___ ___ • ___ ___ 3st Test Date ___ / ___ / ___

Dosage (24 hr. total) ___ ___ ___ ___ ___ mg.

Dosage (24 hr. total) ___ ___ ___ ___ ___ mg.

Dosage (24 hr. total) ___ ___ ___ ___ ___ mg.

(Key: 0 = no problem 1 = slight, 2 = moderate, 3 = severe)

1. Dominance: ____eye, ____hand, ____foot.
2. Posture . . . . _____
3. Neck rotation . . . . _____
4. Gait . . . . _____
5. Hand . . . . _____
6. Grip . . . . rt _____ lft _____
7. Fine motor control . . . . . . rt _____ lft _____
8. Diadochokinesis . . . . _____
9. Finger-thumb opposition . . . . _____
10. Visual pursuits . . . . _____
11. Bilateral coordination—UE . . . . _____
12. Crossing midline . . . . _____
13. Stability—UE . . . . _____

(1 = Mixed dominance)

14. Stability—trunk . . . . _____
15. Classic Romberg . . . . _____
16. Sharpened Romberg, EO EC . . . . _____
17. Overflow movements . . . . _____
18. Neck righting . . . . _____
19. Rolling . . . . _____
20. Asym. tonic neck reflex . . . . _____
21. Sym. tonic neck reflex . . . . _____
22. Tonic labyrinthine reflex . . . . _____
23. Protective extension . . . . _____
24. Seated equilibrium . . . . _____
25. Body image

= Index score ☐

Total score obtained _____

Divide by number of items tested and scored

SUMMARY

I. PHYSICAL ASSESSMENT: ☐   Norm   .50 Min   .90 Mod   1.30 Severe   3.0

_____

_____

_____

_____

II. ABNORMAL MOVEMENTS: ☐   0 Norm   1 Min   3 Mod   5 Severe   14

_____

_____

_____

_____

III. CHILDHOOD HISTORY: ☐   0 Norm   2 Min   6 Mod   10 Severe   29

_____

_____

_____

_____

Therapist's signature _____

Date _____

Figure 12-2. *SBC Adult Psychiatric Sensory Integration Evaluation Summary Sheet. From Schroeder Block Campbell. Schroeder Publishing, Kailya, HI.*

almost nothing about his own physical developmental milestones. He described his childhood as being "normal," with no particular scholastic difficulty. When asked about events related to his own birth, Gordon slumped over and seemed to be using his mother's words and tone of voice when he stated that the birth was painful and the pregnancy had not been planned. He also stated how he had always tried to please his mother to make up for the pain she had endured for him.

Assessment Findings

The COTA and the OTR met and discussed the assessment results the next day. The occupational therapist noted that Gordon appeared to have right-side dominance in eye, hand and foot, which most likely contributed to his proficiency in playing the violin. Lordosis of the lumbar spine was present as were jerky neck movements (probably a result of the residual tardive dyskinesia). He exhibited a shuffling gait and had restricted arm movements; however, fine motor strength and coordination of the hand and wrist seemed quite good. Gordon reported he had done some hand exercises in the hospital, which he had learned from his high school violin teacher.

Gordon did not appear to have any visual problem except when his neck jerked, which occurred when he had intentional movement of the head but not when he was relaxed. This was further evidenced by his successful playing of the violin. Bilateral coordination and crossing the midline tasks were accomplished without difficulty. Gordon exhibited the classic **Romberg's sign**, which is an inability to maintain balance with one's eyes closed while holding the arms out and feet together. His trunk and upper extremity strength were somewhat weak. He exhibited some overflow movements in his mouth and chin when exerting his whole body. His neck postures did not appear to have a reflexive basis. Gordon's **protective extension** (extension of upper extremities in space during specific movement patterns that require anticipating precaution) was adequate, as was his equilibrium while sitting.

In discussing the body image drawing, the OTR immediately recognized the likeness of the COTA despite the primitive nature of the drawing. The COTA described Gordon's bizarre, hallucinatory behavior during the drawing session. When questioned further, the COTA indicated that the patient seemed to have problems relating appropriately to women. She questioned whether he had ever had a normal heterosexual relationship. Recalling the family history, she noted that both the mother and older sister dominated Gordon. The assistant was very aware of Gordon's interest in establishing a relationship with her.

Evaluation of socialization skills was informal. Part of this observation had occurred during the formal evaluations. The inappropriateness of Gordon's behavior toward women was the most obvious problem area. His hallucinations appeared to occur only when in the presence of women. He seemed to have normal friendly relations with the other men in the group. Investigation by the social worker indicated that Gordon had been placed in an all-male group home because of his inappropriate behavior with women.

Based on the assessment results the following summary of Gordon's resources and problems was prepared:
Resources:
- Concerned family
- Musical background
- Good level of cooperation
- Desire for help
- Ability to remember instructions
- Bilateral hand capabilities

Limitations:
- Relating to women
- General socialization
- Grooming and hygiene
- Work readiness skills
- Use of leisure time
- Decreased strength in arms, trunk and lower extremities
- Positive Romberg's sign
- Posture
- Tardive dyskinesia symptoms (neck jerk)

Treatment Planning

The COTA assisted the OTR in treatment planning in a session with Gordon. Basic objectives of the center's programs concerned self-care, readjustment to the community, familiarization with community resources, development of work and prevocational skills, and normalization. Gordon's problem areas fit into the guidelines of service provided by the center. With this in mind, the occupational therapy staff and Gordon considered which of his problems required habilitation and which required rehabilitation. Those that required habilitation could be approached developmentally, accepting Gordon at his current level of functioning and working with him to advance to the next level. Areas requiring habilitation were general socialization, relating to women and physical strength. The areas that required rehabilitation would be approached through reeducation.

Long-Term Goals

The following long-term goals were established with Gordon:
- Develop and demonstrate appropriate socialization behaviors.
- Demonstrate independence in all self-care activities.

- Attain long-term employment.
- Develop improved sensory integration.
- Utilize leisure time effectively.

The COTA and OTR talked with Gordon together during this session because both had administered parts of the evaluations. The team related Gordon's problem areas to things that happened during portions of the evaluations. Gordon concurred with their observations and the goals they selected. These goals would be approached and achieved by working on short-term objectives.

Short-Term Goals

The short-term objectives were set to be accomplished in one week. Each week's progress was to be assessed and recorded, and the short-term objectives would be reevaluated and updated if appropriate. The first set of short-term objectives were chosen so that one related to each long-term goal.

- Participate and interact appropriately in a group of men and women for 30 minutes.
- Arrive daily at center shaved, groomed and appropriately dressed.
- Arrive at scheduled activities on time.
- Participate in at least 15 minutes of moderately strenuous group exercise daily.
- Complete five page leisure checklist.

Social Skills

It was agreed that the social skills area would be addressed in a task group run by the COTA and held in the occupational therapy clinic. The format of the group required each participant to work on the same individual project. Through this activity, Gordon would have opportunities to share tools and supplies and also discuss patterns and techniques. The COTA guided this interaction with the future objective of discussion of individual problems and solutions.

Appearance

In preparation for the "grand opening" of the center, the COTA and OTR had completed a checklist of grooming/ hygiene requirements to aid participants in developing self-care skills. Gordon was given a copy of the list, and the COTA reviewed each item with him. She answered his questions such as how to use a fingernail brush and floss his teeth. The COTA checked his progress daily.

Punctuality

During the goal-setting conference, Gordon was given a written copy of the schedule the OTR/COTA team had developed. They stressed the necessity for punctuality, and Gordon earnestly agreed to observe the following schedule. Occupational therapy practitioners' responsibilities are also noted.

9:00 Grooming—COTA
9:30 Task group—COTA
10:30 Refreshment break
10:45 Individual therapy/leisure counseling—OTR
11:30 Exercise group—shared by COTA and OTR
12:00 Lunch
1:00 Sheltered workshop employment
2:30 Refreshment break
2:45 Sheltered workshop employment
4:00 Time card check with workshop foreman

Exercise

Gordon's exercise program would take place within the context of a structured, daily class of both men and women. This program addressed his strength and balance and provided opportunities for heterosexual socialization. The OTR and COTA conferred each day about which exercises would be emphasized and how to grade them to meet Gordon's individual needs.

Leisure Checklist

Areas included in the leisure checklist were socialization, creative interests, exercises, spectator or audience events, and educational programs. He was instructed to find time to complete this form at the group home.

Treatment Implementation

At the end of the first week of his program, Gordon had successfully accomplished the first short-term objective, although he said it had been difficult not to respond negatively to some of the women in the group and not to answer the voice when it spoke to him. In the early part of the week, the COTA had to remind him when he started responding to the voice and redirect his attention to the group activity. She rewarded him with a large bag of pork rinds at the end of the fifth session. He held the bag and expressed surprise and gratitude appropriately, thanking her for both the gift and her interest. In the following weeks, the group was able to begin to identify individual problems and suggest solutions or possible alternatives. Gordon was an active participant. He had been able to use the grooming/ hygiene checklist successfully. He had received praise and compliments from other staff at the center, which reinforced his efforts. As the weeks progressed, he seemed to develop a real pride in his appearance.

The occupational therapy team shared Gordon's short-term objective on punctuality with the other staff members, who agreed to report any deviations from his schedule to them. The sheltered workshop staff said that Gordon had been late from his break three days the first week. After adjustments were made in his paycheck, this behavior corrected itself, and he had not been late during the last two days of the week. The OTR discussed this problem with Gordon and he agreed to continue working on this objective.

During the first week, there was no measurable change in strength or equilibrium. By the fourth week, Gordon demonstrated increased balance by walking back and forth on the balance beam to the cheers of his fellow exercise classmates. His strength increased very slowly, but the length of time he could endure exercise increased 50% by the fourth week.

Completion of the interest checklist indicated that playing the violin and socializing with others were most important. Successful interactions with the COTA and other female group participants appeared to influence this choice; however, he still had occasional lapses of inappropriate interaction. The OTR, working in collaboration with the night recreation coordinator for the group homes, developed a schedule of cultural events that included free concerts, museum visits and plays. Gordon attended several concerts and participated in a museum outing.

Gordon's renewed involvement with his violin was a slow process. He tried to practice in the group home at night, much to the annoyance of the other residents. The recreation coordinator saw his potential and helped him arrange a time and place that was less disruptive to others. After observing Gordon's level of capability in the sheltered workshop, the OTR made an appointment for him with a vocational rehabilitation agency. Following their assessment of his skills and potential, Gordon was assigned to an apprenticeship where he learned the care and maintenance of stringed instruments.

Program Discontinuation

It is anticipated that Gordon will need a structured environment such as the group home and the mental health center indefinitely. Without close supervision, the staff members thought that he would revert to his previous level of dysfunction. He discontinued the occupational therapy program when all short- and long-term objectives had been accomplished. The coordinator of services at the center continued to follow Gordon's case and agreed to initiate a new occupational therapy referral if Gordon's behavior indicated that former problems were beginning to recur.

At the occupational therapy program discontinuation conference, the social worker noted that Gordon, under the auspices of the vocational rehabilitation agency, was now employed at a part-time job in a local music store. The store allowed him to use a listening studio as a practice room, which eventually led to involvement with other musicians and performances. Part of the process required that he learn to use the public transportation system. The vocational counselor also encouraged Gordon to take a class at the adult night school to complete his high school equivalency tests.

Gordon's interaction with his family increased and improved. His parents were proud of his efforts and accomplishments, both personally and with the violin. As a result, they allowed Gordon to spend increasing amounts of time visiting them in their new condominium. He appeared happy and comfortable living in the structured environment of the group home.

Related Learning Activities

1. Study the Manual for the *Scorable Self-Care Evaluation* and practice administering the test to a peer.

2. Visit a sheltered workshop that provides employment for the mentally ill. Observe at least two workers and describe the types of work they are doing and the goals they are achieving.

3. Obtain literature from a local vocational rehabilitation facility. Determine the services available for the mentally ill.

4. Identify specific activities that could be used to accomplish goals related to Gordon's social skills. (Did you include opportunities for sharing tools and supplies? Were the activities structured to encourage discussion of patterns and methods?)

5. Discuss the roles of a recreation coordinator for group homes with peers and identify areas where the services may overlap with the roles of occupational therapy personnel.

References

1. Miller BF, Keane CB: *Encyclopedia and Dictionary of Medicine, Nursing and Allied Health*, 5th Edition. Philadelphia, WB Saunders, 1992.
2. Clark EN, Peters M: *The Scorable Self-Care Evaluation*. Thorofare, New Jersey, SLACK, Inc., 1990.
3. Van Schroeder C et al: *Schroeder Block Campbell Adult Psychiatric Sensory Integration Evaluation*. Kailua, Hawaii, Schroeder Publishing, 1983.

The Young Adult With Rheumatoid Arthritis

Robin A. Jones, BA, COTA, ROH
Sheryl Kantor Blackman, OTR

Introduction

Arthritis is a condition characterized by inflammation of the joints, with osteoarthritis and rheumatoid arthritis being the two main types. The cause and cure is unknown.[1] **Rheumatoid arthritis (RA)** is a chronic systemic disease that produces inflammatory changes that occur throughout the connective tissues of the body and lead to progressive deforming arthritis. It is classified as a **collagen disease** (pertaining to connective tissue and bones) and results in progressive limitations and deformities that interfere with one's ability to carry out daily activities of living.[2] Pain, inflammation, swelling, redness and structural changes in the affected joints are seen.[3] The onset of rheumatoid arthritis is most common between the ages of 20 years and 40 years of age, affecting men and women equally; however, women are more likely to develop symptoms severe enough to warrant medical intervention. Infants and the elderly may also be affected. The condition tends to be intermittent and one of the most disabling among the rheumatic diseases.[2]

Individuals with this disease are likely to experience psychosocial reactions due to factors such as chronic pain, fatigue, boredom, role losses and immobility. These factors, coupled with distorted body image and loss of independence, may lead to irritability, mood swings and depression.[1]

KEY CONCEPTS

Characteristics of arthritis	Energy conservation
Interdisciplinary home program	Work simplification
Assessment tools and activities	Intervention activities
Exercise program	Adaptive devices
Activity configuration	

ESSENTIAL VOCABULARY

Rheumatoid arthritis

Collagen disease

Boutonnière deformities

Subluxation

Crepitations

Rheumatologist

Joint preservation

Orthoses

Thenar eminence

Exacerbation

Case Study Background

Barbie, a 30-year-old woman, was diagnosed with rheumatoid arthritis at age 25. Predominately, she had bilateral involvement in her elbows, wrists, hands, knees and metatarsal phalangeal joints, with her major complaints being pain and swelling of both hands and feet. Both hands were showing early signs of **boutonnière deformities** (proximal interphalangeal [PIP] flexion with distal interphalangeal [DIP] hyperextension) at the second, third and fourth fingers. Mild volar wrist **subluxations** (partial dislocation of a joint) were present bilaterally; however, they did not interfere with functioning. **Crepitations** (dry, crackling sounds or sensations) at the shoulders and elbows were evident, with the right side greater than the left. A small, subcutaneous nodule, which was frequently irritated, was noted on her right elbow. There were no systemic manifestations; however, Barbie complained of mild dryness in her mouth. The patient's condition was persistent, and it progressively interfered with her daily life-style. She had decreased her activity and had difficulty caring for herself, her husband and their active 3-year-old daughter. Barbie was forced to take sick leave from her job.

The patient's **rheumatologist** (a physician specializing in rheumatic diseases) started her on a bi-monthly treatment of gold therapy; however, she eventually began using prednisone™ because of the persistence of the arthritis and lack of response to nonsteroidal, anti-inflammatory agents.

Barbie continued to see her rheumatologist; however, consultations with another rheumatology specialist were suggested because her status was diminishing so rapidly. The laboratory data and x-ray study reconfirmed the diagnosis of active rheumatoid arthritis with mild structural changes, but no extra-articular disease was clinically evident. The consulting rheumatologist's finding was as follows: "The client was doing poorly and losing ground, despite a reasonable medical program." The physician recommended a thorough review of her disease process with a good multidisciplinary rehabilitation program. Active physical therapy and occupational therapy programs were strongly advised.

Barbie was seen in an outpatient arthritis clinic and was screened by a registered occupational therapist (OTR) and a registered physical therapist (RPT). It was determined that she could benefit from an inpatient stay at the rehabilitation facility. Due to the location of the facility and her responsibilities for her young child, Barbie chose to have her therapy at home. A home interdisciplinary program was initiated including nursing, occupational therapy, physical therapy and social work. The team thought that this was not the ideal course of treatment. Due to the patient's concern for her family, however, it was agreed that therapy would continue in her home. (Home care was covered under the patient's insurance policy.)

Assessment

In assessing management of this patient in the home setting, the OTR and COTA determined that the OTR would be involved in the first visit and at least once a week thereafter. It is important to note, however, that specific patterns of supervision may be mandated by agencies, regulatory bodies and third-party payers.[4] The patient was to be seen for one hour, four times per week, for six weeks. All sessions were approximately one hour, except for the initial evaluation, which was nearly two hours. The OTR was involved on a weekly basis for supervision purposes, and the COTA visited daily.

Before scheduling the initial evaluation, the OTR received the physician's orders for the following services:
- Range of motion evaluation and program
- Joint protection and teaching for all daily living skills: self-care, child care, homemaking, avocation, vocation and community activities
- Work simplification evaluation
- Splinting evaluation
- Adaptive equipment/assistive devices evaluation
- Education to diagnosis, management and therapeutic process

The precautions were to avoid sustained resistance, as the patient's joints were currently inflamed.

Together, the OTR and the COTA began the evaluation process through data collection, with each responsible for specific areas of the evaluation. The OTR was responsible for selecting the evaluation process for assessment of the following skill areas and performance components: activities of daily living, sensorimotor, cognitive and psychological. The OTR evaluated passive range of motion, active range of motion, upper extremity function and musculoskeletal status. The COTA administered a nine-hole peg test, grasp and pinch test (one time only within limits of pain), sharp/dull, two point discrimination, and position sense tests. It should be noted that an entry-level COTA would need direct supervision until he or she displayed competence in the ability to complete these evaluation procedures independently. A joint OTR and COTA assessment for activities of daily living, work activities and leisure activities was conducted.

Barbie was interviewed using a structured format to gather information about her social history and personal goals. The OTR initiated the interview, and the COTA completed the assigned areas. Communication between the OTR and the COTA was ongoing, with data jointly interpreted. The OTR wrote the evaluation documentation and discussed it with the COTA, therapy team and the patient.

Treatment Planning

A treatment plan outline was developed by the occupational therapist, in collaboration with the patient, and given to the assistant. The program planning outline shows the long-term goals established for Barbie, as well as the roles of the OTR and the COTA in relation to the goals (Figure 13-1).

Treatment Implementation

The COTA began occupational therapy treatment after the OTR completed and formally documented the initial evaluation. Under the direction of the occupational therapist, the assistant started an upper extremity exercise program. The OTR wrote a specific routine designed to meet Barbie's range of motion needs as shown in Figure 13-2. The COTA followed this program format, which took approximately ten minutes to complete. It was recommended that Barbie perform this program two to three times a day in addition to her usual self-care routine. The Arthritis Foundation suggests not replacing self-care completion by an exercise program.[5]

Training in principles of joint protection began immediately, as integration of these concepts is often difficult to incorporate into previously learned routines. The following principles of **joint preservation** were utilized:[6]

- Avoid deforming postures
- Avoid deforming forces
- Maintain range of motion
- Maintain muscle strength
- Conserve energy
- Respect pain

In teaching these principles, written tools were used along with demonstration and practice to assure compliance. All areas of activities of daily living, work and leisure were addressed.

Long-Term Goals	Staff Roles	Role Delineation* OTR	COTA
1. Independent use of bilateral orthosis at rest and for functional task completion and good application of joint protection.	1. • Fabricate bilateral resting orthoses. • Fabricate bilateral gauntlet orthoses. • Independent donning and doffing of orthoses. • Help patient tolerate wearing orthoses when performing functional tasks.	X X	X X X X
2. Inependent with and/or without equipment in all self-care, home/child care, and work tasks (individual modification of activities dependent on stage of fluctuating disease process).	2. • Assess need for and provide necessary equipment. • Fabricate assistive devices. • Train in use of equipment and assistive devices. • Independent use of adapted techniques for performance.		X X X X
3. Independent with daily exercise/graded activity program when active and inactive disease is present.	3. • Develop a home exercise/graded activity program that incorporates patient's needs and interests. • Incorporate performance of daily exercise/graded activity into patient's routine.		X X
4. Application of joint protection, work simplification and energy conservation techniques 75% of time with self-care, home/child care, vocational/avocational tasks, and community skills.	4. • Instruct patient in joint preservation techniques. • Monitor and facilitate patient application of joint preservation during daily routine (ie, ADLs, homemaking, child care, vocational/avocational, and leisure activities).		X X

*Note: This plan indicates task assignment for the purpose of this case study only.

Figure 13-1. *Program Planning Outline.*

When one has arthritis, it is important to carry out a regular program of exercise. The following program is designed to put your joints through all necessary motions. Exercise should be performed twice a day, and each exercise should be repeated five to ten times. If pain lasts over one hour after exercise program is developed, discontinue. This is usually a good indication that you have done too much. Please do not hesitate to call if you have any questions. Good luck and keep up the good work.

1. Activities of Daily Living Warm-up: DO FIRST THING IN THE MORNING. Touch your hands to shoulders, mouth, nose, eyes, top of head, up and over head, behind neck, behind back, knees, ankles, and toes. You can do this while lying in bed if painful when sitting, and modify accordingly. Repeat before sleeping at night.

2. Bend elbows so hands are as close to shoulders as possible and straighten toward knees. Be sure to keep elbows at your side.

3. Keeping elbows at your side, hold a stick in your hand and turn it upward toward the ceiling, then down toward the floor.

4. Rest forearm on table top and lift wrist off table. Help with other hand, if necessary, to keep forearm on table.

5. Place palm flat on table; raise each finger toward ceiling, one at a time, and hold each finger up for five seconds. Return finger to table before proceeding with next one; be sure palm is flat on table.

6. Place palm on table and bring fingers, one by one, toward thumb side. Make a fist; then open and begin again, bringing fingers, one by one, to thumb.

7. Make an "O" with your thumb and each successive finger.

8. Make large circles with thumb in both directions.

9. Hold pencil in hand and try to touch with fingertips. Remember: pencil should be at crease between fingers and palm.

DO THE FOLLOWING ONLY WHEN ACTIVE DISEASE IS NOT PRESENT

1. Heavy rubber band exercises of biceps and triceps for strengthening.

2. Bring arms to shoulder height; place three-pound weight on upper arm and hold for five seconds. Take weight off, let arm down, and repeat.

Please contact us if you have any questions or problems.
R. Jones, COTA/L

S. Kantor, OTR/L

Figure 13-2. *Arthritis home exercise program.*

Because Barbie complained of pain, due in part to structural changes, orthotic management was initiated. The OTR saw Barbie during the second week of treatment intervention and fabricated bilateral resting orthoses and wrist gauntlet **orthoses** (devices, such as a splint, to prevent deformity and/or improve function).[7] The latter is shown in Figure 13-3 (A COTA with experience may demonstrate adequate skill to fabricate these orthoses independently). The entry-level COTA assisted with adapting the straps so that Barbie could put them on and remove them independently. The COTA also monitored her use of the orthoses.

After the OTR and COTA discussed Barbie's progress over the past three treatment sessions, the OTR suggested the following changes in the exercise program:
● Review specific hand exercises because the patient demonstrated a poor understanding of the method.
● Be more specific with joint preservation instruction

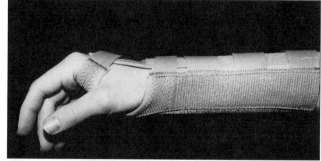

Figure 13-3. *Wrist gauntlet orthosis.*

and identify instances when the patient does not follow identified techniques.

For example, the COTA had observed that Barbie was starting to incorporate the joint preservation techniques in basic skills such as carrying her purse on her shoulder and lifting objects and closing and opening drawers with both hands. However, the COTA also observed that Barbie was sitting in chairs that were too low and using poor body mechanics when picking up her daughter. Although Barbie did plan ahead, she often tried to complete too many projects in too short a time.

Both positive and negative feedback were required for Barbie to adapt properly her life-style to include joint preservation.

The COTA continued with the treatment program and adjusted it accordingly. Use of the resting and gauntlet orthoses were added to the patient's daily routine, as needed. When increased pain was present in the wrist and hands during the day or night, Barbie was encouraged to cease activity and put her resting splints on. If functional tasks were being completed, the wrist gauntlets were used to allow her hands to move freely, but still remind her to be careful not to put too much stress on her painful joints. The COTA noted redness at the **thenar eminence** (fleshy part of the hand at the base of the thumb) when using the gauntlets and reported this to the OTR who directed the necessary modifications.

Activities of daily living became the major focus of Barbie's treatment program. Because of her age and family and work responsibilities, Barbie indicated to the COTA the importance of these skills in maintaining her current life-style. The patient's concern over longevity often interfered with her confidence and capacity to care independently for

herself, her child and her husband. The COTA voiced Barbie's concerns and anxieties in a discussion with the occupational therapist. It was agreed that the focus for the next two weeks would be on daily living skills, with emphasis on home and child care issues, while continuing to incorporate joint preservation techniques. The patient's major complaints of pain during early morning and late evening hours indicated to the COTA that Barbie was overexerting herself in the morning, from caring for herself and her child and breakfast preparation for her husband, and in the evening, from dinner preparation, bathing herself and her child and completing housework. Housework tasks had accumulated, as Barbie was working five days a week before the recent **exacerbation** of the illness (an increase in the severity of the condition).

On days when Barbie experienced extreme pain, she had difficulty with all self-care and child care activities; however, she forced herself to complete these chores, which resulted in increased pain. After further discussion between the OTR and the COTA, it was decided that an activity analysis would be beneficial. The COTA gave Barbie an activity configuration form and assisted her in filling in her specific activities. Tasks that were often painful and difficult to complete were highlighted. A sample activity configuration is shown in Figure 13-4.

Tasks that were analyzed included buttoning, writing, carrying and bathing her child and managing keys and the car door. Although other areas required analysis, these tasks were chosen for the purpose of this case study. The task

Hours	Monday-Friday Activities	Saturday Activities	Sunday Activities
Awakening Time:			
Early morning			
Mid-morning			
Late morning			
Early afternoon			
Mid-afternoon			
Late afternoon			
Early evening			
Mid evening			
Late evening			
Bedtime			

Figure 13-4. *Activity configuration. Adapted from the Activity Configuration Form, Rehabilitation Institute of Chicago, Chicago, Illinois.*

analysis consisted of the following steps:[8]
1. Identification of tasks by the COTA in collaboration with the patient
2. Description of task components, including activity characteristics
3. Identification of solutions by COTA, OTR and patient

The objective was to find less painful methods for task completion through the use of equipment, modification of tasks, joint preservation techniques, and adaptation of clothing and environments. For example, buttoning was painful in the morning. By using a button hook, Barbie could complete the task with less pain. The COTA placed an elastic strap on the button hook, which prevented her from using a tight grasp.

A second area analyzed was bathing her daughter. This task had previously been undertaken at night when Barbie took care of her own hygiene needs. It was recommended that Barbie bathe herself and her daughter in the morning since patients with arthritis frequently report that this is beneficial in relieving morning stiffness. Barbie had always bathed her child while on her knees, leaning over the bathtub. The COTA suggested that instead, she sit on a chair placed next to the tub and that she obtain a lightweight, hand-held shower for rinsing the child. Barbie's daughter enjoyed these changes in her bath routine and spoke of the experiences as "the new bath game." The task of bathing became more enjoyable for both mother and daughter. Further equipment needs were assessed and a long-handled brush was suggested for cleaning the tub after use.

Lifting her daughter in and out of the tub caused Barbie a great deal of pain, so the COTA suggested that Barbie's husband assume this responsibility. Because her husband was not always available, however, an alternate plan was to allow the child to crawl over the edge of the tub with assistance.

Meal preparation was a third area analyzed, as Barbie needed to prepare two meals each day, five days a week, and three meals on weekends. The patient reported that cutting food, opening containers and bending to remove objects from lower cabinets were her major areas of difficulty. The COTA suggested alternative methods for holding a knife and instructed Barbie in the best method for using an adapted container opener along with a rubber pad for added stabilization. The need to reorganize the kitchen cabinets was also discussed in conjunction with her joint preservation training.

Although Barbie seemed to enjoy her role as a home-maker, she indicated that she hoped to return to active employment outside the home. The COTA and Barbie jointly completed an activity configuration for work-related tasks. After further discussion with the OTR, it was decided that the COTA would visit the patient's work site. Barbie worked in a food processing plant, and components of her job included carrying heavy objects to an oven and a great deal of writing. The COTA noted that the gauntlet orthoses

would not be durable enough for her job and discussed the possibility of an alternate orthosis with the OTR. A more durable leather and elastic wrist orthosis was selected for use at work only and was purchased by the patient.

Throughout the course of Barbie's treatment program, the OTR had been in daily communication with the COTA and continued to see the patient once a week to assess progress and coordinate any necessary adjustments in the program.

The OTR arranged a job-site visit with Barbie's employer during the last week of occupational therapy treatment to suggest some modifications in Barbie's work routine, such as performing writing tasks at intervals rather than during a concentrated period of time.

Barbie progressed well in therapy and found it rewarding to involve her daughter in more of her own self-care. Notable changes in her attitude were evidenced by fewer complaints of pain when completing daily self-care and child care tasks. Barbie's husband was very supportive and agreed to share in laundry, grocery shopping and driving responsibilities.

Although Barbie was able to drive, securing her daughter in the special car seat, which was required by state law, was both difficult and painful. The COTA and Barbie discussed the situation and found a solution that incorporated good body mechanics and joint preservation principles. Opening the car door was difficult for Barbie due to pressure placed on the joints of her hand. It was decided that the use of a plastic-coated dowel rod to depress the door latch would be an effective solution. The COTA developed a light, plastic built-up key holder (Figure 13-5), which was easier for

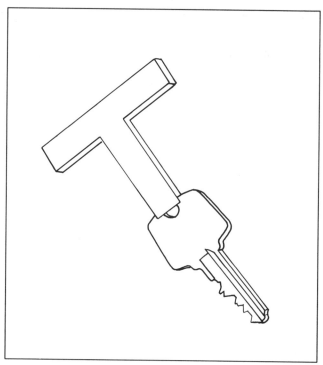

Figure 13-5. *Built-up key holder.*

Barbie to grasp and turn, thus enabling her to turn the key in the car door and the ignition.

Program Discontinuation

During the OTR's fifth visit, she and the COTA discussed the degree of progress that had been achieved with Barbie and the need for further occupational therapy treatment intervention. It was mutually agreed that Barbie had made significant progress toward returning to a more active life-style and that occupational therapy treatment would be discontinued as planned. The follow-up program was discussed, and both Barbie and her husband reviewed the home exercise protocol, all literature provided, the use of equipment and adaptations, and resources for purchasing replacement equipment. The patient was encouraged to contact her physician if her disease or functional status changed. Further assessment for occupational therapy treatment would occur at that time.

The discharge evaluation was handled jointly by the OTR and the COTA. With input from the assistant, the therapist evaluated the musculoskeletal components, and the COTA completed the functional skills assessment. Results indicated that the patient had achieved all goals determined in the initial evaluation. Both the OTR and the COTA recommended that Barbie become involved in the Arthritis Foundation because it provides a variety of beneficial programs and support groups.

Barbie and her employer agreed that she would return to work three days a week and upgrade to five days when she was able. Her daily schedule would be adjusted to allow for her to perform her writing at selected intervals rather than long blocks of time.

Conclusion

The roles of the OTR and COTA in treatment intervention fluctuate with each patient, based on specific needs. In looking at role delineation, an entry-level COTA will require additional supervision to perform various aspects of the evaluation and treatment program. Constant communication is necessary to develop and implement a thorough treatment program. A continuing literature review to identify new approaches and treatment techniques is valuable in providing comprehensive care. In evaluating this case study, it is important to understand that the COTA and the OTR played important roles in the patient's progress. It is the hope of the authors that the field of occupational therapy will continue to grow and maintain a high quality of care during the further development of the OTR and COTA role delineation.

Acknowledgments

The authors wish to express their gratitude to Sheri Intagliata, MS, MPA, OTR/L; Patricia Conlon, OTR/L; Kathleen Burroughs, OTR/L; Mary Andre, OTR/L; and Jeffrey Blackman for their guidance and support in developing this case study.

Related Learning Activities

1. Develop a series of cards illustrating examples of the basic principles of joint preservation. Use simple stick figures to show the right and wrong ways to perform the tasks.

2. Identify community resources for patients with arthritis and their families.

3. Request information about self-help devices specifically designed for individuals with arthritis from The Self-Help Device Office, Institute of Physical Medicine and Rehabilitation, 400 East 34th Street, New York, NY 10016.

4. Write for general information and a listing of publications available from The Arthritis Foundation, 3400 Peachtree Road, Atlanta, GA 30326.

5. List craft activities that should be avoided by people with arthritis. Indicate why.

References

1. Trombly CA: *Occupational Therapy for Physical Dysfunction*, Third Edition. Baltimore, Williams & Wilkins, 1989, pp. 28-29.
2. Miller BF, Keane CB: *Encyclopedia and Dictionary of Medicine, Nursing, and Allied Health*, 5th Edition. Philadelphia, WB Saunders, 1992.
3. Spencer AE: Functional restoration: Neurologic, orthopedic, and arthritic conditions. In Hopkins H, Smith H, (Eds): *Willard and Spackman's Occupational Therapy*, 7th Edition, Philadelphia, JB Lippincott, 1988, pp. 503-504.
4. Supervision guidelines for certified occupational therapy assistants. *Am J Occup Ther* 44:1089-1090, 1990.
5. Arthritis Health Profession Section of Arthritis Foundation: *Arthritis Teaching Slide Collection Manual*. Atlanta, Georgia, Arthritis Foundation, 1980, p. 5.
6. Watkins RA, Robinson D: *Joint Preservation Techniques for Patients with Rheumatoid Arthritis*. Chicago, Illinois, Rehabilitation Institute of Chicago, 1974, p. 16.
7. Melvin J: *Rheumatic Disease: Occupational Therapy and Rehabilitation*, 2nd Edition. Philadelphia, FA Davis, 1982, p. 329.
8. Hopkins HL, Smith HD, Tiffany EG: Therapeutic application of activity. In Hopkins H, Smith H, (Eds): *Willard and Spackman's Occupational Therapy*, 6th Edition. Philadelphia, JB Lippincott, 1983, p. 226.

Part D
ADULTHOOD

The Adult With Multiple Sclerosis

Donna Jensen, OTR
Ronna Linroth, COTA, ROH

Introduction

Multiple Sclerosis (MS) is the most common **demyelinating** (destruction of the sheath that surrounds the spinal cord and brain) disease of the central nervous system. Approximately two thirds of those who have this disease experience their first symptoms between the ages of 20 and 40 years. The cause is currently unknown. MS attacks the myelin sheath, a fatty substance that surrounds and protects the message-carrying nerve fibers of the brain and spinal cord. Where myelin has been destroyed, it is replaced by **plaques** of hardened tissue called sclerosis. This sclerotic condition occurs in multiple places within the nervous system, thus accounting for this condition's name. Initially, nerve impulses are transmitted with minor interruptions; later plaques may completely obstruct impulses along certain nerves.[1]

The symptoms, severity and course of multiple sclerosis vary considerably among those affected. For many, the course of the condition results in a series of attacks, known as **exacerbations** or relapses and partial or complete recoveries referred to as **remissions**.

Symptoms and Groupings

Depending on the location of the sclerosed patches, symptoms may include one or more of the following:[2]

1. Fatigue
2. Visual disturbances, such as double vision or **nystagmus** (involuntary, rapid, rhythmic movement)
3. Impaired sensation
4. Impaired bladder and bowel function
5. Weakness or **paralysis** (loss or impairment of motor function)
6. **Spasticity** (resistance to stretching by a muscle due to abnormally increased tension, with heightened deep tendon reflexes)

KEY CONCEPTS

Types and characteristics of multiple sclerosis

Assessment tools and activities

Intimacy aspects

Work simplification

Energy conservation

Home exercise program

Memory aids

ESSENTIAL VOCABULARY

Demyelinating

Plaques

Exacerbation

Remission

Nystagmus

Paralysis

Spasticity

Tremors

Ataxic

Goniometer

7. Incoordination
8. Disturbances in equilibrium
9. **Tremors** (trembling movements)
10. Slurred speech
11. Swallowing difficulties
12. Cognitive dysfunction

In general, multiple sclerosis may be broken down into five broad groupings based on the level of symptoms and the potential for disability. The following are listed in order of increasing involvement:[3]

Benign sensory MS: May go undiagnosed, as patients in this disease category will experience only a few attacks of the disease during their lifetime. These episodes are often sensory in nature and are not particularly disabling.

Benign remitting/exacerbating MS: Flare-ups occur more often; however, they cause little disability over time.

Chronic relapsing/progressive MS: Tends to be rhythmic, with each new episode bringing about increasing disability.

Chronic progressive MS: Produces symptoms that do not fluctuate and gradually lead to progressive degrees of disability.

Acute progressive MS: The symptoms rapidly lead to significant disability. Because outcome studies indicate that more than two thirds of all persons diagnosed with multiple sclerosis are ambulatory after 20 years, it is important to recognize the pattern in each individual's disease in designing treatment plans.

Case Study Background

Toni is a 35-year-old woman who was diagnosed with chronic, progressive multiple sclerosis four years ago. Her symptoms can be traced back for almost eight years. She is married and the mother of two sons, ages four and nine years. Toni had been employed as the manager of a florist shop until one year ago. The loss of her job has been a financial strain on the family's limited resources. Their attempts to restore their 50-year-old home had created a number of larger-than-expected debts.

Historically, Toni's initial symptoms presented as double vision, numbness, foot drop on the right side, and considerable fatigue. These symptoms would come and go without warning, but became more frequent and severe over time, resulting in a diagnosis of multiple sclerosis by the neurologist.

Toni's current status is marked by the following: an **ataxic** gait (impairment of muscle coordination), balance problems due to weak trunk musculature, weakness in her hip flexors, and mild bilateral upper extremity tremors. Toni is able to transfer independently in all situations, and she can walk less than ten feet without a walker. She is able to use stairs but experiences difficulty. She demonstrates mild, short-term memory loss. Her double vision has cleared; thus she is able to read most print.

Toni was admitted to the neurology floor of a major hospital with the following presenting problems: reduced mobility, recent increase in the number of falls, significant fatigue and increasing incontinence.

Referral

Toni was referred to the occupational therapy department as a routine part of the interdisciplinary team approach to rehabilitation. She had been seen by occupational therapy personnel previously for assistance with work-related problems. Treatment consisted of teaching energy conservation techniques, environmental planning for work simplification and making suggestions for positioning to minimize fatigue.

Assessment

After a review of the medical chart, the occupational therapist conducted an intitial interview with Toni and oriented her to the services of the department. Through questioning, the OTR learned more about Toni's perspective of her present functional level. Data were also gathered to establish an objective baseline status, and the process of goal setting for appropriate intervention was initiated.

The OTR's interview questions related to the following areas:

1. Social history and home situation, including accessibility of housing; type and amount of help in the home; and quality and quantity of social interaction
2. Currently identified or anticipated problems, especially those that precipitated the admission to the hospital
3. Abilities and deficits in activities of daily living, home management, child care, sexual functioning and leisure interests and participation patterns
4. Work status
5. Changes in cognitive or visual status

Based on Toni's responses, the OTR determined which specific or additional evaluation methods to use beyond those normally used to assess a neurologically impaired patient.

The OTR continued the assessment with an evaluation of Toni's general posture and positioning, noting both sitting and standing balance and the ability to accept challenge in those positions. Head and trunk posture were observed at rest and with upper extremities used for task engagement. The latter assessed the impact of an activity on the patient's stability in both a standing and a seated position. A mild increase in upper extremity tremors was noted while Toni was standing.

Upper extremity passive and gross active range of motion were evaluated using a **goniometer** (device used to measure angles) and were within normal limits. Muscle tone was assessed by using the Modified Asworth Scale. Toni was graded at zero, showing no increase from normal. Mild tremors were exhibited throughout the various testing procedures, but they did not interfere with task accomplishment. Muscle strength was evaluated in both upper extremities following the Daniels and Worthingham system. Strength was graded at 4 plus/5 proximally and 4/5 distally, with functional movement patterns. Grip strength was measured using a dynamometer at 45 lb on the right and 40 lb on the left. (Kellor's norms for females of the patient's age are 57 to 60 lb on the right and 52 to 53 lb on the left).[4] Palmar pinch strength was measured with the pinch meter at 12.5 lb on the right and 11 lb on the left. (Norms for a woman of Toni's age are 13 to 14 lb on the right and 12 to 13 lb on the left). It was noted that Toni was right-hand dominant.

Toni was asked to address an envelope to assess her handwriting skill. Cursive writing was performed at average speed and was slightly enlarged but legible. Mild evidence of tremor was seen.

For the next assessment, Toni completed the nine-hole peg test for fine coordination. Her score was 19 seconds with the right hand and 20 seconds with the left. (Corresponding norms are 14 to 20 with the right hand and 15 to 20 seconds with the left).[5]

Coordination was further assessed by performance of finger-to-nose pattern with vision occluded, rapid simultaneous and alternating hand motions (open-close fists; drum fingers on table), and object manipulation. These functions were mildly affected by tremor.

A modified Mini-mental State Examination, including a brief version of the Boston Naming Test and the Symbol Digit Modalities Test, was administered to detect cognitive impairment.[6-8] Toni scored 27 of a possible 30 points; scores at or above 24 points are generally considered functional. Because of the brief administration time of 10 to 15 minutes, inattention and some types of memory deficits prevalent in people with MS are not detected with this test.

Since Toni reported no sensory loss or changes and there was no evidence of burns or related injuries, a sensory evaluation was deferred.

When asked to read the first paragraph of a recipe printed in standard (newspaper-sized) print, Toni had functional vision for reading. The neurologist's report contained in the medical chart also provided the OTR with visual acuity information.

Throughout the evaluation, behavior as it affected the therapist and patient interaction, was noted. The OTR recorded that Toni displayed a positive and hopeful attitude, a high level of cooperation, and interest in learning adaptations and compensatory techniques. When asked to describe

her fatigue level, Toni reported that she usually tires in the afternoon and takes about a 45-minute nap. Tolerance for the evaluation tasks was noted at 45 minutes. Results of the various tests were shared with Toni, and an appointment was made for her to complete a self-care and meal preparation evaluation with the COTA.

After a discussion of Toni's hygiene and bathing routine, The COTA assessed her dressing skills. Although there was a slight problem with small buttons, Toni had compensated by selecting clothing with zipper closures, large buttons or "pull-over" designs. The assistant recommended that Toni stand at a support, such as a wall, when pulling up her pants to compensate for her balance problems and to sit to put on and tie her shoes. Application of makeup was enhanced by having the patient stabilize her elbows on the bedside table to decrease tremors. A two-pound wrist weight was tried to reduce tremors, but Toni indicated that it felt awkward. Rather than using eyeliner that required very precise application, Toni chose a darker shade of mascara.

In the course of discussing grooming and self-care tasks, Toni related that she no longer felt attractive. Further discussion revealed that Toni had some sexual concerns. The COTA provided her with information about common problems that occur with decreased sensation and lubrication in women with MS. Together they discussed some alternative positions, commercial lubricants and other aspects of intimacy such as closeness and touching. Toni appeared to be much relieved to discover her sexual changes were a result of MS symptoms rather than a personal "fault." Referral information was provided in case further counseling was needed. Toni was encouraged to enlist the suport of her husband by discussing her feelings with him. After the treatment session, the COTA selected written materials about the sexual issues discussed to share with Toni in a later session.[9,10]

Meal preparation was also assessed. To determine Toni's ability to calculate accurately, the COTA asked her to reduce quantities by half in a new recipe with ten ingredients and five to six steps. Since this was an unfamiliar environment, Toni had mild problems remembering where various items were located; however, given adequate time, she was able to problem solve, substitute appropriately and observe safety precautions. The COTA suggested that she "check off" ingredients as they were used to help her keep track of steps with a minimum of effort. Work simplification and energy conservation techniques were also discussed and demonstrated. Toni reported that her kitchen cupboards were mounted high, leaving the two upper shelves unreachable without use of a step stool. A plan was established to rearrange the cupboards, placing the most frequently used items within the easiest reach. She indicated that she would also conduct a through cleaning to eliminate items that were unnecessary or rarely used. Toni agreed to use a cart to transport hot or heavy items. Recommendations to remove small rugs and to obtain a more sturdy step stool with hand rails were welcomed, as

Toni was very concerned about her recent falls and wanted to prevent them in the future.

The COTA also conducted a bathroom assessment to evaluate safety and level of independence in toilet transfers and bathing. Toni was able to step in and out of the bathtub with standby assistance for balance problems. On the second attempt, she utilized a grab bar and was independent. Performance of the toilet transfer had similar results, with Toni achieving independence using grab bars and an elevated toilet seat. Use of a shower stool and more moderate water temperature was also recommended to minimize fatigue factors while showering. Resources for funding of adaptive equipment were discussed and the COTA referred Toni to the Social Services Department for follow-up assistance.

Treatment Planning

The OTR prepared a report that summarized the results of the evaluations. The COTA contributed the results of the assessments she had conducted and also made recommendations for the treatment plan.

Treatment Goals

The following treatment goals were established:

1. Demonstrate independence in dressing, bathing and toileting, utilizing adaptive equipment.
2. Exhibit consistent use of energy conservation and work simplification techniques for activities of daily living, homemaking and child care.
3. Demonstrate independence in meal preparation.
4. Demonstrate knowledge of and engagement in three appropriate stress management techniques.
5. Demonstrate skill in use of techniques to compensate for short-term memory loss.
6. Participate in an upper extremity home program for maintenance of strength independently.

The following treatment plan is organized numerically to correspond to the six treatment goals stated in the previous section.

1. Activities of daily living:
   a. Further hygiene, grooming and dressing training to assess carryover of the techniques taught in the evaluation session.
   b. Tub and toilet transfers training to assure safety and carryover, and to reinforce techniques. Provision of transfer methods to compensate for memory loss. Provision of written recommendations for equipment to assure bathroom safety (shower stool, toilet grab bars, tub grab bars and an elevated toilet seat).
   c. Provision of written materials on sexuality issues for individuals with MS.

2. Energy conservation and work simplification training utilizing videotape, discussion, problem solving activities, and practice in typical situations. The main principles (applicable in Toni's case) are:
   a. Sit to do work tasks whenever possible.
   b. Rearrange storage areas so frequently used items are within easy reach.
   c. Use a cart or slide heavy or hot items rather than carrying them.
   d. Alternate periods of activity with periods of rest.
   e. Delegate tasks to family members, including the selection of appropriate tasks for her 4-year-old and 9-year-old sons to perform.
   f. Establish a routine and the necessary communication structure for household tasks (written lists, a chalkboard and charts).
   g. Explore employment of a home health aide for doing heavy household tasks, such as extensive cleaning, yard work and laundry, to enable Toni and her husband to have more energy and time for parenting and for their leisure and social pursuits as a couple.

3. Further meal preparation training with incorporation of work simplification and energy conservation principles, as well as safe use of a walker in the kitchen.
   a. Review meal planning, grocery list preparation, meal service and cleanup activities and incorporate compensatory principles.
   b. Assess feasibility of a powered triwheeled unit for kitchen tasks. (This could also be used for shopping and leisure activities.)

4. Stress management group participation daily during hospital stay to identify how stress affects MS patients and their symptoms.
   a. Identify personal sources of stress and typical responses.
   b. Participate in practice of alternative stress management techniques, including progressive muscle relaxation, imagery, meditation, deep breathing and assertiveness skills.

5. Training in compensatory techniques for memory loss.
   a. Organization of the environment so that important items are readily accessible and are stored in a consistent location (purse, keys, checkbook, etc.).
   b. Development of a comprehensive calendar organization system where all personal and family appointments and plans are recorded when made. Important names, phone numbers and dates are also recorded. Toni's medication schedule is maintained here as well. A daily "to do" list is also a necessary component of this system and should include entries to ensure smooth management of the children's activities.

Personal Data

Name _____

Address _____

City_____ State _____

Zip Code _____Phone _____

Credit Card Numbers_____

1._____

2._____

3._____

4._____

5._____

6._____

7._____

8._____

Insurance Policies

Company_____ Number_____

Home _____

Health _____

Car _____

Life _____

Other_____

Other Document Numbers_____

_____

Driver's License_____

Checking Account_____

Savings Account _____

Retirement Plan_____

Car Registration_____

Safety Deposit Box_____

Passport _____

Social Security_____

Other_____

Dates to Remember

January_____

_____

March _____

_____

May _____

_____

July _____

_____

September_____

_____

November _____

_____

Frequently Called Numbers

Attorney_____

Bank _____

Child Care_____

Counselor _____

Dentist_____

Doctors _____

_____

Florist _____

Insurance Agents _____

_____

Garbage Collection_____

Pharmacist _____

School_____

Other_____

Friends and Relatives

_____

_____

_____

_____

_____

_____

_____

_____

_____

_____

_____

_____

_____

_____

_____

_____

_____

_____

February_____

_____

April_____

_____

June _____

_____

August_____

_____

October _____

_____

December _____

_____

Form developed by Sally E. Ryan

Figure 14-1. *Memory Aid Sheet.*

For the week of: _____

Sunday _____	Things To Do:_____
_____	1._____
_____	2._____
Monday _____	3._____
_____	4._____
_____	5._____
_____	
Tuesday _____	
_____	
_____	
Wednesday _____	Calls to Make:
_____	Name: _____
_____	#
Thursday _____	Name: _____
_____	#
_____	Name: _____
Friday _____	#
_____	Name: _____
_____	#
Saturday _____	
_____	
_____	

Figure 14-2. *Modified Memory Aid Sheet.*

6. Provision of an upper extremity home exercise program, utilizing graded exercises with Theraband to maintain upper extremity strength. (The program encompassed all of the major muscle groups of the upper extremity and was to be performed daily.)

Treatment Implementation

Because Toni was scheduled to be released from the hospital two days after completing the occupational therapy evaluation, it was decided to focus her treatment on items 4, 5 and 6 of the treatment plan—learning and practicing stress management techniques, developing compensatory techniques for memory loss, and learning a home exercise program. Toni was referred to the Multiple Sclerosis Achievement Center to work on the remaining items in the treatment plan. The OTR provided treatment for items 4 and 6, and the COTA provided treatment to assist Toni in developing a system that would help her keep track of her many responsibilities in view of her memory problems.

During the treatment sessions, the COTA introduced a variety of planning calendars for Toni to review. She selected one frequently used in business that would accommodate all of the necessary information and had an extra section for notetaking. A memory aid sheet was also recommended (Figure 14-1). The sheet was adapted to a shorter format of essential items for use outside the home (Figure 14-2). Toni's degree of impairment did not warrant use of a calendar with electronic alarms to remind her of appointments, medications and other important items.

The assistant also told Toni about the availability of memory compensation devices as listed below:

- Car finders—electronic mechanism available from the DAK Corporation
- Sounding devices to locate keys and other personal items
- Telememo Data Bank—wristwatch series available from the Casio Corporation for phone numbers and appointments and Seiko memory watches
- Dictation tape recorders
- Electronic schedule planners, such as the notebook computer from TRY Corporation; Toshiba Memo Note II Memory Aid Calculator, and others manufactured by Sharp and Sharper Image, which can store longer

messages than Telememo watches
● Memory telephones

Toni thought that many of these items would be useful if her memory problems increased and that a memory telephone would be a good investment to make now, as it would be a time saver as well as a memory aid. She also liked the idea of using a chalkboard for daily "to do" tasks. Her husband visited the clinic during one of the treatment sessions and familiarized himself with the various techniques to help Toni compensate for her memory loss. He also indicated his willingness to assist with other aspects of her treatment, including monitoring the home exercise, energy conservation and stress management programs, and helping with kitchen reorganization plans. In anticipation of her discharge, he had already arranged to purchase used adaptive equipment for the bathroom. Toni was given a videotape and printed materials that outlined energy conservation and work simplification techniques. Additional printed materials on sexual information and referral sources were also provided. Both the OTR and the COTA emphasized the need for Toni to carry out her routine activities as independently and safely as possible.

Program Discontinuation and Discharge Planning

The interdisciplinary rehabilitation team thought that Toni could benefit from an ongoing supportive maintenance program. She was referred to the Multiple Sclerosis Achievement Center located in the community. This agency would provide a maintenance rehabilitation program that included occupational, physical and recreational therapy; support groups and individual counseling facilitated by a chaplain; and social services. Although an interview was quickly arranged, there was an anticipated admission delay of four to six months due to the long waiting list. In the meantime, Toni was encouraged to use the services of the local Multiple Sclerosis Society chapter community programs. The swim program, support groups and social opportunities were described and written materials were provided.

Editor's Note

Additional information may be obtained from the National Multiple Sclerosis Society, 205 East 42nd Street, New York, NY 10017.

Related Learning Activities

1. List specific energy conservation and work simplification activities that Toni could use in caring for her children.

2. Visit an electronics store and ask for a demonstration of some of the memory aids described in the chapter.

3. Using a catalog from a large department store, identify clothing that is available for people with problems similar to those of Toni.

4. Write to the local chapter of the Multiple Sclerosis Society and request information on available services.

References

1. Wassermann L: *Living with Multiple Sclerosis: A Practical Guide.* New York, National Multiple Sclerosis Society, 1978.
2. Miller BF, Keane CB: *Encyclopedia and Dictionary of Medicine, Nursing, and Allied Health,* 5th Edition. Philadelphia, WB Saunders, 1992.
3. Schapiro RT: Methodology for the rehabilitation of multiple sclerosis. *Impulse* (Riverside Neurosensory Center, Minneapolis) Summer, 1990.
4. Kellor M, Frost J, Silberg N: Hand strength and dexterity. *Am J Occup Ther* 22:77-83, 1971.
5. Goodkin DE, Hertsgaard D, Seminary J: Upper extremity function in multiple sclerosis: Improving assessment sensitivity with box and block and nine-hole peg tests. *Arch Phys Med Rehabil* 69:850-854, 1988.
6. Beatty WW, Goodkin DE: Screening for cognitive impairment in multiple sclerosis: An evaluation of the Mini-mental state examination. *Arch Neurol* 47:297-301, 1990.
7. Dick JPR et al: Mini-mental state examination in neurological patients. *J Neurol Neurosurg Psychiatry* 47:496-499, 1984.
8. Naugle R, Kawczak K: Limitations of the Mini-mental state examination. *Cleve Clin J Med* 26:277-281, 1989.
9. Carrera MA: MS: The right to a sexual life. *MS Quarterly Report—Summer.* New York, Eastern Paralyzed Veterans Association, 1979.
10. Barrett M: *Sexuality and Multiple Sclerosis.* New York, National Multiple Sclerosis Society, 1982.

The Adult With Aids

William Matthew Marcil, MS, OTR

Introduction

In the decade or so since its existence was made known, acquired immunodeficiency syndrome (AIDS) has had a profound effect on modern society throughout the world. Before 1981, no one had ever heard of this disease, and nothing was known about its etiology, treatment or cure. The only thing that was certain was that a diagnosis of AIDS was tantamount to a death sentence. The disease has so far claimed over 100,000 lives in the United States alone. The number of infected individuals is estimated to be in the millions throughout the world.

During the short time since the discovery of AIDS, much has been learned about this remarkable disease. It is now known what causes it, how it is spread and how to prevent its spread. A number of techniques are available to identify those who have been exposed to the disease, and numerous drugs have been developed to combat the host of opportunistic infections that accompany it. In fact, the amount of knowledge obtained about AIDS is unprecedented in the history of medicine. The only thing lacking is a cure.

ESSENTIAL VOCABULARY

Human immunodeficiency virus

Persistent generalized lymphadenopathy

Kaposi's sarcoma

Pneumocystic carinii pneumonia

Mycobacterium avium intracellulare

Cytomegalovirus

Herpes simplex virus

Varicella zoster virus

Prophylactic

Monogamous

Toxoplasmosis

Subluxation

Decubiti

KEY CONCEPTS

Characteristics of AIDS and HIV

Current trends

Disease prevention

Roles of occupational therapy personnel

Home health practice

Assessment activities

Bathing and dressing program

Adaptive equipment

Pool and sports program

Etiology

AIDS is actually the final stage of infection by the **human immunodeficiency virus** (HIV), which has a tendency to be attracted to the T4 helper lymphocyte, the first line of defense of the immune system. Once it has gained entrance to the body—usually through intimate contact with the blood of an infected individual via sexual intercourse or sharing of contaminated hypodermic needles—the virus seeks out the T4 cells, attaches itself to the outer membrane, and gains entrance to the inner core. Having reached the inner core of the cells, the virus remains dormant for an unspecified length of time until it is triggered or activated. Using an enzyme (reverse transcriptase), HIV is able to make a template of the lymphocyte's genetic program, allowing it to reproduce. As it multiplies, the virus feeds off its host and eventually kills it; the host then explodes, releasing thousands of new viruses that continue the cycle. This process causes a "domino effect" in the immune system and eventually renders the body incapable of fighting off infection from other organisms.

Initially, the infected individual is unaware of the infection. This stage is known as HIV positive, asymptomatic (without symptoms). As the immune system is gradually depleted, the individual develops enlarged lymph glands for a period of six months or more. This stage is known as **persistent generalized lymphodenopathy** (PGL). The next stage is commonly referred to as AIDS-related complex (ARC) or pre-AIDS. At this time the individual begins to become chronically ill and exhibits frequent, drenching night sweats, fever, diarrhea and weight loss, and perhaps some opportunistic infections. The term ARC has questionable clinical usefulness as a diagnostic category, and it is being used less often in the literature. The final stage is AIDS, which is typically manifested by the presence of specific opportunistic infections and infectious diseases such as the following:[1]

1. **Kaposi's sarcoma** (KS): a malignant tumor of the connective tissues that support blood vessels and that also produces visible lesions under the skin, although visceral lesions may also be present.
2. *Pneumocystis carinii* **pneumonia** (PCP): a lung infection caused by an airborne protozoan.
3. Neurologic involvement causing **AIDS dementia complex** (ADC).
4. **Mycobacterium avium-intracellulare** (MAI): an infectious disease involving lungs, skin and lymph nodes, as well as other sites.
5. **Cytomegalovirus** (CMV): a herpes-type virus producing enlarged cells similar to infectious mononucleosis.
6. **Herpes simplex virus** (HSV): an inflammatory skin disease that results in the formation of small vesicles (sacs containing liquid).
7. **Varicella zoster virus** (VSV): a variety of chickenpox in children and shingles in adults.

Although AIDS is the final stage of HIV infection and eventually results in the premature death of the infected individual, it is important to note that death can occur in any stage of the disease process as the result of complications. Figure 15-1 shows the stages of the condition and possible outcomes.

As the immune system is depleted, all body systems are vulnerable to attack by *opportunistic disease*. An opportunistic disease or infection is one that is commonly found in the environment but is governed by the immune response. When the immune response is impaired, these infections are allowed to infiltrate and proliferate within the body. Thus, the individual who is immune impaired, as in AIDS or from chemotherapy, is likely to exhibit symptoms of the skin and cardiopulmonary, gastrointestinal and genitourinary systems. The neurologic system is subject to secondary infections, as well as direct HIV infection, and the individual can exhibit blindness in addition to the following signs and symptoms:[1]

1. *Dementia*: loss of intellectual function
2. *Hemiplegia*: paralysis on one side of the body
3. *Radiculopathies*: diseases of the nerve roots
4. *Ataxia*: failure of muscular coordination and/or irregular muscle action

It should be noted that the majority of deaths from AIDS are not caused directly by HIV, but rather from the opportunistic infections that eventually overwhelm the body.

Current Trends

Today, the individual with HIV infection is, in a sense, more fortunate than his or her predecessors of just a few years ago. The development of drugs such as azidothymidine (AZT) (Ziduvodine and Retrovir) and Dideooxynosine (DDI) can retard the proliferation of HIV. *Pneumocystis carinii* pneumonia, once the most lethal of the opportunistic infections, can now be controlled with the drug pentamidine. In fact, currently over 100 drugs and modalities are available to treat the opportunistic infections caused by the disease. The drugs, despite their cost, can allow individuals to live longer in lieu of a cure or vaccine. A number of vaccines are currently under study and one, VaxSyn, which has been tested in 36 healthy volunteers, shows some promise, although its effectiveness has not been proven.[2]

Early detection of HIV infection is paramount if the disease is to be controlled. The sooner the virus is detected, **prophylactic** (an agent that tends to ward off disease) administration of AZT or DDI can prevent rapid

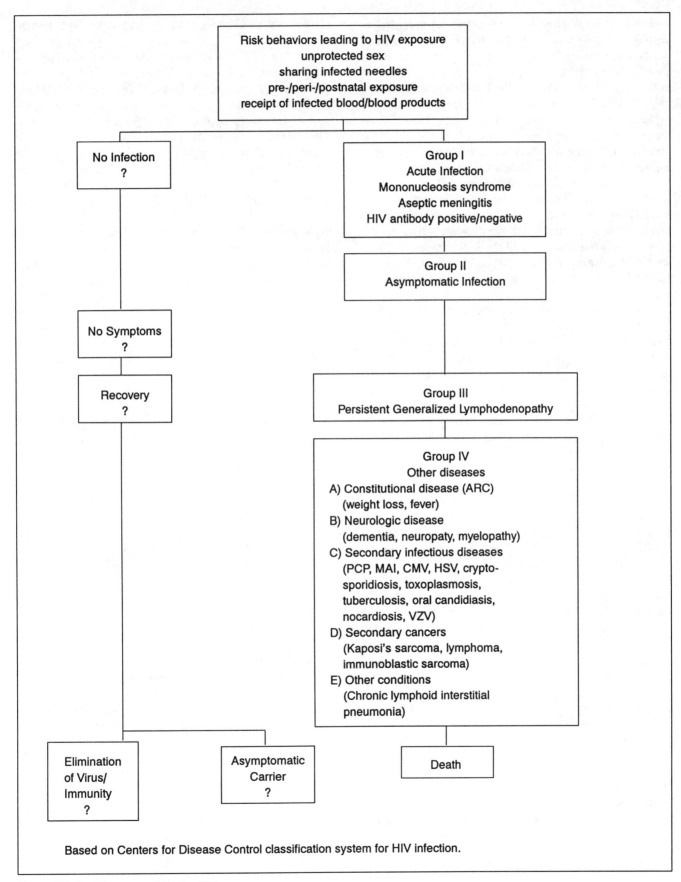

Figure 15-1. *Possible outcomes following HIV exposure.*

replication of the virus and thus retard its progression. Testing methods, such as the enzyme-linked immunoadsorbent assay (ELISA) and the Western Blot test, are able to detect the presence of antibodies to HIV in an individual's blood. The Single Use Diagnostic System (SUDS) also detects antibodies to the virus but within 20 to 30 minutes. The polymerized chain reaction (PCR) is the only test that can currently detect the presence of the virus itself. The value of this test is that it may take up to six weeks for the body to develop a detectable number of antibodies, and individuals tested using standard assays may test negative for antibodies when, in fact, they are actually infected. Although the development of these tests is a great step in diagnosing the disease, testing procedures have been and most likely will continue to be a source of debate and litigation regarding an individual's right to privacy, insurance issues and bias against those who are known or thought to be HIV positive.

It is important to note that no one is immune from HIV infection. Although certain groups, such as homosexual men and intravenous drug users (IVDUs), are at higher risk than is the general population, anyone is vulnerable to infection. The disease is spread through intimate contact with blood, semen, vaginal secretions and breast milk. In short, any body fluid that contains white blood cells should be considered a source of infection. To prevent the spread of infection, individuals should abstain from sex or practice safe sex using condoms and spermicides containing nonoxydil 9, in a **monogamous** relationship (marriage or cohabitation with one person) or with a limited number of partners (preferably known to be HIV negative), avoid the sharing of hypodermic needles, and follow universal precautions as outlined by the Centers for Disease Control (CDC).[3] These recommendations are important because one cannot tell if another individual is HIV positive merely by looking at them. To prevent the spread of HIV, it is important to assume that everyone is infected and then act accordingly.

It should also be noted that the best method of disease prevention is the simplest: handwashing. The regular, methodical washing of hands is the most effective means of preventing the spread of communicable disease and noscomial infections (those originating in a hospital). This advice is not unique to working with the person with AIDS (PWA), but rather to working with any patient. Hands should be washed before and after working with every patient, after contact with mucous membranes, after sneezing or blowing one's nose, after toileting and before and after eating. This routine is especially important when working with a person with AIDS. Although the risk of contracting HIV from the patient is miniscule, the risk of passing an infection to the patient is extremely high.

The Role of Occupational Therapy Personnel

All persons with a chronic or life-threatening illness are subject to impairment of their occupational roles. The person with AIDS is no different; however, these individuals often face the added burden of social rejection, ostracism and stigmatization by their disease. It is the job of occupational therapy practitioners to assist these individuals in the acquisition of new occupational roles or the relearning of previous ones in the areas of activities of daily lving, work and play/leisure if the individual's quality of life is to be enhanced. While other professions, such as medicine, nursing, pharmacology and nutrition, are involved in the treatment of the AIDS patient and are certainly important in helping the person with AIDs to stay alive, occupational therapy is the only profession that can help these individuals live productive, meaningful lives within the confines of their disease.[4] To live without being able to interact with and master one's environment is not really living. It is existing.

To be sure, the basic tenets of occupational therapy practice remain intact when working with AIDS patients. Due to the nature of their illness, these individuals will display symptoms common to other disease processes and can be treated traditionally. Some areas, however, must be given special attention.

The OTR or COTA working with the patient with HIV/AIDS cannot be judgmental before assuming the case. AIDS is not a disease that affects only homosexuals and drug addicts. It is a disease that affects people and each individual is entitled to the best possible care. How these individuals became infected does not matter; how they will function in their daily lives does matter.

Occupational therapy personnel must have a basic knowledge about HIV—how it manifests itself and how it is spread.

Case Study Background

Jim is a 35-year-old black man who was diagnosed with AIDS after seeking medical treatment for chronic headaches. The headaches were found to be caused by a **toxoplasmosis** infection, which closely resembles mononucleosis in some forms and involves cerebral edema.[1] A month after his diagnosis the edema caused a cerebral vascular accident (CVA), which resulted in a a flaccid hemiparesis (slight or incomplete paralysis of one side). Jim was living in another state at the time of his stroke and returned to his hometown shortly thereafter to be closer to his family. He was referred for home health care services through a local visting nurse association.

Assessment

On the initial meeting with the occupational therapist, Jim was living in a second story, walk-up apartment. He had home health aide services around the clock. His mother visited him two to three times a week to take care of his laundry and housecleaning needs. Other family members visited infrequently. An exception was his sister-in-law who was present at the evaluation and expressed great concern for his care. She stated that Jim had recently become diabetic as a side effect of one of his medications, and he required a nurse to come to his apartment each morning to administer his insulin. His sister-in-law thought it would be easier if the therapist could show Jim how to administer his own insulin using only one hand.

Using an occupational history outline, the therapist learned that Jim was an accountant and was the only one in his large family to earn a college degree. He described himself as a hard worker who had always enjoyed school and work in order to make his life better. He stated that he felt cheated by the disease because "I was the only one in the family to get out of this place; now look at me." Jim wanted to return to work or at least to be able to do more for himself and not have to depend on others. He also described himself as a "gourmet chef" and enjoyed cooking. Basketball and swimming were other hobbies. Through questioning and discussion, the OTR determined that Jim had a good understanding of his disease and its likely progression.

The physical assessment revealed that Jim had a flaccid left upper extremity proximally, with a 1 cm **subluxation** (partial dislocation) of the shoulder. He complained of shoulder pain with passive movement. Distally, he exhibited increased flexor tone with minimal flexor synergy noted at the elbow. He was able to bear partial weight on his left leg. His sitting balance was fair. No cognitive, perceptual or sensory impairments were present. Jim became fatigued quickly during most activities. A herpes infection on his groin and buttocks made it difficult for Jim to sit comfortably for any length of time.

The performance assessment revealed that Jim required maximum assistance for all transfers, moderate assistance for bathing and maximum assistance for upper extremity dressing; he was dependent in lower extremity dressing. He was able to ambulate short distances with an ankle-foot orthosis (AFO) and a "quad" cane with contact guard. Jim is right-handed but had difficulty performing object manipulation tasks using only one hand. He had previously been able to carry out his own home management tasks, but he was no longer able to perform any aspect of these tasks.

Before he became ill, Jim had been very active and followed a regular daily schedule. Since his stroke, he reported that he spends his entire day in bed sleeping or watching television.

Toward the end of the interview and evaluation, Jim confided to the therapist that although it was inconvenient for him to have the nurse come to his apartment early each morning to administer his insulin, and that he would like to do it himself, he did not think that it would be wise to have needles around the house because his sister-in-law was an IV drug user. He thought that she wanted to obtain needles from him. The therapist thanked Jim for the information and eliminated self-administration of insulin as a possible goal. The therapist then told Jim what he thought he was capable of accomplishing through occupational therapy treatment. The therapist also stated that he would return the next day to review the treatment plan with him and to begin therapy.

Treatment Planning

The OTR met with the COTA to discuss the case and to outline a tentative plan of treatment. The next day the occupational therapy team visited Jim's home and, after the COTA was introduced to Jim, they presented the plan to him for his input and approval. Jim's home health aide was also included in this session to ensure consistency. The following goals were agreed upon:

Short-term Goals

- Increase right upper extremity (RUE) strength from "good minus" to "good plus" using progressive resistive exercises and functional activities daily.
- Reduce left shoulder subluxation by using a subluxation sling and proprioceptive neuromuscular facilitation (PNF) techniques daily.
- Provide a left hand resting splint for day and night wear.
- Increase comfort and prevent **decubiti** (ulcers occurring over bony prominences as a result of pressure[1]) by providing a wheelchair gel cushion and a water mattress for daily use.
- Independent transfers on and off the toilet will be accomplished using assistive devices.
- Transfers in and out of the bathtub will be accomplished with minimum assistance and assistive devices.
- Independence in upper body dressing will be demonstrated each morning using assistive devices.

Long-term Goals:

- All transfers will be performed with supervision and contact guard only.
- Independent dressing will be completed at least three times a week with occasional minimum assistance.

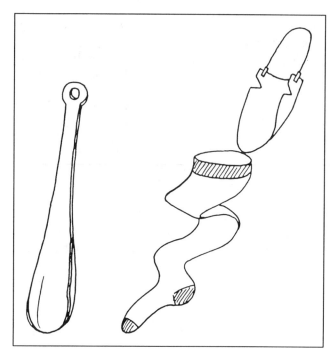

Figure 15-2. *Long handle shoe horn and stocking aid.*

- Planning and assistance in the preparation of at least three meals a week will be demonstrated using assistive devices.
- Weekly participation in at least one activity of choice at a local health club will be accomplished.

The treatment period was planned to include the nine weeks allowable by Medicaid with the option of recertification at the end of that period. The frequency would be reduced gradually over the course of the certification period. Jim would be seen five times per week for the first two weeks, three time a week for the next four weeks, and twice a week for the final three weeks (5W2, 3W4, 2W3) for a total of 28 visits. It was agreed that the OTR and the COTA would alternate visits for the first three weeks; the COTA would make independent visits for the remaining treatment times, with OTR supervision every fifth visit, barring any complications.

Treatment Implementation

After receiving the physician's order for the splint and durable medical equipment (DME), the OTR obtained a subluxation sling, an overhead trapeze for Jim's bed, a shower bench, a tub-mount grab bar, a wheelchair gel cushion and a water mattress for his bed.

During the first two weeks, the COTA saw Jim three mornings a week for a bathing and dressing program. Working with both Jim and his aide, she instructed them in bathtub transfers using the shower bench. Since the tub did not have a permanent shower attachment, she obtained and installed a hand-held model so that Jim could shower himself. A tub-mount grab bar was installed to assist in safe transfers. This device also proved to be helpful for toilet transfers, as the tub was in close proximity to the toilet. A long-handled bathbrush was also introduced to help Jim wash his back and lower legs and feet. Jim said he was "thrilled" at being able to shower again, and he exclaimed, "This is the first time I've been in a bathtub in two months. I feel like a human again!"

Jim was also instructed in one-handed dressing techniques for his upper extremities. Although this technique was difficult for him to perform initially, he insisted on doing as much as he could by himself. The COTA instructed the aide to encourage this activity and requested that he not help Jim with this aspect of dressing unless Jim requested assistance. Because of Jim's inability to manipulate his shirt buttons with one hand, the COTA showed him how to use a button hook.

On the alternating days, the OTR visited Jim for treatment of his left arm and to practice bed and wheelchair transfers. The shoulder cuff sling helped to stabilize Jim's shoulder and reduce both the subluxation and the pain. The splint was fabricated and maintained Jim's hand in a functional position. The OTR instructed both Jim and the aide in the wearing schedule and how to clean the splint.

The overhead trapeze was installed over the bed and enabled Jim to pull himself into an upright position on the edge of the bed in preparation for transferring. The OTR instructed Jim and his aide in proper transfer techniques from the bed to the wheelchair and back to the bed again. Both the gel cushion and the water mattress helped to relieve Jim's discomfort. He reported that he was able to sit for longer periods of time in his wheelchair and to sleep better; thus, fatigue was reduced and Jim exhibited more energy for daily living tasks.

At the conclusion of the first two weeks, Jim was able to transfer in and out of the bathtub and bathe himself with only minimum assistance from his aide. He was also able to transfer on and off the toilet independently. By using the overhead trapeze, he required only contact guard to get out of bed and into his wheelchair. He had also mastered all aspects of his upper extremity dressing. In addition, these activities had increased the strength in his right upper extremity to "good" and, although he had an occasional "bad day," his endurance level was showing signs of improvement. Jim stated he was now ready for "new challenges," and the OTR/COTA team discussed the next set of goals with him. All agreed that Jim would begin to dress his lower extremities, begin simple meal preparation and make plans to leave his apartment for a short outing.

The COTA showed Jim ways to put on his pants, shoes and socks using one hand. A dressing stick, sock aid and long-handled shoehorn were used to facilitate this process.

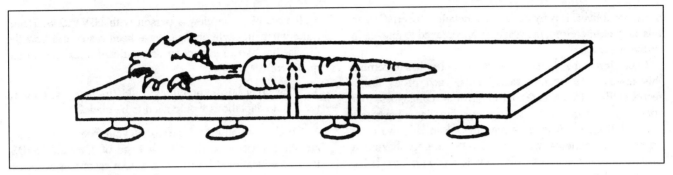

Figure 15.3 *Adapted cutting board.*

The sock aid and shoe horn are shown in Figure 15-2. Jim had difficulty putting on his left sock and shoe and required minimum assistance.

Jim was also taught new ways to work in the kitchen while sitting in his wheelchair. The COTA demonstrated various techniques to allow Jim to participate in meal preparation using one hand and various adaptive devices to make the tasks easier for him. Jim was amazed that he could still make elaborate vegetable garnishes with only one hand by using a board with a nail in it to stabilize the item while cutting (Figure 15-3). The OTR incorporated neuromuscular facilitation techniques, such as diagonal patterns of movement, weight bearing and range of motion when engaged in activities, which allowed him to gain more functional use of his left arm. Jim assisted in cooking a dinner for his mother in honor of her birthday, displaying his skills with great pride. He was also pleased that two of his brothers joined them in the family celebration.

By the end of the fourth week, Jim was able to dress himself with only minimum assistance with his left shoe and sock. He also planned his dinner each day and assisted in its preparation using his new-found abilities. At this time, the OTR and the COTA began to address the final goal of taking Jim out of his apartment to visit the health club.

Because of the difficulty of getting Jim down the 14 steps from the second floor, as well as other obstacles such as car transfers and pool safety, another individual would need to be involved in addition to the OTR, the COTA and the aide. The COTA contacted the local AIDS organization, which provided Jim with a "buddy" to help with this outing and other activities. After instruction in car transfers, the group arrived at the health club. The therapist and the assistant instructed Jim and the others in pool transfers and safety techniques. Because the COTA was a woman, she could not assist Jim in the men's locker room so the aide and the "buddy" were instructed in undressing and dressing techniques, the goal being to conserve Jim's energy for the pool and other activities at the club.

Jim declared, "I'm ecstatic!" as he entered the pool. The water provided him the ability to stand unsupported and allowed him greater freedom to move his affected left side. Because Jim was anemic, he could only remain in the cool water for about ten minutes. A short wetsuit was obtained, which allowed him to remain in the pool for up to 30 minutes in subsequent visits.

After the pool session, Jim went to the gymnasium and tried "shooting baskets" with one hand. Although he wasn't successful at first, he enjoyed the challenge. He met another man who was parapelgic (paralysis of the legs and in some cases the lower part of the body).[1] He and Jim began a friendly rivalry in a game of "twenty-one," while the aide and Jim's buddy recovered the wayward basketball. The rivalry soon grew into a new friendship, which gave Jim further incentive to attend the club each week.

Program Discontinuation

By the end of the eighth week, Jim was participating in as much of his self-care as he could and engaging in activities at the health club every Friday. Although he still did not have functional use of his left arm, he demonstrated steady improvement. At this time the OTR and the COTA recommended that Jim continue his therapy on an outpatient basis. Jim was already receiving weekly medical care at the AIDS clinic of a local hospital, and arrangements were made for him to continue his occupational and physical therapy programs there.

Jim was pleased with the progress that he had made in such a short time. He was reluctant to end his relationship with the occupational therapy team, but he realized that he had to "keep on truckin'." The following week, after the OTR and COTA reviewed Jim's accomplishments with him, he was discharged from occupational therapy home care services.

Conclusion

This chapter has presented some of the salient facts about HIV/AIDS, and the role that occupational therapy practitioners can play in assisting persons with AIDS to live meaningful lives. It is by no means a detailed dissertation on this subject; therefore, the reader is encouraged to engage in further research.

Education is the single best weapon society has to combat this disease. As health professionals, each of us has a responsibility to educate ourselves, our colleagues, our friends and acquaintances, and our families about this dreaded disease if it is to be prevented. Similarly, we must educate our patients with HIV/AIDS. Merely having a disease does not automatically provide one with knowledge about the disease.[5]

It is not only important to be knowledgeable about AIDS as a health care provider; you the reader will also be confronted with it at some point in your life, be it on a personal level, through an infected friend or family member or perhaps you, yourself will test positive for HIV. AIDS is no longer confined to large metropolitan areas such as New York and San Francisco.[6] It is everywhere and can be found in hospitals, schools, nursing homes and throughout the community. The rapid and steady increase in the number of infected individuals increases the chances that occupational therapy practitioners will encounter this disease in the course of their career.[7,8] One cannot choose to ignore it on the assumption that one will never encounter it. Ignorance is no longer bliss. Ignorance is dangerous.

Editor's Note

A number of individuals with AIDS will likely receive hospice services as their disease progresses; therefore, the reader is referred to Chapter 25 for additional information. Chapter 16 should also be consulted for additional information about hemiplegia.

Related Learning Activities

1. Visit an AIDS organization in your community and obtain information about the educational materials and services they provide.

2. If possible, interview a person with HIV/AIDS. Determine what life-style changes have been made and how the disease has had an impact on occupational roles and current quality of life.

3. What other leisure activities could Jim have participated in? What adaptations would need to be made?

4. Conduct an informal survey of your peers and family members relative to their knowledge of HIV and AIDS. Provide educational information and/or resources as necessary.

5. Because this chapter contains a number of medical terms, definitions and acronyms that may be unfamiliar, make a listing of them for study to reinforce your understanding.

References

1. Miller BF, Keane CB: *Encyclopedia and Dictionary of Medicine, Nursing, and Allied Health*, 5th Edition. Philadelphia, WB Saunders, 1992.
2. Study says AIDS vaccine safe but its effectiveness unclear. *Minneapolis Tribune* January 15, 1991, p. 2.
3. Centers for Disease Control: Update: Universal precautions for prevention of transmission of human immunodeficiency virus, hepatitis B virus, and other bloodborne pathogens in health care settings. *MMWR* 36: (Aug. 14), 1987.
4. Marcil WM: *AIDS: Occupational Therapy Can Make A Difference.* (videotape) Buffalo, New York, William Marcil Associates, 1989.
5. Marcil WM, Tigges KN: *The Person with AIDS: A Personal and Professional Perspective.* Thorofare, New Jersey, Slack, Inc., 1992.
6. Burda D, Powils S: AIDS: A time bomb at hospital's door. *Hospitals* 5(1):54, 1986.
7. Where will AIDS go in the 90s? *OT Advance* Jan. 7, 1991.
8. Marcil WM: The Role of Occupational Therapy with the Patient with AIDS. Paper presented at the American Occupational Therapy Association Annual Conference, Indianapolis, April, 1987.

The Adult With a Cerebral Vascular Accident

Barbara A. Larson, OTR, ROH
Patricia M. Watson, OTR

Introduction

Cerebral vascular accident (CVA) or stroke is a complex dysfunction caused by a lesion in the brain. It results in an upper motor neuron dysfunction that produces **hemiplegia** or paralysis of one side of the body, limbs and sometimes the face and oral structures that are **contralateral** (affecting the opposite side) to the hemisphere of the brain where the lesion has occurred. Thus, a lesion in the *left* cerebral hemisphere, or left CVA, produces hemiplegia on the *right* side of the body, and vice versa. When referring to the patient's disability as right hemiplegia, the reference is to the paralyzed body side and not the locus (place) of the lesion.[1]

Hemiplegia is the classic sign of neurovascular disease of the brain. It is one of many manifestations of neurovascular disease, and it occurs with strokes involving the cerebral hemisphere or brain stem. A stroke or cerebral vascular accident results in a sudden, specific, neurological deficit. It is the sudden onset of this neurologic deficit—seconds, minutes, hours or a few days—that characterizes the disorder as vascular. Although hemiplegia may be the most obvious sign of a cerebral vascular accident and a major concern of therapists and assistants, other symptoms are equally disabling. These include the following: sensory dysfunction, **aphasia** (impairment in using and understanding spoken and written language) or **dysarthria** (imperfect speech articulation), visual field defects and mental and intellectual impairment. The specific combination of these neurovascular deficits enables a physician to detect both the location and the size of the defect.[2]

ESSENTIAL VOCABULARY

Hemiplegia

Contralateral

Aphasia

Dysarthria

Infarction

Coordination board

Dyspraxia

Subluxation

Proprioception

Sterognosis

Work simplification

Energy conservation

Dynamometer

KEY CONCEPTS

Characteristics of stroke	ADL activities
Assessment activities	Sensory motor/perceptual activities
Adaptive equipment	Home program

Of significance in treating the patient with a stroke is the recognition that treatment goals directed toward the patient's psychosocial dysfunctions are an important component of rehabilitation. Common emotional reactions after a stroke are anxiety, denial and depression. These responses are compounded by cognitive deficits that affect language, the ability to plan and use logic, memory, and judgment and perceptual and visual deficits. Resulting behaviors exhibited by the patient include impatience, irritability, frustration, overdependence, insensitivity to others and inflexible thinking. Poor social perception, owing to the effects of the stroke, can cause aggravation that results in angry outbursts. Difficulties with communication can result in a buildup of annoyances and angry feelings. These behavioral reactions and misinterpretations of environmental events can lead to a breakdown in social and family relationships.[3]

Although the incidence of cerebrovascular disease has been decreasing for the past 25 years, stroke is still the third most common cause of death in the United States. The incidence of stroke rises rapidly with increasing age. In the 80-year-old to 90-year-old age group, the mortality rates approach the corresponding incidence rates. In the United States, the incidence of stroke is greater for men than women, and for blacks than whites. Cerebral **infarction** (occlusion of the arterial supply or venous drainage as in the case of a thrombus or embolism)[4] is the most common form of stroke, accounting for 70% of cases. Hemorrhages account for another 20% of strokes and 11% remain unspecified. An idea of the prevalence of stroke can be gained by looking at the results of a study conducted in three states: out of every 100 persons who survive a stroke, 10 return to work without impairment, 40 have mild residual disability, 40 are disabled and require special services, and 10 need institutional care.[2]

Case Study Background

Recently, Helen, a 62-year-old homemaker, became ill while preparing dinner. She experienced a severe headache and numbness of her left side. Her husband notified the paramedics who transported her to a nearby hospital where her vital signs were stabilized. After examination and tests, Helen was diagnosed as having a right CVA with resulting left hemiplegia.

Helen's physician referred her to occupational therapy for evaluation and treatment six days after the CVA. The occupational therapy staff consisted of two registered occupational therapists (OTRs) and one certified occupational therapy assistant (COTA). The department was responsible for providing services to both medical and surgical patients in this 300-bed hospital.

Assessment

Upon receipt of the referral, the occupational therapist initiated the data-gathering process. The OTR began by reading the patient's chart to obtain information about her medical, social and work history; vital signs; medications; and special precautions. She spoke with nurses providing care for Helen to find out their observations of the patient and to receive an update on her medical status.

The OTR then interviewed Helen at the bedside. During this first contact, the therapist informed the patient of the occupational therapy referral and briefly described the therapy services; thus, from the beginning, she was included in the rehabilitation process. This visit also provided the therapist with an opportunity to make initial observations of the patient's mental status and attitude toward therapy.

The OTR learned from review of the patient's chart that Helen had enjoyed good health before the stroke. The interview information indicated that she resided with her husband in a small, two-story home in the suburbs. While raising her four children, she had worked part-time as a department store clerk. Since her retirement five years ago, Helen had enjoyed traveling with her husband and spending time with her children and grandchildren, who lived nearby. She also volunteered once a week at a senior citizen center, assisting in the congregate dining program.

Helen was scheduled for an occupational therapy evaluation the next morning in the clinic. During the first one-hour session, the occupational therapist began by outlining the evaluation process. Then the OTR assessed Helen's position in the wheelchair. The patient was in a slouched posture, leaning slightly to the left. Placing a firm seat and back support in the wheelchair and issuing a lapboard provided the necessary stability for maintaining an improved posture. Once the patient was placed in a more optimal position for performance, through use of the equipment shown in Figure 16-1, the evaluation continued. The OTR assessed upper extremity range of motion, muscle strength, sensation, coordination, muscle tone and edema.

During the afternoon of the same day, the COTA saw Helen for an additional half hour. The COTA used a functional **coordination board**, which included buttons, zippers, snaps and Velcro closures to observe Helen's skill in using the unaffected upper extremity. A leisure interest survey was also completed, providing the COTA an additional opportunity to interview the patient.[5]

Early the next day, the OTR visited the patient's room and assessed upper extremity hygiene and dressing skills. When Helen came to the clinic later that morning, the OTR continued administering other evaluation procedures. Perceptual motor, visual and cognitive assessments were used to detect problems with body image, problem solving, sequencing, presence of field cut and **dyspraxia** (the inability to perform motor functions). During the evaluation, Helen was pleasant and cooperative, quickly completing tasks, unaware of her errors. A homemaking evaluation was completed that afternoon by the OTR. This assessment gave the therapist an opportunity to gain information on Helen's judgment and reliability with more familiar activities.

On the next day, the OTR and the COTA met to discuss the evaluation results and plan the treatment. The results were as follows:[6]

Positioning: Helen displayed fair trunk balance. She was able to attain a vertical posture with minimum assistance and remain in midline with cueing. After the wheelchair insert was provided, the patient was able to maintain this position when reaching away from her body about 12 to 14 inches.

Upper extremity functioning: The patient's unaffected right side displayed strength and range of motion measurements within normal limits. Helen was right-handed and results of coordination testing revealed speed of coordination to be within functional limits. Her left affected extremity had minimum spasticity present in the biceps, but this did not interfere significantly with function. Passive range of motion was within normal limits with no complaints of pain during movement. No shoulder **subluxation** (partial dislocation of the joint) was evident but mild edema was present in the hand. Sensation was intact in the areas of **proprioception** (ability to identify the position of body parts in space) and **stereognosis** (ability to identify objects and forms through the sense of touch). Her responses to surface pain, light touch and hot/cold stimuli indicated impairment in these areas.

Synergy patterns: Helen demonstrated a flexion synergy with the strongest components being elbow and shoulder flexion. She was able to flex and abduct her shoulder one-third through the full range of motion and flex her elbow two-thirds through the normal range. She was able to partially extend her elbow and wrist with gravity eliminated. Helen demonstrated the ability to flex her fingers but had no functional grasp.

Mental status: The patient was oriented to time, place and person. She was talkative and had a bright affect. She exhibited moderate impulsivity, decreased insight into her problems, impaired problem solving, decreased attention span and poor concentration.

Visual/perceptual motor: Helen demonstrated left-sided unilateral neglect but did attend to the left, once cued. Mild problems with figure-ground and spatial orientation were also evidenced. These appeared on more complex assessment tasks, which included locating a number in the telephone directory and completing a three-dimensional cube design.

Leisure survey: The patient indicated she liked to be with people. She expressed interest in handicrafts such as ceramics and needlework. She enjoyed cooking and entertaining,

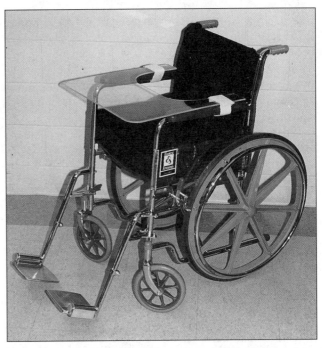

Figure 16-1. *Wheelchair adapted for seating stability. Courtesy of Ann Forrest Clark, Polinsky Medical Rehabilitation Center, Duluth, MN.*

as well as attending movies and sharing gardening chores with her husband.

Activites of daily living (ADLs): The evaluation revealed that Helen needed cues to complete thorough hygiene. She had attempted to use her left arm to assist with tasks after cueing. She demonstrated an ability to learn and follow through after cues and suggestions for dressing techniques were provided. Helen required only minimum assistance with her upper extremity dressing. She was dependent in putting on her brassiere. The patient needed moderate assistance with putting on and pulling up lower extremity garments and was dependent with stockings and shoes. Upper extremity dressing and hygiene were performed from a seated position, and lower extremity dressing was accomplished from a supine position.

Homemaking: The initial evaluation was completed with the patient working from a wheelchair. She demonstrated moderate impulsivity and poor planning when propelling the chair. Initially, she had difficulties with problem solving and displayed lapses in judgment and reliability, but demonstrated an ability to learn from cues provided by the OTR.

Treatment Planning

After the evaluation was completed and the OTR and the COTA had collaborated on the evaluation results,[5] the occupational therapist attended a team conference. This meeting included the OTR, staff members providing care for the patient, physician, nurse, physical therapist and social worker. It was determined that Helen would be treated by physical and occupational therapy for two weeks, with a team meeting held during the second week to discuss her progress. The rehabilitation goal was to return Helen to her home environment with increased independence in functional living skills and provision of support services if necessary.

Helen was scheduled to receive occupational therapy services three times a day. The COTA would see Helen for daily morning dressing sessions and one 30- to 60-minute afternoon period for group sessions or homemaking training. The OTR would treat the patient each morning during a 60-minute functional restoration session. The patient's goals for occupational therapy were established as follows:

Long-term Goals (To Be Established Within Two Weeks)
- Patient will consistently use left upper extremity to assist with a single active motion in daily skills.
- Patient will complete an adapted cutting board project, incorporating use of left upper extremity in this task within one week.
- Patient will demonstrate compensation for left neglect, requiring only one reminder during any treatment session.

Short-term Goals
- Patient will dress self with minimal cuing following 5 treatment sessions.
- Patient will demonstrate good judgment and problem solving skills after four sessions of homemaking training.
- Patient will consistently use the left upper extremity to assist with a single active motion in daily skills by the end of two weeks.
- Patient will complete an adapted cutting board project, incorporating use of the left upper extremity in this task, without cueing by the end of two weeks.
- Patient will demonstrate compensation for left-side neglect, requiring only one reminder during any treatment session by the end of three weeks.

Short-term goals will be reviewed and new goals established or current goals revised, on a weekly basis.

The occupational therapist discussed the treatment goals and plans with both Helen and her husband and incorporated their suggestions. Helen's record, which included problems, evaluation results and the treatment plan, was kept on file in the occupational therapy clinic. The OTR and the COTA updated the file three times a week. This proved to be the most effective means for providing consistency in treatment.

Treatment Implementation

The COTA saw Helen daily for dressing training. Initially, they worked on upper extremity hygiene and dressing.

The patient sat in her wheelchair facing a mirror while at the sink and proceeded to brush her teeth, wash her face and upper torso, and apply deodorant. The occupational therapy assistant instructed Helen to slow down and become more thorough with hygiene. The COTA demonstrated and provided written and illustrated step-by-step procedures for putting on either a front button or a pullover blouse. After three sessions, Helen was able to recall the correct sequence for dressing her affected, left upper extremity first. She was able to put on and take off her brassiere independently after the COTA adapted it with a front Velcro closure. As the patient's balance improved, she progressed to lower extremity dressing. At that time, she was independent with light hygiene. During dressing training, the COTA attempted to enhance Helen's awareness of her affected side while having her utilize the present function. The COTA assisted her in dealing with acceptance of the change in her body so that it could be reintegrated into the performance of tasks. As a result of this training, the patient progressed to complete dressing independence. She demonstrated an improved ability to problem solve and spent appropriate amounts of time in performing tasks, slowing down instead of accomplishing them hurriedly.

The OTR initiated a program to improve Helen's left upper extremity function, maintain her right upper extremity strength and remediate her visual perceptual motor problems, including left neglect, impulsivity, decreased attention span, concentration and problem solving.[5] The therapist used an approach to treatment that incorporated bilateral upper extremity tasks. The COTA and the OTR collaborated so that during treatment sessions, all problems would be addressed by the use of various modalities. The therapist used clasped hand activities such as large peg board games, ball and bean bag toss and a punching bag, incorporating trunk rotation into the movements. Left upper extremity weight bearing was used as Helen worked on simple mathematics problems and progressed to check writing, record keeping and use of a calculator. Visual perceptual motor needs were addressed as she worked on paper and pencil activities, including the use of the telephone directory, writing short pieces of information and engaging in problem solving with hypothetical emergency situations.

The COTA conducted an afternoon CVA treatment group, which met twice each week. The focus of the group was to aid integration of sensory, motor and perceptual skills for improved performance in daily tasks. The peer support also enhanced social skills necessary for resuming former life-style patterns. The occupational therapy assistant instructed the patients in self-range of motion for regaining specific body part movement and awareness. The group also engaged in card and board games to address visual and perceptual problems while facilitating social interaction as well.[6] Helen was an active participant in all of these activities.

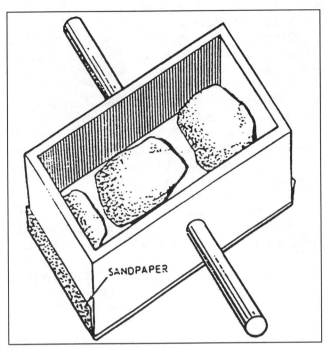

Figure 16-2. *Bilateral sander. From Craft Techniques in Occupational Therapy. Published by US Dept. of the Army, U.S. Government Printing Office, August 1971. Reprinted with permission.*

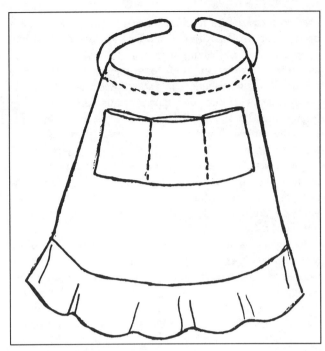

Figure 16-3. *Hoop apron.*

During the one-on-one session, the COTA worked with Helen on individual activities that addressed goals more specifically. The patient sanded an adapted bread board using both hands and an adapted sander. The bilateral sander is illustrated in Figure 16-2. Using the present arm movement, Helen sanded at a downward angle, which eliminated gravity. After working through the synergy pattern, she sanded on an inclined plane, thus providing resistance to shoulder flexion and elbow extension. The patient also worked on completing a rubber link doormat. This activity encouraged bilateral upper extremity use, increased perceptual skill, improved concentration and maintained right arm strength when she worked with a weighted wrist cuff. To address Helen's avocational interests, the COTA provided her with a short-term embroidery project on large mesh canvas. The patient worked on this evenings and weekends, placing the project on her bedside table and stabilizing the work with her left arm and hand.

Twice each week during an afternoon session, Helen participated in homemaking training with the COTA. Initially working from the wheelchair, she progressed to performing tasks while standing at the counter. A narrow based "quad" cane was used for ambulation. As she improved, the patient progressed from opening cans to using the stove top safely. Following the package instructions, the patient successfully baked a cake in the oven. The skills acquired during training enabled Helen to compile a grocery list, sequence tasks properly, and independently prepare a light meal. Although fine motor skill was absent, she used

the weight of her left hand to stabilize objects. A hoop apron with pockets, shown in Figure 16-3, and a utility cart on wheels were used to transport items.[7] The COTA incorporated **work simplification** and **energy conservation** techniques into the sessions. She specifically encouraged Helen to follow these basic principles:[7]

1. Sit while working whenever possible.
2. Slide objects across the counter or table.
3. Keep frequently used items within easy reach.
4. Prepare one-course meals.
5. Plan intermittent rest periods during one's daily routine.

The OTR and the COTA met daily for approximately 15 minutes to review Helen's current status and to update her file when indicated. Both encouraged her husband to attend occupational therapy sessions so he could become more involved in his wife's recovery process. Helen's husband, a retired salesman, appeared somewhat anxious about his wife's illness but was attentive and offered support whenever possible.

After two weeks of intensive therapy, Helen demonstrated much improvement. Her left upper extremity progressed through components of flexion and extension synergies and had gained relative independence from synergies. Upon reevaluation, she demonstrated antigravity movement of her affected upper extremity. She had developed voluntary movement, using her left arm to assist in single sequence activities during daily tasks. Helen regained an active grasp, which measured 2.5 pounds on the **dynamometer** (device used to measure the force of muscle strength.) She developed some isolated finger movement, including partial opposition, yet she would need more therapy to strengthen and refine the motion. With returning hand function, the edema was diminished. The patient was not yet able to manipulate objects smaller than a tennis ball. Because of improvement in Helen's balance and upper extremity function, the lapboard and wheelchair insert were no longer necessary.

Helen was independent with light dressing and light hygiene but required minimum assistance with bathing. She needed a shower seat and a handheld shower head, minimum transfer assistance, and stand-by supervision during the shower.

Using an adapted bread board, a hoop apron with pockets and a utility cart on wheels, Helen had become more independent with light meal preparation. She required less cuing, had slowed down her performance and was demonstrating improved problem solving ability. The patient was able to ambulate 20 feet using a narrow based "quad" cane but did require stand-by supervision. Helen was independent in her bed mobility, requiring only stand-by assistance for bed-to-wheelchair transfer. The patient displayed self-cued awareness of the left side of her body, indicating she had learned compensation for left neglect. Her attention span had improved greatly, allowing improved task performance.

The OTR and the COTA were responsible for daily documentation and recording of charges for their treatment sessions. Each recorded pertinent performance data and noted any changes during the treatment periods. Notes were written using a problem-oriented approach to charting.

Discharge Planning

Before the final team meeting, the OTR and the COTA met to review Helen's progress and to identify further needs. Helen had expressed concern about her ability to function in her kitchen and bathroom at home. She was open to suggestions for improving the arrangement but was having difficulty describing the floor plan. With input from the COTA regarding other areas of progress and concerns, the OTR prepared a progress report to present at the team meeting.

In the team meeting, it was decided that the OTR would make a home visit during the additional week Helen would be hospitalized. The OTR suggested that the patient accompany her. After the team discussed progress to date, they decided that Helen would be discharged to her home the next week. It was recommended that the patient return for additional physical and occupational therapy treatment on an outpatient basis twice a week after discharge. Both Helen

and her husband agreed to this plan.

Helen became very apprehensive at the prospect of returning home, even for a single visit. She expressed concern about her ability to manage in the home atmosphere and thought she would be a burden to her husband. With encouragement from the team members, however, Helen and her husband participated in the home visit. After the home assessment, the OTR suggested several ways that Helen might manage her home more easily. The therapist also gained information that would assist her in focusing more specifically on what was required for the patient to have increased independence once she returned home. The home visit also allowed Helen a brief opportunity to practice some of her hospital-acquired skills. She was cooperative during the visit, secure in the knowledge she would return to the hospital for further treatment.

After the home visit, the OTR and COTA planned treatment for the final week. Dressing training was discontinued, as Helen had become independent in this area.[5] Practicing one-handed techniques, organizing her work more specifically and learning appropriate safety measures were the focus of her current homemaking training tasks. Her husband would assume responsibility for the laundry and heavy cleaning chores, with other family members assisting him as necessary.

Helen's husband had observed his wife's occupational therapy sessions quite regularly. During the last week of inpatient treatment, he became an active participant in her program by assisting her with activities, such as range of motion and providing cues for the proper energy conservation techniques. He encouraged his wife during the final homemaking sessions as she practiced one-handed techniques, such as pouring liquids and breaking an egg, using the function of her left upper extremity to assist her.[7]

The COTA and the OTR collaborated on the development of Helen's home program. The therapist prepared a left upper extremity active range of motion guide with diagrams and written instructions. She also suggested activities such as washing and drying dishes, dusting furniture and objects, folding laundry and getting dressed. These light resistive tasks incorporated grasp and release motions during daily functional activities, reinforcing compensation for left neglect. The COTA identified equipment that Helen would need at home, including adapted bathroom items previously mentioned, as well as an adapted jar opener, a long oven mitt and a hoop apron. Her husband agreed to purchase these. Diagrams and written information on work simplification and energy conservation techniques were also included in the program.

Home safety was discussed with Helen. She was encouraged to remove scatter rugs, to use nonglare, nonskid floor wax, and to store things within easy access to eliminate unnecessary bending or reaching.[7]

During the final days of treatment, the OTR continued

working with the patient, using activities to improve Helen's left upper extremity function. The COTA engaged the patient in completing the rubber link doormat, with her left hand and arm more actively involved in the process.

Program Discontinuation

Before the program was discontinued, both the OTR and the COTA encouraged Helen and her husband to gradually begin resuming their involvement in community activities. They discussed the possibility of Helen visiting the senior citizen center to begin reacquainting herself with friends and activities. She was interested but appeared hesitant and expressed the desire to have more improved function of her left arm and hand before returning to the center. To reinforce what she had learned in the hospital and to gain confidence in her skills, Helen was urged to visit family members and accompany her husband on short outings to the shopping mall.

By the time his wife was discharged, Helen's husband demonstrated comprehension of the home program and was a willing participant in her ongoing rehabilitation. Having been provided with specific treatment suggestions and community resource information, they both felt prepared to deal with situations they might encounter. The COTA and the OTR, as well as other members of the treatment team, looked forward to Helen's continued progress. As her functional abilities improved, she would regain her self-confidence and experience an enhanced quality of life.

Related Learning Activities

1. Working with a peer, brainstorm to develop a list of energy conservation activities for a person with a CVA.

2. Study rehabilitation catalogs and determine the equipment that might be useful to increase independence for someone with a stroke.

3. Contact the local office of the state health department about community resources for patients with stroke.

4. What additional craft activities could Helen have participated in, assuming that she expressed an interest?

5. Make an outline of changes that would be necessary in Helen's treatment if she was aphasic.

References

1. Pedretti LW: Cerebral vascular accident. In Pedretti LW, Zoltan B (Eds): *Occupational Therapy Practice Skills for Physical Dysfunction*, 3rd Edition. St Louis, Mosby-Year Book, 1990, p 603.

2. Ryerson SD: Hemiplegia resulting from vascular insult disease. In DA Umphred (Ed): *Neurological Rehabilitation*, 3rd Edition. St Louis, Mosby-Year Book, 1985, p. 474.

3. Versluys HP: Psychosocial accommodation to physical disability. In Trombly CA (Ed): *Occupational Therapy for Physical Dysfunction*, 3rd Edition. Baltimore: Williams & Wilkins, 1989, p. 27.

4. Miller BF, Keane CB: *Encyclopedia and Dictionary of Medicine, Nursing, and Allied Health*, 5th Edition. Philadelphia, WB Saunders, 1992.

5. Entry-level role delineation for OTRs and COTAs. *Occup Ther Newspaper* 35(July):8-16, 1981.

6. Hopkins H, Smith H (Eds): *Willard and Spackman's Occupational Therapy*, 6th Edition. Philadelphia: JB Lippincott, 1983, ch 22.

7. Klinger JL: *Mealtime Manual for People with Disabilities and the Aging*, 2nd Edition, Camden, New Jersey, Campbell Soup Co., 1979, pp. 6, 56, 72, 84.

Part E
THE ELDERLY

The Elderly With Parkinson's Disease

Kathryn Melin-Eberhardt, BA, COTA
Javan E. Walker Jr., MA, OTR

Introduction

Parkinson's disease or Parkinsonism is a chronic disorder characterized by involuntary tremulous motion beginning in the hands at rest. Movements become slow as the muscles become rigid, causing a masklike face, and the torso tilts forward. Onset is between the ages of 40 and 80 years of age, with an incidence of 20 per 100,000 people. The disease progresses to severe physical limitation, and the intellect may be ultimately compromised. It is a chronic disease of the nervous system that often produces rather remarkable clinical symptoms. In addition to the masked facial appearance, symptoms include rigidity, either "cogwheel" or "lead-pipe"; rhythmic **tremor** (involuntary trembling) of the hands with a pill-rolling motion; and stooped posture. The affected person demonstrates an involuntary tendency to take short accelerating steps when walking, which is referred to as **festination**, an abnormal slowness of movement known as **bradykinesia**, and absence or poverty of movement called **akinesia**. A resting tremor occurs only when the patient is at rest and disappears when there is voluntary movement. Fine motor incoordination, contractures, fatigue and weakness make activities of daily living (ADL) difficult without assistance. There is poor standing balance in late stages of the disease, which along with a tendency toward rapid propulsion and difficulty in stopping, makes ambulation very dangerous. The gradual loss of joint range of motion, which affects the rest of the body, also inhibits oral articulation, causing the patient to demonstrate slurred speech referred to as **dysarthria** and drooling, due to excessive salivation.[1,2]

ESSENTIAL VOCABULARY

Tremor

Festination

Bradykinesia

Akinesia

Dysarthria

Substantia nigra

Graded resistive activities

Postural balance

Adaptive devices

Body mechanics

KEY CONCEPTS

Characteristics of Parkinson's disease

Community-based practice

Activities of daily living

Gross and fine motor coordination

Sensory integration/perceptual skills

Cognitive skills

Craft and leisure groups

Home program

Recovery from Parkinson's disease rarely occurs, and the duration is indefinite. The condition can be induced by certain chemicals, such as "MPTP," a by-product of the street drug "MPPP," a meperidine (Demerol) analog. This suggests that parkinsonism might have an environmental origin. The injury to the body occurs in the **substantia nigra** region of the upper brainstem where the neurotransmitter dopamine is normally produced. Therefore, efforts at drug treatment include use of the dopamine precursor levodopa, as dopamine itself cannot cross the blood-brain barrier. Thirty percent of persons with Parkinson's disease fail to respond to use of this drug.[3] Use of levodopa causes significant side effects such as uncontrolled movements of the tongue, oral or buccal muscles and jaw[4]; depression; and nausea.[3] Other drugs being tested include Deprenyl and tocopherol.

Rehabilitation management by a treatment team composed of the registered occupational therapist (OTR), certified occupational therapy assistant (COTA), physical therapist, and physician can do much to assist the patient faced with this disabling condition. As the disease progresses and breathing problems are encountered, a respiratory therapist often provides treatment as well.

Case Study Background

Willie, a 70-year-old widowed janitor, had been diagnosed with Parkinson's disease five years ago. Although he was still able to ambulate safely, he was forced to retire from his job, due to the increasing physical difficulties related to his disease process. An active man who enjoyed athletic activities, he has begun to attend the George Washington Carver Older Adult Center in his neighborhood.

The center is staffed with a social worker, activity therapists, and counselors as well as a COTA. The local hospital provided the COTA with an OTR supervisor who spent one afternoon each week evaluating patients and developing treatment programs for the COTA to carry out on a day-to-day basis.

Willie's primary interest in coming to the center was to give him social contacts and allow him to remain active. At his last visit to his physician, however, he complained about increased problems when performing household chores around his apartment, and he reported difficulty with some self-care activities. The physician referred Willie to the occupational therapy department at the rehabilitation hospital, which also provided services to the Carver Center. When the OTR received the referral, she called the COTA and asked her to initiate the screening process that they had developed collaboratively and report her findings to the therapist the next day.

Screening

During the initial interview, the COTA explained the role of occupational therapy to Willie and began obtaining some information that was indicated on the standard evaluation form. She asked about the architecture of his home, emphasizing the stairs and kitchen and bathroom layout, as well as the characteristics of other rooms. Knowing that he lived alone, she inquired about what type of help he had or thought he needed in taking care of his apartment and doing his shopping and laundry. Other questions focused on his goals, knowledge of his disability and awareness of his prognosis. After the initial screening, the COTA organized all of her screening data and reported it to the OTR.

The next Monday the OTR visited the center and analyzed the screening data, which the COTA had submitted to her. She then decided on the evaluation tools that would be used and arranged a meeting with the assistant to discuss those parts of the evaluation that the COTA would complete.

Evaluation

The OTR identified four areas of evaluation: ADL, sensorimotor components, cognitive components and psychological components. Because the COTA had received outstanding training, the therapist felt comfortable having her assist in assessing the patient in several areas, including further data collection using a structured format, observing the patient, and administering structured testing in several areas.

Before conducting the evaluation, the OTR discussed her concerns with the COTA and explained the other areas that she wanted the COTA to focus on, such as using her observational skills during the evaluation to further assess the patient's functional motor skills. She stressed the importance of the COTA assisting the OTR by reporting her observations to her after the evaluation. The areas indicated for COTA evaluation were ADL, upper and lower extremity status, fine motor and gross motor coordination, and strength and endurance during the activities of daily living evaluation. Cognitive skills and some sensory integration skills were also to be observed and evaluated.

COTA Evaluation

The COTA set up an appointment with Willie to complete her portion of the evaluation. She began by having him fill out a structured interview form that gathered additional data about his family history, self-care abilities, school and work history and his leisure interests and experiences. The COTA performed her assessment in the following areas:

Activities of Daily Living:
- Grooming
- Head/neck and oral hygiene
- Feeding and eating
- Dressing: upper and lower extremity
- Functional mobility: transfer skills (bed, toilet, tub)
- Functional communication: telephone and writing skills
- Balance and endurance while sitting and standing related to ADL

Upper and Lower Extremity Status:
- Observation of active/passive range of motion in functional activities during the ADL evaluation
- Testing of gross and fine motor coordination with structured tests
- Observation of strength and endurance during functional activities

Cognitive skills:
- Orientation: time, place and person
- Observation of comprehension and attention span
- Observation of cognitive integration

Sensory Integration/Perceptual Skills:
- Observation of body integration during ADL
- Observation of perceptual functioning

After completing her evaluation, the COTA summarized the data and reported the findings to the OTR. They both looked at the data, and the COTA indicated her recommendations at that time, based on her own evaluation data. The OTR then set up an appointment with the patient to complete the evaluation.

OTR Evaluation

The OTR evaluated the patient's neuromuscular status, concentrating on active and passive range of motion and the presence or absence of tremors and rigidity. She performed a manual muscle test and made an assessment of his fine motor and gross motor capabilities. She also noted that the patient did not appear to experience any pain or discomfort while the evaluation procedures were being carried out.

As part of her assessment, the OTR queried the patient about his emotional status, and further explored his leisure skills and interests after his retirement and the death of his wife.

When all the evaluations were completed, the OTR analyzed the data collected, synthesized it and documented her findings and recommendations in the patient's chart. It was determined that the patient was experiencing decreased range of motion in upper and lower extremities, problems with gait and balance, tremor and some difficulty with articulation. He did have a positive attitude and was willing to work on his problems. His leisure skills, which included attending local baseball games, playing cards and board games and hiking, appeared appropriate for his age and situation. His ADLs indicated beginning problems in main-

tenance of personal hygiene, dressing, feeding and eating, home maintenance, shopping and communication when writing. The therapist prepared a report and sent a copy of the evaluation findings to the referring physician.

Program Planning

The OTR, with the assistance of the COTA, began to develop long-term and short-term goals for a program of treatment to be carried out by the assistant. The three areas identified were a daily pattern of functional activities at the center and at home to maintain active range of motion, to preserve the present level of strength and endurance and to continue a life of productivity.[2,5]

Goals were developed for independent ADL, sensorimotor skills, strength and endurance and cognitive and psychosocial skills.

Long-term Goals
- The patient will demonstrate independence in functional activities to prevent further deterioration of daily living skills within two months.
- The patient will demonstrate maintenance and/or increase of fine and gross motor coordination in functional activities within two months.
- The patient will demonstrate maintenance of cognitive and psychosocial skills through biweekly participation in craft and leisure groups.

Short-term goals were also identified that related to each of these. The OTR and COTA began to discuss how to develop a treatment program that would involve the patient in activities at the center and at home and would meet his therapeutic goals. It was significant that both the therapist and the assistant had perceived Willie as a highly motivated patient who was capable of working independently in the treatment program. The OTR stressed that movements should be rhythmic and that adjuncts such as music, clapping, counting out loud or a metronome may be useful during some aspects of treatment. After further discussion, both the COTA and the OTR agreed on the following program for the COTA to carry out:

Activities of Daily Living Skills

Grooming and hygiene: Work with the patient in a group activity; assist in personal grooming skills.

Feeding/eating: Assist the patient as needed during the noon meal and provide large-handled, weighted utensils for feeding at home and at the center to decrease tremors.

Dressing: Assist the patient in developing fine-motor skills in activities such as buttoning and zipping by using a button hook and zipper pulls.

Functional mobility: Even though bed mobility is still intact, standing balance has decreased. Work on challenging activities such as ball catching in a group. Patient may need further assistance with transfers to tub, toilet or car. This area will be evaluated further.

Functional communication: Focus on ability to use telephone accurately in an emergency and maintenance of a legible signature.

Psychosocial Skills

Self-concept/self-identity: Work with patient in small groups and one-to-one, focusing on feelings about his disability including his facial features, tremors and gait. Recommend participation in a support group.

Community involvement: Involve patient with members of agencies and programs, such as a telephone reassurance program, that focus on safety measures and safety while living alone.

Interests: Work with patient individually and in a group to discuss leisure skills and their role in his life. Interest in hiking may not be possible due to progression of disease; encourage daily strolls in the neighborhood. Involve in group card and board games and encourage continued attendance at baseball games.

Neuromuscular and Motor Components

Range of motion: Involve patient in range of motion exercise that can be performed at the center or at home.

Gross motor skills: Work with the patient on cone-stacking activities and games, sitting or standing, to improve gross motor skills. Involve in sports activities at the center such as shuffle board, pitching horseshoes, and relay games.

Fine motor skills: Work with patient on craft activities that require fine-motor skills such as 1-inch mosaic tile work, copper tooling, stenciling or leather work.

Strength and endurance: Work on **graded resistive activities** (tasks that require increasing degrees of resistance), which should include a woodworking project, using a hand saw to cut out pieces; project should require sanding.

Postural control: Ensure that **postural balance** (maintaining equilibrium in different positions) is incorporated in all of the activities.

Therapeutic Adaptations

Assistive or **adaptive devices** may be needed for daily living skills activities. These devices could include a buttonhook, zipper pulls, adaptive silverware, or plate guards and equipment for tub and toilet transfers.

Prevention

Energy conservation, work simplification and proper **body mechanics** (specific methods for lifting, reaching, etc.) should be stressed in performing all activities.

Home Program

In addition to a home treatment program including the

activities identified, the OTR and COTA will make a home visit to determine whether modifications need to be made to ensure that the program is effective in the patient's environment.

Treatment Implementation

Because the treatment program established for Willie was carried out over a long time, the following brief excerpt is provided to acquaint the reader with some of the specific treatment activities.

The treatment plan was implemented the next day by the COTA. Willie joined the craft group at the center and selected a mosaic trivet project constructed with 1-inch tile. While waiting for the glue to dry before applying grout, he started work on an oak book rack. Because Willie had not used a hand saw for a long time, the COTA suggested that he practice first on a piece of pine. This technique also provided a way to grade the activity, as pine offers less resistance than oak wood. Involvement in these activities addressed the treatment objectives in the areas of range of motion, fine and gross motor skills, and strength and endurance.

The COTA observed Willie while he was eating lunch and determined that a plate guard would be needed. She asked Willie to try eating with a 6-ounce wrist cuff on his right hand. He agreed and stated "This really helps get rid of some of my shaking."

During the afternoon, Willie participated in a leisure skills discussion group and later joined some of the group members in walking around the neighborhood. The COTA gave Willie a copy of the recreational calendar of events sponsored by the center and encouraged him to attend the baseball outing and participate in shuffleboard that week.[2] She also made an appointment with him so that she and the OTR could evaluate his apartment. Before Willie left the center for the day, the COTA instructed him in a home range of motion program which emphasized crossing the midline. The assistant recorded observation and progress notes, and called the OTR to report this information as well as to verify a date and time for the home visit.

The home visit was conducted the next Monday morning. The COTA observed Willie while he was washing his face, brushing his teeth and shaving. The latter activity presented some new problems not observed in the initial evaluation. Willie was using a small manual razor, and the COTA suggested that he try a heavier electric razor which she had brought along. Willie stated "I'm going right out to buy one of these!" The COTA also observed Willie while he put on a long-sleeved shirt with front buttons. Noting his frustration in fastening the buttons, she instructed him on how to use a buttonhook (Figure 17-1). With some embarrassment, Willie stated that the only other dressing problem he had was zipping up his pants. He was surprised to see how easily the problem was solved with the use of a zipper pull. The OTR had brought portable grab bars for the bathtub and the toilet and after observing Willie's transfer techniques. She installed the equipment and had the COTA instruct him in using it correctly and safely. Due to trunk and lower extremity rigidity, the OTR also recommended that an elevated toilet seat be used.

Both the OTR and the COTA noted that Willie's general housekeeping was less than adequate so, with Willie's permission, arrangements were made with a neighborhood church to have a volunteer youth group come in to do heavy cleaning every two weeks for a nominal fee that was used to support church activities. The OTR recommended that Willie join a group at the center, which the COTA led, to learn work simplification and energy conservation techniques related to daily cooking and housekeeping tasks. In addition, he was encouraged to join the local Parkinson's disease patient support group that also met at the center. Because Willie lived alone, he agreed to be enrolled in a telephone reassurance program sponsored by a local senior citizens group.

Program Discontinuation

Because of the nature of this progressively debilitating disease, no program discontinuation was anticipated. Instead, the OTR and COTA conducted frequent reassessments of the patient's progress, and continually adapted the program to his gradual loss of independence. It was anticipated that they would contact a therapist in a nursing home if and when it became necessary for Willie to transfer to an intermediate care facility.

At the present time, however, Willie is doing quite well. His spirits have improved as a result of his continued ability to maintain an independent existence. Although he recognizes his present level of difficulty, he has expressed appreciation to the occupational therapy staff for their assistance in maintaining his sense of dignity by helping him to remain independent.

Acknowledgment

Appreciation is offered to Barbara O'Keefe, MA, OTR, College of St. Catherine, for her content suggestions and modifications.

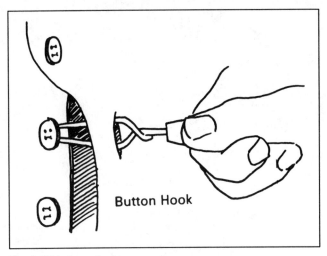

Figure 17-1. *Button hook.*

Related Learning Activities

1. Write to the American Parkinson's Disease Association, 116 John Street, New York, NY 10038, and request copies of their free brochures.

2. Attend a meeting of a Parkinson's disease support group in your community. Identify local resources available to patients.

3. Depending on the patient's interests, what are some other functional activities that could be used to increase or maintain strength, endurance and gross and fine motor skills?

References

1. Okamoto G: *Physical Medicine and Rehabilitation*. Philadelphia, WB Saunders, 1984, pp. 181-182.
2. Spencer EA: Functional restoration-specific diagnosis. In Hopkins H, Smith H (Eds): *Willard and Spackman's Occupational Therapy*, 7th Edition. Philadelphia, JB Lippincott Co., 1988, pp. 481-483.
3. Kottke FJ, Lehmann JF: *Krusen's Handbook of Physical Medicine and Rehabilitation*. Philadelphia, WB Saunders, 1990, pp. 780-782.
4. Weiner WJ, Klawans HL: Lingual-facial-buccal movements in the elderly I: Pathophysiology and treatment. *J Amer Geriatr Soc* 21:314-320, 1973.
5. Miller BF, Keane CB: *Encyclopedia and Dictionary of Medicine, Nursing, and Allied Health*, 5th Edition. Philadelphia, WB Saunders, 1992.

The Elderly With Alzheimer's Disease

Ilenna Brown, COTA, ROH
Cynthia F. Epstein, MA, OTR, FAOTA

Introduction

Alzheimer's disease, first described by the German physician Alois Alzheimer in 1907, is a neurologic brain disorder that causes both intellectual and physical decline and eventually, death. Early stages of the disease are characterized by a gradual, and sometimes imperceptible, decline in many areas of intellectual function with accompanying physical decline. Initially, only memory may be noticeably affected. There may be difficulty learning new skills or problems with tasks requiring abstract reasoning.

As the disease progresses, impairment in both language and motor ability is seen. Inability to find the right word or words to describe things and increasing difficulty understanding explanations known as expressive and receptive **aphasia** become evident. Changes in personality and outbursts of anger may be seen. Late in the illness, varying symptoms such as **incontinence** (lack of bowel and/or bladder control), inability to walk and inability to recognize people are characteristic. Alzheimer's disease usually leads to death in about seven to nine years.

In the last few years, several theories as to the possible causes of Alzheimer's disease have been considered. Research is in progress investigating the possibility that it may be caused by an infectious agent that may lie dormant in the human body. **Genetic** (hereditary) and environmental factors may then trigger the disease in later life.[1] Another study points to a link between Alzheimer's disease and distortions of blood vessels in the brain.[2]

KEY CONCEPTS

Characteristics of Alzheimer's disease	Environmental adaptations
Nursing home practice	Mealtime program
Assessment tools and activities	OT and activities program
Action plan	

ESSENTIAL VOCABULARY

Aphasia

Incontinence

Genetic

Embolism

Plaques

Geriatrician

Figure-ground discrimination

Form constancy

Mental Status Questionnaire

Dyadic

An estimated 1.3 to 1.8 million Americans over 65 years of age have Alzheimer's disease. Another 80,000 or more in their 40s and 50s also contract it. To date, there is no cure for Alzheimer's disease, and death occurs probably not from brain deterioration itself, but from physical infirmities such as pneumonia and pulmonary **embolism** (occulsion of a blood vessel that can accompany the disease).

A final diagnosis of Alzheimer's disease rests on the presence of neurotic **plaques,** which are patches or flat areas and neurofibrillary tangles in the structure of the brain. Researchers continue to explore new methods of verifying Alzheimer's disease in its early stages, but at present a brain autopsy is the only way of making this determination, and these examinations are not routinely performed. Currently, clinical observation, the absence of any other causes for the condition, and a compatible CT (computerized axial tomography) scan are the basis on which a diagnosis of Alzheimer's disease is made.[3,4]

Case Study Background

Born on April 6, 1910 in New York, Gertrude is the oldest of four children, two of whom are still living. Gertrude never married and lived by herself, employed as a secretary, until her retirement at age 65. She then went to live with her sister and her husband, where she was a productive member of their household. Four years later, her sister noticed that Gertrude was becoming increasingly forgetful, often misplacing personal belongings or leaving pots unattended on the stove. Additionally, Gertrude could not concentrate on an activity and did not seem to enjoy participating in family discussions the way she had in the past. Her sister attributed these problems to Gertrude's "getting older," not recognizing them as possible symptoms of early Alzheimer's disease.[1]

Four more years passed and the home situation had significantly worsened. The sister's husband became ill and was hospitalized. When he returned home he required a great deal of time and care. Gertrude had become a serious management problem for her sister. She was withdrawn, spoke very little and often had sudden outbursts of temper over seemingly inconsequential matters. She would frequently leave the house and then not be able to find her way home. One day Gertrude walked out of the house without putting on her shoes or stockings. At this point, her sister recognized the seriousness of the problem and, feeling unable to cope any longer, took Gertrude to a **geriatrician,** a physician who specializes in working with older people.

Gertrude was diagnosed with Alzheimer's disease. The physician referred the family to a community support group, which was sponsored by the local chapter of the Alzheimer's Disease and Related Disorders Association, to help them

cope. As the family realized the severity of the problem and the increasing demands of Gertrude's illness, they began to consider nursing home placement. They visited many facilities, seeking one that would be supportive of patients with this disease. Guidelines provided by the support group helped the family identify important services, such as occupational therapy, that should be available in the nursing home.

The nursing home selected was well known in the community for its supportive care to Alzheimer patients. They even had a special family council, where families met together with staff to plan special events for the patients. Because of its excellent reputation, the facility had a waiting list. The family decided it was worth waiting and obtained homemaker assistance plus the help of the sister's grown children and grandchildren. This strategy allowed Gertrude's sister to manage her invalid husband and Gertrude at home until a bed became available in the nursing home.

During the month of waiting, Gertrude became progressively worse. At the time of her admission, presenting problems were increased confusion and forgetfulness, rapid mood changes and catastrophic reactions involving a refusal to participate in activities of daily living such as bathing, dressing and undressing.[4]

Assessment

A referral for occupational therapy evaluation was made by the physician upon the patient's admission. As part of the screening process, the occupational therapist (OTR) assigned the occupational therapy assistant (COTA) to perform the preliminary chart review. Using a structured reporting format, the COTA gathered information on the patient's educational and occupational history, her leisure interests and prior living situation. With this information, the OTR met with the family to obtain a more comprehensive picture of the patient's functional level before admission.

In assessing a patient with Alzheimer's disease, the caregivers provide an important source of information, as the patient is usually not a reliable informant. The family reported that the patient's increasing forgetfulness, unsteady gait and increasing incontinence had made home management unfeasible. They indicated that she had never been very social, but was, at times, pleased to be involved in small homemaker chores such as folding linen and paring vegetables.

The evaluation procedure was carried out over a week and a half so that the patient would not become overly stressed or agitated. The procedure utilized formal evaluation tools administered by the OTR and observational assessments performed by the COTA and OTR.

The evaluation covered performance of selected physical and psychological daily living skills as well as sensorimotor, cognitive and psychosocial components. In daily living, the patient was incontinent of bowel and bladder, unable to perform self-care activities without physical assistance and unable to self-feed when presented with a meal tray. She had difficulty transferring in and out of bed. The patient could verbally make her needs known, but at times would be unable to express herself coherently. She could not make appropriate decisions regarding performance of activities of daily living such as when to brush her teeth or hair, when to go to the bathroom or when to go to sleep.

In the sensorimotor area, the patient's range of motion and muscle strength were essentially within normal limits for her age and status. She ambulated with an unsteady slow gait, stooped posture and almost absent arm swing. Visually, she was able to follow an object, but visuospatial deficits were noted in **figure-ground discrimination** (differentiating objects and shapes from their background) and **form constancy** (recognition of objects and forms as the same in different sizes, positions or environments). There was an identified hearing loss, greater in the left ear. The patient had been fitted for a hearing aid, but she refused to wear it. When engaged in purposeful tasks, Gertrude tired easily, sustaining only three to four minutes of activity. Difficulty was also noted in right-left discrimination and in such tasks as writing, buttoning and cutting.

Selected cognitive assessment tools were used to help develop baseline data. The patient's short attention span and tendency toward agitation limited the testing. Because the COTA had begun visiting the patient daily and was establishing a supportive relationship, it was decided to incorporate selected aspects of the cognitive assessment into these visits. The COTA was able to assist in administering some of the structured test material and reported her findings to the OTR. It was also possible for the OTR to observe the COTA as she worked with the patient during the assessment process, thus providing additional important information.

The patient was given a 10-item test, called the **Mental Status Questionnaire (MSQ)**, which is used to assess orientation and recent and remote memory. A rating of six to eight errors indicates moderate to severe chronic brain syndrome. The patient made eight errors, only answering two questions correctly.

The FROMAJE test was then given.[3] This test covers seven areas: function, reasoning, orientation, memory, arithmetic, judgment and emotional state. The test follows a structured interview format and utilizes information from family members, the patient, and current caregivers such as nursing, social service and occupational therapy staff. The COTA was able to perform portions of this assessment under the direction of the OTR. A rating of 13 or more on this test indicates severe dementia or depression. The patient scored 19. During this portion of the evaluation, it was noted that the patient became highly agitated and at times physically abusive when presented with problem-solving tasks that were beyond her capabilities.

Psychosocially, the patient was noted to have signs of depression, including lethargy, withdrawal from social interactions, suspiciousness and sudden mood swings. Gertrude would not participate in any group activities and was highly selective in her **dyadic** (one-to-one) interactions, requiring maximum encouragement and support from caregivers to obtain meaningful responses.

The evaluation results were summarized in a written report, prepared by the OTR. This report, which was to form the basis for the treatment plan, identified the following problems, which occupational therapy would address:

1. Incontinence
2. Relocation in new environment
3. Dependence in self-care activities of daily living
4. Lack of purposeful activity
5. Poor physical endurance
6. Depression
7. Significant cognitive deficits

The treatment plan would include the use of specific activities and therapeutic methods in the areas of activities of daily living skills training as well as sensorimotor, cognitive and psychosocial treatment. In addition, the treatment plan incorporated specific training for other staff caregivers.

The occupational therapy treatment plan was one component in Gertrude's overall plan of care. To realistically develop a comprehensive plan, the OTR and COTA met with the full team to develop the program plan.

Program Planning

A postadmission team conference was held with family, patient and staff involved in the case. Due to the patient's cognitive and behavioral problems, the conference was conducted in two stages. The initial part of the meeting took place without the patient's involvement. At this time, team members reviewed findings and presented their suggested goals for the team's information and consideration. After discussion, the following long-term goals were identified:

● Encourage patient's optimal functioning within the nursing home environment.
● Establish an activities of daily living maintenance program that could be periodically reevaluated and adjusted.
● Maintain patient's functional physical capacity within the limits of the disease process.

The OTR presented and discussed the occupational therapy program plan and goals with the team. The COTA, designated as the person responsible for primary treatment, explained the initial occupational therapy treatment objectives in relation to the goals. These objectives, in order of priority were as follows:

- Reestablish patient's continence in conjunction with nursing.
- Adapt and stabilize physical environment to enhance patient's cognitive performance.
- Establish structured plan for patient's performance of self-care activities.
- Identify feasible work and leisure activities for patient's participation.
- Involve patient in purposeful activities on a regular basis.
- Provide in-service for nursing staff on unit to ensure carryover of structure and environmental adaptations for the patient.
- Integrate patient into small group exercise program in conjunction with activities department.

The team accepted the occupational therapy goals. Specific objectives for interdisciplinary goals were incorporated into the treatment plan for each respective discipline. It was agreed that the initial team focus would be the reestablishment of continence and independence in eating. The COTA would work with the nursing staff on the unit to provide in-service regarding the procedures and structure for guiding the patient.

Gertrude was present for the last part of the conference. Because of her cognitive deficits, the goals established were discussed in very general terms and focused on the team's desire to help her feel more comfortable and independent in her new home.

In accordance with the team plan, the initial occupational therapy treatment plan had a primary focus in the area of activities of daily living skills. The OTR identified techniques, media and activity sequence. Input and discussion between the OTR and COTA helped to refine and formalize the initial plan. A primary key to facilitating the activities of daily living skills for this patient was the stabilization and adaptation of the environment. To accomplish this goal, the team must be involved in the occupational therapy treatment plan. Specific responsibilities and actions were developed as shown in Figure 18-1. A similar action plan was also developed for each of the short-term goals.

As the patient progressed, an activities of daily living skills maintenance program was to be instituted. This approach would require that nursing aides understand and demonstrate the ability to provide Gertrude with needed structure and sequence so that she could perform the activities of daily living tasks under their supervision. In accordance with the guidelines developed by occupational therapy, a care plan card was to be made by the COTA for each general daily living skills area. These cards would contain environmental guidelines to assure stabilization, such as key phrases to use when guiding the patient in an

activity and special approaches that would help the patient refocus if she became agitated or confused with the task at hand. The plan also required that the COTA provide in-service to the aide staff so they would understand how to use the cards when working with the patient.

In conjunction with the activities department staff, headed by another COTA, a plan was developed to integrate the patient into a small exercise group. This strategy was to be accomplished by having both COTAs co-lead the group while Gertrude became acclimated to the setting. The group leaders would also reinforce the patient's work and leisure roles in this group structure. The initial plan was to have Gertrude hand out name tags to each group member when they met and collect them at the conclusion of the meeting.

It was hoped that this plan would allow the patient to become more independent and comfortable in her new environment and the staff to be more capable of carrying over the specifically designed structure. The OTR and the COTA were then to develop a monitoring plan to be carried out after the patient was discharged from the occupational therapy treatment program.

Treatment Implementation

After long-term and short-term goals had been established and the program plan developed, a treatment program based on these goals was initiated by the COTA. Gertrude was now familiar with the occupational therapy assistant by sight, although she could not remember the COTA's name. To establish structure, the patient was treated at the same time five days a week, and a routine was followed as strictly as possible. In addition, the physical environment was simplified.

In light of the environmental problems presented, the COTA worked with the staff to make certain changes. The bathroom door in the patient's room looked very similar to other doors in the room, and Gertrude was unable to distinguish among them. To give the patient visual cues, a sign reading "Toilet," along with a picture of a woman of the type seen in many public rest rooms, was affixed to the bathroom door.

Gertrude shared a room with another woman, and she frequently confused her bed and closet with those of her roommate. The room was rearranged so that Gertrude's bed, with the bedspread from home, was nearer the door. Her dresser from home was brought in, as well as a small lamp and doily, which were placed on top. To help Gertrude remember where her clothes were in the dresser, the COTA made labels and affixed these, along with appropriate pictures, to each of the drawers.

The patient was seen daily in a corner of the day room, which contained a table and two lounge chairs. Each day,

Staff	Action Plan for Stabilizing and Adapting Environment
OTR/COTA	1. Assess patient's room in light of her limited cognitive abilities and existing environmental barriers. Develop plan to modify room.
COTA	2. Draw up plan.
OTR/Nursing/ Housekeeping/Maintenance	3. Meet with supervisors from nursing, housekeeping and maintenance. Request assistance from their staff in modifying the patient's room, using the plan developed by the occupational therapy department.
OTR/COTA/ Social Service/Family	4. Meet with social service and family to request help in bringing familiar objects and furnishings for the patient's room.
COTA	5. Analyze self-care activities, including toileting, so that the modified environment would facilitate patient's motor and cognitive daily living skills performance. Begin to implement plan.
COTA	6. Contact other departments for assistance as needed (ie, maintenance to make sign for toilet and housekeeping to move furniture).
OTR/COTA	7. Meet periodically to discuss and document progress. Modify plan as needed.
OTR/Team	8. Keep team supervisors informed of progress and ongoing needs.
OTR/COTA/Team	9. Meet with the team, including family, as needed, to ensure continuity and continue stabilization of new environment.

Figure 18-1. *Action plan.*

after the COTA greeted Gertrude, she offered her a glass of juice, which she seemed to enjoy. During this initial part of the treatment session, the COTA attempted to engage the patient in conversation. It was difficult for Gertrude to respond to questions that required anything but a "yes" or "no" answer. She had problems finding words and would often make statements such as, "Well, of course, you know, don't you?" or "What day is it you want to know? Well, you know," rephrasing the question asked of her. The COTA would then respond, supplying the answer, "Yes, I know. Today is Wednesday." In this way, the patient was given the opportunity to answer herself, and was also given the correct information without being placed under stress.

After this initial period of several minutes, a plan to reinforce Gertrude's adapted environment was implemented. Each day, the patient was taken to her room. She was given a flower to place in a vase on her dresser, and she was complimented on how beautiful her room looked. She was then shown where her bathroom was and was made aware of the word "toilet" on the door. After Gertrude used the bathroom, she was again reminded of how beautiful her room looked with the flower on her dresser, her bedspread and special lounge chair nearby. The COTA then escorted Gertrude back to the day room. At subsequent intervals during the day, nursing staff accompanied the patient to the bathroom; thus a team approach was used to meet the goal of reestablishing continence.

Mealtime for Gertrude was another problem. Meals were given to the patients on trays. Paper plates and cups and plastic utensils were used. The patient's response to receiving a tray full of food, plates and cups was to sit and look at it. She appeared unable to feed herself. When staff members urged her to eat, she would say, "I'm not food." The occupational therapy department worked in conjunction with the dietary department and nursing staff to normalize and simplify the patient's mealtime. Instead of paper goods and plastic utensils, Gertrude was provided with ceramic dishes and stainless steel utensils. Nursing aides no longer placed a full tray of food in front of the patient but, rather, gave her a small portion of food on a plate or in a bowl, and handed her the appropriate utensil. The rest of the meal was placed outside of the patient's visual field. Gertrude was able to eat when presented with one item at a time.

Based on a previous discussion with Gertrude's sister, it was thought that the patient might agree to participate in concrete, meaningful tasks that took place in her immediate environment. The job of sorting mail was chosen. Because room numbers appeared on the envelopes as part of the patient's address, Gertrude was directed to sort the mail by these numbers. The patient responded positively to this activity, feeling that she was being helpful to others. She was very pleased to discover her own mail mixed in with the other envelopes, as the abstract concept that the nursing home was now her home was still not clear to her. Even after several weeks, Gertrude continued to be surprised when she discovered an envelope with her name on it.

Another activity in which Gertrude became involved was helping to serve juice to the other patients in the afternoon. The COTA structured the task so that all the juice was poured into cups that were set on a cart for Gertrude, who would then push the cart to each patient in the day room and say, "Juice?" and hand the patient a cup. The activity proved satisfying to the patient, as it provided a concrete task for interaction with others in a nonthreatening way. In subsequent weeks, this activity was carried out in the morning in conjunction with nursing staff. An attempt was made to increase the complexity of the task by having Gertrude pour the juice, but the addition of another step interfered with the patient's ability to interact with others, so it was discontinued.

During the treatment period, the COTA and OTR held weekly meetings to discuss the patient's progress and ways in which the treatment program could be modified or enhanced. The COTA reported observations related to the patient's ability to perform simple activities, make her needs known and participate in activities of daily living.

The COTA worked closely with the nursing staff throughout Gertrude's treatment program to help them incorporate the structured and sequenced approach needed to effectively manage her. With the environmental adaptations in her room and with supervision and verbal cuing, Gertrude was eventually able to dress herself. Because the patient responded well to verbal encouragement, the nursing staff was able to dress Gertrude's roommate, while at the same time offering Gertrude the supervision and positive feedback she needed to be independent in morning care. Through the activities of serving juice and sorting mail, the patient began to feel useful and needed. Nursing staff began to see her as an asset rather than the difficult behavior and management problem she had been when she entered the nursing home.

Toward the end of the treatment program, the COTA visited the patient three times a week instead of five. The nursing staff worked with Gertrude on the other two days, using the care plan cards developed by the occupational therapy assistant. The COTA met with the members of the nursing department at the end of each week to discuss problems that had arisen, offer suggestions, and clarify areas on the care plans that were unclear.

In the activities area, the COTA worked cooperatively with the head of the department, also a COTA, to help integrate the patient into a small group exercise program. Gertrude was initially resistant to becoming involved with this group. During the first several days, she observed the other patients. By the end of the first week, with encouragement from both COTAs, the patient was performing some exercises. She much preferred the beginning and end of each session when she distributed and collected name tags with the assistance of the COTA, as this task made her feel special and important.

After several weeks of co-leadership, the activities direc-

tor was able to work independently with the patient in the group. Gertrude had responded positively to the group setting and performed her assigned tasks with satisfaction.

By using this method, a smooth transition was established from the occupational therapy treatment program to a continuation of structured supervision by the nursing and activities staff. The patient became used to associating a structured, positive approach with nursing and activities tasks as well as with occupational therapy. Thus, this patient received the kind of supportive environment that would enhance her optimal functioning.

Program Discontinuation

The monitoring program, formulated jointly by the OTR and the COTA, was presented to the team as part of the occupational therapy program discontinuation. This program provided for periodic review of the patient's performance in the areas where treatment had been provided. A structured checklist was completed by the COTA every three months after discharge. If regression occurred, the OTR would perform a reevaluation.

The occupational therapy department would also work cooperatively with the activities department about the patient's performance in work and leisure activities. If the COTA in charge of activities noted any changes, a request for reevaluation would be made to the occupational therapist.

The care plan cards were reviewed as part of the team conference. The nursing department integrated the use of these cards into the daily plan of care for the patient. It was agreed that if the nursing staff noted any problems with the patient's performance, a request would be sent to the OTR for a reevaluation.

The occupational therapist prepared a discharge summary with the assistance of the COTA. The summary documented the patient's progress, treatment outcomes and the follow-up plan. The treatment program was then terminated and the monitoring plan was implemented.

Conclusion

This case study of a patient with Alzheimer's disease residing in a nursing home illustrates the effectiveness of the team approach to patient care. The involvement of the family and the social services, activities and nursing departments in the occupational therapy intervention program was the key component of its success. The development of a specific maintenance program for this patient allowed the OTR and the COTA to monitor the status after direct patient treatment services were discontinued. This case points up the importance of ongoing communication and interaction between the OTR and the COTA as they work together to provide optimum patient treatment.

Related Learning Activities

1. Discuss the FROMAJE evaluation with an experienced OTR and determine the sections appropriate for a COTA to administer.

2. Practice administering the Mental Status Questionnaire. Ask an experienced therapist or assistant to observe you and to provide constructive feedback.

3. Identify community resources for patients with Alzheimer's disease and their families.

4. Use a medical encyclopedia to learn more about expressive and receptive aphasia.

5. Plan an in-service education program on "Alzheimer's Disease and the Role of Occupational Therapy" for a group of nursing assistants. Include specific examples of activities and appropriate visual aids.

References

1. Alzheimer's Disease *OT Week* 2(32):2, 1990.
2. Health Update *Geriatr Rehabil Prev* 2:(4) Fall, 1990.
3. National Institutes of Health, Office of Scientific and Health Reports: *Alzheimer's Disease—A Scientific Guide for Health Practitioners*. Bethesda, Maryland, US Department of Health and Human Services, 1984, p. 3.
4. Mace NL, Rabens PV: *The 36 Hour Day—A Family Guide to Caring for Persons With Alzheimer's Disease*. Baltimore, Johns Hopkins University Press, 1981, pp. 38, 71-108.
5. Snow T: Assessing mental status. *AOTA Gerontology Special Interest Section Newsletter* 1:1, 1983.

The Elderly With a Hip Arthroplasty

Dairlyn Gower, BS, COTA
Marcia Bowker, OTR

Introduction

Hip **arthroplasty** is the surgical replacement, formation or reformation of the hip joint. It is performed to restore motion and preserve the necessary stability to a stiffened or painful joint to ensure function. Arthroplasty of the hip is usually necessary because of degenerative joint disease, rheumatoid arthritis or other disease processes or trauma.

Surgical procedures vary depending on many factors, including severity of joint involvement, previous hip surgery and preferences of the physician. Three types of surgical intervention may be used: 1) cup or mold arthroplasty, 2) total hip arthroplasty, and 3) total hip surface replacement.[1] Complications resulting from surgery can include infection, joint dislocation and blood clots.[1] Treatment implementation can also vary depending on the type of surgery performed, as well as the individual's age, general health and motivation.

Total hip arthroplasty (THA), the procedure discussed in this case study, is often necessary as a result of a chronic disease or condition. THA can improve the patient's quality of life by decreasing pain and by increasing range of motion and mobility. The prognosis is generally good after an approximate seven to ten day hospitalization (although these time frames can differ based on various factors) and a two to three month recovery period. An individual who is independent before undergoing a total hip arthroplasty should continue to be independent after surgery. In some instances, the patient may prefer to have some assistance if total independence is not a high priority.

KEY CONCEPTS

Characteristics of total hip arthroplasty

Questionnaire and checklist

Action plan

Implementation strategies and activities

Adaptive equipment

Program discontinuation

ESSENTIAL VOCABULARY

Arthroplasty

Prosthesis

Acetabulum

Methyl methacrylate

Anterolateral

Posterolateral

Trochanter

Protocol

Work simplification

Energy conservation

In the surgical procedure, a metal **prosthesis** (replacement part, an artificial substitute) replaces the worn head and neck of the femur; a high-density polyethylene socket component replaces the worn **acetabulum** (socket in the hip that receives the head of the femur). The components are attached to the bones of the pelvis and femoral head by means of **methyl methacrylate**, a self-curing, acrylic resin adherent, which is applied in a paste form and becomes bonelike when hardened. A new technique that can be used in place of this fixation method is referred to as biologic fixation or bony ingrowths. In this technique, the replacement socket and head prostheses are fabricated with a specially textured attaching surface that allows the new bone to "form" around the prothesis for a more permanent attachment. Individuals who are younger and demonstrate maintenance of heathly bone (as seen through an x-ray film of the long bone) are generally the best candidates. Although it requires a weight-bearing restriction varying from 6 to 12 weeks after surgery, it is thought to be a more secure attachment.[1,2]

Surgical procedures vary for hip arthroplasty. The procedure can be performed **anterolaterally** (in front and to one side) or **posterolaterally** (in the rear and to one side).[2] Regardless of the approach, success of recovery relies on the compliance of the patient for approximately the first three months after surgery. Specific instabilities resulting from the anterolateral approach include hip external rotation, extension and adduction. Instabilities resulting from the posterolateral approach include movement over 90 degrees of hip flexion, adduction and internal rotation.[2] With both approaches, patients are strongly advised not to cross their legs until they have physician authorization. If patients do not adhere closely to precautions, they are at risk for interruption of good muscle and soft tissue healing, thus increasing the risk for hip dislocation.

The team members involved in the care of the patient with hip arthroplasty usually include the following: primary physician, orthopedic surgeon, nursing staff, occupational therapy and physical therapy personnel, dietitian, pharmacist and social worker.[2] The role of the team is to facilitate the healing of the **trochanter** (a process on the femur) and soft tissues and to facilitate the development of a capsule around the joint for future stability, as well as to teach proper body mechanics, mobility, positioning and methods related to carrying out every day activities during the recovery period.

Case Study Background

Carl was born June 22, 1918 in Duluth, Minnesota. A self-employed plumber, he is married and has adult children. At the age of 57, Carl had a rapid onset of osteoarthritis. Because of right hip pain and stiffness, he began experiencing difficulty fulfilling his job requirements, which included getting in and out of his truck and lifting, twisting and pulling at odd angles. By 1982, Carl had become semiretired, doing only minor plumbing jobs with the assistance of one of his sons. His wife continued to be involved in the business, managing records and the bookkeeping system.

The next year, the family physician referred Carl to an orthopedic surgeon who discussed the option of a total hip arthroplasty with him. Carl chose not to have surgery at that time because he didn't want to have it until it was "necessary." He was also concerned about the expense and lost time from work during recovery.

One year ago Carl, at age 72, was experiencing extreme hip pain, decreased joint mobility (especially limited hip abduction), stiffness and a painful gait. Carl, his wife and the orthopedic surgeon decided it was time to have THA surgery. Being able to play "a good game of golf" was Carl's primary source of motivation. Surgery was scheduled during the winter to ensure that Carl would have adequate recovery time before the golf season.

Assessment

The orthopedic surgeon made a referral for occupational therapy services according to standard postoperative orders of the facility. The **protocol** (specific plan of action) used for occupational therapy evaluation, planning and treatment was originally developed by the OTR and the COTA. This protocol identifies general precautions and procedures for performance of activities of daily living but is flexible enough to be easily adapted to the patient's individual needs, life-style and home situation, as well as the specific surgical procedure.

Using a structured questionnaire and checklist, the COTA performed a preliminary chart review. The chart review allowed the COTA to screen for possible complicating factors that may impair the patient's progress (ie, preexisting conditions of rheumatoid arthritis, cancer, cardiac or pulmonary disorders or dementia) and to consult with the OTR regarding any specialized evaluations that may be needed to establish realistic goals, such as active range of motion (AROM), strength and cognition.

On the fifth day after surgery, the COTA scheduled an initial visit with Carl. The primary purpose was to explain the purposes of occupational therapy intervention and gain information about living arrangement, physical layout of the home, household activities generally performed, previously pursued leisure activities, abilities in self-care and an inventory of specific patient concerns. The questionnaire and checklist used is shown in Figure 19-1.

This inventory is designed to provide your occupational therapist with information about your home living environment and activities. With this information, your therapist is able to identify what area he/she can best serve you in preparation for your return home.

Personal Care

Can you dress yourself? _____ Areas of difficulty_____
_____

Can you feed yourself?_____ Areas of difficulty_____
_____

Can you perform bathing/grooming tasks independently?_____
Were you independent in the above areas prior to your hospitalization?_____
Areas of difficulty_____
_____

Is there someone available to help at home?_____ If yes, who?_____
_____

Physical layout

Do you reside in an: _____Apartment   _____House   _____Other
Is there an elevator?_____
Number of floors _____   Steps inside house_____   Steps into house_____
Location of: Bedroom_____   Bathroom _____
Tub _____   Shower _____   Combination _____
Any areas of particular concern regarding physical layout?_____
_____

Household responsibilities

Which of the following activities are you currently able to perform?
_____Cooking   _____Grocery shopping   _____Cleaning   _____ Laundry
_____Dish washing   _____Pet care   _____Trash carryout   _____Snow shoveling
_____Care of lawn   _____Gardening   _____Maintenance   _____Other
_____

Meal preparation

Are you able to prepare meals?_____ Areas of difficulty_____
_____
How many meals do you prepare daily?_____ For how many people_____
Is there someone available to help?_____
Are the following available for your use?
_____High kitchen stool   _____Kitchen cart   _____ Microwave   _____Other
_____

Transportation

Do you drive? _____   Is there someone available to drive, if necessary?_____
Who? _____

Employment

Are you employed? _____   Retired _____
Type of occupation_____
Present work status_____
Work duties (include use of stairs, lifting, bending)_____
_____
_____

Recreation

List hobbies/recreational activities _____
_____
Activities discontinued because of medical condition_____
_____

Figure 19-1. *Home Activity Inventory.*

Program Planning

Once Carl had demonstrated general competence in ambulation in physical therapy, the OTR and the COTA established an individualized plan for occupational therapy treatment. The long-term goal for Carl and others undergoing this type of surgery was to return home, demonstrating independence in all activities of daily living with all movement precautions observed. Overall functional independence is expected to be the same, if not improved, after a total hip arthroplasty, as the patient should now be demonstrating an increase in pain-free range of motion. General short-term goals that are expected to be achieved during the hospital stay should be, but are not limited to the following:

● Demonstrate understanding of specific precautions and bending restrictions
● Demonstrate independence in lower extremity dressing through utilization of adaptive equipment
● Demonstrate independence in basic homemaking skills (ie, simple meal preparation, work simplification, and energy conservation)
● Demonstrate independence in functional mobility tasks (ie, shower/tub and toilet transfers)

The action plan developed jointly by the OTR and the COTA for Carl's treatment appears in Figure 19-2.

Treatment Implementation

Standing orders at the hospital where Carl was a patient indicate that occupational therapy is to be initiated on the fifth to sixth day after surgery, unless otherwise indicated. Physical therapy was initiated the first day after surgery. Carl's treatment program included therapeutic exercise, mobility training and gait training. During the first three days Carl used a walker and then advanced to using crutches.

On the fifth day, the COTA visited Carl in his room as previously discussed and also outlined the treatment protocol for a total hip arthroplasty. Carl's wife was present for a portion of this time and stated that she would like to attend her husband's treatment sessions to gain a better understanding of his occupational therapy program.

On the morning of the sixth day, the COTA gave Carl and his wife a copy of of the precautions and limitations he must follow. All items were discussed and procedures were demonstrated whenever possible. Questions were answered and Carl and his wife indicated that they understood the importance of observing the precautions and limitations during the performance of all daily living activities. This listing is shown in Figure 19-3. The COTA also provided them with a copy of the booklet *Daily Activities After Your Hip Surgery, Revised.*[3]

Post Surgery	ACTION PLAN
Day 5	Initial OT contact; explain occupational therapy and treatment protocol; assessment using activity inventory; consult with OTR
Day 6	**AM Treatment Session:**
	Provide patient with and discuss list of precautions and limitations and *Daily Activities After Your Hip Surgery*—revised edition; instruct patient in lower extremity dressing
	Assistive devices: sock aid, dressing sticks, reacher, elastic shoe laces, long-handled shoehorn
	Instruct patient in tub/shower and toilet transfer
	Assistive devices: raised toilet seat or commode chair, tub chair, long-handled bath brush, grab bars
	PM Treatment Session:
	Instruct patient in basic home management, work simplification and energy conservation techniques
	Assistive devices: utility cart, high stool, crutch or walker bag/pail, firm, sturdy arm chair
Day 7	Patient demonstrates dressing techniques; patient repeats back precautions and limitations; discuss and clarify any questions or concerns patient or family members may have

Figure 19-2. *Action plan developed by the OTR and COTA for Carl's treatment.*

The COTA brought a variety of assistive devices, including a reacher, elastic shoelaces, a long-handled shoehorn, dressing sticks and a sock aid to Carl's room. Some of these items are shown in Figure 19-4. Using the dressing devices, she

After hip surgery there are positions that could cause dislocation of your hip. Special precautions must be followed for approximately six to eight weeks after surgery or until your doctor tells you otherwise.

1. When ambulating, don't put more weight on your surgical side than was specified by your physical therapist and doctor.
2. Do not bend at the waist or hips more than 90 degrees.
3. Do not lift the knee on your surgical side higher than your hip.
4. Do not cross your legs, even at the ankles.
5. Do not turn toes outward while standing.
6. A firm, sturdy chair with arm rests is recommended for sitting.
7. Use assistive dressing devices to dress lower extremities.
8. Consult with your physician regarding resuming sexual activity.
9. Other precautions specific to you:

Figure 19-3. *Total hip arthroplasty—precautions.*

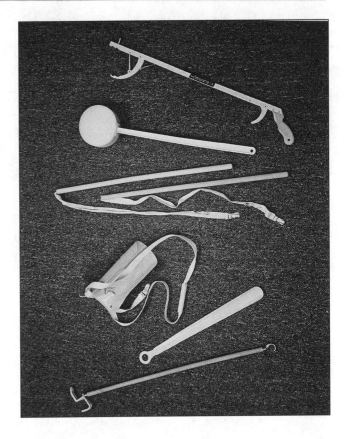

demonstrated how to do lower extremity dressing tasks such as putting on underwear, pants, socks, antiembolism stockings and shoes. Use of sock aid is depicted in Figure 19-5.

Carl chose to use the reacher, dressing sticks and sock aid, as they worked well for him. His "loafer" style shoes were easy for him to put on without any assistive devices. After practicing, Carl was able to do lower extremity dressing safely, without flexing his hip beyond 90 degrees and without rotating his hip. Although Carl had already been taught how to assume a standing position in physical therapy, the COTA reminded him to extend his surgical hip and leg and to use his arms to push up on the chair arm rests as shown in Figures 19-6 and 19-7, being careful to observe other precautions as well.

Next, Carl, his wife and the COTA went to the occupational therapy bathroom area to learn shower/tub and toilet transfers. Carl indicated that the shower in their home had a 3-inch step at the entrance. Carl was shown a number of assistive devices, including a tub chair, grab bars and a long-handled bath brush. Carl decided that he would like to have a grab bar installed in his shower, not only because of his current situation, but also as a long-term safety device. He stated that he had a chair at home that he could use in the shower. Carl was instructed to walk to the step of the shower and turn so that he was facing away from the shower stall. He was then told to reach for the chair, sit and lift his legs into the shower stall. Carl thought the long-handled bath brush would "come in handy" at minimum cost.

The COTA talked with Carl and his wife about toilet use

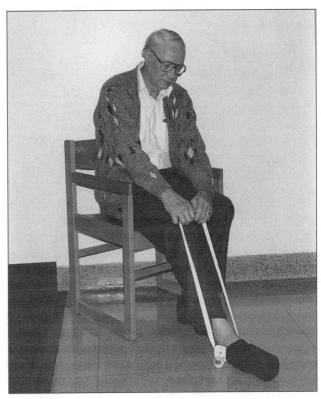

Figure 19-5. *Use of a sock aid.*

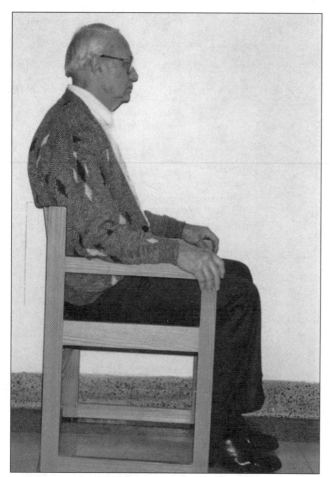

Figure 19-6. *Assuming a standing position from a chair.*

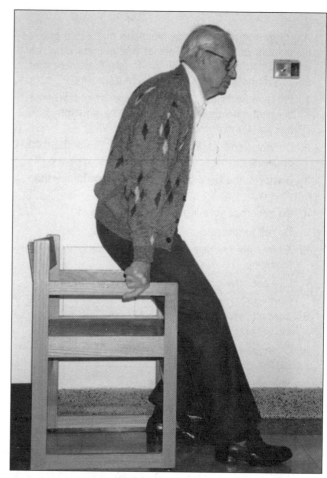

Figure 19-7. *Assuming a standing position from a chair.*

and learned that the toilet in their home was low. Using a toilet of this type would cause hip flexion beyond 90 degrees. Carl would need to use an over-the-toilet commode chair or a sturdy raised toilet seat. His wife indicated that a commode chair could be borrowed from a relative who was no longer using it. The COTA taught Carl to "back up" to the commode chair until he could feel the back of his knees touching it. He was then instructed to reach to the arm rests, extend his surgical hip and leg, and sit down as he had been taught previously. To stand, the COTA emphasized that Carl must again extend his surgical hip and leg and push up on the arm rests until a full standing postion was reached. This activity concluded the morning treatment session, and the time of afternoon treatment was confirmed.

That afternoon, Carl and his wife met the COTA in the occupational therapy kitchen. Instruction was provided in basic home management, **work simplification** (methods for making tasks easier to accomplish), and **energy conservation** techniques (methods for reducing exertion). Although Carl's wife normally assumed most of these tasks, she was employed in their plumbing business, four hours a day, four days per week between 10:00 AM and 2:00 PM. Thus, Carl would have to prepare his own lunch and clean up and perform other

activities of daily living independently.

During this treatment session, the COTA also demonstrated specific tasks such as using a reacher, sliding items on a countertop, transporting items on a utility cart and using a bag or a pail in conjunction with a walker or crutches. Effective methods for removing and storing items in the refrigerator were also stressed, as well as using a high stool to sit on during meal preparation and dish washing. Carl was then asked to make a sandwich and a bowl of soup and clean up, incorporating the techniques he had been taught. He completed these tasks successfully, requiring only infrequent reminders. Carl also indicated that he already had a utility cart and an ice cream pail at home for transporting items.

More general work simplification and energy conservation techniques were discussed with Carl, and important safety factors were stressed. Emphasis was placed on the following principles, which must be adhered to at home:

1. Rearrange commonly used items to avoid excessive bending and reaching.
2. Remove clutter, cords and scatter rugs to prevent tripping.
3. Rest periodically and whenever needed to avoid fatigue.

4. Sit in a firm, sturdy armchair.

5. Use assistive devices as required.

6. Observe all precautions and limitations when engaging in daily living activities.

At the conclusion of the afternoon treatment session, Carl, his wife and the COTA agreed to meet the next day to review the treatment activities and procedures and to answer questions. The COTA summarized and reported Carl's progress to the supervising OTR who determined that his program would be discontinued on the next day if dressing goals were continuing to be met independently and the patient demonstrated a thorough understanding of the precautions and limitations.

On the seventh day after surgery, the COTA saw Carl in his room. He was able to demonstrate lower extremity dressing techniques and the effective use of assistive devices. He was able to verbally list the precautions and limitations that he must observe and related them to specfic tasks and activities. Carl had several questions that the COTA answered and several that she helped Carl to answer for himself. Upon completion of this fourth treatment session, the COTA verified treatment and documentation with the OTR, who co-signed the note and placed it in Carl's medical chart.

Program Discontinuation

Treatment was discontinued after the fourth treatment session. The OTR and the COTA met with Carl and his wife and again stressed the importance of following the precautions and limitations discussed in occupational therapy, as well as those addressed by physical therapy, nursing personnel and his physician. The COTA suggested that they refer to the booklet *Activities Following Your Hip Surgery*,[3] to obtain additional information. She also indicated that both she and the OTR would be available by telephone if they needed any assistance with unanticipated problems. They also reminded them of Carl's six-week appointment, which had been scheduled with his physician. The OT team emphasized that if, at that time, there continued to be limitations in performing activities of daily living, Carl would again be referred to occupational therapy. The Occupational Therapy Orthopedic Rehabilitation Discharge Note shown in Figure 19-8 was completed and entered in the medical chart.

Six months after his surgery, Carl was able to complete minor plumbing jobs independently for friends and family members. He had also achieved his number one objective of playing golf without pain, something he had not been able to do for years. His only regret was that he hadn't had the surgery several years earlier when it had first been discussed.

Conclusion

This case study discusses the treatment given to a patient after a total hip arthroplasty. There are a variety of factors to consider in the treatment of THA, including the type of surgical procedure performed and the individual situation of the patient. Although treatment precautions and protocols

Patient: _____   Date of Initial Contact:_____

Diagnosis: _____   Today's Date:_____

Physician: _____   MR #: _____

Living Situation:_____

ADL Status: Homemaking:_____

    Bathing: _____

    Dressing: _____

    Bathtub and Toilet Transfers:_____

Instruction in Work Simplification and Energy Conservation Techniques Completed:_____

Precautions Reviewed:_____

Adaptive Equipment Recommended:_____

    Provided: _____

Assistance Available During Recovery:_____

Additional Comments: _____

Figure 19-8. *Occupational Therapy Orthopedic Rehabilitation Discharge Note.*

are similar, it is imperative to follow the physician's orders for each individual's unique situation regarding weight bearing, hip mobility and positioning. Precautions apply to participation in all activities of daily living.

Once a COTA has had adequate experience working with this type of patient and treatment protocol, the occupational therapy assistant can usually implement the treatment program with minimal general supervision. The entry-level COTA requires closer supervision from the OTR. In all cases, consultation should take place with the supervising occupational therapist after reviewing the medical chart and in preparation for discharge.

Acknowledgments

The authors would like to acknowledge the following individuals for their contributions and assistance: Mr. and Mrs. Carl Eisenach, Starr White, Frank W. Budd, MD, Mary Jo Lepisto, COTA, Geralyn Heitkamp, COTA and Diane Kaiser, OTR.

Related Learning Activities

1. Study the list of precautions and limitations that must be adhered to following a total hip arthroplasty. Practice demonstrating these techniques to a peer.

2. Using the same precautions and limitations, draw stick figures to illustrate the principles. As a second activity, incorporate the figures into small posters that would be useful for teaching patients.

3. Make a list of as many work simplification and energy conservation techniques as you can think of. Compare this list with those recommended for Carl. What additional ideas did you arrive at that might be useful to a person recovering from hip arthroplasty?

4. Locate adaptive/assistive devices that may be useful to a patient with THA and practice using them for your own daily living tasks.

References

1. Brashear HB, Raney RB: *Shand's Handbook of Orthopedic Surgery*, 9th Edition. St. Louis, Missouri, CV Mosby, 1978.
2. Pedretti LW: *Occupational Therapy: Practice Skills for Physical Dysfunction*, 2nd Edition. St. Louis, Missouri, CV Mosby, 1985.
3. Platt J: *Daily Activities After Your Hip Surgery*, Revised Edition. Rockville, Maryland, American Occupational Therapy Association, 1990.

Chapter 20

The Elderly With Hearing and Visual Impairments

Barbara (Bobbie) Hansvick, COTA
Marietta Cosky Saxon, OTR

Introduction

A functioning sensory system allows a person to perceive and to interact with others and with their environment. It effects the person's ability to maintain competent behavior, appropriate self-esteem and relationships with others. The sensory changes that occur as one ages are a normal part of the aging process. As people grow older, they will experience some type of sensory loss owing to changes in the body's ability to receive and process sensory stimuli.

Review of the literature suggests that one can make certain generalizations about sensory change in the elderly person.[1] *First* all sensory processes show a decline with age. *Second*, all senses do not age equally. That is why one may see an elderly person with only visual impairments and other elderly individuals who have impairments of vision, hearing and equilibrium when all are the same age. *Third*, and of high importance, is that sensory losses do not always lead to disability. In fact, the majority of elderly people are able to learn how to compensate for certain sensory losses and can continue to function independently in their home environment. Finally, sensory losses occur gradually and have a cumulative effect. For example, the average age for Americans to require bifocal glasses is 43 years of age.[2] Other sensory changes also occur when people are in their forties and generally progress slowly into old age. This gradual onset allows the individual to adapt to the changes and learn to use intact sensory functions and environmental supports to compensate for the overall sensory losses.

ESSENTIAL VOCABULARY

Acuity

Glare

Paranoia

Arrhythmia

Fibrillation

Tachycardia

Hypertension

Sclerosis

Anemic

Hypotension

Regimen

KEY CONCEPTS

Characteristics of sensory impairments

Occupational therapy role

Medical assessment

Functional assessment

Occupational performance

Intervention strategies and activities

Adaptive equipment

Program discontinuation

This chapter presents information on visual and hearing impairments and the role of occupational therapy personnel in helping the elderly person adjust to these impairments.

Sensory Impairments

Vision

One's visual functioning can be affected in many ways. The more common impairments that occur among the elderly are the following:[1]

1. Reduced visual **acuity** (acuteness or clearness).
2. Reduced ability to focus on people or objects. (Most elderly tend to be farsighted.)
3. Reduced capacity to adjust to changes in illumination, ie moving from a sunlit area to inside a building requires extra time for the elderly person's eyes to adjust.
4. Decreased resistance to **glare** (harsh or very bright light).
5. A shift in color vision; as the lens of the eye ages, it yellows. Colors such as yellow, orange and red are more easily discriminated than violet, blue and green.
6. Impaired depth perception.

Most elderly people experience some type of visual impairment.

Hearing

The hearing impairments experienced by the elderly person are fewer in number, but are considered the most devestating of all sensory losses because they isolate individuals from other people and their environment. Feelings and behaviors commonly exhibited by people with hearing deficits include isolation, anger, suspicion, depression, rejection and **paranoia** (a mental disorder characterized by systematized delusions and projection of personal conflicts based on supposed hostility of others). These feelings and behaviors can lead to social and emotional problems. The more common hearing impairments among the elderly include the following:[1]

1. Hearing loss that interferes with social interactions
2. Impaired discrimination of sounds that interferes with ability to identify
3. Difficulty in hearing higher frequency consonants: z, s, g, f, and t

It is estimated that one third of all people between ages 65 and 74 are affected by some kind of hearing loss.

Occupational Therapy Role

The educational background and clinical training of occupational therapists (OTRs) and occupational therapy assistants (COTAs) prepares these practitioners to play a unique role in helping the elderly person to learn to compensate for sensory changes and possible deficits. The individual is first assessed to determine whether the sensory loss interferes with daily functioning and/or emotional well-being. If physical or emotional functioning is affected, the elderly person is taught how to compensate and adapt to the changes or losses in sensory functioning. This is accomplished primarily in two ways. First, the person is shown how to capitalize on their sensory assets or on the secondary functioning that is still intact to help compensate for the loss. Second, the individual is educated relative to methods for adapting his or her environments. For example, tape strips placed on stairs will assist the visually impaired in judging distances correctly and alarm clocks with low frequency buzzers will serve as "reminders" for people with hearing loss.[1]

The following case study presents an elderly woman who has visual and hearing impairments, as well as some typical physical problems, often experienced by people her age. The entire occupational therapy process will be discussed as the OTR and the COTA help the individual prepare to live as independently as possible.

Case Study Background

Martha was born May 16, 1914, in Jamesville, North Dakota. One of eight children, she has three brothers and four sisters. When she was young, her family moved to a small rural community in Minnesota where they farmed. Martha completed a high school education and married her husband Albert in 1942. Following two stillborn births, her only child, William, was born. Her primary work role was a homemaker; however, she was employed part-time for approximately five years as an assistant to the cook at the local elementary school when her son was older.

Before his death 12 years ago, Albert and Martha had sold their home and moved into a townhouse so they would be free to travel with fewer concerns about the upkeep of a large space and yard. Martha currently resides there. She reported that there are three steps into her home with the living areas located on the ground floor. There is also a basement for laundry, utilities and storage. Before admission to the hospital, she was living alone with no support services. Her son lives in the area, but has intermittent contact because of frequent business trips. He is divorced and the father of three children who reside with his former wife who lives nearby. The grandchildren see Martha infrequently, primarily on holidays.

For approximately the past two years, Martha has been having increased problems with short-term memory, vision and hearing deficits and decreased ability to care for herself.

Before that time, she had been moderately active, attending church services and participating in volunteer projects, including preparing clothes for the needy and serving as a hostess for various church functions. Chronic concern and anxiety about medication regulation for congestive heart failure have required repeated admissions to the hospital.

Medical History

Martha was admitted to the emergency room of the local hospital recently as a result of an angina attack. After medical evaluation, she was sent home with no change in medications.

The patient has a significant history of **arrhythmia,** (abnormal heartbeat) both atrial **fibrillation** (involuntary muscle contraction) and venous **tachycardia** (abnormally rapid heartbeat), currently controlled with digoxin and quinidine. The patient also has **hypertension** (persistently high blood pressure) that is controlled with triamterene. There is a history of aortic **sclerosis** (hardening of tissue) without any significant clinical disability. A history of lupus reaction from procainamide has been documented, so use has been discontinued. Arthritis is controlled with tolmetin. The patient also is taking Premarin for hormone replacement and iron for osteoporosis. Records of a recent hospitalization indicate that an **anemic** (reduced red cells and level of hemoglobin in the blood) condition was resolved.

Medical Findings

The patient has had arrhythmia over the past two years. That condition, coupled with her other medical problems, led to the conclusion to end the cycle of hospital admissions brought about by poor home support and her inability to cope with these problems independently.

At the time of hospital discharge, Martha reported that she was "feeling better." She indicated that the major problems in her home situation were because of decreased vision and hearing. It was decided to transfer her to a community convalescent and long-term care facility for assessment of her daily living skills before a decision was made regarding the best living environment. Martha indicated that she had made inquiries at a senior citizen apartment complex, with the encouragement of her son.

Assessment

Martha was seen initially by the OTR to conduct an interview and complete a functional assessment. The following results were recorded:

1. *Range of motion*: Within normal limits for age for both upper and lower extremities.
2. *Strength*: Good (4 plus) strength in both shoulders and normal (5) strength in elbow, wrist and fingers.
3. *Coordination*: The nine hole peg test was used to assess finger dexterity and coordination.[3] Scores were within normal range.
4. *Sensory functioning*: The patient was given the Functional Low Vision Assessment shown in Figure 20-1.[4] The results indicated difficulty in reading small print, impaired visual acuity (which interferes with her ability for self-care and produces anxiety when alone at home) and impaired depth perception. Difficulty negotiating rough terrain, stairs and curbs was both observed and reported. The patient currently wears bifocal glasses. Hearing impairments were also identified. A referral was made to the patient's physician for more intensive vision and hearing tests. (A hearing aid was later ordered and fitted.) These visual and hearing impairments appeared to decrease self-confidence and had lead to social isolation.
5. *Cognition*: Chart review indicated the patient had reported being forgetful at times. During the occupational therapy assessment, however, she was alert and cooperative and displayed only minor relocation disorientation. Her memory appeared to be intact, and she was able to follow directions and communicate appropriately with others.
6. *Endurance*: The patient tires easily due to congestive heart failure and dehydration. She was able to tolerate a 60-minute evaluation session with a few short rest periods and encouragement from the therapist. The patient displayed postural **hypotension** (lowered blood pressure) and dizziness when she moved too quickly from one position to another. Endurance was further assessed by the COTA as a part of a comprehensive daily living skills assessment.

Occupational Performance

The COTA saw Martha in the occupational therapy clinic to assess her daily living skills. Martha reported she was independent in feeding, hygiene, dressing and bathroom transfers to tub and toilet. Martha was asked to put on and take off pajamas to demonstrate dressing and undressing skills. She was able to complete this activity without assistance, but she did become fatigued and complained of being dizzy during lower extremity dressing.

Martha reported that she performed most of her homemaking tasks. These skills would be assessed in a homemaking and kitchen evaluation before discharge.

The patient stated that she could no longer participated in the leisure activities she enjoys, such as sewing, needlepoint, reading and volunteer work. Her major current pastime is watching television. The COTA asked Martha to read a portion of the local newspaper aloud. Martha could read the headlines, but not regular size print. In demonstrating writing, her signature was "shaky," but legible. Other activities found on the Functional Low Vision Daily Living

Patient's Name _____

Date _____

Diagnosis _____

Date of Onset _____

Date of Last Eye Exam and Location _____

Glasses: (   )   Yes (   )   No (   ) Bifocals   Date Changed _____

Symptoms _____

Patient's Understanding of the Loss _____

_____

What Patient Wants to Achieve _____

_____

Expectations of the Caregiver _____

_____

Medications Currently Using _____

_____

Complicating Factors _____

_____

Depth Perception: (   ) Normal   (   ) Impaired

Comments _____

Visual Field: (   ) Normal   (   ) Impaired

Comments _____

Color Identification _____

_____

_____

_____

Near Vision: at 12" - 14" from eyes (date and print size) _____

_____

_____

_____

Magnification Needed (date and degree) _____

_____

Aids Currently Using _____

_____

Figure 20-1. *Functional Low Vision Assessment. From Physical and Occupational Therapy in Geriatrics 3:55-61. 1983, Haworth Press. All rights reserved, developed by Lucy A. McGrath, OTR.*

Skills Checklist[4], shown in Figure 20-2, were also administered to Martha. She was able to accomplish them with minimal problems, with the exception of identifying money. This checklist also served as a guide for planning and carrying out treatment.

The OTR and the COTA reviewed their findings and recommended that the patient would benefit from occupational therapy intervention. The OTR obtained orders for treatment from the physician.

Treatment Planning

Within the first week of admission to the long-term care facility, a care conference was held to communicate evaluation results, plan a course of treatment and discuss possible discharge options for Martha. All team members were present, including representatives from occupational therapy, physical therapy, dietary, social services, recreation and chaplaincy. Martha and her son were also present. After evaluation results were shared, it was decided that certain areas would be addressed as collaborative efforts among several team members. Hygiene goals would be the focus of OT and nursing; leisure skills and use of adaptive equipment would be the responsibility of OT and recreation; and general endurance and safety with transfers would be addressed by OT and PT. In addition to these collaborative efforts, each treatment discipline had their own specific treatment plan. The long-term objective of all treatment plans was to address the discharge plan: "the patient will be discharged to live independently in a supported living situation for the elderly." The occupational therapy treatment plan, developed collaboratively by the OTR, the COTA and Martha, is shown in Figure 20-3.

After development of the treatment plan, it was decided that the COTA would provide primary treatment with periodic supervision and review provided by the OTR. Since the OTR had advanced training in gerontology and the sensory changes that occur during aging, she would conduct the patient education sessions related to sensory changes.

Treatment Implementation

Treatment consisted of two sessions per day, five days a week. The morning session was 45 minutes long and focused on one-to-one instruction with the COTA. During the afternoons, Martha attended the cardiovascular conditioning group for 30 minutes. This group is conducted for six to eight patients by the COTA. Patients are monitored for their endurance levels by taking their radial pulses before and after the exercises. Pulse rates are monitored more

frequently if a patient exhibits signs of distress or fatigue or has specfic physician orders for monitoring. Recreational activities were planned on a regular basis, and three small group offerings were incorporated into Martha's schedule. She also participated in a session on patient education conducted by the OTR. Ten of the morning sessions are described in the following section.

Session 1

The patient was asked to plan a menu for a meal and make an ingredient list for preparation of the food the next day. She was also asked to fill a grocery bag with canned goods and other kitchen items. The COTA observed that Martha had difficulty reading labels and organizing tasks to conserve energy. She was given magnifying glasses to see which ones met her reading needs. Martha also read portions of a large print cookbook and noted where a copy could be purchased. Methods of packing groceries to distribute weight evenly and transporting groceries in the kitchen by using a cart were discussed and demonstrated, emphasizing the need to conserve energy. These principles would be reinforced and related to other tasks she would perform in her future living environment.

Session 2

To further assess Martha's safety, endurance and judgment in occupational performance skills, she was asked to prepare the meal she had planned during the previous day. Martha prepared eggs, coffee, juice and a packaged muffin mix. She used large print measuring cups and spoons, a stove with brightly marked on/off controls and magnifying glasses for recipe reading to compensate for her visual loss. A large print, low-tone timer was used to time the baking. These adaptations provided adequate cuing to assure Martha's safety when preparing a simple meal. The COTA also recommended that she use oven mitts instead of hot pads to reduce the potential for accidental burns. Martha displayed low tolerance for the activity. During the course of the meal preparation, she required several rest periods. She was unable to complete the clean-up portion of the task because of the slow pace of her work, need for rest and the time limitation of the session. Martha showed no deficits in eating skills, and increased socialization was observed as she offered to share the meal with another patient in the clinic kitchen at the time. At the conclusion of the session, Martha agreed to meet with the COTA and a member of the nursing staff in her room at 8:00 AM the next morning.

Session 3

The focus of this session was to further assess and provide instruction to Martha in dressing, grooming and hygiene tasks. Martha exhibited independence with tasks, provided there was adequate safety equipment and lighting, and she was familiar with the location of needed supplies and

DATE														
Daily Living Skills														
Identify Dials:														
Washer														
Thermostat														
Oven/Stove														
Pour Hot Liquids														
Medication Labels														
Identify Pills														
Use Telephone:														
Dial														
Phone No.														
See Clock														
Read Calendar														
Discriminate:														
Tub/Bathroom														
Equipment														
Identify Money:														
Bills														
Coins														
Read:														
Regular Print														
Mail														
Newspaper														
Write Letters														
Sign Name														
Recognize Familiar People														
See the TV														

THERAPIST SIGNATURE _____

Comments: (date) _____

_____

Scale: I = Independent
    S = Supplements vision with auditory/tactile/memory cues (adequate)
    C = Relies completely on auditory/tactile/memory cues (adequate)
    R = At risk; not adequately using cues
    D = Dependent on other people

Figure 20-2. *Functional Low Vision Daily Living Skills Checklist. Adapted from Physical and Occupational Therapy in Geriatrics, Vol. 3(1), Fall 1983, by Haworth Press.*

Precautions: Postural hypotension and congestive heart failure

Problem		Goal	Treatment Activity
1. Decreased physical endurance	LTG*: STG*:	Improve physical endurance. a. Patient will tolerate cardiac exercises to a 3.1 MET level.	Attend cardiac exercises daily, monitor pulse, pallor, breathing patterns, and percentage of participation.
		b. Patient will demonstrate energy conservation/work simplification techniques during functional tasks in OT clinic which can be carried over to independent living.	Pulse and indicators of fatigue will be monitored during daily living skills activities, ie kitchen tasks, light homemaking tasks. Obtain floor plan of new apartment from social worker and review with patient regarding energy-saving techniques.
2. Hearing and visual impairments that are interfering with independent living.	LTG: STG:	Improve compensatory skills to enhance remaining auditory and visual functioning. a. Patient will be independent in light homemaking tasks displaying safety principles and sound judgment.	Prepare simple meal, make a bed, discuss grocery shopping, ie reading labels, carry groceries safely, transportation, laundry, budgeting, money management.
		b. Patient will demonstrate correct and consistent use of assistive devices.	Teach correct use of hearing aid, ie batteries, setting, etc., use of magnification devices.
3. Decreased social interaction.	LTG: STG:	Improve social interaction, especially with peer group. a. Patient will demonstrate an understanding of sensory changes in self and how this affects her interaction with others.	Provide education information about sensory changes in the elderly population.
		b. Patient will have an auditory and visual examination.	Refer to nursing for physician's orders and scheduling.
		c. Patient will attend three small group activities conducted by the recreation department.	Report back to OT with reactions, problems, concerns, and progress.

*LTG, long-term goal; STG, short-term goal.

Figure 20-3. *Occupational Therapy Treatment Plan.*

clothing. In making transfers in and out of the tub, she used a grab bar successfully. Martha said that she would like to have one at home. When performing hygiene and grooming tasks, Martha exhibited some difficulty in finding items, possibly because of her new surroundings and the inadequate lighting, which made easy identification difficult. This problem was particularly evident when she was selecting clothes. The COTA discussed these concerns with the OTR. They decided to make special note of the lighting arrange-

ment when they reviewed the floor plan of Martha's new apartment to identify additional lighting needs.

Session 4

The COTA consulted with the nursing staff to determine their instructions regarding medications, including number, frequency of administration and patient compliance with the **regimen** (regulated plan). They expressed concern about Martha's accuracy and her history of anxiety about medications. A nurse joined the COTA to present a joint instructional session on her home medication program. The nurse stressed the importance of adherence to the medication program and instructed Martha regarding the purpose of each of her medications. The COTA introduced assistive tools and ideas. Martha's medications were labeled with black labels with white print to make them easier to distinguish and read. Martha was given a large print chart of her medications, including the name of the drug and the frequency of administration. Medications were set up in a pill organizer.

Session 5

Before the fifth session, the COTA and OTR met and discussed Martha's treatment and reviewed the progress notes. The apartment floor plan was also assessed. The focus of this session was to explain the floor plan to Martha and to make recommendations. The discussion emphasized energy-saving principles and the following safety considerations:

- Furniture arrangement to assure easy access and clear walkways
- Hot water temperature setting not to exceed 130 degrees
- Use of accoustical materials to absorb background noises
- Centrally located telephones with amplified signal and enlarged numbers on the dial (both available from the local phone company)

Session 6

The main objective of this session was education. The OTR met with Martha and discussed the sensory changes that normally occur in an elderly person as a result of the aging process. The emotional issues, such as anger, frustration, low self-esteem and tendencies to isolate oneself as a result of the sensory losses were discussed. Martha stated she was often fearful of being left alone, yet too self-conscious about her visual and hearing impairments to reach out to others; therefore, she began to withdraw from social events. The OTR asked Martha to participate in three small group activity sessions conducted by the recreation department. The OTR and the COTA would monitor her response to these activities through discussion with Martha and the recreation staff. Martha reported that she felt slightly apprehensive as she left the treatment session, yet she expressed an interest in the recreational activities, indicating that she was "happily looking forward to doing something fun with the rest of the folks!"

Session 7

This session focused on the area of light housekeeping. Although Martha would have assistance for major housekeeping tasks in her new apartment through a community

service, she would still need to be able to complete the daily tasks necessary for basic home maintenance. The COTA saw Martha in her room where she could simulate her home environment as closely as possible. Martha removed the bedding from the bed and remade it with clean linens. She also did some dusting and arranging of her personal items on the bedside table and the dresser. While Martha performed these tasks, the COTA observed that Martha used many unnecessary steps. She instructed her on the procedure for making a bed by only walking around it once, instead of going back and forth. Other work simplification suggestions were also made, such as using a lightweight electric broom to vacuum small areas while seated. During these activities, Martha's pulse was monitored and although elevated was within the normal range. She required rest only once during the session, indicating a significant improvement when compared to the initial sessions. Martha reported that she was feeling much stronger because of her participation in the cardiovascular conditioning program. The COTA reported that initially the patient tolerated the 2.8 MET (metabolic equivalent tables, which report measurements of energy expenditure) level with 70% participation, but was now tolerating the 3.1 MET level at 85% participation. More information on METs is shown in Figure 20-4.[5]

Session 8

For this treatment session, the COTA secured Martha's monthly bills and bank statements from her son, with Martha's permission. The assistant discussed them with Martha who then wrote the necessary checks and prepared her bank deposit and withdrawal forms. These were familiar activities for Martha, and she exhibited a good grasp of the fundamental skills necessary to complete these tasks efficiently and correctly. A page magnifier was provided to aid her in reading figures. The COTA then demonstrated how to keep a budget using a notebook with large line intervals. Although Martha did not have any current financial problems, she had voiced a need to "keep closer track of her money." She indicated that her son would continue to balance her checkbook each month, so she "wouldn't have to worry about that!"

The final portion of this session was devoted to identifying and handling money. Martha was given a compartmentalized coin purse and a divided, sectioned wallet to make sorting money by denominations easier. Martha adapted to handling, organizing and storing her money quickly by using these items.

Session 9

The OTR met with Martha again and provided her with written information about materials available from the local county extension office. This community resource for the elderly (and others) provides a variety of educational materials on numerous topics, ranging from proper nutrition and

A MET is a measure of energy expenditure. A MET is a numerical value that describes how much work you are doing according to the amount of oxygen your body needs as you perform a given task.

1 Liter Oxygen Consumption - 3.5 METs

For example, you utilize. . .
1 MET

2 METs

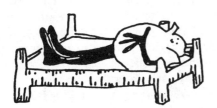

Lying Relaxed

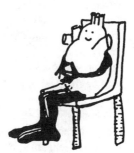

Working with Both Arms

3 METs

6 METs

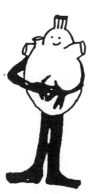

Walking on a Flat Surface

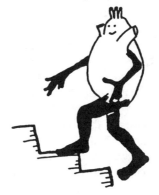

Climbing Stairs

Factors that influence energy expenditure include:
—speed of movement
—body weight
—stress and emotion, tension, pressure
—competition, anxiety
—part of body exercising

It is important to balance your activities (in terms of their MET requirements) throughout the day.

Figure 20-4. *Metabolic Equivalent Table (MET). From Bear P, Radomski MV, Smith AC: Take It To Heart, 2nd Edition. Coon Rapids, Minnesota, Mercy Medical Center, 1985.*

volunteer services to legal services and tax preparation. Martha was encouraged to use these resources after discharge. Martha was also given the name of a contact person and the telephone number of the senior citizen center near her new apartment. Occupational therapy time would be arranged for Martha to meet with a center representative if she requested it.

This session also focused on the use and care of hearing aids. The OTR provided Martha with a large print information sheet that detailed basic hearing aid care and use. The following points were stressed:[6]

1. Changing the batteries
2. Cleaning and proper placement of ear molds
3. Checking ear molds for cracks
4. Setting the on/off switches and volume control
5. Precautions: Remove while bathing and sleeping; keep away from hot surfaces; and avoid using hair spray with hearing aid in place

During the latter part of this session, the COTA introduced Martha to several craft activities that she could continue after discharge. Martha chose to work on ceramics and selected a greenware vase to begin cleaning.

Session 10

Martha had requested a meeting with a representative of the senior citizen center, which the COTA scheduled during this session. The OTR also met with them. Martha was pleased to learn about all of the activities the center offered, and she stated she was "very excited to hear they had an ongoing ceramics program!" Thus, she could continue her new-found hobby. At this time, Martha also spoke of the recreational activities she had been involved in. She noted that since she had been at the center, she had learned to participate in activities in smaller groups in areas where there was less likely to be background noise. She also reported that positioning herself with her back to a window decreased visual interference from glare. Martha stated that she is better able to communicate with her son now that they both understand the nature of her hearing deficit and the various compensatory techniques used to deal with it. Martha indicated that she was anxious about being discharged, but that she was looking forward to living in her own apartment.

Program Discontinuation

Since Martha's admission referral was for assessment of and planning for independent living, discharge planning was begun at the initial care conference. During the course of treatment, the occupational therapy department had maintained close contact with the social worker and the nursing department regarding Martha's potential for safe, independent living, including the services and assistive devices necessary. The medical team concluded that Martha was capable of independent living once she had attained additional skills and demonstrated an understanding of her sensory losses and how to compensate for them. Martha had visited the apartment complex with the social worker, and her son was pleased to learn that an apartment would be available when she was discharged.

Before the discharge conference, the OTR and the COTA met to review Martha's progress and formulated recommen-

dations that would assist in maintaining her abilities in the assisted living arrangement. Because the COTA had been Martha's primary therapist, she attended the discharge conference with the other staff, Martha and her son. During the conference, the COTA reported reviewing the floor plan and the ideas regarding furniture placement and other environmental considerations. It was recommended that Martha be involved in the selecton of household items to be moved. Another recommendation was that Martha participate in organized events conducted at the facility. The occupational therapy department would contact the activity coordinator and provide information about helpful compensatory techniques and assistive devices. An added recommendation was that arrangements be made for major housekeeping tasks to be carried out by a service, as these activities were too strenuous for Martha. The nursing staff suggested that a visiting nurse monitor Martha's compliance with medications monthly. It was believed that adherence to these recommendations would decrease Martha's anxiety, dependence and overutilization of her physician and medical services.

Conclusion

This case study demonstrates how intervention at an early stage can prolong independent living and interrupt the progressive isolation and deterioration of the elderly that can occur due to sensory impairments. Early intervention allows the elderly person to gain knowledge about the aging process, as well as community resources and assistive devices that may be helpful (see the Resource Guide, Appendix B). This case also highlights the effective teamwork that can be achieved between the OTR and COTA when both are comfortable and knowledgeable in their roles. Formal education, experience and the professional/technical role delineation[7] provide the latitude for the COTA to be the primary therapist for this type of patient. This team approach increases efficiency and effectiveness by allowing the OTR to focus on more complex, acute cases while the COTA focuses on more chronic cases. Of primary importance in this working relationship is that the OTR provide necessary clinical information, supervision and feedback. The COTA must seek necessary assistance and report progress and concerns regularly. This relationship can encourage growth for both team members and enhance their understanding of their unique roles.

Acknowledgments

The authors express their thanks to the Occupational Therapy Department at St. Mary's Rehabilitation Center, Minneapolis, Minnesota, for their assistance and direction during the development of this case study. Special thanks is also given to Sibyl Drake, Anoka Technical College, for her technical assistance and advice in the preparation of this manuscript.

Related Learning Activities

1. Visit a local library and determine available services for the hearing and visually impaired.

2. Obtain copies of some of the catalogs found in the listing of resources in Appendix B. Become familiar with the different types of devices that are available to assist people with sensory impairments.

3. Contact the local telephone company and obtain information about special equipment available for customers with vision and hearing impairments.

4. Visit an elderly individual with a sensory impairment. Discuss what life-style and environmental adaptations have been made.

5. Simulate a visual impairment by using clear glasses, spread with petroleum jelly. Carry out your usual activities for two hours, noting any difficulties you experience. Add cotton balls and earmuffs to simulate a hearing deficit and continue recording difficulties.

References

1. Davis LJ, Kirkland M (Eds): *The Role of Occupational Therapy with the Elderly*. Rockville, Maryland, American Occupational Therapy Association, 1986.
2. Christenson, MA: *Aging in the Designed Environment* Binghamton, New York, Haworth Press, 1990.
3. Mathiowetz V et al: Adult norms for the nine hole peg test of finger dexterity. *Occup Ther J Res* 5(1):24-38, 1985.
4. McGrath LA: Functional low vision assessment. *Phys Occup Ther Geriatr* 3(1):55-61, 1984.
5. Bear P, Radomski M, Smith AC: *Take it to Heart*. Coon Rapids, Minnesota, Mercy Medical Center, 1985, p 29.
6. Lewis SC: *Elder Care in Occupational Therapy*. Thorofare, New Jersey, Slack, Inc., 1989.
7. Entry-level role delineation for registered occupational therapists (OTRs) and certified occupational therapy assistants (COTAs). *Am J Occup Ther* 44:1091-1102, 1990.

Section III
CONTEMPORARY MODELS OF PRACTICE

Work Hardening

The Role of the COTA as an Activities Director

Traumatic Brain Injury

As evidenced by the preceding section, occupational therapists and occupational therapy assistants work in a variety of settings, providing services to individuals with varying abilities and disabilities. Building on this foundation, this segment provides more in-depth, comprehensive information about intraprofessional roles within specific practice models.

Work capacity assessment and work hardening, the role of the COTA as an activities director and head injury were

selected as examples because they represent areas where demand for services is increasing. The reader should note the variety of different skills, tasks and responsibilities assumed by members of the intraprofessional team in these practice models and the complementary nature of the team members' working relationship in the context of specific case studies. The level of independence exercised by a COTA providing therapeutic activities services is an important emphasis.

Work Hardening

Jeffrey Engh, COTA
Sallie Taylor, MEd, OTR

Introduction

The profession of occupational therapy has historically viewed work as an integral component of therapeutic intervention as evidenced through philosophy, theory development, practice and research. Work has been defined broadly to include one's typical paid employment as well as homemaking, child care, parenting, elder care, student efforts and volunteer work.[1]

Since their inception in the early part of this century, work therapy programs have been utilized by individuals with deficits including mental illness, congenital handicaps, chronic physical illness, sensory loss and brain injury. Occupationally injured workers and soldiers also receive treatment.

This chapter focuses on a basic understanding of one aspect of therapeutic intervention in this area—work hardening, as it relates to return to competitive employment. A model of practice format has been used to provide a framework for learning about the systems that support practice, the populations served and methods of intervention. Equipment needs, resources and promotional activities are also presented. A case study details specific OTR and COTA roles in this area of practice.

Definitions and Benefits

Work hardening is very likely the fastest growing area of service delivery in occupational therapy.[2] It offers almost unlimited opportunity for the COTA to work in partnership with occupational and physical therapists, physicians, marketing specialists, insurance representatives and officers of companies in the business community.

ESSENTIAL VOCABULARY

Work hardening

Graded activities

Exercises

Functional status

Rehabilitation question

Job site visit

Baseline evaluation

Job capacity evaluation

Occupational capacity evaluation

Work capacity evaluation

Job simulation

Work conditioning

KEY CONCEPTS

Definitions and benefits

Medical and business components

Identifying and interacting with the client

Goal-setting and evaluating work performance

Terminology and equipment

Program components

Intervention strategies and activities

Work hardening is a well-coordinated, multidisciplinary, therapeutic intervention, individually designed for each worker. The objective is to move the injured worker from a submaximum level of performance to a level of functioning adequate for entry or reentry into the competitive work force. The program is guided by physiologic principles of **graded activities** (increasing levels of resistance; simple to complex; slow to rapid) and **exercises** to increase endurance, strength and positional tolerance for activity—particularly activity needed by the worker to perform the job. The work hardening rehabilitation model has demonstrated success and growth over the past 12 years. As a result, the length of time employees receive Workers' Compensation has decreased. Formerly, an injured employee may have been unable to work due to a job-related injury for several years. Work hardening programs have had a dramatic effect in assisting with a more progressive and timely return to work, satisfying the needs of the employee as well as the employer.

There are many benefits of early return to work. The worker's family generally does not experience the tremendous disruption brought on by the sudden change in loss of employment. It is rarely necessary to alter roles within the family unit because of the employee's inability to work and the resultant decrease in family income. The injured worker's employer also experiences less disruption, as it is usually not necessary to hire a replacement worker. A reduction in the number of lost work days results in reduced costs.

The majority of work hardening programs focus primarily on facilitating the return of the injured worker to the job. If the limitations resulting from the injury make that impractical, the work hardening staff will assist the individual in identifying abilities and limitations relative to other jobs within the company or the competitive labor market.

The System: Medical and Business Components

Work hardening has evolved as a direct response to a variety of needs and demands from the medical and business community—each with its own goals and priorities. Work hardening is perhaps unique in that the traditional application of the medical model, with the physician acting as the case coordinator, often does not work best with this population. The main "product" when treating an individual receiving Workers' Compensation generally is improvement in the **functional status** (level of ability to perform tasks and carry out roles). In current practice, this information is usually obtained by the individual providing treatment. The OTR or the COTA takes on the role not only of clinician, but of coordinator of up-to-date information on the

injured worker. The physician often relies on the rehabilitation professional to provide the necessary information regarding when to terminate medical intervention. The physician is also frequently "shopping" for rehabilitation services that will provide the most comprehensive and up-to-date treatment and information regarding the patient.

In the business community, the worker's change in functional status takes on a different priority. Rapid return of the worker to the job becomes a matter not only of good medical management, but of cost reduction. Expenses associated with on-the-job injury (ie lost days, decreased productivity, medical expenses and Workers' Compensation claims) all result in decreased profits for the employer. The cost of each case is most often reflected in the premiums paid for insurance coverage. In addition to these obvious costs, the employer requires the worker to function at a competitive level, viewing an increase in function as an increase in productivity.

In recent years, "overseers" or third-party administrators have been utilized to manage Workers' Compensation claims, particularly for lengthy or involved cases. These professionals are usually referred to as "rehab nurses." They often provide recommendations about what specific rehabilitation services might be indicated and, occasionally, who should provide them, thus becoming the link between the medical community and the employer.

Identifying and Interacting with the Client

Work hardening is a highly competitive service in most parts of the country. The total number of therapists offering services in any one location has made cost for services a major factor for potential clients. Client satisfaction with services is a critical factor as well. The service plan must be organized to meet the needs of the customer. Unlike most businesses, work hardening programs have numerous clients to satisfy. Often the COTA will find it challenging trying to satisfy these sometimes conflicting needs. Therefore, an overall plan should be established for each referral to the program.

Patient-Client

The patient-client is the most immediate and important. (The term "client" is in common usage.) The majority of those receiving work hardening services have sustained an injury while on the job. Most of these injuries are orthopedic, although a number are the result of brain injuries (see Chapter 23).

Interactions with individuals in a work hardening program take on a different dimension because the workplace is frequently the "clinic." Business-like courtesy should be expected of all involved parties. Common work behaviors, such as meeting appointments on time, being prepared for the assessment and treatment sessions and taking adequate time to explain procedures and answer questions, are important. They provide a foundation for the worker's formulation of expectations relative to self and the rehabilitation provider. Damage can occur in the therapist-client relationship when these basic expectations are not met. Many technically fine work hardening programs have been seriously hurt through negative reporting by a displeased client. The primary goal of the staff is to show the workers that their needs and care are of the utmost importance.

Physician-Client

The worker's referring physician is also a primary client of the work hardening program. Physician satisfaction with the treatment the individual receives and satisfaction with the staff's methods, timeliness and accuracy of communication are important factors in continued utilization. Flexibility in coordinating the work hardening program with the physician's overall treatment plan is also a factor.

Employer-Client

The individual's employer is another important client. The employer-client is key in the overall management of each case. The employer is ultimately responsible for authorizing treatment and for paying the costs of services for the injured employee. The employer must be informed of the worker's progress and degree of compliance, at least in general terms, while the employee is participating in the program. Timely and accurate written and telephone communication is essential.

Insurance Carrier-Client

Insurance carriers or their representatives (rehabilitation case managers) are also viewed as clients. As the injured worker is treated in the program, providing timely written reports, supplemented by periodic telephone calls to the claims adjustor or the case manager, is essential. Information about treatment techniques utilized, progress achieved and expected time frames in the rehabilitation process should be clearly communicated. When it becomes necessary to receive authorization for further treatment and/or testing, the well-informed insurance carrier is more likely to approve the added expense.

With so many clients to serve, occupational therapy personnel appropriately and necessarily devote a considerable part of the treatment day to insuring that all of the program's clients are well served by the program.

The Rehabilitation Question

When an injured worker is referred to a work hardening program, it is very important that the staff, the referral source and the patient have a clear understanding of the objective of referral. This statement of the objective, the **rehabilitation question,** is designed to pull together all the information necessary to establish an ultimate goal of the service. In most cases, where the referral is made by a physician, the treatment goals and precautions are established before treatment begins. This is not always the case when the referral is made by an insurance carrier or an employer. In these instances, it will be especially helpful for the work hardening team to state the program expectations as a rehabilitation question before the initial evaluation takes place.

The following brief excerpts illustrate how the rehabilitation question can be applied in a variety of cases:

- If the individual was referred because of low back strain, the rehabilitation question may be stated as: "Can the worker recover sufficiently to return to his or her job?"
- If the worker has been referred to work hardening simply for training in proper body mechanics, the rehabilitation question may be rephrased to ask: "Can improved mastery of proper body mechanics techniques enable the worker to perform the job more safely?"
- If the worker has been severely injured, the referral may be to assist the individual in maximizing his or her abilities through transferring to another job in the competitive labor market, the rehabilitation question becomes: "What is the highest level of performance that may be reasonable to expect the worker to give on a consistent, 'day in, day out' basis in the competitive work force?"

While all three of these examples focus on individuals who have back injuries, each question is quite different, based on the severity of the problem. The formulation of the rehabilitation question reminds the work hardening staff that the primary focus of the person's treatment program is return to work. The application of the rehabilitation question generally makes it easier to formulate the long-term and short-term goals.

Goal Setting

Establishing realistic goals for the client is one of the most important steps in establishing a treatment program. Generally in occupational therapy, the goals are set at the time of evaluation. Long-term goals and outcomes, however, should be considered at the time of referral with this population. The long-term goal is usually stated from the rehabilitation question. The short-term goals tend to be statements of performance achievements expected within a short time frame, usually one week. When establishing these goals, it is important to include client input. The client's collaboration with the staff in goal-setting helps to ensure a commitment to accomplishment and clarifies expectations for all parties. The system also points out that work hardening is indeed a process of moving incrementally at the client's own pace toward clearly defined goals. Progress is closely monitored, usually weekly, and is generally measured quantitatively. Range of motion, minutes tolerated and weight lifted are examples. The goals are adjusted, based on weekly results, until the rehabilitation question has been answered and achieved.

Evaluating Work Performance

Accurate evaluation of the individuals' strengths and limitations relative to employability is the most important component of any work hardening program. The many parties involved with any Workers' Compensation claim require different information from the person providing treatment. The physician needs up-to-date reports on physical status; the insurance carrier values documentation regarding disability determination; and the employer requires a realistic prognosis as to when the injured employee can safely return to work. The OTR and the COTA must address these requirements in the evaluation, treatment and documentation conducted for every client if the case is to be resolved successfully.

To be successful in evaluating a worker's ability to perform a specific job or the demands of a particular occupational group, an accurate description of the job demands must be obtained. The treatment goals will be established based on that information.

Job Site Visit

Conducting a **job site visit** is the most useful and reliable approach in evaluation. Through observation of the work in progress, the practitioner not only evaluates the physical requirements, (weight lifted, work range and position), but also obtains information about the environmental factors, including temperature, work pace, physical layout and, on occasion, the relationships of the employee with co-workers and supervisors. When possible, the job site visit should be arranged before the evaluation or within the first several treatment sessions. Most often the visit is coordinated with the safety/health department of the employer.

Because of the relatively short amount of time that can be spent at the job site (most employers prefer as little time as possible), it is important to obtain information quickly. To accomplish this goal, basic equipment should be brought to the site and organized in a case or bag for easy access. Typical equipment that might be included is listed here.

- Tape measure for evaluating surface heights
- Large goniometer to measure surface angles and bending
- Strain gauge
- Graph paper to draw diagrams
- Safety goggles and ear plugs
- Stopwatch to measure frequency

When arranging the job site visit, it is helpful to ask if any special equipment is needed, such as a hard hat. It is also a good idea to wear rubber-soled shoes, as it may be necessary to walk on slippery or uneven surfaces.

Documentation is an important aspect of the job site visit, with notes made on all observations, including reports from workers and supervisors. Names of persons providing information should be recorded. The findings are documented either in the evaluation or in a separate report.

When it is not possible to conduct a job site visit, a job description can be obtained via telephone from the employer, the client and the rehabilitation case worker (if one is involved). Each of these reports should be documented in the evaluation.

Related Resources and Methods

It is often helpful to use the *Dictionary of Occupational Titles* (DOT)[3] to gain a basic understanding of the physical demands of a particular occupational group. The DOT is a listing of job titles and descriptions compiled by the US Department of Labor. Used with its companion volume *Classification of Jobs* (COJ),[4] an overall view of the physical demands and aptitudes can be obtained for most job titles. Use of these references is discussed in greater depth in a following section.

The type of evaluation conducted for an injured worker is determined by the needs of the referral source. Most often, the assessment is performed to provide a baseline measurement of the worker's functioning at that given time in recovery. Based on these findings, a program is established to eliminate the areas where abilities fall short of job demands. In a few cases, when the worker has been disabled for an extended time, the goal may not be to determine when a worker can resume employment but whether it is realistic for the worker to return to competitive employment at all. The evaluation becomes a determination of the individual's maximum functional capacity and may not involve specific remediation of limitations. The information obtained is most often utilized in determining permanent disability and/or establishing vocational goals that meet physical limitations.

Terminology

Because of the vast increase in work hardening programs during the past decade, a wide variety of assessment terminology is being used. Since the 1970s, the Commission on Accreditation of Rehabilitation Facilities (CARF) has provided guidelines for the types and titles of evaluations conducted under the auspices of accredited work hardening programs. The four primary types are listed here:[5]

1. **Baseline evaluation**: A baseline assessment of functional ability to perform work activities; includes the physical demand factors detailed in the *Dictionary of Occupational Titles*.
2. **Job capacity evaluation**: An assessment of the match between the individual's capabilities and the critical demands of a specific job.
3. **Occupational capacity evaluation**: An assessment of the match between the individual's capabilities and the critical demands of an occupational group.
4. **Work capacity evaluation**: An assessment of the match between the individual's capabilities and the demands of the competitive environment.

Each evaluation is designed to compare the worker's performance to a specific group of population norms. Due to the growth of CARF-accredited programs, this listing of evaluations is rapidly becoming the accepted terminology.

Equipment and Resources

A study of the earliest work hardening programs in the United States showed that programs typically used a combination of standardized tests and "low tech" and "high tech" equipment in therapeutic intervention.[2]

Standardized tests have set procedures for administration. When properly administered, they allow comparison of the individual's performance with a set of established normative values. These norms give an indication of how well the patient's performance compares with that of a previously tested group. The Bennett Hand Tool Test, the Purdue Peg Board Test, the Minnesota Rate of Manipulation Test and selected components of the Valpar Test System were among the most commonly used standardized tests.

"Low tech" equipment generally consisted of a variety of tasks devised by the work hardening staff, such as graded lifting and carrying activities. Many of these tasks simulated actual job components for individual workers in the work hardening program. The WEST II Lifting Apparatus was a common "low tech" testing device found in many of the early work hardening programs. Figure 21-1 depicts a COTA observing the performance of an individual using a wheelbarrow and a shovel in a simulated situation.

The most common "high tech" equipment item was the Baltimore Therapeutic Work Simulator shown in Figure 21-2. The COTA is observing the individual's ability to lift a specified amount of weight (a job requirement) and noting whether proper body mechanics are being used.

Since a 1991 demographic study on occupational therapy work hardening programs,[2] much new equipment is available. Certainly, much of the technology that has been used

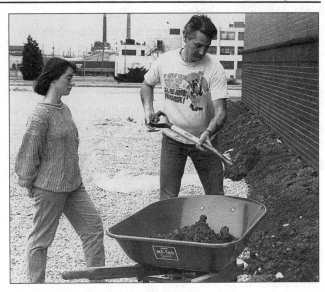

Figure 21-1. *Observation of work performance.*

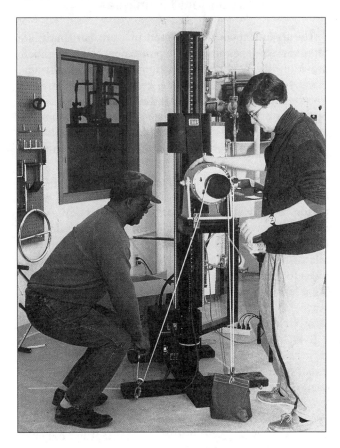

Figure 21-2. *Lifting with Baltimore Therapeutic Work Simulator.*

only for research purposes will be adapted for clinical application, particularly in the areas of measurement and analysis of lifting.

Most "high tech" equipment is quite expensive and may become outdated rather quickly. The most successful work hardening programs will be those in which the staff:

- Has carefully identified the areas of performance that are desirable to measure.
- Has studied the available products that will accomplish the desired measurements.
- Has selected items that address the needs of the specific work hardening program. Sometimes "low tech" items will adequately accomplish the job of "high tech" items.

It is imperative that the work hardening staff establish good working relationships with manufacturer's or equipment sales representatives. The salesperson will keep the staff apprised of available new items. It is important to learn of new developments early so that money for needed equipment can be budgeted for timely purchase.

Treatment Techniques

The treatment techniques used in work hardening are often varied, depending on the professional staff members providing the service (occupational therapy or physical therapy) and the location of the center (hospital-based or free-standing). The one constant in all programs tends to be the use of job simulation as a treatment technique. The treatment program is established based on the limitations of the individual found in the initial evaluation compared to the physical demands of the work situation. When establishing a treatment program, care should be taken not to treat only the diagnosis, but to treat the whole person. For most people, work is a "full body experience" and any attempt to bring about a successful return to employment must recognize and treat all the work-related needs of the individual. Attention should also be given to the length of time the worker has been experiencing a less than normal activity level. Often, a decrease in range of motion and strength is present because of inactivity and may not be directly related to pathology.

It is important to design a realistic success-oriented program. This goal is often difficult to accomplish in the initial phases because the individual being may not recognize the gain. Whereas the therapist and assistant are looking for increases in flexibility, lifting ability and strength, the worker may be experiencing the same level of discomfort. In such cases, it is important not only for the worker to perform tasks but also to record progress. To assist with this procedure, charts and graphs may be used to record daily performance.

When a worker begins a work hardening program, the first several sessions usually focus on improving strength, flexibility and symptom control. Special attention is paid to how the worker performs the activities. Education is provided to reduce risk of further injury or pain through teaching proper body mechanics. Once these basic techniques are learned, conditioning and flexibility activities are generally incorporated within the worker's level of tolerance. Most initial sessions range from one hour to several hours daily, depending on the physical level of the individual.

The initiation of **job simulation** (replication of actual work tasks) as a part of the worker's therapy program should begin as soon as the individual is able to tolerate it for short periods. Job simulation that a worker has attempted and failed because of increased pain or other symptoms can have disastrous effects on the individual's motivation or "worker behavior." Often the simulation is broken down into the critical job demands and may involve several components of one activity. The duration of each simulation is monitored and increased as the worker's toleration increases. Gradually, job simulation replaces the initial strengthening and conditioning program. Sessions at this point are increased and generally range from three to eight hours daily.

Because work hardening is designed to replace the patient role with the worker role, it is essential to include worker expectations in the program. Behaviors that are expected in the employment setting should be expected in the work hardening program. These behaviors include punctuality, following directions and maintaining an adequate productivity level. Reporting of levels of achievement in relation to these traits is often as important as the gains made in physical abilities.

Program Components

Through growth and experience, return to work programs added services that complement the work hardening program. Today in many instances, programs that offer work hardening treatment have an expanded "product line," including work conditioning, body mechanics training and symptom management.

Work Conditioning

Work conditioning is a relatively new term that identifies a course of treatment that differs somewhat from work hardening. As with work hardening, the final outcome of the service is successful return to work, but the program uses different methods to prepare the worker to return to the job place. **Work conditioning** may be defined as the biomechanical rehabilitation process of building physical conditioning to a level similar to the job demands. Unlike work hardening, work conditioning does not use job simulation as a primary treatment technique, making it difficult to monitor and assess some of the worker behaviors. Generally, the work conditioning program focuses on building the worker's flexibility, strength and endurance. For the employee who has not worked for a long time, loss in overall strength and stamina places that employee at risk for further injury or reinjury once normal activities are resumed. A short program of work conditioning may be prescribed to address these general endurance issues. A work conditioning program is a natural extension of a physical or occupational therapy program and is generally designed and managed by an occupational therapist, a physical therapist or an exercise physiologist.

Recently, work conditioning has been used by some industries as an injury prevention measure. Employers have found that when it becomes necessary to move workers to new or different positions, those who have moved to positions of greater physical demands show higher injury rates than those who have been performing regularly at higher demands. To help reduce these risks, some programs are providing a two- or three-week course of general conditioning before beginning the new job demands.

Body Mechanics Training

The majority of industrially related injuries involve the back. Although back discomfort can have many different etiologies, the most prevalent injuries are strains to the low back. Both the prevalence and the enormous cost associated with this injury make its prevention a major priority in the workplace.

Most work hardening programs have a strong body mechanics training emphasis. The worker who masters good body mechanics will have a reduced risk of reinjury after he or she returns to work. If the program has also incorporated flexibility and back strengthening components, the worker's risk for reinjury will be significantly reduced.

The application of body mechanics training becomes a viable answer for the worker who has had several back injuries or has become symptomatic once again, paricularly when the job requires the performance of physical tasks of lifting, bending or prolonged postures. Medical examinations generally reveal no new injury or negative findings with this population, and medical management becomes noneffective. A patient with this type of history is an excellent candidate for a program of body mechanics training and usually does not require other services. The length of time the patient is followed varies, but generally the training takes place over two weeks. Initial treatment focuses on review and practice of general body mechanics principles and moves to incorporating these principles into performing specific job tasks. Thus the worker acquires new habits in the clinic setting that will translate directly into the work role.

Symptom Management

The injured worker frequently expects to be free of pain before returning to the job. In a work hardening program the individual learns that instead of being pain free, he or she may expect to be able to carry out symptom management effectively by the time a regular work schedule is resumed. Clients are taught to manage discomfort through education about the causes of pain relative to their specific injury, the physiology of natural healing, and ways to pace work through managed rest breaks. Although it is unrealistic to expect to be pain free, it is appropriate to be reasonably comfortable during work. Perhaps most significantly, it is important for the worker to realize that he or she has some control over the degree of comfort or discomfort being experienced. A psychologist, therapist or COTA who has completed specialized training in pain management may lead the symptoms management educational program.

Marketing

The COTA is often as effective as the occupational therapist or the program director in marketing a work hardening program. The person who can identify the client's interest in work hardening services and is able to promote the benefits of the program with professionalism and enthusiasm can be a successful salesperson. In presenting the program to a prospective referral source, the marketing person must always keep in mind what the prospective "purchaser" wants and how work hardening can address those needs. Many programs now have professional sales people representing their product lines, with members of the work hardening staff serving as consultants.

A sales call to a physician's office, an insurance agency or an employer's company provides an initial opportunity to describe the work hardening program. When possible, it is desirable to bring the potential client to the treatment center. Few people who take the time to visit a work hardening program fail to be impressed by the staff, the process and the outcomes of a well-managed program.

Cost-Effectiveness

Employers and their insurance carriers or administrators generally consider work hardening programs a good investment as long as the charges for services are reasonable and the length of time of treatment is limited. Competition for dollars from business and industry is high. The organizations with the flexibility and the creativity to modify existing programs and to design new, effective programs that return the injured worker to the job quickly—or (better yet), keep that worker on the job—will be the programs that survive over time and win in this competitive service area.

Case Study

Background and Referral

John is a 35-year-old firefighter, employed in a large metropolitan area. He has been working with the department for 13 years and was referred to the work hardening program three weeks after he had sustained a lumbar strain. John is married and the father of two school-aged children. There is a family tradition of employment with the local fire department dating back to his great-grandfather who served as the chief.

Review of the medical records revealed that this was John's second back injury. Approximately two years earlier, he had experienced a lumbar strain when he was hit by rubble from the wall of a falling building. As a result, John was unable to work for five weeks. Treatment consisted of bed rest and medication.

The COTA conducted the initial interview with John, focusing on his history since his previous injury, including any treatment received. John reported intermittent discomfort over the past two years, although it was not severe enough to cause him any lost work time. Self-administered treatment had consisted of rest and applications of a heating pad to the lumbar area. He stated that his most recent injury occurred while assisting a man who was escaping from a second story window during a fire. When lowering the person, he experienced a "dull ache" in the central portion of his lower back, which increased during the next few hours so that he was no longer able to continue working. John visited a physician early the next day and was referred for two weeks of physical therapy, emphasizing use of pain reduction and increased flexibility modalities. Referral to the work hardening program followed this acute phase of treatment.

Assessment

The COTA and the OTR collaborated in conducting the work performance evaluation. While the OTR completed the interview and biomechanical testing (manual muscle, full body range of motion and coordination testing), the COTA prepared for the functional test of lifting and job simulation. The lift test was was conducted utilizing the West II lifting frame. Using the standard protocol, John's lifting ability was 15 lb initially; weight was added in 5-lb increments until the range (inches above floor level) and additional resistance prevented continuation.

A job simulation was carried out by the COTA based on the job-site evaluation he had completed earlier that day revealing the following physical demands:
- Lifting and carrying loads greater than 100 lb.
- Climbing and standing on ladders with loads greater than 100 lb.
- Pushing and pulling weights greater than 100 lb.
- Climbing up and over uneven surfaces.

Specifically, the simulation included lifting and moving of weight between surfaces of varying heights and short periods of climbing on and off ladders and platforms.

Both the OTR and the COTA monitored John's body mechanics in the lifting test and simulated work tasks.

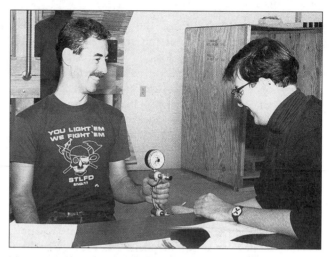

Figure 21-3. *Dynamometer used to measure grip strength.*

Dynamometer readings were also taken to measure grip strength as shown in Figure 21-3.

Results revealed normal body strength. It was noted, however, that John was limited by discomfort in the low back during manual muscle testing in this area. Restrictions in back flexion, side bending and rotation were noted; the hamstrings were shortened bilaterally. Overall pain was reported at level 5 on a 1 to 10 scale, with 10 indicating maximum pain. John's work range was limited below waist level because of pain with forward bending and squatting. His maximum lifting ability was 50 lb from knee to shoulder level. John was limited to climbing the ladder without weight and was not able to climb onto a 2.5 ft platform.

Impact on Role Performance. During an interview with the OTR, John spoke of his uneasiness about continuing employment as a firefighter. While he was receiving Workers' Compensation benefits, his unemployment status affected on his role as the "family provider." He expressed frustration and fear about his future employment role if he could not return to his job, as he had no other formal training.

Treatment Planning

The COTA visited the job site to determine specific work requirements, as well as personal clothing and equipment required for fire fighters. This information was reported to the supervising occupational therapist, and John, the OTR and the COTA established a treatment plan focusing on the following goals:
1. Demonstrate ability to use proper body mechanics without prompting within one week.
2. Climb and jump from a 3-foot platform successfully five out of five attempts within two weeks.
3. Demonstrate ability to carry a minimum of 100 lb up and down a 12-ft ladder three out of three attempts within three weeks.
4. Reduce level of pain discomfort while engaged in simulated work tasks for eight hours to a level of 1 on a 10-point scale within three weeks.

Treatment Implementation

The COTA initiated John's treatment program the following day. His early program emphasized flexibilty, including stretching and "warm-up" exercises and general conditioning. Despite physical evidence that John was continuing to experience some pain, he was compliant with the treatment regimen and appeared to be committed to achieving the mutually established goals. Since the job site visit had revealed that John was required to wear a fire-proof coat, boots, helmet, oxygen tank and face mask (the latter occasionally), the COTA obtained these items from the firehouse, so that work simulation activities would parallel those on the job as closely as possible. The total weight of the clothing and equipment could exceed 30 lb.

Once John demonstrated the necessary level of physical conditioning and flexibility, the program emphasis shifted to specific job simulation activities. His treatment sessions were increased to eight hours daily, and activities were chosen that corresponded to those discussed in the goals in the previous section. Initially, he had difficulty lifting 60 lb; however, by using the West lifting frame, John was able to gradually increase his lifting ability to 100 lb and to successfully carry this weight up and down a 12-ft ladder. His ability to climb and jump from a 3-ft platform proved to be an easier task, and John was able to perform this job skill successfully the first week of treatment. This achievement proved to be a great psychological "boost" for John, and the COTA noted that he seemed to have renewed confidence in his abilities.

As John continued to experience success in the work hardening program, his initial fears regarding his role as the family provider disappeared. He expressed appreciation to the treatment team and exhibited renewed self-esteem. A visit to the clinic by his supervisor was an added incentive and had a positive impact on John's performance in reaching goals.

Program Discontinuation

At the conclusion of the third week of treatment, John's discomfort dropped to a level 1, following a full day of job simulation. The OTR and the COTA met with John to review the extent of his progress and encouraged him to continue some of his favorite leisure pursuits, including bowling and gardening, to maintain his level of conditioning and flexibility. He was referred back to his physician for a final medical assessment and returned to work full time.

Follow-Up

The COTA conducted the formal follow-up for John at the work site two weeks after his return to work. He indicated that he had experienced little or no discomfort and reported that he was performing his stretching and "warm-up" activities daily. He also stated that he thought the body mechanics principles he had learned would be very beneficial in preventing further problems. John concluded the follow-up visit by stating how pleased his wife was that he had resumed gardening responsibilities because she viewed the work as "too hard!" They had also rejoined their weekly bowling league and looked forward to this opportunity to exercise as well as socialize with friends.

The COTA conducted a one-year follow-up with John, which included a job site visit, an interview and completion of a one page questionnaire. A report of the follow-up information was sent to John's physician, his employer and the insurance representative. This information was also used in the work hardening program's research study about outcomes of therapeutic intervention.

Summary

Work hardening is a specialized area of occupational therapy practice that provides a system of therapeutic intervention to assist individuals in returning to the competitive employment market. In addition to the injured worker, program clients include the referring physician, the employer and the insurance carrier's representative. Components of a work hardening program are work conditioning, body mechanics training and symptom management. Goals are established through development of the rehabilitation question at the time of referral and evaluation. Treatment emphasis is job specific and is based on information gathered at the job site. Progress is monitored by improvements in the client's ability to perform job simulation activities and exhibit work behaviors. Specific equipment and methods are used to return workers to the competitive work force. Examples of OTR and COTA roles are presented to illustrate the intraprofessional team approach.

Note to Reader

Several important references should be available in every work hardening program. *The Dictionary of Occupational Titles* (DOT)[3] and its companion publications, *Dictionary of Occupational Titles Supplement* and *Classification of Jobs According to Worker Traits* (COJ).[4] These books provide useful information on more than 20,000 jobs found throughout the United States. The DOT and the DOT Supplement provide an alphabetical listing of all occupational job titles, brief descriptions of job titles by industry and an analysis of requirements placed on the worker who performs the job.

Classification of Jobs According to Worker Traits, is used in conjunction with the DOT and the DOT Supplement,[4] provides information about the worker trait factors associated with each of the job titles listed in the other volumes. These factors include information relative to environmental exposures, such as extremes of temperature, noise, fumes and hazards. It gives specific information regarding physical demands of each job, such as lifting, carrying, climbing, seeing, hearing and handling. General educational level or required training and aptitudes, such as intelligence or manual dexterity, are also included. Interests and temperaments are described for each job listing as well.

The National Institute of Occupational Health and Safety (NIOHS) publishes a manual, *Work Practices Guide for Manual Lifting*,[6] which is also an important reference in work hardening. It provides a great deal of information about identifying high-risk lifting tasks; the principles applicable to reducing injuries in high-risk lifting jobs are also described.

Related Learning Activities

1. Locate catalogs that feature work hardening equipment and become acquainted with the wide variety that are available.

2. Visit an occupational therapy clinic that offers a work hardening program and interview at least one client. Determine the following:
   a. Nature of injury
   b. Symptoms and problems (perceived or real)
   c. Therapeutic activities engaged in
   d. Personal feelings about injury in terms of impact on role

3. Discuss the various treatment approaches used in work hardening programs with a peer.

4. Interview a vocational specialist regarding how workers with cognitive deficits are placed in the work environment.

5. Participate in a body mechanics program and practice injury prevention techniques.

References

1. Reed KL: *Models of Practice in Occupational Therapy*. Baltimore, Williams and Wilkins, 1984.
2. Wyrick J et al: Occupational therapy work hardening programs: A demographic study. *Am J Occup Ther* 45:109-112, 1991.
3. United States Department of Labor: *Dictionary of Occupational Titles*. Washington, DC, United States Department of Labor, 1986.
4. United States Department of Labor: *Classification of Jobs According to Worker Traits*. Washington, DC, United States Department of Labor, 1986.
5. Commission on Accreditation of Rehabilitation Facilities: *National Advisory Committee Recommendations for Work Hardening Programs*. Tucson, Arizona, Commission on Accreditation of Rehabilitation Facilities, 1988.
6. Department of Health and Human Services: *Work Practices Guide for Manual Lifting*. Cincinnati, Department of Health and Human Services, Ohio, 1981.

The Role of the COTA as an Activities Director

Sally E. Ryan, COTA, ROH

Introduction

The position of activities director, coordinator or supervisor is one for which the certified occupational therapy assistant (COTA) is well qualified. With an educational background in human development throughout the life span, disabling conditions, the teaching/learning process, group dynamics and activity analysis, as well as an understanding of every individual's need for purposeful, meaningful activity, the COTA is able to carry out activities programs of exceptional quality.

Activities directors are employed in a variety of settings including community centers, large apartment and condominium complexes for the well and the disabled, group homes and institutions for the mentally retarded and the chronic mentally ill, and long-term care settings for the elderly and others. Since a large number of COTAs are employed as activities directors in long-term care facilities, this chapter focuses on principles and applications for those settings. Although in many cases the majority of people residing in these facilities are elderly, a growing number of younger individuals are also residents. Activities planning must meet their unique needs and interests, and special measures must be taken to ensure that these individuals do not feel isolated due to age. The activity director is often in a position to help develop these social partnerships.

KEY CONCEPTS

Definitions

An **activities program** may be defined as an on-going plan for providing meaningful activities, which is determined in relation to the individual needs and interests of those involved. Such programs are designed to provide a variety of opportunities for individuals to participate in activities, with the goal being to promote their physical, mental and social well-being.[1] The term *resident* is used in keeping with the terminology adopted in the current Medicare and Medicaid standards for long-term care facilities.[2]

An **activities director** is employed by the facility and is directly responsible for planning, scheduling, implementing, documenting, managing and evaluating an activities program. The program is designed with the overall goal of meeting the individual resident's needs for healthy activity that will assist in maintaining optimum levels of functioning and quality of life.

An **activities consultant** is a qualified individual who is employed by the facility to provide guidance to the activity director about all aspects of the activities program. This person may also provide consultation to other staff members and departments as requested by administration. Occupational therapists, experienced occupational therapy assistants, therapeutic recreation specialists and social workers often provide consultative services.

Legislation and Regulations

The Department of Health and Human Services establishes requirements for Medicare and Medicaid programs in long-term care facilities, which include specific regulations for activities departments and personnel. These regulations have been modified as a result of new legislation. All required changes were implemented October 1, 1990, with the exception of changes related to assessment, which were implemented April 14, 1991. Details of these changes may be found in the *Federal Register*, Vol. 54, No. 249, Section 483.15: Level B Requirement.[2] Complete copies of all regulations are available from state health and human services offices.

Many of the legislative changes center around the Nursing Home Reform Amendments of the **Omnibus Budget Reconciliation Act** (OBRA) of 1987, which were designed to improve the standards of nursing homes "from the bottom up" and became law in 1990.[3] Establishment of these amendments "is an attempt to set minimum standards across the country for all nursing homes that receive federal aid."[3] These new standards address the following:[2,3]

1. Rights and quality of life
2. Preadmission screening
3. Assessment and quality of care
4. Training of nurse's aides
5. Annual resident review
6. Facility survey and certification
7. Enforcement

Experts have noted that the new standards for resident assessment are one of the most important provisions of the law. Residents rights are protected relative to free choice and "freedom from chemical and physical restraints used for (control), involuntary seclusion, discipline or staff convenience."[3] Further, the new requirements mandate that individuals be assessed in terms of strengths as well as weaknesses, level of initiative and involvement and personal preferences, with an emphasis on resident outcomes.

In addition to these federal regulations for skilled nursing care facilities (SNFs) and intermediate care facilities (ICFs), most state health departments and licensing agencies have specific regulations for activities programs. The activities director must have a complete understanding of all of these regulations before initiating an activities program.

Job Descriptions

The director and all employees of the department must have a job description that specifically outlines all responsibilities and expectations. The following items should be included:[1]

1. Job title, supervisor and supervisees
2. Qualifications, including formal education and training and any specialized training that might be required such as remotivation, reality orientation and reminiscence techniques, cardiopulmonary resuscitation (CPR) and first aid
3. Licensure and/or certification requirements
4. Other skills such as effective written and verbal communication and related public relations activities.
5. Required participation in continuing education and professional activities
6. Specific activities responsibilities such as assessing individual resident activities needs; planning, scheduling, implementing, documenting and evaluating the activities program. Definitive time lines should be included, eg, weekly, monthly or quarterly
7. Participation in the care planning process including specific requirements for attending meetings and frequency.
8. Staff and volunteer recruitment, training, supervision, evaluation and termination
9. In-service education training responsibilities for staff and volunteers
10. Reports to be prepared and frequency
11. Procurement of supplies and equipment

12. Orientation activities for new employees and residents in the facility
13. Other responsibilities such as coordinating barber and beautician appointments and making arrangements for voting
14. Methods and frequency of evaluation; conditions of probationary employment

Job descriptions should be reviewed and modified as necessary, at least on an annual basis. Sample job descriptions for activities directors are often available from state health departments.

Developing an Activities Plan

The first step in developing an activities plan is **data collection** about the likely participants. The medical record and the resident preadmission history will provide information regarding the primary and secondary diagnosis, precautions and limitations, physician's approval for activities participation, the resident's birth date, nationality, social history and the name of a family contact.[1]

Another step in the data collection process is to determine the interests of the residents. A structured questionnaire or interview may be used to seek information in specific areas of activities. One method is to divide potential activities into the following eight **activity categories**: physical, social, creative, productive (work substitute), educational, leisure, spiritual and democratic community activities. These are described further in the accompanying box.

Another method of categorizing activities is in terms of their potential to be supportive, provide maintenance, or provide empowerment. The following definitions are drawn from the Standards of Practice of the National Association of Activity Professionals (NAAP):[4]

Supportive activities "promote a comfortable environment while providing stimulation or solace" to those individuals who "cannot benefit from either maintenance or empowerment activities." Such activities are usally provided to those individuals who may be severely cognitively or physically impaired or those unable to participate in a group program. Examples include providing soft background music; placing plants, pictures, and other colorful objects in the resident's room; and providing olfactory or tactile stimulation.

Maintenance activities provide the individual with opportunities to maintain physical, cognitive, social, spiritual and emotional health. These areas are delineated under the eight activity categories discussed in the previous section.

Empowerment activities "emphasize the promotion of self-respect by providing opportunities for self-expression, choice, and social and personal responsibility." These activities differ from those designed to provide maintenance

Eight Activity Categories

Physical activities: These activities might include participation in exercise groups, sports and games such as lawn bowling, shuffleboard and badminton, and daily walks.

Social activities: Activities in this category include parties, picnics, meals at community restaurants and "tea time." The primary goal is to provide an opportunity for patients to interact socially. Family members should also be invited to some of these events.

Creative activities: Crafts, calligraphy, creative writing, and oil and watercolor painting are examples of creative activities. Such endeavors provide an outlet for creative expression, and although they often are presented in a group setting, socialization is not required.

Productive (work substitute) activities: Many people have a need to be engaged in a productive activity. Work on community service projects, such as filling fund raising packets for the American Cancer Society or stuffing envelopes for a local charity, should be provided. Other work-related activities include writing and producing a facility newspaper, rolling bandages for the Red Cross and baking items for a bazaar. Productive, volunteer endeavors such as these allow the participants to continue to make a meaningful contribution to society.

Educational activities: Opportunities for lifelong learning are virtually endless. Photography clubs, music appreciation groups, book review and discussion groups are examples. Individual activities such as learning to speak a foreign language or to operate a microcomputer should also be included.

Leisure activities: Almost everyone needs time to read a good book, write letters, listen to the radio or view a favorite television program. Quiet strolls in the park or just sitting on the patio observing and enjoying nature can be meaningful, refreshing pastimes.

Spiritual activities: Spiritual needs can be met in a variety of ways such as participation in Bible study groups, a choir or regularly scheduled religious services in the facility as well as the community. A missionary group also often assists in fulfilling spiritual needs.

Democratic community activities: Living in a residential community affords members many opportunities to assume roles in determining the future of their community. These empowering activities include organizing forums for discussion and resolution of issues of mutual interest, forming a resident and staff council to discuss problems and concerns and to establish policies, writing editorials for the facility newspaper, and organizing activities related to political and social issues that impact on the quality of life of the participants.

because they focus on opportunities for individuals to "redevelop a sense of purpose in their lives." Examples may be found under the categories of creative, productive and democratic community activities, as well as others.

Whatever methods are used to categorize activities, it is important to assure that every resident has an opportunitiy to particpate in meaningful activities that are of interest and based on individual needs, strengths and goals. Activities that require decision making should be emphasized as well. Etta Solashin, Professor Emeritus of Social Work at the University of Minnesota notes that "decision-making is the core of independence."[5]

If potential participants fill out a questionnaire, an interview should also be arranged to verify and expand the needed activity information. If residents are reluctant to discuss items on a questionnaire, a more generalized approach may be used by asking open-ended questions such as:

1. What activities did you enjoy before coming to the nursing home?
2. What are some of the things you did during your spare time this week?
3. If you were the activities director, what do you think would be an important activity to provide?

The interviewer should provide added cues as necessary to keep the responses to questions on target. Speaking with family members and other staff is also recommended to gain as much additional input as possible, especially if the resident is cognitively impaired or uncommunicative. Figure 22-1 provides an example of a form that may be used.

Once the data are gathered, the information must be tabulated and categorized and priorities established in terms of available staff, volunteers, space, existing supplies and equipment, community resources and operating budget. For example, if the category of creative activities indicates that many residents are interested in arts and crafts, a general session should be scheduled daily. Perhaps a small number are interested in knitting. While they could participate in the general group, they may also enjoy forming a knitting club that meets once a week to work on a special project, such as knitting hats and mittens for a children's home or homeless people in the community.

Initial activity planning can best be accomplished by setting up a "mock" weekly calendar with dates on the left, including Saturday and Sunday, and the eight major categories of activities listed across the top. Enter the large group activities first—those in which residents indicated the greatest interest, such as crafts, movies, concerts and games. Next, enter the small group activities, such as baking, gardening, and oil painting. Determine which of these activities existing staff and volunteers can supervise and identify additional needs. Be sure that necessary space, supplies and equipment are available. Look for gaps in the plan and be creative about introducing new activities. It is

also important to determine whether activities are primarily active or passive in terms of degree of participation. Every effort should be made to schedule activities such as picnics, shopping tours and visits to museums and zoos, so that residents maintain contact with the community. Some individuals will prefer not to join groups; therefore, time must be set aside for individual activities participation.

Activities needs cannot be totally met by a program that only schedules events Monday through Friday during the usual daytime working hours. Flexibility is necessary, and every effort should be made to provide some activities in the evenings and on weekends. Arrangements can usually be made for the staff members assigned to take compensatory time off during the regular work week. The proposed activities plan should also be evaluated to assure that at least some of the activities are held at a time when family members can participate and efforts should be made to encourage them to do so.

Once the mock plan is developed and staffing patterns are established, it is important to look at timing of the events. Consideration must be given to "set" activities such as meals, routine nursing care, physicians' rounds, occupational and physical therapy schedules and visiting hours.

Public Relations

Effective **public relations** is an important component of activity planning. When the final monthly plan is developed, it must be communicated as widely as possible. Copies should be provided to administration and all departments in the facility, as well as to each resident at least seven days in advance. Large weekly posters should be made and posted in prominent locations throughout the building. Individual posters should also be made to advertise special events such as a concert or a bazaar. If a public address system is available, use it to make daily announcements of forthcoming events. Flyers can be mailed to family members when events are scheduled in which they may participate. The community should also be informed through providing local newspapers with press releases of activities of interest, such as a resident's 100th birthday, or an announcement of the individuals who received "ribbons" for their entries in the county fair.

Related Planning Principles

Activities planning must always occur at least one month in advance. Failure to do so will produce undo stress for the director, staff and volunteers and will result in unmet resident activities needs. Even the most thorough planning will not be flawless. The activities director must have alternative plans to draw upon when, for example, the high school band does not show up for a concert or a torrential rainstorm ruins picnic plans. Flexibility, adaptability and resourcefulness are important attributes of the successful activities director.

Name _____ Room _____ Admit Date _____

Date of Birth _____ Age _____ Hometown _____

Marital Status _____ Children _____

_____ Grandchildren _____ Great Grandchildren

Siblings _____ Do any live nearby? _____

Ethnic/Cultural Background _____

Languages Spoken _____ Religion _____

Education _____

Occupations _____

Work History _____

Registered Voter _____ Veteran _____ Branch of Service _____

Clubs and Organizations _____

Interests: (Code - S = small group; G = large group; I = individual)

Note: Interviewer should give examples in each category below.

● Physical activities _____

_____

● Social activities _____

_____

● Creative activities _____

_____

● Productive activities _____

_____

● Educational activities _____

_____

● Leisure activities _____

_____

● Spiritual activities _____

_____

● Democratic governance activities _____

_____

● Typical Day Profile _____

_____

_____

● Typical Week Profile _____

_____

Life Goals _____

_____

Previous Living Arrangement _____

Diagnosis _____

Reason for Admission _____

Physician _____ Functional Limitations/Strengths:

Mobility _____ Vision _____

Hearing _____ Comprehension _____

Orientation _____ Behavior _____

Attention Span _____ Other _____

Contact Person _____ Phone _____

Address _____

Figure 22-1. *Activity Interest Questionnaire. S. Ryan, 1991. Used with permission.*

Individual activities plans should be developed for every resident and be included in the total **resident care plan**. Problems and needs are identified and specific objectives are established along with methods for accomplishing the goals. Copies of both state and federal regulations should be obtained to be sure all required information is included. A brief example of a plan is provided in the box:[4]

A card system should be developed for each resident's individual activity plan. The resident card should also have information on the primary and secondary diagnosis, limitations and precautions, physician's permission to participate in activities, birth date and other pertinent social history facts. Preferences should also be noted, such as small group versus large group participation and afternoon activities versus morning or evening activities. Locating the card system in a central place, such as the activities department office, will allow all staff members convenient access to it. Additional information on patient care planning and specific activities plans appears in the section on records and reports.

Implementing the Activities Program

Once initial planning has been completed, the activities program is implemented, often gradually over several weeks. As activities take place, the activities director must carefully monitor all aspects to ensure that the programming is effective in helping to meet resident's goals. The following items are of particular importance:

1. General attendance and degree of participation
2. Adequacy of staff and volunteer coverage
3. Adequacy of space, furnishings, equipment and supplies
4. Adequacy of lighting, ventilation and temperature control devices and general safety
5. Effectiveness of communication with other departments

Problem/need: Few social contacts; rarely participates in any group activities

Capabilities/strengths: Articulate; knowledgeable about current event and sports

Activity goal: Participation in one small group event weekly

Approach: Invite to current events group or sports group as a resource person; offer a choice and structure role to be as nonthreatening as possible; stress that others are interested in the information the individual could share

---

6. Timing of events in relation to other activities taking place in the facility
7. Specific ways to improve the activity and the degree of participation the next time it is presented

Keeping a clipboard close at hand is a good idea so that observations relative to the issue presented in the preceding section may be recorded immediately. It is also important to seek critiques from participants as well as staff members and volunteers. An activities planning committee should be established to review past events and make recommendations for future activities.

Another helpful method is to break activities down into very specific **activity components**, particularly if they tend to take too much time or participation is less than expected. An example would be the weekly songfest. This activity is made up of at least twelve distinct parts:

1. Furniture arrangement
2. Transportation for non-ambulatory participants
3. Introduction of song leader and pianist
4. Distribution of song sheets
5. Use of an overhead projector with enlarged words to songs
6. Use of clapping and marching activities
7. Distribution and use of rhythm instruments
8. Playing "name that tune" game
9. Collecting and storing supplies and equipment
10. Returning nonambulatory residents to their units
11. Rearranging furniture
12. Documenting participation

Resident Motivation

A successful activities program involves much more than planning and carrying out a variety of activities. It must also include the creation of an atmosphere that is warm, friendly, caring and as nonthreatening as possible; an atmosphere that offers decision making opportunities and promotes independence; and an atmosphere where residents are offered encouragement and support but are never coerced or forced to participate. These are very important motivational factors.

The main activities room should serve as a central gathering spot for those who just want to get away from their room for a while. Space should be provided for people to observe the activities taking place, particularly new residents. Serving coffee and tea is a method to comfortably include observers in the activities group. It encourages socialization and may increase motivation to become directly involved in the activity.

Motivation comes from within, but it can be enhanced by showing a genuine interest in the residents. Sometimes writing a short personal note to invite an individual to participate will be a motivating factor. Others will be motivated or drawn to activities because they can be assured of some degree of success and they feel "needed" by the other group members. For example, a person who is not interested in working on the mosaic mural in the dining room may be willing to spend hours sorting tile so that the others can work more efficiently.

Records and Reports

A system of regular documentation must be established, in keeping with the requirements of federal, state and facility regulations. The general categories of documentation include resident care plans, activities plans, activities notes, activities schedules and participation records. The latter must be maintained for all group and one-to-one activities and should be a part of the resident's permanent record. Confidentiality must be maintained for all resident records and reports. Records should also be maintained for all staff members and volunteers, indicating hours worked as well as major responsibilities. Budget reports must be prepared regularly, and the administration of the facility may require monthly summary reports of the activities program as well as an annual report. The activities director will also be responsible for developing and maintaining an activities policies and procedures manual. It is also advisable to keep records of supply needs and an inventory of equipment and furnishings.

Resident Care Plans

One of the main purposes of resident care planning is to assess needs and problems in a systematic way. Specific goals are established and methods are identified for accomplishing them. The resident care plan must be completed 21 days after admission and must include a comprehensive activities assessment. Comprehensive resident care plans promote a coordinated effort in providing medical as well as multidisciplinary services for the individual. Effective care planning must include the resident, the family and significant others, as well as the primary health care providers in the facility. Resident care plans must be reviewed and revised regularly. Medicare and Medicaid regulations require the use of a standardized assessment called the Resident Assessment System, which includes a minimum data set (MDS) and 18 resident assessment protocols (RAPs) to provide a framework for planning.[6] The activity assessment must reflect information from the MDS. After admission, the minimum data set is used as a means of updating the staff relative to the resident's status, particularly during times of change.

Activity Plans

Activity plans are developed, evaluated and updated on a regular basis, usually monthly. They are a part of the resident's clinical record. The activity director must allocate specific blocks of time each week for this task to assure that all plans are always up to date. To assist in this process, a system should be developed for staff and volunteers to record daily their

---

12/5/Yr. Mr. Jones began a mosaic flower pot project and worked one hour.

S. Smith, Volunteer

12/7/Yr. Resident finished mosaic project and said he didn't like it; expressed interest in making a wooden jig saw puzzle for his granddaughter.

M. Jones, Act. Aide

12/8/Yr. Resident worked on puzzle and stated he was a little "nervous" about being the discussion leader for the current events group.

S. Smith, Volunteer

---

observations of individual residents. A notebook with a page for each resident is a simple way of collecting the information. A microcomputer may also be used. An example of the way these observations might be written is shown in the box.

In addition to contributing to the activity plan, observation notes such as these will also assist the activity director in evaluating the resident's degree of progress in attaining goals.

Activity Notes

Activity notes are included in the resident's clinical record and should be written whenever change is noted or at least once a month. A good activities note should include a summary of the kinds of activities the person has been participating in, the frequency of participation and the time involved. Notes should reflect maintenance, progress or decline. Quotations may be used. All notes must be dated, written legibly in ink and signed. Use of abbreviations should be avoided unless the facility has an approved list of abbreviations for use in records. Activity notes must be objective, accurate and complete. They should relate directly to the activity plan and the total resident care plan.[1]

Sample Activities Note:

3/21/Yr. Mr. Johnson is actively participating in woodworking activities every weekday morning for one to two hours. He frequently takes a nap after lunch and participates in the weekly photography club and the current events group in the afternoons. He has been discussion leader of the current events group on three occasions. He also visits the library frequently and stated that "Reading is one of my greatest pleasures." He is maintaining the level of activity noted last month.

Jane Doe, COTA, Activities Director

Participation Records

Participation records should be maintained on a daily basis to provide an overall view of activity trends and fluctuations. Such records will reflect individual resident inactivity as well as overactivity and are a barometer of interest in specific activities. These records may also be used to provide justification for hiring additional staff members. Graph paper may be used to develop a simple participation recording form. The names of all residents are listed on the left-hand side and the different activities are listed across the top. To save space, use a coding system such as "C" = crafts, "B" = Baking and "G" = Gardening. It is important to remember that if people come to the activity area and fall asleep, they have not participated!

Activities Schedules

Activities schedules are generally the monthly calendar of events. These schedules should be filed, as they provide specific information on the variety of activities offered and when. The schedules may also be coded to indicate whether activities require active or passive participation and the number of staff members and volunteers that are needed for each activity. Review of past schedules is a great help in planning for future events.

Activities Reports

Summary reports of the activities program are written regularly as required by the administration and at least annually. A typical report might include information about the number of residents participating in the eight major activity areas (physical, social, creative, productive, educational, diversional, spiritual and democratic community) with a breakdown of individual and group activities. New or unique events may be highlighted. Budget information should be included in the categories of income, expenditures, and cash on hand. The number of staff and volunteers should be noted as well as consultation services received. In-service training programs for staff and volunteers should be briefly described.

Policy and Procedure Manual

The activities director is responsible for developing, reviewing and revising the departmental policy and procedure manual. A policy may be defined as a statement that describes how basic objectives can be met. Policies are not subject to frequent change. Procedures are methods for carrying out the policy and are subject to modification as need arises. For example, the policy and procedures for conducting a birthday party might be written as shown in the box:[1]

Staffing Needs

The literature yields little information on the topic of staff requirements. This author believes that the employment of

---

SUBJECT: Birthday parties

POLICY: A monthly birthday party shall be held in the facility.

PURPOSE: To honor all residents who are celebrating a birthday during that month.

RESPONSIBILITY: The activity director shall be responsible for planning and carrying out the party.

PROCEDURES:
1. Written invitations will be sent to all residents celebrating a birthday during a given month. Invitations will also be sent to family members.
2. The date, time and location of the party will be advertised at least two weeks in advance. All residents and staff are invited.
3. Corsages and boutonnieres will be provided for those being honored.
4. Cake, ice cream and beverages must be ordered from the dietary department at least one week in advance of the event. Provisions for those on special diets must be accommodated.
5. Prizes may be awarded to the youngest and the oldest residents who are celebrating their birthday.
6. Musical entertainment will be provided.

---

one full-time activity director for every 50 to 60 residents should be an absolute minimum in skilled and intermediate care facilities. Individual state regulations and licensing agencies may specify other minimums for activities personnel. It should be kept in mind that providing a minimum number of activities personnel may not allow maximum services to be provided in meeting the residents' individual activity needs and enhancing their quality of life.

As more individuals become actively involved in the activities program and increased needs are identified, it may be necessary to increase the staff size. Before hiring additional personnel, a specific job description must be developed that includes most of the items described in the beginning of this chapter. Administration must approve all new staff positions. Plans and procedures must also be developed for orienting and evaluating new employees and providing for their continuing education.

Volunteers

Although **volunteers** are a most important asset to any activities program, they should never take the place of paid staff under any circumstances. Rather, they should be used to enhance the program.

Before a volunteer program is initiated, legal and insurance issues must be considered to assure that adequate liability safeguards are provided. Volunteers should be recruited, screened and trained as needs arise to assist in increasing the effectiveness of the program. They can often provide some of the extra services that help personalize the program, particularly in relation to individual needs. Volunteers can carry out a variety of tasks including letter writing, resident and departmental shopping, leading songfests, teaching creative activities and typing. Volunteers may be recruited through facility posters, more formal advertising in church and synagogue bulletins, high school and college newspapers and general announcements at neighborhood events. All volunteers must have specific job descriptions and hours and should participate in an orientation and training program. It is important to recognize volunteers for their contributions at least annually. Certificates or pins should be presented at a special gathering in their honor.

Program Management

As a departmental manager, the activities director must develop systems and approaches that will provide for the most effective and efficient delivery of activities services to meet the goals of the residents, the department and the health care facility. Failure to do so may result in decreased motivation and interest on the part of workers and participants.

It is the responsibility of the supervisor to develop and utilize objective tools such as job descriptions and evaluation forms to measure employee performance. The supervisor should also encourage the staff to participate in self-evaluation activities on a regular basis. Individual job performance goal setting should be a collaborative process between the supervisor and the supervisee. When specific deficits in performance are noted, the supervisor should be constructive in the criticism given by providing guidance, resources and opportunities that will assist the worker in skill improvement.

Above all, an effective supervisor must be caring, honest, objective and open in relationships and be willing to carry "a fair share" of the work load. A person who provides a strong role model and demonstrates a sincere interest in the well-being of those they supervise is indeed effective (see Chapters 2 and 3).

Financial Planning Role

The activities director is responsible for financial planning for the department and must have skills in developing and managing a budget. The main categories that must be considered in budgeting are salaries, nonexpendable equipment, expendable equipment and supplies, maintenance and repair, travel and professional development. Projected income and cash-on-hand figures should also be included.

Salaries. Salaries are generally the largest budget item. In planning, consideration must be given to actual salary amounts as well as post-probationary raises, merit and cost of living increases, overtime costs and annual bonuses. Social security contributions, health care benefits, retirement plans and life insurance costs must also be included.

Nonexpendable Equipment. Purchases of major items, such as stereo systems, tables and desks, are included in this category. Before requesting new equipment, it is wise to check with other departments such as housekeeping to see if the needed items are in storage or available from another area of the facility.

Expendable Equipment and Supplies. This category of budget planning is likely to result in mistakes due to false assumptions or inaccurate information. The big problem lies in determining just exactly what is "expendable." According to my own *Ryan Rule*, "Anything smaller than a large bread box that is not bolted down, kept under lock and key or constant surveillance is eventually expendable." Table looms, radios, coffee pots and hand tools are among the items that frequently disappear.

Interdepartmental Activities. Another aspect that makes budget planning difficult is "who pays for what" when several departments participate in an activity. For example, when a picnic is held in the park, is the cost of food charged to the dietary department or the activities department? If a nurse's aide is designated to assist with the activity, are the hours worked charged against the nursing budget or the activities budget? Matters such as these must be resolved with administration. Once these questions have been answered, more accurate planning can occur. One method is to keep track of actual expenses for three months, multiply that amount times 4 and add at least 12% to cover inflation and margin of error.

Maintenance and Repair. Routine maintenance is required for sewing machines, powered woodworking tools, typewriters and all audiovisual equipment. Departmental painting and redecorating may also be included in this category.

Travel. Expenses incurred for bus rentals for resident outings are generally the largest item in this category. If the facility has a vehicle for resident use, determine if any charges are made to your department. Reimbursement of employee and volunteer mileage for errands and shopping should also be covered in this budget category.

Income Sources. Cash donations, bazaar receipts and bake sale proceeds are examples of income sources. The activities director must have a clear understanding of exactly what the administration's expectations are for income-producing activities. Although some activities may be self-supporting in terms of revenue generated, it is an unreal expectation to expect an activities program to generate enough income to cover expenses. Activities programs should *never* be forced to exploit resident endeavors to raise money.

Professional Development. In light of the many rapid changes in health care policy, coupled with new research, legislation and resulting changes in the provision of services, it is important for activity directors and activities personnel to have opportunities for professional development. Costs for continuing education courses and workshops, conventions, conferences, meetings, books, journals and related travel and per diem are items that should be covered.

Continuing Education

We live in an age where change occurs very rapidly, particularly in our health care delivery systems. The activities director, in collaboration with administration, staff and volunteers, and with necessary outside consultation, must identify the continuing education needs and develop a plan to meet these needs. Such a plan must include the required financial support. For example, many facilities require all staff members and volunteers to take a first aid course, and some require specialized training in cardiopulmonary resuscitation (CPR). As residents' needs change, staff members may also need to be trained in the techniques of reality orientation, remotivation and reminiscence therapy. The activities director and everyone involved in the delivery of activities services must be given opportunities to participate in continuing education courses and workshops to assure that existing skills are maintained and new ones acquired. Continuing education is important to provide necessary activities services, to enhance those services and to be responsive to the changing needs of the residents.

Interdisciplinary Role

Most health care facilities view the activities director as a department head and an integral member of the health care team. The activities director should participate in all department head meetings and patient care planning conferences, as the delivery of effective activities services depends on cooperation from and coordination with a number of other departments. Efforts should be made to develop both structured and informal communication channels that will assure quality resident care and the achievement of goals.

Consultation

A consultant is a person who is employed by a facility on a contractual basis to provide indirect service. Consultants

may be used to give information, assist in strategy development and problem resolution, to clarify issues and to advise.[7] Typically, a consultant is employed by administration to provide services to a department or several departments in relation to specific concerns. Consultative services may be as short as a one-time visit or may extend over several months or years depending on the nature of the consultation required. It is important to understand that a consultant works "outside" the facility and brings expertise and an objective viewpoint to the facility.

The activities director might use a consultant to assist in providing information about and interpretation of federal and state regulations regarding activities programming. Other areas in which a consultant might offer assistance include continuing education and general community resources, activity suggestions for nonparticipating residents, establishing resident care planning goals and suggesting ways to improve departmental management procedures. A consultant can also be a valuable resource for developing strategies for improved communication with another department or individual.

It is very important to note that when an occupational therapist (OTR) is employed as a consultant it does not mean that occupational therapy services are being provided. Further clarification is found in the official position paper of the American Occupational Therapy Association entitled *Roles and Functions of Occupational Therapy in Long-Term Care: Occupational Therapy and Activity Programs.*[8]

Coordination of Occupational Therapy and Activities Services

In recent years, I have become increasingly concerned about the apparent "division" in some long-term care facilities that provide both activities and occupational therapy services. These services may not be coordinated and there may be little effort to reinforce the resident's goals in occupational therapy in the activities program. Informal observation and feedback from individuals working in the field present an interesting contrast in terms of "what is" and "what could be." A number of nursing homes and other long-term care facilities employ occupational therapists and assistants on a contractual basis to provide direct services under what is often viewed as a medical, rehabilitation model, frequently oriented primarily to physical dysfunction. The same facility may also employ COTAs to deliver activity services under a more holistic, humanistic, supportive and maintenance model. Unfortunately, communication between the two services may be minimal. For example, a person with hemiparesis may be working on coordination activities in occupational therapy and treatment could be reinforced by a COTA in the activities department, but this coordination may not take place in many instances. It is imperative that these efforts be coordinated and that the service providers critique their respective models and methods of service delivery to assure maximum benefits to the recipients that are also cost-effective.

New Model for Long-Term Care in the 1990s

The **Lazarus Project** provides a model that should be considered as a possible solution to the problems in long-term care facilities that extend beyond those discussed previously. The model outlines the politics of empowerment based on a community model of democratic governance where residents, staff and administration participate equally in creating an environment that is responsive to *all member needs*, thus improving the quality of life for those residing in these facilities.[9] The COTA serving as an activity director or a direct OT service provider can have a marked influence in bringing about the necessary changes in the 1990s and beyond, using the innovative principles stressed in this important work.

The Lazarus' Vision

It seems fitting to leave the reader with a vision for the future in which the profession can play a vital role. While members of other age groups may be served by nursing homes, the needs of the frail elderly deserve particular attention. Therefore, the vision statement from the Lazarus project is shown in Figure 22-2 to provide a vehicle for study, reflection and challenge and a catalyst for implementing needed change.[9]

Summary

The role of the COTA as an activities director offers many challenges and opportunities. Skills in assessing activities needs, planning, implementing, documenting, managing and evaluating programs are essential. An activity director must also have strong interpersonal, leadership, supervision and management abilities. The need for qualified activities personnel in long-term care facilities for the elderly and others is increasing, and the educational background of occupational therapy assistants provides them with excellent preparation for such positions; however, employment of a COTA or OTR consultant does not mean that occupational therapy direct services are being provided.

Recent federal legislation is emphasized and provides a foundation for following topics. Discussion of specific documentation needs and financial and other management tasks provides the reader with basic information. Interdisciplinary roles and consultation are a focus as well. The need for

---

The Lazarus Project Vision

The Lazarus Project believes that frail elders can be contributing members to society. It is through contribution that individuals exercise power and are able to live a life of meaning and dignity. Empowerment happens when communities are created—communities which govern themselves by drawing on the diverse strengths of members to address common problems.

The Lazarus Project believes this kind of community can be created in nursing home environments. This requires a broad, holistic understanding of health. This concept of health includes the ability to have authority in one's life, to shape one's environment, and to extend influence within a broader public world.

Aging is a public issue; it is not simply an individual experience. When people become older and more frail, their ability to be contributing members to society changes. In a society that measures worth in terms of contributions and influence, the loss of physical and cognitive capacity quickly defines frail elders as "a problem." One of the ways the public has chosen to address this "problem" is to separate itself from chronically ill and disabled elders by "institutionalizing" the aging.

The authors of the Lazarus Project believe that the focus on the medical and service missions of long-term care institutions views residents as incapacitated rather than as contributors. When this assumption becomes embedded in the institution's governing system, it can lead to a loss of power for all involved—the residents, the staff, administrators, and families. This loss of influence constrains an institution's ability to effectively respond to the problems of aging.

Figure 22-2. *The Lazarus Project Vision.*

---

coordination between activities services and occupational therapy services is addressed and culminates with a brief discussion of a model for service delivery in the 1990s and beyond in which COTAs can play a vital part, regardless of their specific roles in the provision of long-term care services.

Acknowledgments

Appreciation is extended to Nancy Kari, MPH, OTR, and Peg Michels, MA, for sharing material from the Lazarus Project. Special thanks is also given to Shirley H. Carr, MA, OTR, FAOTA for her critique and helpful comments and to Pamela Hayle, Therapeutic Activities Programmer, for providing information and forms. Penny Boulet, COTA, is also acknowledged for providing resources.

Related Learning Activities

1. Visit a long-term care facility that has an activities program. Review the calendar of events and determine the variety of offerings in terms of the eight major categories identified in the text.

2. Practice using the form in the text as an interviewing guide with at least three people over age 70.

3. Assume that a group of six residents is interested in participating in a baking group. Plan this activity in detail, breaking it down into specific components.

4. Discuss the following question with a peer: "How does an activities program differ from and occupational therapy direct service program?"

5. Read the mission statement of the Lazarus Project. Discuss implications with a classmate.

References

1. Minnesota Department of Health: *Functional Model for an Activities Program*. Minneapolis, Minnesota, Minnesota Department of Health, 1978.
2. Medicare and Medicaid programs: Requirements for long-term care facilities. *Fed Regist*, 54:249, 1989.
3. Saltz DL: Celebration marks reform of nursing homes. *OT Week*, 4(41):12-13, 1990.
4. National Association of Activity Professionals: *Standards of Practice: Section A—Standards of Care*. Washington, DC, National Association of Activity Professionals, 1990.
5. Solashin E: Unpublished remarks, television interview. Minneapolis, Minnesota, 1975.
6. American Occupational Therapy Association: *Resident Assessment System*. Rockville, Maryland, AOTA, 1990.
7. Pochert L: Our new role challenge: Occupational therapy consultation. *Am J Occup Ther* 24:1-2, 1970.
8. Rogers JC :Roles and functions of occupational therapy in long-term care: Occupational therapy and activity programs. *Am J Occup Ther* 38:799-802, 1983.
9. Kari N, Michels P: The Lazarus project: A politics of empowerment. *Am J Occup Ther* 45:719-725, 1991.

Chapter 23

Traumatic Brain Injury

Adair Robinson, MA, OTR
MAJ Melissa Sinnott, PhD, OTR

Introduction

Traumatic brain injury (TBI) is one of the leading causes of death and disability among young adults, particularly males between the ages of 15 and 24 years of age. Over 750,000 patients with head injuries in the United States require hospitalization each year. The survivors experience feelings of devastation because of the dramatic changes in their abilities and their lost potential to achieve previous life goals. Family members and significant others experience feelings of devastation about "losing" the person who was their loved one. Even if the injury does not result in death, the loss is almost as great because the injured person experiences so many changes. Members of the family are often frustrated and exhausted by the personal and financial demands placed on them. They must learn to cope with the irrevocable changes in the person with traumatic head injury and provide the necessary care, perhaps for the remainder of their respective lives.

The brain is the command center of the central nervous system. It controls involuntary functions, such as heart rate and respiration. It also controls volitional movement, the five senses, thinking and emotions. Traumatic brain injury causes a disruption in one or, more typically, many of these functions. The severity of the head injury can range from a concussion to coma to death. The complexity and broad range of the patient's problems present a challenge to the therapist, assistant, family and patient. Individuals who sustain more severe head injuries need occupational therapy services to help regain lost function or to learn to compensate for a permanent loss of function.

KEY CONCEPTS

Characteristics of traumatic brain injury

Patterns of brain injury recovery

Rancho Los Amigos Scale of Levels of Cognitive Functioning

Intervention strategies and activities

Transdisciplinary medical management

Model of Human Occupation

Coma stimulation approach

Environmental control model

Skill building model

Strategy substitution model

ESSENTIAL VOCABULARY

Coup/Counter-coup

Torque

Infarcts

Coma

Cognitive domains

Psychomotor retardation

Volition

Habituation

Performance

Personal causation

Multisensory input

Occupational therapy plays an integral role in the rehabilitation of traumatic head injury survivors. This chapter describes the various levels and stages of head injury, the treatment models and methods and a case study of a head-injured patient.

Neuroanatomy of Head Injury

Several different things happen to the brain structures when an individual has a traumatic brain injury. The following brief anatomic review provides the reader with a context for these occurrences. The brain is a semisolid structure nested in the cranium and attached to the spinal cord at the base of the skull. A thin cushion is created by the three layers of membrane and cerebral spinal fluid that surround the brain in the cavity of the cranium. The effect of rapid acceleration and deceleration on the brain can cause a **coup** and a **counter-coup**. The coup and counter-coup are the points at which the brain actually makes impact with the hard skull. The impact results in a bruising of the brain tissue called a lesion. The momentum of force may also cause shearing of the brain tissue, as the brain rotates in the cavity of the skull. Shearing causes **torque** or rotation at the brain stem resulting in predictable impairments related to brain stem functions. In addition, to coup, counter coup, and shearing, the momentum of injury may cause multiple vascular **infarcts**, a term used to refer to blockages of arterial supply or venous drainage resulting in the death of tissue[1] of the major and tiny vessels supplying the brain. Medical management at a trauma center focuses on the reduction of intercranial swelling, which can cause further damage to delicate brain tissues.

Understanding what happens to the brain in a traumatic brain injury is necessary to identify the variety of potential deficits resulting from such an injury and differentiates traumatic head injury from other neurologic conditions, such as stroke. A person who has experienced a stroke generally has a more focal brain lesion with an attendant set of deficits lateralized to one side of his or her body. In contrast, a person who has sustained a traumatic head injury will generally have several brain lesions and a much more diverse set of deficits. Traumatic brain injury does not spare motor functions, although the emphasis in this chapter is on the cognitive, perceptual and behavioral *sequelae*, a term used to describe abnormal conditions brought about by another event.[1] A comprehensive evaluation is essential for identifying the patient's strengths and weaknesses.

Patterns of Recovery from Brain Injury

Before discussing the occupational therapy assessment, it is important to know the stages of recovery after head injury.

The majority of patients will experience some period of loss of consciousness requiring life support intervention. Patients with a moderate to severe degree of injury will be in a **coma**, defined as an unarousable, unresponsive state with absence of primitive reflexes. Unlike the dramatic "awakenings" recently depicted on television and in movies, patients come out of comas very gradually. The Rancho Los Amigos Scale of Levels of Cognitive Functioning describes eight stages of recovery that patients progress through as they become increasingly responsive and interactive within their environments.[2] It is important to note that the Rancho Scale is a guideline for the recovery process. Patients will vary in the length of time they spend in each stage or appear to miss a stage. The scale is presented in Figure 23-1 and discussed in the section on assessment.

In addition to classifying patients by the Rancho Los Amigos Scale, one may also describe their performance abilities in terms of **cognitive domains**. These domains are hierarchical and require a patient to achieve increasing degrees of arousal and cognitive proficiency. Figure 23-2 presents a brief introduction to and definition of the cognitive domains, based on the work of Sohlberg and Mateer, which will be referred to in this chapter.[3]

The Rancho Los Amigos Scale and cognitive domains indicate that there is both a continuum and a variety of cognitive, perceptual and behavioral deficits that a patient experiences after sustaining a traumatic head injury. The role of the COTA and the OTR is to assess the patient's cognitive level and treat his or her cognitive deficit areas during rehabilitation.

Occupational Therapy Intervention

Assessment

Given this background about head injury recovery and cognitive functions, the COTA and the OTR collaborate to prepare an assessment plan. They establish a preliminary

I	No response
II	Generalized response
III	Localized response
IV	Confused-agitated
V	Confused, inappropriate, nonagitated
VI	Confused-appropriate
VII	Automatic appropriate
VIII	Purposeful and appropriate

Figure 23-1. *Rancho Los Amigos Scale of Levels of Cognitive Functioning.*

1. *Orientation:* The level of arousal resulting in awareness of self, environment and time.

2. *Attention:* The concentration of mental effort on sensory and/or mental events to include sustained attention, selective attention, divided attention, alternating attention and processing capacity.

3. *Memory:* The ability to store, retain and recall information for use in cognitive processes. Memory classifications include immediate, short-term, long-term, new learning and one's general fund of knowledge.

4. *Visual processing:* The ability to recognize and/or synthesize visual information; to assign it meaning. This process includes part/whole recognition, recognition of gestalt (a unified whole; a pattern or configuration having specific properties that can be derived from a summation of the parts),[1] sequencing, and processing speed.

5. *Language:* Many forms of human thinking, problem solving and information storage and retrieval are mediated by language.

6. *Reasoning and problem solving:* The thinking processes that result in the transformation of information by inference, judgment, deduction, abstraction and synthesis. The results are concept formation and logic.

7. *Executive functions:* The mediation of cognitive skills, such as organization, establishing priorities and hypothesis testing.

Figure 23-2. *Cognitive Domains.*

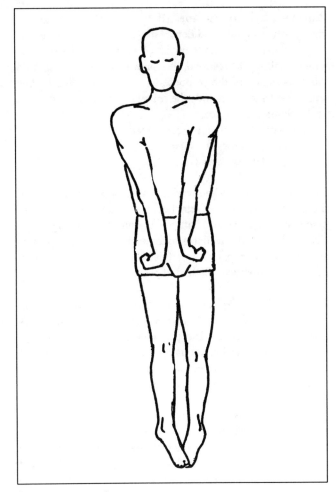

Figure 23-3. *Decerebrate posture.*

assessment plan after reviewing the patient's medical record and interviewing ward staff and the family. The medical record supplies a rough estimate of the patient's level of cognitive functioning and concurrent medical, physical and speech limitations. The ward staff interviews focus on descriptions of their observations and interactions with the patients. Based on this subjective and objective data about the patient, the OTR and the COTA identify the appropriate areas to assess.

The following standardized and nonstandardized assessments may be used based on the Rancho Los Amigos levels and concomitant cognitive domains. The role of the COTA in conducting assessments is determined by the need for using particular standardized or structured assessments and the COTA's demonstrated level of competence in relation to the specific problems presented and the tools used. It is the responsibility of the OTR to provide adequate supervision and to interpret the results of those assessments delegated to the COTA. Specific examples may be found in the case study presented later in the chapter.

Rancho Level I. At this level the patient is unresponsive to the environment, but will require occupational therapy intervention for the following:

1. Positioning
2. Maintenance of passive range of motion
3. Splinting

The therapist must assess the patient's head and limb position, skin integrity and muscle tone. Patients may exhibit decerebrate posturing in which hips and shoulders extend, adduct, and rotate internally; elbows and knees extend; the forearm is hyperpronated; the wrist and fingers flex; and the feet are inverted and in plantar flexion. The head retracts and the trunk extends.[1,4] This posture may be seen in Figure 23-3. Spasticity and flaccidity are also noted.

It is a good practice to contact family members of patients at this level to inform them of the role of occupational therapy practitoners in therapeutic intervention.

Rancho Level II. The patient who is at this level begins to respond to noxious stimuli. The therapist will assess the patient's protective reactions and responses to deep pain, light, sound and smell. A coma stimulation program is initiated at this stage and is discussed in depth later in the chapter.

Rancho Level III. At level III the patient will begin to change quite rapidly and demonstrate a variety of stimulus-response reactions. The therapist or assistant will assess the patient's ability to respond, the quality of the response and the consistency of the response to a variety of stimuli. The assessment should include the following components:

1. Name recognition
2. Recognition of significant others
3. Visual/auditory tracking
4. One-step commands

Rancho Level IV. When working with patients at this level, the therapist and the assistant assess orientation to person, place, and time; level of attention; and object recognition. Few commercially available assessment tools are appropriate for use with patients at this level. Documentation of behaviors is the ideal method of assessment.

Rancho Level V. At this level the therapist and the assistant assess orientation, attention, memory, motor performance and visual processing. The patient generally displays **psychomotor retardation** and lacks the ability to sustain his or her attention to complete standardized assessments. The OTR and the COTA must use creativity to structure simple repetitive tasks that informally assess the patient's skill level. Again, documentation of behaviors is the ideal method of assessment.

The following standardized tests are readily available and are suggested for use at this level, keeping in mind that that the patient's attention span may prevent completion of the assessment in one session.

1. Box and Block Test
2. Benton Facial Recognition Test
3. Benton Three-Dimensional Block Construction
4. Motor-Free Visual Perceptual Test
5. Rivermead Behavioral Memory Test

Rancho Level VI. The patient begins to demonstrate greater ability to sustain attention, demonstrate carry-over tasks from day to day, and participate in activities of daily living. Assessment focuses on orientation, attention, memory and visual processing. A functional screening tool is used to identify the patient's level of competence in basic activities of daily living, which include money management, use of community resources, meal preparation and knowledge of safety. Assessment also includes basic visual-perceptual and visual-motor skills. The patients are able to complete a wider variety of standardized assessments because they have acquired the prerequisite motor and attention skills. The following are some of the tests that may be used:

1. Kohlman Evaluation of Living Skills (KELS)
2. Bay Area Functional Performance Evaluation (BAFPE)
3. Test of Visual Perceptual Skills

4. Beery-Buktenica Test of Visual Motor Integration (VMI)

Rancho Level VII. At this level the patient's problems are much less obvious. The occupational therapy assessment focuses on memory, reasoning and problem solving, and executive brain functions. The patient is ready for a variety of standardized prevocational assessments. The purpose of assessment is to identify the patient's residual limitations and need to acquire compensatory skills. Reasoning and problem solving are primarily assessed through functional activities that will be reviewed more extensively in the treatment section of this chapter. Assessments include the following:

1. Minnesota Rate of Manipulation Tests
2. Purdue Pegboard Test
3. Grooved Pegboard Test

Rancho Level VIII. Patients' problems at this level are primarily in the domain of memory and social skills. The therapist and the assistant assess the patient's vocational potential by assessing the patient's effective compensation for residual memory, reasoning and problem solving, and executive function deficits.

A variety of work-based assessments may be considered (see Chapter 21). The patient may also be referred to a vocational rehabilitation agency or be engaged in a structured trial of work therapy.

Case Application

Background

Kevin is a 23-year-old man whose life was dramatically changed by a motor vehicle accident in which he sustained a traumatic brain injury. He was only weeks away from graduating from college at the time of the accident one year ago. For the past nine months, Kevin has been involved in an intensive mutlidisciplinary therapy program to prepare him to resume independent living.

Having been in a coma for approximately one month, Kevin has a resulting memory gap for events in his life surrounding the accident and details of his initial hospitalization at the trauma center.

Kevin was admitted to a rehabilitation hospital for cognitive rehabilitation. At the time of his admission his outstanding problems included mild left hemiparesis, double vision, seizure precaution, questionable paranoia and cognitive deficits.

Kevin has worked diligently, and somewhat dogmatically, in his therapies. The focus of physical therapy was to help him develop coordinated gross motor skills. He walked with a gait deviation characterized by hip circumduction, head tilt and decreased reciprocal arm swing. It is doubtful that Kevin will ever be able to run without falling, but he is now able to hop, jump and skip without losing his balance. Kevin was an avid soccer player before his accident. He has talked with the physical therapist about coaching a community youth league. Kevin has responded positively to this idea because he misses the social and fitness benefits of recreation.

Inpatient Intervention

Occupational therapy intervention initially focused on facilitation of left hand function. This goal was a priority for Kevin because he is left-hand dominant. He practiced fine motor assembly tasks, writing and typing. The COTA supervised Kevin in a daily task group during which he completed a series a graded craft projects. The COTA structured Kevin's choices of crafts. As his hand skills, attention to details of work quality, and direction-following ability improved, he was guided toward increasingly complex projects. He began with a small wood project that required static prehension of the pieces during sanding, staining, and glueing. He progressed to a tile trivet to work on repetitive grasp and release of small half-inch tiles, and precision placement of tiles. Next, Kevin completed a leather stamping and lacing project to work on hand-eye coordination. Finally, the COTA guided Kevin in the selection of a ceramic project, which was designed to help Kevin develop his ability to modulate the pressure he applied as he cleaned the greenware. His fine motor skills have plateaued without reaching a competitive work speed, but he is now able to perform precise tip-to-tip prehension tasks and feels confident about his work.

At the time of admission, Kevin was able to perform basic personal activities of daily living such as bathing, grooming and dressing; however, during the initial assessment, the COTA noted that it took Kevin an inordinate amount of time to accomplish these tasks as he was frequently distracted and disorganized and repeated unnecessary task components. The COTA worked with him to increase his speed and organization. A checklist and a household timer, positioned by his bed, helped Kevin to attend to the tasks and decrease the time it took to perform specific tasks, such as styling his hair and brushing his teeth. The occupational therapy assistant also helped Kevin coordinate his clothes to decrease the time spent in selecting outfits.

Participation in age-appropriate activities had been significantly curtailed since the accident. Kevin's network of social contacts gradually disintegrated as his hospitalization continued. When his girlfriend stopped visiting, Kevin verbalized a great deal of anger toward her. He did not recognize the changes in his personality; consequently, he could not understand why she wanted to end the relationship. For a short time after this incident, Kevin seemed to lose his motivation to participate in occupational and physical therapy and was mildly depressed. He would refuse to socialize with fellow patients, and he required more structure and rewards for performance from staff members. Kevin used his memory deficits as an excuse for being late or missing appointments. He gradually resumed a more active role in treatment planning and was friendlier toward fellow patients; however, he still tends to make excuses when he experiences frustrations, instead of thinking about alternative problem-solving strategies.

Outpatient Intervention

When Kevin was transferred to out-patient status he returned to his parents' home. They were supportive of his needs and continued to reinforce the goals of therapy. Kevin essentially became the focus of the family's activities. His parents reported that he generally did not initiate activities without their guidance. He had acclimated so well to the hospital structure that the treatment team had neglected to address Kevin's lack of initiation, a very common problem after a head injury. His parents also reported that his sleep requirements increased to approximately ten hours per day, a common development because patients are exerting a phenomenal amount of energy to carry out their daily activities. The OTR provided Kevin's parents with information about abnormal behavior patterns so that they could be better prepared for these occurrences.

Kevin depended on his parents for transportation and finances. He would sometimes say that it was upsetting to be "treated like a high school kid" again. To reduce his feelings of dependency, the COTA, working with Kevin and his mother, developed a schedule of household chores that Kevin could perform. The COTA retaught Kevin laundry procedures. He also practiced cooking favorite family recipes at the hospital and made them for the family on weekends. It was agreed that Kevin would be responsible for one evening activity each week for the family. The treatment team collectively decided that Kevin was not ready to be trained in the use of public transportation because three bus changes were required to get to the hospital, and he was easily frustrated when he became lost in the hospital. Being lost in the city would only compound his level of frustration.

Kevin experienced the following cognitive deficits: specific visual spatial, memory, reasoning and problem solving, and executive function. He was chronically late to his therapy sessions and very rigid in his daily routine. Any deviation in the therapy schedule seemed to disorganize him. Kevin was opposed to carrying a calendar, tending to disregard his tardiness. A sign-in/sign-out sheet provided him with tangible evidence of his tardiness and eventually helped him to internalize an awareness of time and benefits of using external memory aids.

The OTR took an active role in compensatory memory training. She worked with Kevin daily to fill in the calendar and review upcoming events. She also trained him to use an auditory cuing watch to reinforce the written schedule. She also taught him a series of other applicable strategies, such as list making, categorization and visual association. Through graded practice activities, Kevin relearned problem solving approaches to visual-spatial problems. He and the OTR practiced with puzzles, three-dimensional assemblies, map reading and designing floor plans. Computer-based exercises were used to augment functional visual-perceptual activities.

Deficits in the area of reasoning and problem solving were evident each time Kevin encountered a novel task. He required external cues to help him identify problems and potential solutions. The OTR trained Kevin to use a few problem solving *algorithms,* which are sets of rules with a

---

Upper Extremity Function:
Range of motion
Muscle tone
Equilibrium reactions
Motor integration
Coordination and dexterity
Strength
Endurance
Sensation

Spatial Perception:
Proprioception
Kinesthesia
Body scheme
Position in space
Directionality

Visual and Visuomotor skills:
Visual acuity
Visual fields
Tracking
Scanning
Convergence
Divergence
Saccades
Nystagmus
Hand-eye coordination: tracing, drawing, writing
Reading

Visuoperceptual Skills:
Visual discrimination: size, shape, color
Figure-ground
Visual-spatial: part/whole, spatial operations, gestalt
Form constancy
Visual closure

Behavior, Cognitive, and Memory Skills:
Confusion
Frustration tolerance
Fatigue tolerance
Cognitive domains: orientation, attention, memory, visual
    processing, language, reasoning and problem solving,
    executive function

Community Living Skills:
Activity of daily living skills: time, telephone, money management,
    cooking, etc
Leisure skills
Prevocational skills
Driving

Figure 23-4. *Rehabilitation Hospital Occupational Therapy Checklist.*

finite number of steps, when he encountered novel tasks. Together they worked through a series of simulated problems and he was encouraged to use the algorithm approach in solving actual problems in the task group. Kevin continues to need help with reasoning and problem solving tasks. His greatest difficulty is knowing which algorithm or memory strategy will work best for him. He tends to use the same strategy regardless of the task goal, a function of his rigid thinking style.

Treatment in speech therapy focused on the restoration of linguistic and social language skills. The objective was to decrease Kevin's tangential speech tendencies by increasing his awareness of this tendency and providing him with self-monitoring strategies. All members of the treatment team reinforced this goal during their daily interactions with him. The OTR and the COTA encouraged Kevin to discuss feelings, issues and current events during their treatment sessions to practice social conversation. Since Kevin was egocentric, he had to be encouraged to engage in pleasant social exchanges, such as asking others about their weekend. After telling about his weekend activities he frequently would not reciprocate by asking about the therapist's weekend.

The rehabilitation hospital included a psychosocial support group as a part of its cognitive rehabilitation program. In this group setting Kevin and other patients discussed their personal experiences of adjusting to living with a disability with the clinical psychologist and the social worker. The OTR and the COTA were not present during this group, but communicated informally with the co-leaders about the behaviors they noted during their treatment. This group gave Kevin a forum to talk about his anger and frustration. He received support from fellow patients who had the same diagnosis, but varying sets of coping mechanisms. The group frequently discussed adaptive and maladaptive coping techniques.

After six months of combined therapies, the treatment team decided that Kevin was ready to begin vocational exploration. He is currently involved in a patient work therapy program at a local greenhouse. In this setting, under the supervision of a trained layperson, Kevin practices good work behaviors and receives the incentive of a minimum wage salary. The treatment team and Kevin's parents are optimistic that Kevin will be able to receive vocational retraining and return to work in a less structured and autonomous setting.

Assessment

When Kevin came to the rehabilitation hospital he was functioning at a Rancho Level V—confused, inappropriate and nonagitated. Together the OTR and the COTA reviewed the Rehabilitation Hospital Occupational Therapy Assessment Checklist and decided which assessment areas needed to be addressed and the division of labor. The checklist is shown in Figure 23-4.

Kevin required an assessment in almost all of these areas with the exception of reasoning and problem solving, executive function, community management skills, prevocational skills and driving. He was not yet ready to be assessed in these areas. (See Chapter 26 for information about driver training with a head-injured patient.)

Both the COTA and the OTR were present during Kevin's first visit to the occupational therapy clinic. They explained to Kevin that they would be working as a team. The initial session lasted an hour, during which the COTA measured Kevin's upper extremity passive and active range of motion, grip and pinch strengths, and sterognosis and administered the Box and Block Test. He received verbal directions and demonstrations about how to elicit his maximum performance. A practice trial was permitted for the dexterity test to familiarize Kevin with the test procedures.

During a one-hour afternoon occupational therapy session, the OTR interviewed the patient to assess his orientation to person, place and time and his ability to provide a personal history. The therapist directed questions to determine his ability to recall personal past experiences and well-learned facts with accuracy. Kevin's ocular-motor skills and visual fields were assessed using confrontation testing and a line bisection activity, respectively. Visual-motor and dexterity skills were assessed using a block construction test.

The next day the COTA and the OTR worked together to assess Kevin's equilibrium reactions in seated, kneeling and standing positions. The COTA wanted to know Kevin's balance abilities before he performed an activities of daily living (ADL) evaluation. The therapist and the assistant also assessed central nervous system sensations with identification of body parts, imitation of positions to anticipate problems Kevin might experience with a functional dressing task. They assessed his hot/cold and sharp/dull perception to ensure safety in the shower and during shaving. The next morning the COTA observed Kevin performing his morning grooming and hygiene to assess his level of independence and need for ADL training.

During the second afternoon, the COTA assessed visual perceptual and visual processing skills using the Motor-Free Visual Perception Test. This test is performed as a generic screening to identify perceptual deficits, as well as unilateral neglect and sustained attention. The OTR further assessed orientation, attention, memory and visual processing with subjective procedures, asking the patient to write the alphabet, match objects and pictures, and sequence and execute one- and two-step commands. The Rivermead Behavioral Memory Test was administered to assess the patients level of orientation, selective and sustained attention, object and face recognition, and supervision needs for remembering his schedule.

Treatment Planning

The next step in the intervention process was for the COTA and the OTR to score and discuss the results of the assessments, complete an observations list and formulate a treatment plan that established priorities.

The COTA noted that Kevin's range of motion was within normal limits, but he lacked average grip strength and was clumsy as he performed a grasp and release test (Box and Block Test). The patient incorrectly identified small objects on the *stereognosis* assessment, a test of one's ability to identify objects through the sense of touch. His performance on the Motor-Free Visual Perceptual Test showed many left-sided errors, and difficulty with the visual-memory, form constancy and visual closure subtests.

The OTR also noted that Kevin had decreased balance in kneeling and standing positions. His fine motor skills were influenced by changes in motor integration, psychomotor retardation and generalized decreased strength. The occupational therapist attributed stereognosis errors to decreased attention to fine details and limited self-correction. Kevin was consistently oriented to person and place, but not to time and date. He was able to follow simple two-step commands accurately, but was occasionally confused by phrases such

as, "to the right of," "two from the end," and "adjacent to." He made more errors following three-step commands. He was not able to recite the alphabet correctly or recall the names of the COTA and the OTR.

Together, the occupational therapy assistant and the occupational therapist listed their observations of Kevin's behaviors. They had observed that he was distracted by other people in the clinic and often thought that their conversations were directed at him and would answer. He did not make eye contact with the COTA or the OTR when they were talking to him. He required frequent redirection with verbal prompts and demonstrations to complete picture matching and sequencing tasks. Kevin seemed to fatigue after 20 minutes of activity. As he was leaving the clinic, it was noted that he could not find the exit.

The OTR and the COTA identified the four treatment areas based on the occupational therapy initial assessments: hand skills, orientation, attention and ADLs. They established the following short-term and long-term goals:

Short-term goals:
- The patient will increase gross manual dexterity on grasp and release tasks by 10% in two weeks.
- The patient will consistently refer to environmental cues to answer orientation questions in two weeks.
- The patient will use environmental cues to negotiate to/from appointments within the hospital in two weeks.
- The patient will sustain task orientation, without external cues, for task duration of 15 minutes in two weeks.
- The patient will perform personal hygiene and grooming tasks according to a checklist within two weeks.

Long-term goals:
- The patient will be able to assemble and disassemble small tasks using fine motor prehension patterns and hand-held tools in one month.
- The patient will be able to document independently his daily schedule in his appointment book in one month.
- The patient will be able to follow visual and verbal directions to locate novel places within the hospital in one month.
- The patient will be able to perform tasks in a high stimulus environnment without demonstrating decreased tolerance to extraneous sensory stimuli in one month.
- The patient will be able to prepare a light meal with minimum staff asistance for sequencing in one month.

Treatment Implementation and Models of Treatment

There are many models of treatment, but this chapter describes only the medical management model and occupational therapy models used with Kevin at the trauma center and the rehabilitation hospital.

Transdisciplinary Medical Management

The advantage of the transdisciplinary medical management model is that multiple disciplines work in conjunction to achieve continuity of care for the duration of the admission and to anticipate rehabilitation needs and provide efficient discharge planning.

From the time of his admission to the trauma center,

Kevin's case was medically managed with a transdisciplinary model. This approach involved coordinated medical treatment that recognized the unique skills and knowledge domains of the physicians and allied health professionals on the treatment team. Initially, the transdisciplinary model was essential to meet Kevin's multiple life support needs. Each team member worked collaboratively with the other disciplines. The function of occupational therapy in the intensive care setting was to provide coma stimulation, passive range of motion, positioning devices and splint fabrication. The occupational therapist and the COTA assumed the role of primary therapy providers. They also assumed secondary roles as educators, providing instruction to the nursing staff and the family about the methods being used. Input from the occupational therapy team was highly valued because they were often the first to observe changes in the patient's cognitive function. Their primary intervention focused on illiciting responses from the patient in contrast to disciplines primarily focused on providing essential patient care for basic needs.

Interaction with the treatment team was both oral and written. The OTR and the COTA documented the patient's responses in the medical record to communicate to other team members. Because the trauma center was busy 24 hours a day, information about Kevin's performance during occupational therapy sessions had to be documented in a central location so that all team members on all shifts could read it. In turn, the OTR and the COTA obtained valuable information from the patient record, such as respiratory and cardiac function, electroencephalogram (EEG) and magnetic resonance imaging (MRI) findings.

As Kevin improved medically and moved from the intensive care unit (ICU), the transdisciplinary model facilitated his integration into postacute rehabilitation. Occupational therapy intervention in the ICU had maintained good joint mobility in the patient and established a system of communication between the therapist and the patient. The postacute rehabilitation continued until Kevin was discharged to the rehabilitation hospital where the transdisciplinary model is also used, although for slightly different reasons.

The transdisciplinary model is regarded as essential at the rehabilitation hospital because of the complexity of the problems that patients experience after a traumatic head injury. The model encourages treatment by professional specialists who share their expertise with the treatment team. The underlying premise of the model is that the treatment team will work in a collaborative manner to reinforce treatment in a variety of settings using a variety of therapeutic devices. Thus the model simulates the "real world" as it prepares the patient to carry over skills from setting to setting and from therapist to therapist.

Model of Human Occupation

The model of human occupation provides a meaningful context for understanding the occupational therapy treatment of traumatic brain injury.[5] The chrraracteristics and components of this model recognize the complex myriad of problems encountered throughout the various stages of

recovery from brain injury. The model was used to explain the impact of brain injury on Kevin's occupational behavior, including work, play and daily living or self-maintenance activities.

This model viewed Kevin as an open system, comprised of multiple, interrelated structures and functions that when organized into a whole, allowed him to interact with his environment. Kielhofner, Igu and Burke identified three major hierarchical subsystems: **volition, habituation,** and **performance.**[6]

The volition subsystem oversees the entire human system and symbolizes the need for exploration and mastery of the environment. Kevin's volition subsystem was severely impaired by his brain injury and was evidenced by his family's observations about his difficulty initiating activities without guidance. Values and interests are major elements of volition. Kevin's prior interests (soccer and a girlfriend) and his values (being independent from his family) were threatened. He could no longer fully pursue these interests and values. **Personal causation,** which refers to the sense that one can effect change in the environment, was also influenced by the brain injury. This influence was most evident in some of the behavioral sequelae of Kevin's injury and in his adjustment to living with a disability.

The habituation subsystem includes roles and habits that influence and guide occupational behavior. After Kevin's injury, his roles shifted dramatically. As a student and boyfriend, he had been preparing for a number of age-appropriate roles to include worker and spouse. In his recovery, Kevin was forced to be dependent on the hospital staff and his family; his girlfriend broke off their relationship, and his transition from student to worker role was derailed. Kevin's habit structure was markedly affected by the brain injury. His residual cognitive and memory deficits made the organization of habits and the degree of flexibility/rigidity applied in that habit structure difficult to modulate.

Kevin's most overt deficits were in the performance subsystem in skills needed to perform purposeful behavior. His brain injury left him with difficulties in the three types of performance skills: communication/interaction, process and perceptual motor. The initial focus of Kevin's occupational therapy treatment was facilitating return of function in his left dominant hand. Kevin's deficits in fine motor skills and visual spatial functions were perceptual motor problems. His communication and interaction difficulties were evident in his memory, reasoning and problem solving deficits and in various executive level functions. Although the focus of Kevin's occupational therapy intervention seemed to be primarily in the performance subsystem, treatment was also provided for deficits in the habituation and volition subsystems. The treatment approaches described previously address problems in all three subsystems.

Coma Stimulation Treatment Approach

The occupational therapist is the health care professional responsible for the coma stimulation program at a trauma center. The purpose of the program is to expose the comatose or semicomatose patient to graded sensory input and to facilitate normalized responses to the input. The program is graded to match the patient's level on the Rancho Los Amigos Scale of Cognitive Function and follows a developmental progression based on the patient's level of orientation and attention.

Multisensory input is used. Initially, the therapist's objective is to elicit a reflexive response to the stimuli. For example, the patient retracting his or her hand from a hot or sharp object. Sometimes a bell, bright light, or ammonia is used as noxious stimuli. After the patient is responding reflexively, the therapy progresses toward the integration of the reflex and volitional responses. Less offensive sensory stimuli are applied. Initially, the patient's performance will conform to a stimulus-response pattern. The patient is given a ball and he or she squeezes it, or the therapist moves to the other side of the bed and the patient visually tracks the therapist's movement. The stimulus must be varied to encourage a variety of response patterns and avoid having the patient become stimulus-bound. This behavior appears perseverative or imitative. It is not desirable because it is stereotypical and will ultimately retard the patient's progress toward volitional performance. The therapist provides common stimuli for the patient to identify and manipulate. Treatment objectives and treatment strategies are summarized in Figure 23-5.

The occupational therapist also assists nursing staff and family members to construct a suitable environment for the comatose or semicomatose patient. Many of these patients are actually overstimulated and suffer from a syndrome known as ICU psychosis. This syndrome involves prolonged disorientation secondary to the milieu of the ICU. The patient becomes disoriented because there is not a day/night cycle on the unit. The lights and noises of monitors and equipment are present 24 hours a day. Patients' sleep cycles usually last only a few hours and they are often fatigued due to inadequate sleep. Occupational therapy personnel can help the staff and the patient's family members by turning out lights and limiting auditory sound for six to eight hours a day.

Environmental Control Model

The general principle of this model is that the patient's environment is controlled and structured by the treatment team to elicit the optimal performance from the patient. This model is frequently used with head-injured patients who are confused, agitated and/or inappropriate. A patient who displays any of these behaviors lacks the internalized ability to predict or organize actions. The patient is merely able to respond as he is bombarded with demands and stimuli from the environment and begins to feel overwhelmed by events and stimuli that seem beyond his or her control. The person thus becomes frustrated, realizing that his or her responses to the environment are less than optimum and yet the response is irrevocable.

The purpose of environmental control is to minimize the confusion, agitation, inappropriate behaviors and frustration by organizing the environment and facilitating positive experiences. The desired end result is to have the patient interact with the environment in an adaptive rather than a maladaptive mode.

In Kevin's case the environmental control model was used to address the goals of orientation and attention. The COTA coordinated Kevin's therapy schedule with the other disciplines and posted it in his room and at the nurse's station. She arranged an escort system so that Kevin would be punctual for all of his appointments. Part of the orientation treatment was to routinize Kevin's day so that eventually he would be able to execute the routine without external guidance. Initially, the occupational therapy assistant took responsibility for orienting Kevin each day to the calendar, weather, names and faces of his treatment team, and his therapy schedule. Each day they played a trivia game to help Kevin regain personal memories. The COTA had obtained the information from family members and made flashcards and a board game based on these facts. She also helped him match his clothes and labeled his drawers. While Kevin was in the clinic participating in a task group, the occupational therapy assistant structured the environment by minimizing the number of distractions. Initially, they worked in a quiet

---

Treatment Objectives

1. Patient will respond to noxious stimuli in reflexive manner.
2. Patient will consistently respond to novel stimuli (ie tactile, auditory, vestibular) by directing sensory receptors (eyes, ears, hands) in the direction of the stimuli.
3. Patient will respond to novel stimuli with directed and overt motor behavior such as reaching, grasping.
4. Patient will consistently execute habitual motor acts in response to stimulus presentation.
5. Patient will reliably identify common objects and facts in a verbal or nonverbal mode.
6. Patient will execute simple 1- and 2-step command consistently.

Treatment Strategies

Present ammonia, sharp pin, loud sound, ice to patient.
Vary presentation of sensory stimuli: size, intensity, rate, sequence, location.

Place novel stimuli within proximity of patient and guide discovery of stimuli such as bubbles, balloons, therapy putty.
Present common ADL objects and guide purposeful use.

Present patient with common objects and orientation questions. Ask yes/no questions.
Vary commands. Ask patient to identify body parts or sensory stimuli.

Figure 23-5. *Coma Stimulation Program.*

room. Next, she introduced more stimuli by opening the door to the room as they worked. The next progression was to work in the busy clinic at a table by themselves. Finally, the COTA and the patient sat at a table with other patients and staff who were free to interrupt the COTA as they worked. The occupational therapy assistant informed Kevin that his job was to remain task-oriented despite distractions. She reinforced his increased attention span with praise. Scheduling reinforcement intervals is another method of environmental control.

The environmental control model was used throughout the course of therapy as Kevin encountered new tasks and required assistance identifying a realistic method of organizing and accomplishing the task.

Skill Building Model

This model was also used quite successfully with Kevin. The underlying principle is related to the old adage "practice makes perfect." Because of his head injury, Kevin experienced a decay in many age-appropriate skills, as well as limitations in his work speed and manual dexterity, secondary to motoric deficits. The COTA helped Kevin acquire personal hygiene and grooming skills through daily practice under supervision. The assistant's role was to redirect him when he became distracted or perseverated. As he progressed, she minimized her intervention by having Kevin perform a self-check using a checklist. His initial tendencies to perseverate were minimized with the use of a kitchen timer.

The COTA used a skill-building strategy called chaining to help Kevin learn his way around the hospital. Initially, Kevin was escorted to and from appointments by staff. The next step was to have Kevin think of the routes as trails marked with "blazes." Together with the COTA, he identified visual blazes that would help him find his way and marked them on a map that he carried with him. Staff intervened only when he made a mistake. This skill was reinforced in the clinic by asking Kevin to refer to his map and verbally give the therapist directions to destinations within the hospital.

Kevin increased his manual dexterity through graded work projects that the COTA provided. She facilitated an increase in his work speed by giving him repetitive tasks with daily performance quotas.

Later in the treatment program, the skill building principles of practice, graded activity, chaining and reinforcement were applied to cooking, money management, visual-spatial problem solving, writing and work therapy.

Strategy Substitution Model

Several different principles apply to this model: strategy appropriateness, strategy durability and generalization. Occupational therapy personnel first identify ineffective strategies that the patient currently uses. The patient is then provided with an alternative strategy. Practice activities help the patient to observe strategy effectiveness in a performance situation. The other purpose of practice is to help the patient internalize the strategy, thus promoting strategy durability. The ultimate goal of treatment is for the patient to be able to generalize the strategy to a new situation.

This model was used in Kevin's treatment program to identify strategies that were and were not helpful for him. Initially, Kevin was unable to maintain his schedule by himself; however, one of Kevin's goals was to be able to use a daily planning calendar. The OTR noted that Kevin did not self-monitor his behavior and had difficulty anticipating events; therefore, he probably would forget to look at a calendar. The occupational therapist initiated a strategy by substituting a cassette recording of his schedule. Because Kevin was frequently listening to a portable tape recorder/player, it seemed likely that he would also listen to his schedule throughout the day. This external aid proved to be a more effective strategy. He learned to use the recorder microphone to revise his schedule when appointments were changed. After several weeks of practice, Kevin had learned the importance of keeping appointments and had received positive feedback from the staff. He was then able to transfer his schedule to a daily planner. The OTR thought it was important for Kevin to use a calendar format, because it is more versatile for long-term planning; however, use of the tape player continued to be reinforced. When Kevin began his work therapy he used the tape player to teach himself the route to and from the hospital using public transportation. The tape described important information such as the bus route number, the landmarks along the way and the final destination. These are examples of strategy generalization.

Summary

Traumatic brain injury is a complex diagnosis with varying degrees of severity and residual dysfunction. Each patient is unique. This chapter provides general information on the causes and stages of head injury and treatment models. The anecdotal case history describes how a head injury is manifested functionally, behaviorally and emotionally. The head-injured patients that the reader is likely to treat will vary greatly; therefore, this information should be viewed as a general reference to assist in planning and implementing assessments and treatment. The most important message of the case history is that the COTA's creativity is invaluable in structuring meaningful activities that help the patient to regain lost skills and feelings of independence. Using creativity and treating the patient as a unique individual are the keys to successful treatment outcomes. It is anticipated that COTAs will find their work with traumatic brain-injured patients to be rewarding because they have the opportunity to significantly enhance the patient's quality of life and resumption of roles.

Editor's Note

The authors have written this chapter in their private capacity. No official support or endorsement by the U. S. Department of the Army or the Department of Defense is intended or should be inferred.

Related Learning Activities

1. Practice administering some of the assessment instruments used by the COTA in the case study. Note any areas of difficulty, and seek assistance from an OTR or a experinced COTA.

2. Describe the various models and treatment approaches presented.

3. Develop a chart delineating the specific OTR and COTA roles and tasks in working with Kevin. Identify and discuss any areas of overlap with peers.

4. Write to the National Head Injury Foundation, P.O. Box 567, Framingham, MA 01701 to obtain information about the services and publications they provide.

References

1. Miller BF, Keane CB: *Encyclopedia and Dictionary of Medicine, Nursing, and Allied Health*, 5th Edition. Philadelphia, WB Saunders, 1992.
2. *Rancho Los Amigos Scale of Levels of Cognitive Functioning.* Rancho Los Amigos, Downey, California, Undated.
3. Sohlberg M, Mateer C: *Cognitive Rehabilitation.* New York, Guilford Press, 1989.
4. Trombly CA: *Occupational Therapy for Physical Dysfunction*, 3rd Edition. Baltimore, Williams & Wilkins, 1989.
5. Kielhofner G. (Ed): *A Model of Human Occupation: Theory and Application.* Baltimore, Williams & Wilkins, 1985.
6. Keilhofner G, Igi C, Burke JP: A model of human occupation. Part 4: Assessment and intervention. *Am J Occup Ther* 34:777-788, 1980.
7. Parenté F, Anderson-Parenté J: *Retraining Memory Techniques and Applications.* Houston, CSY Publishing, 1991.

Section IV
EMERGING MODELS OF PRACTICE

Stress Management

Hospice Care

Driver Assessment and Education for the Disabled

S tress management, hospice care and disabled driver education were selected as emerging models of practice, reflecting the move to reduce health care costs by providing more community-based services. The specific goals of this section are the same as those for section three: to provide the reader with in-depth, comprehensive information about these par-ticular models and the intraprofessional working relationship of OTR and COTA practitioners in these settings. Detailed case studies are presented to illustrate the occupational therapy team approach. In addition, the reader should be able to use the information as a guide for developing similar models of practice or enhancing existing ones.

Stress Management

Terry Brittell, COTA, ROH

Introduction

Stress may be defined as a physical, chemical or emotional factor (trauma, histamine, or fear) to which an individual fails to make a satisfactory adaptation and which causes physiologic tensions that may be a contributory cause of disease.[1]

Occupational therapy practitioners involved in stress management programs should view their role as one of program developer, instructor and group facilitator. The preparation and training of therapists and assistants provide numerous strategies for intervention, such as assertiveness training, occupational performance evaluation, environmental analysis and program development. This chapter provides a basic understanding of how to use these strategies in stress reduction and stress management programs.

Societal Pressures Contributing to Stress-induced Illness

Some labeled the 1980s an "age of anxiety.".[2] Naisbitt and Aburdene suggest in *Megatrends 2000* that the 1990s will be a decade of drastic changes, so much so that this decade will be recorded in history as "the decade of change."[3] Concomitant with accelerated change is a greater potential for stress-induced illnesses. In its efforts to combat such illnesses in the 1990s, the National Institute of Mental Health (NIMH) is concentrating its energy on developing intervention programs in the following four major categories:[4]

1. Education programs to modify personal practices that adversely affect health such as use of tobacco and alcohol and improper or inadequate diet.

ESSENTIAL VOCABULARY

Social conditions

Holism

Maladaptive

Dysadaptive

Context

Individual vulnerability

Loss

Life change

Patterns of response

Isometrics

Aerobic

Dysthymic

KEY CONCEPTS

Societal pressures	Goal attainment scale
Stress management	Stress reduction program
Stress and role competence	Personnel
Stress history outline	Community resources

2. Epidemiologic studies to reduce the prevalence of certain major illnesses, including cancer, HIV infection, AIDS, sexually transmitted diseases, and mental illness.

3. Health and safety programs to increase public awareness in areas such as environmental health hazards and unintentional injuries.

4. Maintenance programs that address maternal and infant health and the quality of life of older people.

In addition to these areas, a number of other **social conditions** need to be addressed because of their stress-inducing potential. Included among these conditions is a trend toward an enlarged population of homeless people, greater poverty, declining access to health care, increased out-of-wedlock births and the stresses faced by some single-parent families. Economic pressures, which have forced more and more families to become two-wage earner families, have led to other stresses resulting from the dual commitment to work and to child care and/or elder care responsibilities. In a society extremely dependent on a wide range of sophisticated, automated technologies, a high school diploma no longer guarantees employment in the 1990s. Higher education has become a greater priority, which places a tremendous financial burden on many families. In contemporary society, work is a primary source of stress-related illnesses exacerbated by an increased emphasis on quality, accountability and "doing more with less."

Other changes also affect stress levels. For example, parents not only place high expectatons on themselves to achieve, but also on their children. These expectations are often compounded by those of teachers and other adults. In addition, dramatic changes in the past two or three decades have blurred gender roles and responsibilities, the family structure and individual and family value systems. These changes have had a profound impact on one's perception of self and on one's capacity to control stressors, as well as to respond to stress.

These examples are only a few of the societal pressures that can contribute to stress-induced illnesses; whatever the etiology, however, the management of stress deserves the attention of the occupational therapy practitioners.

Stress Management Concepts

Stress management programs should be designed within the concept of **holism**. Girdano and Everly describe holism as "the context underlying an approach to control stress and tension that deals with the complete life-style of the individual, incorporating intervention at several levels: physical, psychological, and social simultaneously."[5] The following intervention strategies should be included in a stress management program:

1. Minimize the frequency of stress
2. Develop abilities to become better prepared, psychologically and physiologically, to withstand excessive stress
3. Utilize the by-products of excessive stress arousal, such as body awareness activities and exercise for pure pleasure[5]

Stress is an integral aspect of all practice models. It can be seen as a causative agent in a medical model, a response in a behavioral model, ego damaging in a personality model, delaying in a developmental model, and interrupting and disorganizing in a functional performance model. The model selected dictates the intervention techniques. I advocate a holistic approach for managing stress because it is not only effective, but also is compatible with the basic philosophical beliefs of the profession.

Stress and Role Competence

The ultimate objective of any stress management program is to intervene to promote role competence.[5-7] Consider the following two examples involving psychiatric patients. According to King, psychiatric patients tend to be divided into two major categories: **maladaptive** or **dysadaptive**.[8] The maladaptive patient has not learned the skills and tasks required for role performance. This person needs to learn and practice role specific skills, beginning at the individual's current level of performance and moving toward the degree of performance required at the next functional level. For instance, it is inefficient to spend time and effort teaching a patient to cook if the individual is to be released to a nursing home or other residential facility where meals are prepared and provided by the staff. The maladaptive patient should be taught to do those tasks necessary for survival. On the other hand, the dysadaptive patient is one who functions at least marginally in the community, but who is seen on an acute care-service because he or she cannot cope effectively in the community. This person needs to refine or strengthen existing skills in performing role-associated activities effectively.[8]

McLean provides a structure for viewing the conditions in which stressors are most likely to produce symptoms that affect daily function or push the person beyond the ability to maintain personal control. These three conditions are as follows:[9]

1. Individual vulnerability
2. Context or the environment in which that vulnerability is exposed to a stressor
3. Resulting behavioral symptoms, which may be subtle or complex

According to McLean, two factors help to determine if a

stressor will produce symptoms. The first factor is whether the stressor occurs within the **context** of an external environment. The context includes the social, physical and psychological *milieu* (condition) of the situation and may be either supportive or destructive. The second factor is **individual vulnerability,** which is made up of personality characteristics and personal experience. The history of experience in adaptation or failure at developmental junctures and previous responses when confronted with problems reflect the available choices and vulnerability of each person.[9] Another important consideration for treatment has to be the strength of the stressor or stressors.

As an example of McLean's model, imagine a work situation in which the budget has just been cut, eliminating a prized project that is close to completion with a successful outcome in sight. The stressor is loss. Others in the workplace are sympathetic and offer volunteer time to help complete the project. This context is friendly and supportive. The individual in charge of the project has good time management skills and is feeling in good health. This person's resistance to vulnerability is strong, and few symptoms probably would emerge with this stressful situation. In contrast, a person encountering this same situation who is recovering from a bad case of influenza and who is faced with a large backlog of work, complicated by personal problems, may be at risk. The context is nonsupportive, individual vulnerability is susceptible to damage, and the chances of symptoms occurring are high.

When applying McLean's construct to stress management treatment, goals should focus on the following:

1. Reducing individual vulnerability
2. Strengthening a supportive environment
3. Reducing the power of the stressor

For instance, understanding the relationship between **loss** (death of loved one, laid off job, broken engagement, etc) and **life change** (eg, marriage, new job, relocation) and the processes necessary to establish new routines and goals can reduce individual vulnerability. Using assertiveness skills and developing a support network can strengthen the context. Pain management and stress reduction exercises, such as deep breathing, can decrease the power of the stressor.[9]

Evaluation Tools

The Stress History Outline

The Stress History Outline (SHO) is a standardized, structured interview used to gather data on an individual's perceptions of the pressures that influence his or her life.[10] It focuses on current stressors in seven areas, as well as **patterns of response** used by the individual in the past. A numerical score is assigned to the resulting data, which can be compared to the scores of the average individual. This score can also be aligned with Axis IV of the *Diagnostic and Statistical Manual of Mental Disorders*.[11] The need for intervention is indicated when the individual's score falls into the categories from moderate to catastrophic, or if very high stress is indicated in a specific area. The SHO does not determine the presence of psychiatric illness; rather, it identifies the degree of severity of each of the stressors described here.[10]

Loss: The pressure brought by bereavement over loss and permanent role change prompted by death, birth, employment, divorce, or deterioration accompanying a physical or mental limitation all contribute to creating stress. Loss is a high level stressor, but most people can cope with one or two losses with a strong support network (see life change).

Performance: Any event or condition that pressures the individual to achieve may bring about a stress response. This stress may be self-imposed or imposed by others. If the performance requires greater skills than the individual has mastered, the problem may be in skill acquisition, lack of practice, or the inability to generalize existing skills to new situations. If the stress is self-imposed, the individual needs to reevaluate goals realistically. Situations that lead to performance stress are interpersonal, occupational, family and leisure.

Frustration: These pressures usually come from "double bind" or "no-win" situations where decision making, assertiveness or acceptance are required. Frustration occurs when one is blocked from doing what is desired, whether it is exhibiting a certain behavior or attaining a particular goal.[5] Frustration can result in feelings of anger and aggression causing a stress response.

Fear: This emotional reaction ranges from apprehension to panic, which usually causes a "flight-or-fight" reaction. The person's response may be to an actual or perceived danger. The stress response usually occurs in three phases: initial anxiety surge, panic and the anxiety spiral.[12] A prolonged stress response can deplete the individual to the point of death. Fear decreases with control over any problem area.

Boredom: This response tends to correlate with a decreased activity and interest level and frequently is self-imposed. It may be seen as the inability to respond to stimuli or lack of stimuli. The reaction may be compounded by depression, poor concentration, fatigue, lack of initiative or goals, or laziness. Chemical changes in the brain found with addiction to various substances, severe aggression and rage, and organic changes resulting from disease should be ruled out.

Life change: Appearance of this stressor precedes, accompanies or results from loss situations. Readjustment strategies and new goals must be instituted. Most adults have developed response patterns to life change. Those who have been successful are likely to continue with their adaptive methods. Those who have not been successful require education in adaptive skill behavior.

Environment: Stressors in this category may be compounded by inadequate diet, polluted water, chemical abuse, smoking, lack of exercise or sleep, dust and other atmospheric contaminants, and meterologic conditions such as excessive heat or cold, high altitude, full moon or storms.

In addition to these seven categories of stressors, other factors should be considered such as the individual's personality type (A or B) and resulting behaviors, as well as any patterns of procrastination and general time management skills. Type A behavior is characterized by one's perception of a life event and results in becoming a workaholic or a race horse. These individuals are usually aggressive, extroverted, and have a high competitive drive. They are impatient and task-oriented and seldom take time for relaxation. Type A people are prone to cardiovascular disease and disorders. Behavior of type B people is characterized by being laid back and unconcerned with time pressures or demands. These individuals tend to be more creative in problem solving and take life's problems in stride.

The Goal Attainment Scale

The Goal Attainment Scale (GAS), developed by Kiresuk and Sherman in 1976, uses patient identified problems to set goals and objectives.[13] At the end of the program, the treatment team and the patient determine how many of the goals have been achieved. This is an extremely important therapeutic practice that promotes the patient's active involvement in the process of recovery. Through use of this instrument, the patient identifies three to five problems and determines the ideal solution for each. Patients are then asked to describe a "worst case scenario" so that they can gain a better understanding of their situation. Frequently, they discover that their concerns are not as problematic as they thought when compared with the "worst case" situations they described. Next, they identify what would be a slight improvement and then set a realistic goal that could be accomplished within the scope of the treatment program. Strategies for attaining goals are discussed in treatment sessions.

Stress Reduction Programs

Stress reduction programs usually do not last more than ten hours and are used along with other occupational therapy interventions. Most individuals can benefit from learning stress reduction techniques; however, they often tend to be "Band-aid" methods that offer a temporary solution for problems such as controlling anxiety or combating insom-

nia. Matching various techniques to the particular needs of an individual in a group requires application of the principle of biasing the central nervous system to increase or decrease stimuli. Not every individual can or should adopt all of the techniques, but it is important for patients to practice each technique in a given program before deciding which ones work best.

The major benefits of a stress reduction program are that it increases concentration, decreases anxiety and makes patients more amenable to other therapies. Patients may be referred to a stress reduction program because of high anxiety levels, the inability to relax or feel comfortable with self, or inability to tolerate involvement in a stress management program.

Goals of Stress Reduction

At the conclusion of a stress reduction program, the patient should be able to demonstrate the ability to accomplish the following:

1. *Develop and use guided imagery*: Guided imagery is the process of developing a picture in one's mind that is centered around an environment one has experienced, which represents peace and relaxation, such as a lake, mountains or the seashore.
2. *Relax muscle groups in both lying and sitting positions through isometric and gross motor exercise*: **Isometrics** is a series of body positions that represent force and resistance, such as pushing both hands together. The exercises should be performed very rapidly for 15 to 20 minutes, almost to the point of exhaustion, to be beneficial. Individuals with high blood pressure or diabetes should not engage in isometrics unless approved by a physician. Gross motor exercise refers to exercising large muscle groups through activities such as running, brisk walking, mopping or sweeping a floor, or gardening. Individuals with cardiac and respiratory problems should have physician supervision for such programs.
3. *Maintain a sufficient amount of oxygen for deep breathing exercises*: Deep breathing is learning diaphramatic breathing, which involves moving downward to the lowest part of the lungs and filling with air, filling the middle part until the chest expands, and finally filling the upper part of the lungs with air and exhaling slowly. This exercise is based on the principle that an increased amount of oxygen slows down the heart rate and produces a relaxation response. This practice is contraindicated for individuals with lung disease.
4. *Use aerobic exercise appropriately*: The term **aerobic** means in the presence of oxygen, which includes the total environment—air, nutrition, and exercise. Aerobic exercises are used to increase blood supply and circulation to the extremities.

5. *Use techniques to reduce tension*: These techniques include massage, brushing, stroking, and self-massage.

6. *Engage in progressive relaxation techniques*: Progressive relaxation techniques are also referred to as autogenics. These techniques teach how to focus on bodily sensation and how to relax. They are a series of exercises that involve tensing one's muscles and relaxing them in a specific part of the body or in the total body.

7. *Use thought stopping or refocusing to reduce periods of preoccupation*: Thought stopping involves shouting the words "stop it" in your mind as soon as you are becoming aware of added anxiety or preoccupation. It is a form of refocusing to regain concentration.

The objectives of a stress reduction program are attained through a combination of the following methods:

1. Practice sessions using the techniques previously discussed

2. Mini-lectures, discussions and demonstrations

3. Group activities to encourage group participation and to create an atmosphere of belonging

Typically, participation in stress reduction programs is limited to eight to ten patients who usually meet for one-hour sessions, twice weekly, for three to four weeks. The ultimate goal of the program is for each patient to demonstrate five stress reduction techniques and provide evidence that they are using them in stressful situations.

An entry-level COTA providing services in this type of program will require regular, on-site supervision by an OTR. Once skill levels have been fully developed and refined through experience, the COTA may need less direct professional supervision.

Stress Management Programs

Stress management programs are an effective and efficient form of intervention. They are structured and time limited. Patients appreciate a starting and ending point of treatment and often relate these sessions to continuing education. They play an active role within their own treatment regimen. Participants are advised of their major stressor scores obtained through evaluation instruments such as the Stress History Outline, and they are provided with guidance and opportunities to learn and practice skills and techniques to gain mastery in their deficit areas. At the conclusion of the program, the patient should be able to demonstrate the following:

1. A reduction in stress level from the original score on the Stress History Outline evaluation by 50% or more

2. An ability to use stress reduction techniques, such as guided imagery, isometrics, thought stopping, self massage, etc.

3. Ability to use techniques, methods, and skills to manage the following stressors: life change, fears, frustration, environment, boredom, performance and loss

Figure 24-1 shows a partial list of strategies that can be used in a stress management program. Refer to the references at the conclusion of this chapter for additional information.

Referrals

Patients may be referred to a stress management program by the treatment team, community agencies, physicians and others. Acceptance into the program is determined by evaluation using the Stress History Outline. Criteria for referral include the following behavioral factors:

1. High anxiety levels

2. Inability to relax or feel comfortable with self

3. Reduced problem-solving ability and abstraction skills

4. Severe depression

5. Numerous losses

6. Low frustration tolerance

7. Long history of seeking medical advice

Program Structure

The stress management program is designed to meet the needs of persons who demonstrate a high level of severity on the Stress History Outline, (a score of more than 95.0) or of persons who have a normal stress score, but whose scores are severely skewed in one or more stressor areas, such as loss. People who might be described as disadaptive with regard to problem solving and abstraction skills will also benefit. Individuals who score below the norm may also need intervention to correct problems with boredom and perhaps some degree of depression. The stress management group is a closed group, limited to 10 or 12 members, to ensure that that one can complete the program in the shortest amount of time and, more important, to establish a strong support network among group members. Nine, 2-hour meetings are held over 4.5 weeks. This schedule may be modified by conducting meetings over three months or, in an acute setting, meeting two hours a day for two weeks.

Objectives are attained through a combination of the following:

1. Mini-lectures on management of each of the seven stressors

2. Practice sessions using group discussions, role plays, written exercises, films, physical activities and other techniques

3. Stress reduction methods

Program effectiveness is measured by reviewing pretest and posttest scores of each individual. Recommendations for termination or continuance are based on this information.

Stressor:	Strategy:
Fear:	Provide positive self-talk exercises
	Provide tension control exercises
	Provide imagery training exercises
	Provide briefing/debriefing exercises
	Provide thought-stopping exercises
	Provide description of the origin of fears
Boredom:	Explain the relationship between nonproductive and destructive behavior and boredom
	Explain how the lack of stimuli or lack of motivation to change stimuli can lead to boredom
	Conduct activities that help reduce boredom (physical and intellectual)
	Discuss performance stress and resultant overload with suggestions for reducing this load
	Provide instructions about how to set new goals with alternative steps
Frustration:	Present information on the causes of frustration
	Demonstrate time lining techniques for establishing self-goals and motivation
	Provide assertiveness training techniques and role play exercises
	Provide empathetic listening exercises
	Provide problem-solving/decision-making exercises
	Provide and encourage feedback and suggestions on conflict reduction via role play exercises
Loss:	Present and provide information on various types of losses, such as retirement, income, status, possessions, self-esteem, rape trauma, functions, body parts, etc.
	Present understanding of the stages of grief
	Provide instruction and exercises in how to work out anger
	Provide exercises on how to finish business; closure activities
	Describe methods and activities to help manage loss
Environment:	Facilitate discussion on environmental stressors, including internal and external stressors
	Describe the importance of a balance of work, leisure, sleep and of a further balance in leisure, socialization, recreation and relaxation
	Provide priority-goal setting exercises
	Provide instruction for nutrition management
	Provide instruction and exercises to improve time management skills
Life Change:	Provide discussion on how life change affects all individuals (time and role disruption) and how and when, coupled with additional stressors, may become overwhelming
	Provide understanding or resolving of old roles, going on with life (resolution/closure)
	Provide exercises on setting new goals
	Provide methods to manage life at times of change

Figure 24-1. *Stress Management Strategies.*

Personnel

The occupational therapist serves as a consultant when working with an experienced certified occupational assistant (COTA). The OTR should provide one, 2-hour session weekly to review evaluation scores and treatment plans, to discuss program content or changes, and to complete documentation required by the agency or third-party payers.

Roles assumed by the COTA include serving as program manager, developer, instructor and group facilitator. The scheduling and administration of evaluations is another important responsibility. Other roles include maintaining necessary records through regular documentation and serving as an advocate for each patient through representation of their interests in treatment planning with other team members. In addition, the COTA may be required to collect and maintain data for quality assurance studies.

Termination

At the conclusion of the program, each participant is again administered the Stress History Outline to measure progress or lack thereof. A closure session (often a potluck-type dinner or luncheon) is planned, which is ceremonial. Feelings regarding the value and termination of the group are discussed. Members are encouraged to express feelings to others, individually and collectively, about the importance of the group in their personal growth. Information about home programs and community support resources is provided and a telephone support network is established for those who wish to participate.

Self Improvement, Victim, and Health-Related Groups
- Weight Watchers
- Smoking cessation
- Alcoholics Anonymous, Alateen, Alanon
- Gamblers Anonymous
- HIV and AIDS support groups
- Recovery (for former mental patients)
- Family involvement programs
- Bereavement
- Better Breathers, etc.

Special Interest Groups
- Art expression
- Poetry composition
- Creative writing
- Music appreciation
- Gardening
- Creative dance
- Photography
- Crafts
- Bird watching
- Coin and stamp collection, etc.

Exercise and Sports Groups
- Bowling
- Walking
- Cross country skiing
- Aerobics
- Swimming
- Softball, etc.

Social Clubs/Fraternal Organizations
- Elks, Lions, Moose, etc.
- YMCA and YWCA
- Single parent groups
- Card groups
- Sightseeing groups, etc.

Continuing Education
- Basic literacy, GED
- Assertiveness training
- Adult education short courses
- Local college courses

Community Agencies
- Department of Social Services
- Church/synagogue-related social services
- Association for Retarded Citizens
- Association for the Blind
- Meals on Wheels, etc.

Religious Organizations
- Choir
- Religious History Study
- Couples ad family groups
- Men's and women's groups
- Stress and support groups

Figure 24-2. *Stress Management Resources.*

Community Resources

In any stress-related program, the availability of community resources is vital. The focus of many such programs is wellness education, which may be defined as teaching people how to actively accept the responsibility for their own well-being. The purpose of these community-based programs is to assist individuals in getting involved in the process of arriving at solutions for their problems. The concept of wellness education, using a holistic approach to treatment, has provided the foundation for stress reduction and stress management programs.

With the increased emphasis on prevention and wellness in society, numerous resources are available throughout the country that offer assistance to people on managing stress and potentially stressful situations. A number of examples are presented in Figure 24-2.

Occupational therapy practitioners must be knowledgeable about community resources that can assist the patient in reentry and maintenance in the community. Lacking the necessary means to support community living, the individual must rely entirely on his or her own resources, which may, over time, prove ineffective.

Case Study: Anne

Anne is a 55-year-old married woman who was referred from a community mental health outpatient program to a day treatment program. Her diagnosis, based on the DSM III-R, was as follows:

Axis I	300.40	dysthymic disorder
Axis II	V71.09	no personality disorder
Axis III	278.00	obesity
Axis IV	6	extreme depression
Axis V	3	good

Background

Anne was seen as an outpatient on an "as needed" temporary basis during episodes of depression over a five-year period. She participated in treatment until she felt stabilized, and then discharged herself from services. Her most recent depression began after a series of life events that she found overwhelming. Anne's mother had died recently

Name: _Mrs A._   Assessment Date: _2-19-93_

Birth Date: _3-11-35_ Marital Status: _Married_ Children: _1_

Highest Grade Completed: _12_   Employed: _Homemaker_

Work Location _____   Title: _____

Living Situation: _own home_   Support Person: _Husband_

Question #1: Reaction Indicators:

_____8_____Total Physical   _____9_____Total Emotional

Stress Profile

Questions #	Loss	Performance	Environmental	Frustration	Fear	Boredom	Life change
2			3.0			1.5	
3			5.0				
4	5.0						
5					17.0		
6							13.5
7	0.0						
8				12.5			
9				9.0			
10				9.0			
11						0.0	
12	6.0						
13		2.0					
14		3.0					
15		0.0					
16		10.0					
17			5.0			5.0	
18		2.5	2.5	3.0			
19		0.0	8.5	3.5			
20	5.0	5.0	5.0	5.0	3.0	5.0	5.0
21		5.0	5.0	5.0			
Subtotal	16.5 +	27.5 +	34.0 +	46.5 +	20.5 +	6.5 +	18.5
Total							169.5

Figure 24-3. *Stress History Outline.*

and her father required her daily care and assistance due to several physical disabilities. This situation was compounded when her husband was laid off work and they now have to file for bankruptcy. In addition, both her husband and daughter were currently undergoing psychiatric treatment at the outpatient clinic. Anne had never been hospitalized; however, her husband, who was diagnosed with paranoid schizophrenia and alcoholism, had been hospitalized several times. Anne's husband is also a "brittle" diabetic who does not maintain a therapeutic routine. Her daughter has been diagnosed as **dysthymic** (having mental depression) and is currently in the process of getting a divorce. She resides with her two children in an apartment in Anne's home.

Anne tends to enjoy being the family martyr, frequently taking on others' problems. Her history indicates that she becomes depressed whenever family members become more independent.

She has a rather sporadic work history and has never held a job outside the home for more than one year. Currently, she is a homemaker who does not belong to any community groups, although she stated that she has many friends.

At present, she is being seen monthly in a community mental health outpatient clinic and is receiving 25 mg maprotiline (Ludiomil), BID (twice a day).

Anne is neatly dressed and groomed and appears alert, aware and cooperative. Her remarks are well connected, coherent and relevant; no psychotic or delusional ideas could be elicited.

Levels of Predicted Attainments	Scale 1: (weight 1#)	Scale 2: (weight 2#)	Scale 3: (weight 3#)	Scale 4: (weight 4#)	Scale 5: (weight 5#)
Much less than the expected level of outcome	Never let daughter be independent.	Never having independent social life based on personal need.	Never feeling competent in interpersonal roles without interfering in others' lives.	No communication with others.	Becoming more anxious and depressed.
Somewhat less than the expected level of outcome	I know I should let daughter be independent but I can't let go.	Entire social outlet is based on solutions of other people's personal problems.	Tries to find solutions to everybody else's problems.	Superficial communication with others.	Feels caught between anxiety and depression.
Expected level of outcome	Give advice once per week.	Investigates (try out) leisure activities and select one.	Assists the person with problem solving but not making any decisions.	Develop listening skills including summarizing and responding.	Stress reduction and some stress management techniques.
Somewhat more than the expected level of outcome	Give advice once per month.	To develop competency in one activity.	Able to return problems to rightful owner.	Engage in meaningful give and take conversation, eg dyadic encounter.	Completion of Stress Management Program, demonstrating mastery of techniques.
Much more than the expected level of outcome.	Daughter lives independently and asks mother if advice is needed.	Demonstrating a well-balanced leisure.	Will not play the Ann Landers role.	Give and take communication.	Being able to cope with situations and relationships that cause anxiety and depression.

Figure 24-4. *Goal attainment scale. Used with permission of the Program Evaluation Resource Center, 501 Park Avenue South, Minneapolis, MN 55415.*

Stress Assessment

The COTA administered the Stress History Outline to Anne to determine major stressors and the appropriateness of a stress management program. Her total numerical score was 169, indicating an extreme level of stress.[9] Anne's three major stressors were frustration, 46.5; environment, 34.0; and performance, 27.5 as shown in Figure 24-3.

Through use of a structured checklist, the COTA gathered the following additional data. Anne experiences increased stress and more problems on paydays and personal days, such as her birthday, anniversary and the date of her mother's death. Her performance is most likely to be affected during mornings. She reports that the time passes extremely slowly, and seems to rationalize this feeling by saying, "I'm not a morning person." Recurring physical problems that she considers minor are diarrhea, foot pain, weight, insomnia, poor vision, and intermittent pain from an old back injury. She reports that high blood pressure and fluid retention are her major physical problems.

Anne stated that her fears include failing, losing a loved one, insects (particularly spiders), and failure to be able to identify someone she knows. She indicated that her reactions to physical stress are fatigue, which results in a tendency to sleep more; an irregular heartbeat; labored breathing; hyperventilation; rash; hives; upset stomach; a tendency to eat more; loss of control, manifested by hitting others and throwing things; and frequent urination. Anne's emotional reactions to stress include lack of concentration, crying, argumentativeness, aloofness, memory loss, helplessness, anger, ambivalence, stuttering and indifference. She reported that the life changes that were most difficult for her to readjust to were marriage and caring for her aged parents. The situations Anne finds most upsetting are arguments, "a blaring stereo or TV," loud noises, praise and rewards, financial matters, traveling and doing nothing.

This information was presented to the OTR who verified the scoring of the Stress History Outline. She also studied the results of the structured questionnaire in relation to the medical chart and determined areas where more information was needed.

In an informal interview with Anne, the OTR determined that she had guilt feelings about the resentment she feels toward her mother, who was extremely rigid and overprotective. It was also discovered that Anne tends to be overprotective with her daughter, not allowing her to live her own life. In addition to other findings, the OTR determined that Anne is dysadaptive, with role dysfunctioning in communication and recreator roles. She recommended Anne as a suitable candidate for the stress management program.

Program Planning

The COTA administered the Goal-Attainment Scale[13] to Anne and the following problems were identified:

1. Inability to allow daughter independence in decision making
2. Acting as an "advice giver or Anne Landers" to all acquaintances
3. Few leisure interests
4. Superficial communication with others (maintains secret self)
5. "Caught between depression and anxiety"

Working with the OTR, Anne was able to identify ways that these situations could deteriorate, and she was also able to describe increments of improvement, setting realistic goals with the OTR's assistance. The Goal Attainment Follow-Up Guide for Anne is shown in Figure 24-4.

In further planning, Anne's scores on the Goal Attainment Scale were compared with those of the avarage population. It was noted that she indeed was experiencing an extreme level of stress. The OTR determined that most of the problems identified by this instrument resulted from negative interpersonal relationships. It was important for Anne to learn the difference between assertion and aggression and to develop listening skills to reduce her frustration. It was thought that her performance stress could be reduced by finding a leisure skill and social outlets that involve "doing rather than talking."

Treatment

Anne completed the stress management program carried out by the COTA with good results. Although she was unable to attain all of the goals established, her progress indicated that these goals were likely to be met in the near future. While participating in the program, Anne was also being seen in the mental health outpatient clinic once every two weeks by a psychiatrist. Her medications were reviewed and individual psychotherapy was provided. A social worker provided direction for community involvement and problem solving, building on and supporting the progress Anne was making in the stress management program. Anne was also seen regularly by a community mental health nurse who assisted her with diet and nutrition management.

Summary

This chapter has provided strategies for two types of patient intervention. Stress reduction programs, which are an adjunct to other occupational therapy treatment, are designed to temporarily reduce overwhelming stress responses, making the patient more amenable to other forms of treatment. The program consists of relaxation techniques and exercises designed to reduce anxiety, increase focus and attention, and increase one's productive activ-

ity level.

Eighteen-hour, time-limited stress management programs provide alternative responses to cope with loss, life changes, fear, frustration, environment, performance and boredom. After the initial evaluation, stressors are identified that can cause dysfunction in the patient's life roles as a prelude to teaching the individual strategies that will help manage stress. The patient begins a life style change by focusing on the practice of new stress management techniques. The OTR and the COTA are responsible for decreasing the strength of the stressors through patient education, increasing environmental support, and decreasing vulnerability by providing additional methods for enhancing problem solving and communication skills.

Editor's Note

This chapter, by Terry Brittell, was completed shortly before his death in May 1991. He will be remembered for his leadership in the COTA community and for his years of dedication and service to the profession.

Acknowledgments

I dedicate this chapter to my son Keith who gave me the inspiration, support and strength to complete this work at a difficult time in my life. Through his stamina and perseverance, he exemplified the true meaning of how to manage stress successfully.

Phillip Shannon, MA, MPA, and Lyn Hill, MS, OTR, FAOTA, as friends and professional colleagues are gratefully acknowledged for their continuing support. Their clarifying of ideas, guidance, review of concepts and content, and above all, patience in assisting me in completing this manuscript are valued.

Joseph (Lynn) Salmon, COTA, is also thanked for reviewing this chapter to ensure that the manuscript would meet the needs of entry-level occupational therapy assistants.

Related Learning Activities

1. Review the references and bibliography and select two stress management strategies that you are interested in. Practice these methods and prepare a plan that could be used to instruct patients in use of these techniques.

2. Obtain copies of stress assessment tools and practice administering them to yourself and a peer. Ask an OTR to assist you in determining the accuracy of the scoring.

3. Participate in a discussion with family members or friends about what they find stressful. Determine what methods they use to successfully control stress.

4. Discuss the following factors relative to how they might influence treatment planning with an OTR:

- Internal and external environments that can fixate or regress the functioning level of individuals
- Cultural values of your geographic area
- Engagement in particular purposeful activities to ensure practice to reduce a specific stressor

References

1. *Webster's New International Dictionary, Unabridged.* Springfield, Massachusetts: Meriam Webster, 1989.
2. Naisbitt J: *Megatrends.* New York, Warner Books, 1982.
3. Naisbitt J, Aburdene P: *Megatrends 2000.* New York, William Morrow, 1990, pp 178-240.
4. National Institute of Mental Health: *Health Objectives Planning for Year 2000, Draft Priority Areas.* Bethesda, Maryland, National Institute of Mental Health, 1988.
5. Girdano D, Everly G: *Controlling Stress and Tension: A Holistic Approach.* New York, Prentice-Hall, 1979.
6. Hill L, Brittell T: *The Role Competence Model, Adult Psychiatric Day Treatment Proceedings.* St. Paul, Minnesota, University of Minnesota Press, 1981.
7. Hill L, Brittell T, Kotwal J: A community mental health group designed by clients. *Occup Ther Health Care* 6:(1), 1989.
8. King LJ: Eleanor Clarke Slagle Lecture: Toward a science of adaptive responses. *Am J Occup Ther* 32:429-437, 1978.
9. McLean AA: *Work Stress.* New York, Addison-Wesley, 1979, pp 37-40.
10. Hill L, Brittell T: *Stress History Outline.* Unpublished, 1981.
11. American Psychiatric Association: *Diagnostic and Statistical Manual of Mental Disorders,* 3rd Edition, Revised. Washington, DC, American Psychiatric Association, 1987.
12. Sharpe R, Lewis D: *Thrive on Stress.* New York, Warner Books, 1977.
13. Kiresuk TJ, Sherman RE: Goal attainment scaling: A general method for evaluation of comprehensive mental health programs. *Community Ment Health J* 4:443-453, 1968.

Hospice Care

William Matthew Marcil, MS, OTR
Kent Nelson Tigges, MS, OTR, FAOTA, FHIH

Introduction

Hospice is a medieval term for a place of safety; a place for travelers to stop, eat, sleep and be refreshed on a long journey. The first hospices were used by the crusaders on their way to the Holy Land. The term hospice came into modern usage in the 1960s when Dame Cicely Saunders conceived an idea and implemented a plan to provide a model of health care for people with advanced metastatic disease for whom there was no hope of a cure, and who had a life expectancy of six months or less. Saunders, who was a nurse, then a social worker, and subsequently a physician, recognized that the needs of the terminally ill patient could not be appropriately assessed or met in traditional hospitals or nursing homes, as their model of care was either cure, rehabilitation or long-term maintenance.

Saunders' model for hospice care did not emerge out of, or as, a medical speciality, but rather from a humanitarian model. Saunders opened the first modern hospice, St. Christopher's in England, in 1969. She continues to be the foremost authority on the subject, and most hospices in the United States and Canada are based on her model.

The first hospice to open in the United States was the Connecticut Hospice in New Haven in 1971. The first Canadian hospice, at the Royal Victoria Hospital in Montreal, opened in 1973. In 1970 the National Hospice Organization was incorporated and provides guidelines for developing hospices and promoting the hospice model of care.

ESSENTIAL VOCABULARY

Hospice

Narcotics

Diagnosis

Prognosis

Quality of life

Bereavement

Shiva

Remission

Seculsion

Glioblastoma

Hemiplegia

Vital signs

KEY CONCEPTS

Medical management of pain and symptoms

Diagnostic honesty

Quality of life

Training of the COTA

Role and supervision of COTA

Treatment discontinuation

Case illustration

At the present time there are approximately 3,000 hospices in the United States offering varying levels of care. Regulations for certification of Medicare providers became effective in 1983, and presently most of the nation's health insurance carriers offer hospice coverage.

Tenets of Hospice Care

Medical Management of Pain and Symptoms

The single most significant reason why patients are referred to or seek hospice care is for the severe and unrelenting pain that frequently is associated with advanced cancer. In traditional medical situations, pain alerts the physician that something is wrong and must be investigated. Once a medical workup is completed, a course of treatment is undertaken to resolve the problem. When the problem is corrected the pain ceases. If the pain does not cease, traditional physicians, not understanding the true nature of pain and being reluctant to use moderate or large doses of narcotics, cause patients to suffer unnecessarily.

In the case of advanced cancer, because the source of the pain cannot be removed or treated, the pain itself becomes the major concern of medical treatment. During the past 20 years, hospice physicians have studied and researched the pain experienced by the cancer patient and have developed successful chemotherapy protocols that in 98% of the patients treated, will completely eliminate the pain. When appropriately medicated on either small, moderate or high doses of **narcotics** (drugs that lessen or eliminate pain and cause sedation), hospice patients are free from pain; experience no addiction; and are sufficiently alert to be out of bed, bathe, dress, leave their homes and in some cases return to work. The key to successful pain control is the physician's understanding of the disease, its associated pain and the appropriate use of narcotics.

Diagnostic Honesty

All too frequently, when unfortunate, devastating or life-threatening news is learned, both lay and professional people react in either one of two ways. First, not wanting to admit or accept that they are powerless to change the situation, physicians proceed to bring about cure with all effort, or, failing that, put their efforts into prolonging the patient's life. Second, as no one wants to be the bearer of bad news, with all the best intentions, people respond to the patient's inquiries with a lie. Communications become strained when such situations occur. Eventually, when the patient learns the true **diagnosis** (description of the cause or nature of a condition or problem) and **prognosis** (forecast of the probable course and outcome of a disease or condition), and realizes that he or she has been deceived, communica-

tion may cease. With such deceptions, patients frequently experience the pain of isolation and abandonment.[1]

It is the hospice philosophy that patients not only have the right, but also the need to know the nature, course and outcome of their diagnosis. It is thought that without such knowledge patients cannot make realistic plans for the remainder of their lives. Hospice staff members advocate an open and honest attitude. No matter what question a patient asks, an honest answer is given. In dealing with diagnostic honesty, great caution and sensitivity are always necessary.

Quality of Life

Some advocates believe that the two greatest deterrents to quality of life are physical pain and discomfort. If the pain is controlled and the patient's physical needs are met, then the patient will have quality of life. Hospice philosophy recognizes that quality of living extends far beyond physical pain and discomfort. **Quality of life** is relative rather than absolute. It is a concept that people define individually within the context of their social community. Factors that are inherent in determining a given quality of life include:

1. Excellence of character
2. Achievement
3. Accomplishment
4. Personal/social status
5. Sense of personal well-being

When a terminal illness dashes all hopes for a future, it is not uncommon to see patients either relinquishing their desire to live or struggling to maintain a desire to live. When persons believe that they can no longer be independent, have a purpose, or be significantly contributing members of society, it is little wonder that they display an attitude of helplessness and hopelessness. In either situation it is of paramount importance for hospice professionals not only to be knowledgeable about the components necessary for quality of life, but also to take as much time as needed to help the patient work through the process of identifying what he or she would like to accomplish before death. In the final analysis, hospice measures its success if patients die free from pain and adverse symptoms and with feelings of excellence of character and personal well-being. To accomplish these tenets requires not only appropriate education, but also a composition of team members that are compatible with each other and have a close and respected appreciation for each other's contribution.

Training of the COTA for Hospice Care

As the treatment of the hospice patient is not an entry-level skill for either the registered occupational therapist (OTR) or the certified occupational therapy assistant (COTA), more education and experience must be undertaken before entering practice.[2] For the COTA, the education, training and selection should follow the following protocol:

1. When a COTA shows an interest in working with the terminally ill, the OTR should hold an initial interview with the assistant. This interview is intended to specify the reasons why the COTA wishes to enter hospice practice. As the hospice movement is new and gaining increasing popularity with health professionals, many are eager to be associated with hospice for a variety of reasons. The initial interview acts as a screening process to determine appropriate motives and suitability.

2. If the COTA is considered an appropriate candidate, the next step is to have the assistant complete a thorough review of the literature, summarize fundamental concepts and principles, and present the findings in an oral report.

3. The COTA is then given the charge to prepare for a series of four debates and role plays with the OTR. Topics to be covered are dying/death, spiritual/religious attitude, diagnostic honesty, and grief and **bereavement** (being deprived by death). These topics are dealt with in two categories: first, personal beliefs and values, and second, professional attitudes and intervention.

4. Upon successful completion of these steps, the COTA begins a trial period of accompanying the OTR to team meetings and on assessments and treatments of patients.

5. The assistant then follows a minimum of two cases: one case with the OTR and the other under supervision. Both cases must include all aspects of intervention, e.g. assessment, treatment planning and involvement during death, wake, funeral, burial or **shiva** (a Jewish custom involving gathering of the family and friends after a death).

6. Upon completion of the training program, an exit interview is held to determine if the COTA is still committed to hospice care and if the OTR thinks that the assistant is personally and professionally suited for hospice care.

Role and Supervision of the COTA

As the nature of the prognosis and the needs of the terminally ill patient are considerably different from patients with "traditional" diseases and problems, the role delineation between the OTR and the COTA does not follow the exact pattern established by the American Occupational Therapy Association.[3,4] The following model is presented for COTA involvement in hospice care.

Due to the highly charged emotional nature and personal vulnerability of patients and their families, it is essential that the OTR open every case. The physical, emotional and social status and needs of the patient are determined during the first meeting with the patient and family members. Equally important, the personal, emotional, social and interpersonal dynamics between the patient and family members are also assessed. If appropriate future treatment planning is to occur, it is essential for the OTR to screen, make an initial evaluation and establish short-term goals, and when possible, begin treatment at the first meeting with the patient.[5]

It is not only advisable but also highly recommended that the COTA accompany the OTR during screenings and evaluations. This approach is important for three reasons. First, the assistant is introduced to the patient and the family from the onset and conveys an impression of the close teamwork that will occur between the OTR and the COTA. Second, the assistant will be in a position to observe the interpersonal interactions and dynamics between the therapist and the family members. If the COTA should be assigned to the case, he or she will be in a substantially better position to follow through with the treatment. Third, the COTA can separate either the patient or the family member from the other. It is always advisable to include the family in the initial screening and assessment; however, there are times when it is either recommended or essential to speak to the patient alone and to the family member or members alone. Such situations occur under the following conditions:

1. The family member answers for the patient, and the patient cannot or does not participate in the screening or assessment.

2. The patient is apprehensive about being open and honest regarding personal needs, concerns, fears or goals.

3. The goals or expectations of either the patient or a family member are not compatible or agreed upon.

Depending on the nature and complexity of the case as determined by the OTR at the time of the first visit, the occupational therapist will make one of the following determinations: 1) the OTR will follow the case exclusively, 2) the COTA will be assigned to the case, or 3) the treatment requires that both the OTR and the COTA treat the patient simultaneously.

If the second decision is made, the assistant, often under close supervision by the occupational therapist, will be responsible for carrying out all or part of the treatment plan and continually assessing the patient's status. With advanced metastatic disease, it is not uncommon to observe either a situation where the patient has consistent fluctuations between loss of function and increase of function or a steady physical deterioration. In both situations, it is the responsibility of the COTA to assess such changes and report them to the OTR after each treatment. The occupational therapist will then make the appropriate modifications in the treatment plan.

The treatment and ongoing assessment of patients that experience temporary remission, accompanied by increased physical independence, poses quite a different set of problems for the OTR/COTA team. It is not uncommon for occupational therapy personnel to provide treatment to patients that results in a significant increase in physical independence. While visiting St. Luke's Hospice in Sheffield, England, I had a conversation with noted writer E. Wilkes who stated that after pain and symptom control, it is occupational therapy that provides the single greatest contribution in maximizing patients' quality of life. This contribution can only occur if the occupational therapist and the assistant are practicing from an occupational behavior perspective. Working from this point of view, the occupational therapy team focuses exclusively on maximizing the patient's roles in relation to self-care, work and leisure.

Sometimes medical intervention affords patients a substantial **remission** (lessening or abatement of the symptoms)[6] in their disease process. With appropriate occupational therapy intervention, the patient experiences a significant "improvement" in physical function and independence. In some cases, patients who have been bedridden upon admission to hospice care, have subsequently been able to return to work. In such "miracle" cases, it is extremely important for the OTR/COTA team to maintain an appropriate professional perspective and to remember that the increase in performance and independence is only temporary. If professional objectivity is lost, not only will the patient develop unrealistic hopes, but occupational therapy personnel may experience feelings of failure when the patient begins to deteriorate and dies. Loss of objectivity jeopardizes treatment.

In other cases, when the patient perceives the increased improvement as "proof" of cure, regardless of what has been stated directly, the patient is determined to believe that he or she will be a survivor. In such cases, the COTA responsible for treatment must be careful not to "feed" into the patient's false sense of reality. A fine line must be drawn: encouraging while at the same time not promoting false hope for survival.

After being assigned to a case, the COTA must constantly assess how the patient is perceiving new-found independence. The COTA must then convey this information to the OTR to facilitate clarification between the patient and therapist. In traditional clinical settings, diagnostic and prognostic communication with the patient has been the sole responsibility of the physician. In hospice care, it is the role and responsibility of all professional personnel. Although they may be unfamiliar with such roles, occupational therapists and assistants must be prepared to talk to patients honestly and explain that increased function does not indicate survival.

In still other situations, the OTR may determine that both the occupational therapist and the assistant should treat the patient simultaneously. This type of situation occurs when there are significant interpersonal stressors between the patient and family members. The following are examples of such situations:

1. The patient and/or a family member is excessively apprehensive about adjusting to any change in the established routine of living; they are immobilized by the situation and have few or no outside resources to support them.
2. The patient or family member is totally dependent or independent and goals cannot be agreed upon.
3. The family member, due to a sense of responsibility, becomes unnecessarily overprotective and renders the patient dependent.

No matter how independent the patient desires to become, he or she relinquishes this need out of fear of either upsetting or alienating the family member. When the OTR and COTA treat the patient at the same time, appropriate strategies can be put into place to meet the individual and collective needs of the family.

An important consideration in treating the hospice patient, be it in a free-standing unit or in a home care setting, is **seclusion**. No matter how attractive or familiar the environment, a sense of confinement and isolation can occur over time. Occupational therapy treatment planning should always include the option and feasibility of setting goals that would allow the patient the opportunity to engage in familiar community activities or events.

Treatment Discontinuation

Discontinuation of treatment begins the day that the patient becomes confined to bed and is no longer able to cognitively or physically engage in any aspect of self-care, work or leisure. If the occupational therapist and/or the assistant had minimum involvement with the patient, treatment is discontinued with appropriate "good-byes." If occupational therapy personnel have had a significant role and involvement, the patient should be followed to the time of death. At least one member of the OTR/COTA team should participate in the vigil and be with the patient at the time of death. If the occupational therapist is the only professional person present when death occurs, it is the therapist's responsibility to note the time of death, notify the hospice and carry out the routine procedures of caring for the body and giving support to the family until a nurse or physician arrives. After the death of a patient, occupational therapy personnel assist in seeing the family through the wake, funeral, memorial service, burial and/or shiva. Only then is the case officially closed.

The following two case studies illustrate the role of the COTA in hospice care.

Case Study I—Bill

Bill, a 63-year-old, 6'4", 240-lb man with a diagnosis of **glioblastoma**, a malignant tumor of the brain, was referred for occupational therapy services by his hospice physician. The OTR and COTA made the initial visit together to Bill's suburban home.

After meeting with Bill and his wife to explain the hospice program and the services that could be provided by occupational therapy, the OTR administered an occupational history to Bill. During this time, the COTA talked with his wife in another room to establish a relationship and to obtain information that might assist in Bill's treatment.

The occupational history revealed that Bill was a detective with the local police department, a job he valued and hoped to return to. This desire was evidenced by statements such as "I'm only on sick leave." Bill continued to carry his badge. It was also determined that Bill was an active outdoors man who enjoyed camping and swimming.

A physical assessment indicated that the tumor had left Bill with a flaccid, left-sided **hemiplegia** (paralysis of one side of the body) and a severe sensory loss. Bill was concerned that this condition had made it difficult for him to perform daily living activities such as bathing, dressing and functional household ambulation. This problem, combined with his inability to work, interfered with his role as family provider. The increasing dependence on his wife led to feelings of anger, depression, and being "less of a man."

When Bill asked the therapist what could be done to return function to his left side, the therapist replied that nothing could be done for his hemiplegia. Bill then asked angrily what good was therapy. The therapist told him that although no function could be returned, he could help him use his time in a meaningful way regardless of his condition. Bill accepted this response.

While the OTR worked with Bill in the living room, the COTA talked with Bill's wife in the kitchen. She stated that she was concerned with the amount of care Bill required and that she was frightened she might not be able to care for him much longer because of his size. She also told the assistant that due to the overall design of the house, it was difficult for Bill to move about in his wheelchair and impossible for him to go outside. She added that this confinement was contributing to his depression and causing growing friction between them.

After the two-hour assessment, the occupational therapy team left. While driving back to the office, they compared notes from their separate interviews. Drawing from this information, with emphasis on Bill's occupational roles and interests, the following tentative treatment plan was formulated:

1. Increase Bill's independence in dressing, using one-handed techniques.

2. Increase Bill's ability to assist with bathing and toileting, using adapted equipment as necessary.

3. Increase Bill's ability to assist in bed-to-wheelchair and wheelchair-to-chair transfers.

4. Assist Bill in leaving the home a minimum of one afternoon per week for swimming and socializing.

The OTR and the COTA returned the next day and discussed the treatment plan with Bill and his wife. After explaining how the various activities would be accomplished, both Bill and his wife agreed to the goals and the plan was implemented.

Work on the first three goals was initiated immediately. The OTR and COTA had brought various pieces of adapted equipment, which they had previously determined would help in Bill's self-care. They discussed use of these items with Bill and his wife, and they chose those they thought would be most helpful. Decision-making opportunities such as these allowed Bill to take a more active role in his self-care and transfers and also gave him a sense of control over other events.

The therapist and the assistant then demonstrated proper transfer techniques and body mechanics to both Bill and his wife. This approach assured safety and the prevention of back injuries for Bill's wife.

One-handed dressing techniques that would allow Bill to dress himself were demonstrated. It was agreed that the COTA would see Bill three mornings each week to reinforce the dressing program.

The final goal, assisting Bill to leave his home for short periods, presented the biggest challenge. After inspecting the home and studying the design, construction of a traditional ramp was ruled out. To solve this problem, the OTR and COTA designed a system of portable metal runner ramps and an electric winch, which could be installed and removed in minutes[7]. This technique made it possible to help Bill in and out of the house safely and easily. This system is illustrated in Figure 25-1.

Each Thursday afternoon, the occupational therapy team took Bill to a local health club and spa for a swim, steambath and a shower. Bill looked forward to these weekly outings with great enthusiasm. His depression lifted and he would often state: "It's great to be alive." In addition to the psychological boost, the swimming session provided buoyancy to support Bill's left side. This buoyancy also allowed an increase in passive range of motion that could not be achieved out of the water. Both the therapist and the assistant worked with Bill during these sessions in the pool.

After the visit to the health club, Bill, the COTA and the OTR would stop at Bill's favorite bar and grill for a meal and a drink. Bill would often meet old friends, many of whom he had not seen since he became ill, and would spend time socializing. This time "out with the boys" would prove to be the best therapy for Bill.

Although he never denied that he would soon die, Bill began to believe that he would regain function of his left side. He convinced himself that the swimming, which allowed him to stand, as well as his increased independence in self-care, were sure signs of improvement. This situation

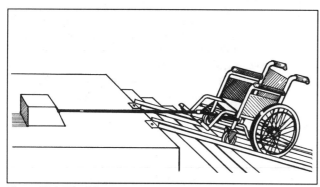

Figure 25-1. *Wheelchair ramp.*

is common among hospice patients and must be dealt with honestly by the therapist and the assistant.

One day, on the way to the health club, Bill asked when he could expect full return of function to his flaccid limbs. The COTA and OTR had to deal with this false hope by stating very frankly that there would be no return no matter how much exercise he undertook.

Bill cried heavily when he heard this information. The treatment team parked the car and allowed Bill to continue crying. When he had composed himself, he said "I didn't want to hear that, but it's better than not knowing for sure. Thanks for being straight with me."

Three weeks later, when the OTR and COTA came to pick Bill up for swimming, his wife, who was crying, met them at the door. Her husband had lapsed into a coma earlier in the day and the hospice physician told her that he would probably die within a few hours. The therapist and the assistant stayed with her to provide comfort and support. Two hours after they arrived, Bill died.

The OTR, after checking vital signs, determined that Bill was dead. The COTA called the hospice to notify them and stayed with Bill's wife offering continued support. Bill's wife was so upset that she was unable to call the funeral home to make the proper arrangements, so the COTA made the call. Both the OTR and COTA assisted Bill's wife in choosing the suit in which Bill would be buried. At the wake, Bill's wife introduced the COTA and OTR to family and friends and at her request, they both served as pallbearers at Bill's funeral.

After the graveside services, a funeral breakfast was held, which both the assistant and the therapist attended. It was here that the case was discontinued. By saying good-bye to both Bill and his family through ritual funeral attendance, the treatment could be considered at an end and closure complete.

Case Study II—John

John, a 72-year-old retired grocer with a diagnosis of lung cancer with subsequent metastases to the brain and spine, was referred for occupational therapy evaluation by the hospice visiting nurse.

The COTA and OTR made an initial visit to meet with John and his wife. John was lying on the couch in the living room when the occupational therapy team arrived. The therapist performed an occupational history and sensory motor evaluation while the COTA observed and assisted.

The occupational history indicated that John was a "homebody" with few interests. However, he did enjoy going for drives in the country or to an occasional movie. Since he had become ill, he had little desire to do anything but watch television because he was "too weak and tired to do anything." His wife stated that although he had generalized weakness of his right side, he was physically able to care for himself, but he chose not to get dressed and received only an occasional sponge bath from his wife if she "nagged" him.

From the information obtained in this first meeting, the OTR and COTA outlined the following program, which would be carried out twice a week by the assistant with input and supervision by the therapist as needed:

Short-Term Goals:
● John will shower and dress daily within one week.
● John will engage in a leisure/social activity of his choice two times a week at home.

Long-Term Goal:
● John will attend a movie or go for a ride in a car with the COTA at least one time.

The following day the assistant arrived at John's home and found him watching television. He asked John if he might be more comfortable sitting in a reclining chair that was by a window. The patient agreed and was assisted in walking to the chair. The COTA then presented the treatment plan for John's approval.

John stated that he would like to shower and dress, but because he was so weak, both tasks were difficult and he was also afraid that he might fall in the shower. He also stated that he had no leisure interests. In regard to the long-term goal, John stated that he did not want to be seen in public in his condition and was happy to stay indoors.

The COTA then explained to John that he could teach him alternate methods of dressing that would allow him to dress himself while expending as little energy as possible. In terms of the shower, the assistant explained that many assistive devices were available to make the process easy and safe. John agreed to "give the plan a try."

It had been previously determined by the COTA and confirmed by the OTR that John could benefit from a long-handled bath brush and an adapted tub seat[7] to aid in showering (Figure 25-2). The assistant removed these items from the car and carefully explained how the equipment could be used. The assistant then asked John if he would like to shower and he replied "You mean right now?" John carefully inspected the tub seat and asked the assistant if he was sure it was safe. When the COTA assured him that it would be, he agreed to try. It should be noted that it is important in hospice practice to engage the patient in activity as quickly as possible because treatment time is at a premium and must be used effectively.

The COTA assisted John to the bathroom and asked his

wife to accompany them. He demonstrated to both of them how to install and remove the tub seat, as well as the proper transfer techniques. John, who was initially skeptical about this activity, remained in the shower for 30 minutes and repeatedly commented regarding how "great" it felt and that he wanted to shower on a daily basis from then on.

After the shower, the assistant demonstrated dressing techniques that John could accomplish easily and independently while seated in an armchair. Once dressed, John looked in the mirror and told the assistant that he felt like "a human again."

The COTA assisted John with his self-care program for the next three days and he became totally independent. While dressing on the third day, John told the COTA that he enjoyed playing poker but had not played since he had become ill, partly because his "poker buddies had stopped coming around," and also because he didn't want anyone to see him "like this." He stated that he would like to play again and the assistant encouraged this activity, indicating that they would discuss it further on the next visit.

After each visit, the COTA recorded accurate notes on the patient's physical and psychological status and any progress achieved in relation to the established goals of the treatment plan. These notes were discussed with the OTR on a weekly basis and also signed by the therapist. Because the self-care goals had been met in a short period of time, the therapist encouraged the COTA to pursue the poker game as a leisure activity leading to social interaction.

At the next meeting with John, the assistant played a few hands of poker with him after he had showered and dressed. During the game, John talked constantly and expressed feelings of remorse about how he missed his weekly poker games with his friends, which allowed him to socialize, relax and "get away from the little woman for awhile." The COTA asked him if he would like to invite his friends over some night for a 'real' game. John was apprehensive and hedged on the answer. The assistant, not wanting to press him and damage the rapport and trust that had been established, told John to think about it and then changed the subject.

The next day, John told the COTA that he had thought about the game and decided he would like to do it. Together, he and the assistant made plans to schedule the game for the following week. The patient became more excited as the planning process continued and called to invite two of his friends that day. He also indicated that he would like the assistant to be present at the card party.

While John remained in the living room, the COTA explained the plan to his wife who was in the den. He asked her if she could make plans to go out that evening. She readily agreed, as she had not been out of the house since her husband had become ill. She immediately went to the living room and informed her husband of her plans to go out. John responded, "Good, that will give me a chance to visit with my friends." This particular interchange was significant because it gave John a feeling of control and a sense of having a "normal" poker game.

The night of the game, while John and the COTA were

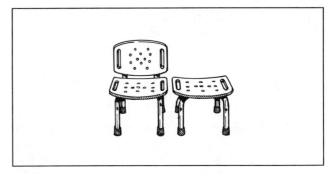

Figure 25-2. *Adapted tub seats.*

setting up, he asked the assistant whether, now that he was able to function independently and was living a relatively normal life, he would be able to "beat" his cancer and resume life as it had been. The assistant knowing the tenet of diagnostic honesty, told him that his cancer was far too advanced to be treated. He also stressed the importance of the fact that it was still possible for John to make the most of the time he had left. John was noticeably hurt by this response and said, "But I thought that I was getting better." The COTA responded, "You have gotten better in terms of what you can do, regardless of your disease, but you can't make your cancer go away." John began to weep and then said, "Well, this isn't going to ruin my night. Nobody is going to bring me down without a fight!"

The poker game was a success and John had "one of the best nights of my life." He was even able to tell his friends that although he wasn't going to live much longer, they were welcome to come by and play cards anytime.

The next week, when the COTA arrived at John's home, he found him on the couch, not feeling well. John told the assistant that he felt weak and didn't want to do anything. When asked if he would like the assistant to stay and talk, he agreed. They discussed the poker game and John smiled at the memories. During the conversation, John had a seizure and lapsed in and out of consciousness. Sensing that John would die soon, the COTA went to inform his wife of the situation. John also sensed that he was dying and took this last opportunity to tell his wife that he loved her and to say good-bye.

While John and his wife were talking, the COTA recognized their need for privacy and left them alone for a brief period. He then called the hospice physician and the OTR to inform them of the turn of events. When he returned to the living room, John was dead. The assistant comforted John's wife and checked her husband's **vital signs** (pulse, respiration and temperature)[6], determining that he had in fact died. The COTA then covered John's body and led his wife to the kitchen where he remained to console her until other hospice staff arrived. Before he left, the COTA removed the bath bench and brush to spare John's wife any unnecessary future visits.

Although John ultimately died, the COTA helped him to achieve a better quality of life in the time that was left to him. Without occupational therapy intervention, John would have remained immobile on his couch and would not have experienced some of life's pleasures.

Summary

The hospice philosophy is the most innovative model of treatment developed in the 20th century. As the hospice model departs substantially from traditional medical and rehabilitative attitudes and values, a reconstruction of the roles of occupational therapy practitioners, particularly the COTA, has been outlined in depth. The tenets of hospice care point out the important elements of medical management of pain and symptoms, the importance of diagnostic honesty, and the need to maintain quality of life for the terminally ill patient. The occupational therapy model of occupational behavior is used as a framework for the delivery of services. The occupational therapy process is modified to some degree because the therapeutic intervention time is limited. Case study examples illustrate the many ways in which occupational therapy can help the terminally ill *live* before they die.

Related Learning Activities

1. Organize a panel discussion with peers relative to:

   a. Different religious beliefs about death and life after death

   b. Various family traditions regarding wakes, funerals, memorial services, burials and shiva

2. Interview an OTR or a COTA who has worked with terminally ill patients to determine:

   a. Roles, functions and goals of treatment and how they compare with those of hospice care

   b. Feelings about working with this type of patient

3. Read a book or article that deals with death, grief and bereavement and present a report to your peers.

References

1. Tigges K, Sherman L, Sherwin F: Perspectives on the pain of the hospice patient: The role of the occupational therapist and the physician. *Occup Ther Health Care* 4:55-68, 1984.

2. Tigges K: Occupational therapy in hospice. In Corr CA, Corr DM, (Eds): *Hospice Care Principles and Practice.* New York, Springer, 1983, pp 160-176.

3. Entry-level role delineation for OTR's and COTA's. *Occup Ther Newspaper* 35:8-16, 1981.

4. American Occupational Therapy Association: Entry-level role delineation for occupational therapists, registered, (OTRs) and certified occupational therapy assistants (COTAs). *Am J Occup Ther* 44:1091-1102, 1990.

5. Tigges K, Sherwin F: Implications of the pawn-origin theory for hospice care. *Am J Hospice Care* 2:29-32, 1984.

6. Miller BF, Keane CB: *Encyclopedia and Dictionary of Medicine, Nursing, and Allied Health*, 5th Edition. Philadelphia, WB Saunders, 1992.

7. Tigges KN, Marcil WM, Alterio, CJ: *Caring for Someone in Your Home.* Buffalo, New York, Mast Health Group, 1992.

Chapter 26

Driver Assessment and Education for the Disabled

Dana Hutcherson, MOT, OTR

Introduction

This chapter provides information about occupational therapy intervention for evaluation and treatment of the daily living skill of driving. Characteristics and credentials of occupational therapy practitioners, administrative considerations for development and implementation of an adapted driving program, a theoretical framework and the intervention process are discussed. Suggested assessment tools and treatment techniques are also presented. The complexity of driving and the intervention process prevents a complete description of these aspects within this text; therefore, the reader is advised to use the resources identified for further information.

Background

In many societies an individual's success may depend on one's ability to travel from the residence to the work place. One's **self-esteem** (respect for or a favorable impression of oneself) may be associated with independence, which may relate to the ability to drive a motor vehicle. This interest in driving affects most age groups that are eligible to obtain a driver's license. Adolescents may view driving as an important factor in their transition to adulthood. Older adults depend on their ability to drive to gain access to basic needs or to maintain their sense of self-worth. Individuals with disabilities are exceptionally challenged when they are

---

KEY CONCEPTS

Characteristics of OT practitioners	Assessments
Credentials	Treatment
Program development and implementation	Discharge and follow-up
	Case illustration
Theoretical framework	

---

unable to provide their own transportation in pursuit of vocational or leisure goals.

Traditional therapeutic programs have increased their services for the past 10 to 15 years in an effort to recognize the value of occupational therapy intervention for transportation needs. These programs incorporate driving and using public transportation as occupational performance areas. The types of services may vary from assessment, training and equipment modification, to research.

In an "assessment only" program, the occupational therapist (OTR) and certified occupational therapy assistant (COTA) conduct in-clinic evaluations of skills and determine the individual's strengths and weaknesses related to driving and knowledge of public transportation services. Generally, a referral is made to another facility that can provide on-the-road testing and training. Some rehabilitation programs provide both clinical and on-the-road evaluations to determine if experienced drivers may return to driving.

Driver retraining may be provided to those experienced drivers who need therapeutic intervention. Often, a new driver with disabilities may need special testing and training. Some rehabilitation programs that provide both clinical and on-road evaluation and training have qualified instructors who work with new drivers. Other rehabilitation programs conduct driver assessment, training, **equipment modification** (alteration of the vehicle and or its controls) and research. A team of OTRs, COTAs, rehabilitation engineers, driver educators and vehicle modifiers provide services while tracking the assessments, training, equipment needs and modifications for specific disabilities. Research from these services helps in the developing training programs that best meet the needs of disabled drivers. Research programs are often located within a university model of driver assessment and training.

Additional models of driver assessment and training include the public schools, commercial driver schools and hospital or rehabilitation facility-based programs. Public schools rarely have the personnel and equipment available to serve special needs students. Commercial schools may have driver educators who are knowledgeable about adapted equipment use, but have little training or knowledge of etiology and assessment of disabilities. The medical model of hospital or rehabilitation facility-based programs provides an advantage with an appropriate assessment and training team approach. Communications between evaluators and trainers facilitate the identification of skill areas for specific training.

All programs' provision of services depend on personnel qualifications, equipment availability and allotted treatment times. These programs may advocate for disabled drivers' rights as well. Further development is needed in the areas of automobile insurance for the disabled, insurance reimbursement for the therapeutic services of driver evaluations and

training, consistent licensing requirements, vehicle manufacturing with the disabled in mind and availability of reasonably priced equipment.[1]

Occupational Therapy Practitioners

Characteristics and Abilities

Occupational therapists and assistants who work with disabled drivers must possess unique characteristics and abilities that promote the best performance from their patients. A thorough understanding of state **driver licensing regulations**, including reexamination, driver restrictions and medical review board procedures is necessary. The OTR conducting predriving evaluations needs a knowledge of traffic safety principles and evaluating driving potential. The evaluator should communicate to the patient the positive and negative findings of evaluations, relate how the evaluation information reflects driving skills, share concerns identified through the predriving phase of evaluation and discuss the skill performance necessary during the behind-the-wheel evaluation to confirm safe operation of a motor vehicle. At the same time, the therapist must convey an understanding of the patient's fear in loss of his or her license and assure the individual that the goal is to provide assistance in reaching the maximum level of independence.

The COTA conducting behind-the-wheel evaluations must maintain an open mind to a patient's potential for driving. Dysfunction in driving during the evaluation phase must be analyzed for cause and potentials for remediation identified. Prognosis in driving potentials can no more be predicated than those in other therapeutic processes, and the patient should be given sufficient opportunity to develop safe performance sklls. Driving evaluators must possess and display confidence in their own skills for an alertness to performance, prediction and reaction to quick-changing situations, while maintaining a calm, collected demeanor.

The therapist or assistant must clearly communicate recommendations for equipment use, **licensure restrictions** (limitations on driving such as day only, use of glasses, etc.) or the most difficult of tasks, the inabilities of a patient to continue or return to driving. The most challenging situations for occupational therapy practitioners may be to inform elderly patients that they no longer possess the skills necessary for safe operation of a vehicle. The challenge increases when the patient must be convinced to use alternative means of transportation and resources are not available for alternatives. Therapists often want the local department of motor vehicles (DMV) to be responsible in refusing licensure; however, the therapist may know more about a patient's abilities than those detected by a DMV inspector during one on-road evaluation.

A thorough activity analysis will guide the therapist and

assistant in the evaluation process. Knowledge of the effects of disabilities on driving is helpful in identifying specific evaluation areas. Knowledge of assessments for visual, perceptual, cognitive and motor skills sets apart the services of an occupational therapy adapted driving program from those offered by many commercial schools and licensing agencies.

Credentials

States vary in the credentials required for driving evaluators and instructors. State agencies that regulate individuals and facilities conducting driver evaluation and training may include the state department of education, state department of commerce, state department of motor vehicles, or rehabilitation service agencies. The Association of Driver Educators for the Disabled has established a program to recognize professional credentials and experience. Practitioners who plan to conduct predriving evaluations are not necessarily required to have proper credentials, but a thorough knowledge of the driving task is essential for analysis of skills performance. Therapists and assistants are advised to receive instruction in the teaching of driver education through a college, university or agency such as the American Automobile Association, National Safety Council or American Association of Retired Persons (AARP).

Administrative Program Development and Implementation

Developing a driving program for the disabled can be extremely frustrating and costly if research, planning, administration and medical support are inadequate. A needs assessment for potential referral sources and patient populations is vital in founding a program that will grow and produce revenue.

The administrator must consider several factors in deciding to develop a driving program versus contracting for services from an already established program. Commitment is essential to finance and support the program; the departmental budget must be able to absorb some expenses; the referral base should be varied for many diagnostic groups and age ranges; and, staff must be trained and interested in providing the service.[2] **Liability** (legal responsibility) and risk management must be documented. Time must be invested to gain knowledge in the proper forms and procedures for meeting commercial and governmental regulations. Long-term and short-term plans for marketing and expenses must be outlined.

Under the guidelines of governing agencies, the program services are designed to meet patient population groups. If new drivers, especially those under certain age limits, are to be evaluated and trained, then special credentials, qualifications of staff and licenses may be necessary.

The patient population will also dictate the equipment needs for an evaluation/training vehicle. Therapists and assistants with little experience in driving evaluations or training may be less threatened by limiting the services to car use rather than a modified van; thus limiting the patient population to those who can transfer or are ambulatory.

Reimbursement (repayment of costs) for services is the most challenging aspect of program implementation. The administrator must pursue as many reimbursement agencies as possible. Examples of these agencies may include the state department of rehabilitative services, local or regional vocational training agencies and school systems that do not have the resources to provide driver training to disabled students. Seeking reimbursement for the older population is particularly difficult. Medicare has been reluctant to identify driving as one of the activities of daily living, and third-party payers have the tendency to follow Medicare's lead. The therapist and assistant must document to the best of their ability the functional skills performance as related to driving. A direct communication and explanation of driving services with the Medicare intermediary may prove helpful.

Theoretical Framework

An **occupational behavior** framework may guide the therapist and assistant in the evaluation and treatment of an individual's ability to drive. As described in the companion volume to this text, the occupational behavior framework focuses on the individual's achievement, roles, play and work.[3]

An individual's achievement is based on the developmental process, influenced by one's abilities, interests, skills and habits. A child who develops the ability to control a tricycle, a bicycle or a scooter is developing skills related to the driving task. Speed control, depth perception, awareness of spatial relations and equipment manipulation are necessary for success in learning to drive. The disabled child must be provided with opportunities to develop these skills. Creative **mobility toys** (wagons, scooters, peddle cars, etc.) or adapted cycles provide sensory motor training related to the driving task.[4,5]

The child's habits carry over to habits of driving. The habit of looking both ways before crossing a street is an essential habit for driving. The child who never experiences independence in crossing the street, whether by wheelchair, crutches or scooter, may have difficulties in learning the task of driving.

As an individual matures, interests and concerns in driving develop with life roles: adolescent, young adult, worker and retirees. Successful driving is identified with the transition from adolescence to adulthood. Successful transition into the worker role often depends on successful driving skills, and the ability to continue to drive becomes a concern with the transition into elderly years.

The experienced driver who acquires a disability may be served through the occupational behavior framework. The OTR and COTA determine strengths and weaknesses related to driving by identifying achievements after an injury or illness. A history of premorbid abilities, interests, skills and habits as related to driving will guide the therapist and assistant in thinking of driving potentials. The patient's roles, leisure activities and work history will influence the occupational therapy practitioner in planning driver assessment and training. For example, the 55-year-old realtor diagnosed with a cerebral vascular accident who was responsible for driving customers during the work day presents a combination of factors identified through the occupational behavior framework.

In summary, the occupational behavior framework works well in guiding occupational therapy intervention for mobility independence. The next section presents an example of this intervention process.

Occupational Therapy Intervention

Referral

Requests for service may be for predriving, clinical assessments, behind-the-wheel assessments, equipment recommendations, driver training and consultation to public or commercial school driver educators for adapted teaching techniques. The OTR and COTA may work together in receiving these orders. The OTR conducts in-clinic predriving evaluations with patients to identify abilities and limitations in behind-the-wheel potentials. The COTA who has secured driving instructor experience and credentials, if required, may assist in the assessment process by observing behaviors during a functional behind-the-wheel evaluation. Orders to provide driver training may be received directly by the COTA conducting the on-road retraining or instruction.

Referral sources may include physicians, rehabilitation agencies schools, parents and self-referrals. Examples of these sources include the following:

1. *Physiatrists*: For patients with spinal cord injury, cerebral vascular accident, traumatic brain injury and other disorders
2. *Pediatricians*: May refer adolescents (in collaboration with schools) for providing special education services
3. *School personnel*: May seek occupational therapy services for equipment recommendations or consultation relative to adapted teaching techniques
4. *Gerontologists*: For patients who need assistance with the effects of aging
5. *State and local departments of rehabilitation and*

independent living centers: Clients seeking assistance in developing mobility independence
6. *Parents*: For children needing special equipment and additional training for successful completion of driver education
7. *Individuals*: To meet needs for independent transporation

Referral information should include the patient's name, age, diagnosis, disabling symptoms and any special equipment needs. A list of prescribed medications and possible effects on driving should accompany the referral information.

The Assessment Process

The assessment process includes screening of the person's need for intervention and evaluation of abilities and disabilities. Treatment plans are based on the findings of the assessment process. Techniques or issues for each step of the assessment process are discussed in the following sections.

Screening

Information is obtained by using observation, interviews and formal reports to determine if occupational therapy intervention would be beneficial to the patient in achieving greater mobility independence. COTAs are a vital link in the screening process, as their work with these individuals in traditional treatment programs often provides necessary information. Tools used by the COTA to assist in the screening process include Driving Questionnaire and the Daily Driving Diary.[6] A number of other screening tools have also been developed by several agencies and rehabilitation centers.[7]

The occupational therapist must have a thorough knowledge of state regulations for driver licensing and educational requirements for new drivers to assure that the appropriate information is collected. The OTR seeks information to identify deficits that may be influenced by occupational therapy intervention. This information may include the following:

1. Proof of licensure status for those with previous driving experience
2. Possession of a valid license or instruction permit to participate in on-road, behind-the-wheel evaluations
3. For some states, the driver education information of individuals under the age of 19 years
4. Biographical data such as past medical history, medications prescribed and effects on driving
5. Persons able to provide support in assisting the patient in driving outside of the occupational therapy intervention process

6. Reimbursement source
7. Additional information that would assist in compliance with state regulations for a driver's license
8. A physician's medical approval for driving assessment

The occupational therapist's decisions for providing services, choosing appropriate evaluations and estimating the duration of intervention are based on this information obtained during the screening process.

Intake Process

Once the patient is accepted for occupational therapy intervention, a formal intake process is initiated. The following factors must be brought to the patient's attention and documented:

1. Legal issues concerning consent for participation
2. Responsibility for risks assumed in participation
3. Consent for information release to referral source and possibly the state department of motor vehicles
4. Final licensure requirements by the department of motor vehicles
5. Expectations for compliance during the program

An informal consent contract, as shown in Figures 26-1 and 26-2, may be necessary to document the patient's understanding of the issues. States may have regulations for driver reevaluation or physician's approval after a change in medical status that influences the patient's need for driver assessment. A form is shown in Figure 26-3. Applications for special permits or record transcripts should also be considered. Figure 26-4 presents an example of the latter. An example of a special permit form may be found in the case study which follows. The COTA may be responsible for the entire intake process.

Evaluations

Predriving Evaluation. Before a functional driving evaluation is administered, the occupational therapist should assess the patient's prior level of functioning as well as the current level of functioning. The therapist uses information from the screening process and additional data through the formal in-clinic evaluations. The data provide objective measures of the patient's abilities and assists the therapist in formulating an approach to the functional driving evaluation and treatment planning process.

A comprehensive occupational therapy evaluation is performed, which focuses on physical, perceptual and cognitive abilities. The following data are obtained:

1. Present type of vehicle, if any
2. Previous driving record
3. Home situation for accesssing a vehicle
4. Neuropsychological tests completed
5. Communication skills for understanding traffic signs
6. General mental status

7. Joint range of motion
8. Muscle strength
9. Coordination
10. Sensation
11. Balance
12. Ability to transfer

The patient's diagnosis may indicate specific types of evaluations to be administered. Deficits or difficulties noted during the predriving evaluations are recorded and presented to the driving evaluator conducting the behind-the wheel evaluations. The driving evaluator attempts to confirm or negate the effects of predriving difficulties on actual driving skills.

Standardized evaluations and driver testing equipment have been used to predict driver potentials for various disabilities. These tests, including psychological evaluations, must be administered by properly trained personnel. An example of such tests is the visual screening test administered to determine the patient's potential for passing the visual requirements of most departments of motor vehicles. Many testing devices are used for measuring a patient's reaction time, depth perception, glare recovery, danger perception, scanning abilities and certain perceptual and cognitive abilities.[8,9] COTAs may assist in the administration of predriving evaluations by conducting these objective assessments, once the required level of competence has been demonstrated.

The OTR administers other standardized assessments helpful in predicting a patient's driving potential, including the Motor-Free Visual Perceptual Test; the Picture Completion, Digit Span, Picture Arrangement, Block Design, and Digit Symbol subtests of the Weschler Adult Intelligence Scale-Revised; the Trailmaking Test, Parts A and B; the Minnesota Rate of Manipulation Tests; and the Minnesota Spatial Relations Test. Driving simulators have also been developed for testing and training disabled drivers.[10-13]

The occupational therapist conducts predriving evaluations to predict potentials of disabled individuals to drive and identify deficits that may interfere in safe operation of a motor vehicle. An example of a form used is presented in the case study, which appears later in the chapter.

Behind-the-Wheel Evaluation. The assessment process must include actual attempts at driving, using adapted equipment as necessary, to determine the patient's abilities to safely operate a vehicle with modifications. If additional modifications are required, the OTR and COTA should collaborate and a follow-up session should be scheduled. A decision regarding actual driving abilities should be made after a functional behind-the-wheel evaluation has been conducted as outlined in Figure 26-5 or after several predriving evaluations have indicated consistent behaviors that interfere in the individual's potential for driving. A COTA who is a certified driving evaluator may conduct the behind-the-wheel evaluation.

Johnston-Willis Hospital
Occupational Therapy Department
Driving Assessment and Educational Program

<u>Consent for Driver Assessment / Education</u>

I, _____ , will be receiving driver assessment and/or training through the Johnston-Willis Hospital Driver Assessment and Educational Program for the purpose of determining my abilities to safely operate a motor vehicle. I agree to participate in the program procedures as prescribed by my Registered Occupational Therapist who is a certified driving instructor.

I will assume all risks to participate in this program and do not hold Johnston-Willis Hospital administrators and staff responsible for any claims which may occur as a result of my participation in this program.

I understand that my completion of this program does not guarantee my reciept of a driver's license from the VDMV.

I also understand that my physician and/or Johnston-Willis Hospital's driving instructor may (based upon their professional judgment) terminate my involvement in the driver's program.

_____	_____
signature of patient	signature of witness
_____	_____
signature of parten/guardian if patient is a minor or unable to sign	title
	_____
	address of witness
_____	_____
Date	relationship to patient

Explanation of authorizing signature: (minor, disability, etc.)

Figure 26-1. *Consent form for Driver Assessment/Education.*

Johnston-Willis Hospital
Occupational Therapy Department
Driving Assessment and Educational Program

<u>Authorization for Release of Information</u>

Patient's Name: _____

                    (Last)   (First)   (Middle)

Social Security Number:_____

Information Released to:

        The Virginia Division of Motor Vehicles
        2300 West Broad St., P.O. Box 27412
        Richmond, VA 23269

The purpose of this release is to provide information to the VDMV in obtaining medical clearance for driving. This will allow JWH staff to complete driver assessment and education and make the necessary recommendations as to the patient's driving skills and equipment needs.

I am permitting the release of the following information:

1. Information and recommendations to physicians and VDMV from my driver's assessment and educational program.

2. Return of information from the VDMV including a copy of my driving record (if applicable, may require a $3.00 fee) to the Occupational Therapy Department for necessary planning and delivery of services.

Date:_____   Signature: _____

                    Witness: _____

Figure 26-2. *Authorization form for release of information.*

DL191 (1/91)

SAMPLE

CUSTOMER'S MEDICAL REPORT

CUSTOMER INSTRUCTIONS

1. Complete this side of report with all the information that applies to you.
2. Sign in the space provided below.
3. Have your physician complete the applicable sections on the back of the form and mail it to DMV.

CUSTOMER INFORMATION

Name		Birth Date	DL/SS Number	
Residence Address		City	State	Zip Code
Mailing Address		City	State	Zip Code

Please describe your medical impairment in detail: _____

_____

BLACKOUT INFORMATION

Have you experienced a blackout, seizure, loss of consciousness, or syncope? ☐ Yes ☐ No

If yes, when did the episode occur: _____

Explain what happened during the episode: _____

MEDICATION INFORMATION

NAME OF MEDICINE	DOSAGE	TIME(S) TAKEN

RELEASE INFORMATION

I hereby authorize _____, a licensed physician to complete this certification and, if necessary, to provide further clarification or information about my physical condition. I consent to the Virginia Department of Motor Vehicles using this information in arriving at a decision concerning my ability to operate a motor vehicle safely.

NOTE: The personal information requested is for the proper identification of your records on file in this office. In accordance with the Virginia Privacy Protection Act of 1976.

Customer's Signature and Authorization (Parent must sign for minor.)	Date

Figure 26-3. *Customer medical report form.*

PHYSICIAN INSTRUCTIONS -- This form must be completed by a licensed physician.

Physician must: 1. Complete all applicable sections.

                2. MAIL the completed form to the Medical Control Section, Driver Licensing and Information Division, Department of Motor Vehicles, P. O. Box 27412, Richmond, Virginia 23269-0001.

    NOTE: THE EXAMINATION MUST HAVE BEEN WITHIN 30 DAYS FROM THE DATE OF THIS REPORT.

PATIENT'S INFORMATION

1. How long has customer been your patient? _____

2. What is your diagnosis? _____

PATIENTS WITH MENTAL OR PHYSICAL IMPAIRMENTS

1. Is there significant physical or mental disorders? ☐ Yes ☐ No   If yes, give details.

_____

2. Medications prescribed: _____

PATIENTS WITH SEIZURE DISORDERS

Is seizure disorder present? ☐ Yes ☐ No   If yes, complete the following:

A. Date of last episode: _____

B. History of previous episode(s): _____

C. EEG Results: _____

D. Medication prescribed: _____

E. Prognosis: _____

HOSPITAL INFORMATION

Has patient been hospitalized as a result of the above diagnosis? ☐ Yes ☐ No   If yes, complete the following:

A. Reason for admittance: _____

B. Dates hospitalized: _____

C. Patient's mental and/or physical ability when released: _____

PATIENT'S WITH VISUAL IMPAIRMENTS

1. The following section should be completed by an ophthalmologist or optometrist.

2. The examination should be conducted without the aid of a bioptic telescopic device.

Visual Acuity Without Glasses	Right Eye	Left Eye	Both Eyes	Horizontal Vision Field	Right Eye	Left Eye	Both Eyes
	20	20	20		°	°	°
Visual Acuity With Glasses	20	20	20	If one eye only	Temporal	Nasal	
					°	°	

PHYSICIAN'S INFORMATION

NAME	SIGNATURE	PHONE NO.
ADDRESS	CITY	STATE	ZIP CODE	DATE

PHYSICIAN PLEASE NOTE:

1. Is it permissible for DMV to release the information on this form to the patient? ☐ Yes ☐ No

2. If you have any questions, please call the DMV Staff Physician at (804) 367-6639 on Monday, Wednesday or Friday between 9 and 11 a.m.

Figure 26-3. *Continued*

DL 20 (REV. 8/85)

DEPARTMENT OF MOTOR VEHICLES

SAMPLE

CITIZEN REQUEST FOR DRIVING RECORD TRANSCRIPT

NAME _____
      (First)   (Middle)   (Last)

DATE OF BIRTH _____   SEX _____

DRIVER'S LICENSE NUMBER _____

ADDRESS _____
                        (Residence/Post Office Box)

        _____
                  (City)   (State)   (Zip Code)

INFORMATION NEEDED FOR:

	INSURANCE		EMPLOYMENT
	PERSONAL USE		EMPLOYMENT: TO OPERATE SCHOOL BUS

SIGNATURE _____

INDICATE BELOW IF YOU WISH TO AUTHORIZE ANOTHER INDIVIDUAL TO OBTAIN A COPY OF YOUR DRIVING RECORD:

☐ I Authorize the Department of Motor Vehicles to furnish a copy of my driving record to:

NAME _____
      (First)   (Middle)   (Last)

DATE OF REQUEST _____

FEE _____

Figure 26-4. *Request for driving record transcript form.*

Findings and Recommendations After the completion of all evaluations, the COTA should summarize the assessment data that have been gathered and report this information to the OTR. The occupational therapist reviews all assessment information and should note the implications of the deficits identified through the various evaluation procedures and use these findings as a basis for planning a strategy of instruction and/or rehabilitation. Data obtained from predriving assessments should be used as a guide for further assessment and training. Caution must be exercised in deciding a patient's driving abilities based entirely on one or two predriving evaluations or even an entire battery of predriving evaluations that show inconsistent behaviors. The COTA and the OTR may collaborate on the development of adapted equipment recommendations that may be required. After this assessment is completed, the findings and recommendations are documented.

Program Planning

The OTR, COTA, the patient and family work together to establish goals and in planning a program for meeting the long-term and short-term goals that address the difficulties noted during the assessment process. In addition to driving, the program may include other therapeutic activities designed to increase physical, cognitive and visual perceptual skills necessary for driving. The program plan may establish time lines for securing modified equipment and follow-up training in its use. Resource information is provided regarding vendors who install necessary equipment and/or make modifications and financial assistance providers. A referral to a rehabilitation agency may also be made if it is thought that the patient could benefit from additional services.

Treatment Implementation

The program plan guides the patient and occupational therapy practitioners in the treatment process, and the COTA may be responsible for implementing the treatment plan. The following activities are some that may be used:

1. Transfer training in accessing the vehicle
2. Wheelchair access by using lifts
3. Manual and electric equipment loading techniques
4. One-handed steering techniques or adapted methods for steering control using devices
5. Bilateral use of hands for performing two different activities at the same time (ie, left hand for brake and gas; right hand for steering)
6. On-the-road driver training using adapted equipment

Training may be provided initially on a small-scale vehicle such as a golf cart, modified with the necessary equipment. In-clinic treatment may incorporate computer activities that require integration of eye-hand coordination, perception of dangers and quick decision-making skills.

Discharge

The program is discontinued any of the following general objectives have been met:

1. Adapted equipment recommendations have been achieved.
2. Patient has achieved preestablished level of performance in meeting long-term and short-term goals.
3. Patient has plateaued in skills development.

The COTA may assist in the discharge process by providing information about equipment needs, skill performance progress or lack thereof and any recommendations relative to needs beyond the present occupational therapy intervention. The OTR includes this information in the discharge summary. This report may also include recommendations for driving licensure or licensure restrictions, if appropriate. The discharge summary is submitted to the referral source to assist the physician or agency in reaching decisions regarding licensure, equipment needs or additional ancillary services.

Follow-Up

Orders for equipment modifications may require equipment training after discharge. If the vehicle modifier is not trained or qualified to provide driver training in the use of adapted equipment, occupational therapy follow-up may be requested to confirm that the patient is able to operate the vehicle safely and to determine whether any adjustments are necessary.

In addition, general follow-up information should be gathered relative to the overall effectiveness of the occupational therapy services provided. Specific information is likely to include the patient's degree of success with driving, difficulties experienced when utilizing adapted equipment, and to what extent occupational therapy services have assisted in providing total independence in driving. This information may be used as a guide for modifying the program.

Case Study

Matthew, a 24-year-old electrician with **traumatic brain injury (TBI)** (wound to the brain from an external source), was referred to occupational therapy by his physiatrist for a

Johnston-Willis Hospital
Occupational Therapy Department
Driving Assessment and Educational Program

<u>Worksheet for Behind-the-Wheel Driving Assessment</u>

Name:_____

A. <u>Preparation for Travel</u> circle the "+" for satisfactory performance; circle the "-" for unsatisfactory performance; circle the "∆" if action was not observed.

+	-	∆	Turn key in Door	+	-	∆	Dimmer Switch, FL HC
+	-	∆	Open Door - Outside	+	-	∆	Operate Turn Signal
+	-	∆	Prepare for transfer	+	-	∆	Operate Horn
+	-	∆	Transfer	+	-	∆	Operate Temp. Control
+	-	∆	Load W/C etc. Time ____	+	-	∆	Operate Radio/Cassette
+	-	∆	Close Door	+	-	∆	Operate Window Knobs
+	-	∆	Adjust seat	+	-	∆	Fasten Seatbelt
+	-	∆	Adjust mirrors	+	-	∆	Start Engine
+	-	∆	Operate Door Locks	+	-	∆	Apply/Release Parking Brake
+	-	∆	Operate Window Washer	+	-	∆	Operate Gas/Brake, FL HC
+	-	∆	Operate Headlights	+	-	∆	Operate Gear Selector

Score Part A: _____ (Subtract total "-" from total "+"s) + (22 - total "∆" s).

B. <u>Driving Performance</u>: circle the "+" for satisfactory performance; circle the "-" for unsatisfactory performance; circle the "∆" if action was not observed.

	JWH Grounds	Residential	Freeway
Steering Control	+ - ∆	+ - ∆	+ - ∆
Hand Control Acceleration	+ - ∆	+ - ∆	+ - ∆
Hand Control Braking	+ - ∆	+ - ∆	+ - ∆
Foot Control Acceleration	+ - ∆	+ - ∆	+ - ∆
Foot Control Braking	+ - ∆	+ - ∆	+ - ∆
Straight Line Driving	+ - ∆	+ - ∆	+ - ∆
Straight Line Backing	+ - ∆		
Stopping Distance Control	+ - ∆	+ - ∆	
3-Point Turn Around	+ - ∆	+ - ∆	
U-Turns	+ - ∆	+ - ∆	
Figure 8 Maneuvers	+ - ∆		
Parking(Straight,Angle,Curb,Parallel)	+ - ∆	+ - ∆	
Speed Control	+ - ∆	+ - ∆	+ - ∆
Left Turns	+ - ∆	+ - ∆	
Right Turns	+ - ∆	+ - ∆	
Following Distances		+ - ∆	+ - ∆
Right-of-Way	+ - ∆	+ - ∆	+ - ∆
Lane Positioning	+ - ∆	+ - ∆	+ - ∆
Lane Changing		+ - ∆	+ - ∆
Passing Other Vehicles		+ - ∆	+ - ∆
Perceptive of Signs, Signals, Markings	+ - ∆	+ - ∆	+ - ∆
Enter/Exit Road and Freeways	+ - ∆	+ - ∆	+ - ∆
Perceptive of Potential Dangers	+ - ∆	+ - ∆	+ - ∆
Emergency Situations	+ - ∆	+ - ∆	+ - ∆
Defensive Driving	+ - ∆	+ - ∆	+ - ∆
Totals	⌐__⌐ max=22	⌐__⌐ max=23	⌐__⌐ max=17
Scores	_____	_____	_____

Figure 26-5. *Worksheet for behind-the-wheel driving assessment.*

driving reevaluation. He was receiving Workers' Compensation because his injury resulted from a fall while on the job. At the time of the referral, Matthew was living in an inner-city apartment, and he was dependent on specialized transportation for travel to and from the rehabilitation center.

Screening

Since Matthew had been seen in the occupational therapy department at the rehabilitation center, he had already undergone screening procedures that included observations, interviews and a review of previous documentation of his rehabilitation program. It was noted that a previous evaluation, earlier in the recovery process, indicated that the he was lacking in vehicle control for lane positioning. Other findings revealed that the patient had improved significantly since his admission to the day rehabilitation program and seemed motivated to attempt driving again. The OTR concluded that the data indicated that Matthew was an appropriate candidate for occupational therapy intervention in driving skills.

Intake Process

The COTA conducted the intake process for the driving evaluation. Program objectives were discussed with Matthew who stated that his main reason for returning to driving was to be able to return to work. The assistant gave him the facility's Consent for Driver Assessment/Education form, which Matthew signed, documenting his agreement to participate in the program. This agreement stated that he assumed all risks involved in his participation and that he understood that participation did not guarantee that he would regain his driver's license. Signing of the form also indicated his agreement to comply with the directions of the therapist/evaluator (see Figure 26-1). The COTA also discussed confidentiality and requested Matthew's permission to send his physician's report and his current medical report to the state's Department of Motor Vehicles upon completion of the driving evaluation (see Figures 26-2 and 26-3). He was told that after receipt of these reports, the DMV requirements for driver retesting and medical approval to continue driving would be received.

During the in-take process, Matthew indicated a memory loss when questioned about specific time periods in his driving experience. The assistant requested a transcript of his driving record, which indicated eight years of driving, a record of maximum safe driving points, and one conviction for improper passing (see Figure 26-4). An application for special parking permits was completed and forwarded to Matthew's physician for approval. The intake interview also revealed Matthew's prescribed medications, which potentially could have adverse effects on his driving, were not administered at high doses.

A review of Matthew's past medical history indicated the following: visual problems requiring glasses since the age of 2 years and required for driving, family history of diabetes and no seizure incidents.

Matthew's driving history revealed that he posessed a valid driver's license, which had not been revoked after his accident, but was due to expire within eight months. He had completed driver education in high school. Matthew reported that he had not driven during the two years since his injury. His vehicle was a five-speed, manual transmission model that was inappropriate for continued use because of his left upper extremity level of functioning. He lived alone in his ground floor apartment, and his vehicle was parked curbside about 40 feet from his door on a flat, paved parking lot. All intake information was recorded on the Predriving Evaluation form and turned over to the OTR assigned to in-clinic predriving assessments (Figure 26-6). After completing the first day of intake activities, the COTA scheduled Matthew for a two-hour assessment session.

Assessment

The OTR met Matthew in the occupational therapy clinic, noting that he ambulated with a straight cane and exhibited severe tone in his nondominant left upper extremity and left lower extremity. The Visual Language Traffic Test and the General Mental Status Examination were administered, with scores of 95% and 100%, respectively. His joint range of motion was within normal limits (WNLs) for all active and passive movements with the following exceptions: active left shoulder flexion 0 to 10 degrees; shoulder abduction, 0 to 10 degrees; elbow flexion, 0 to 10 degrees;, and elbow extension, supination, pronation and wrist flexion, all 0 degrees. Therefore, functional limitations were severe in his left upper extremity. The OTR conferred with the physical therapist assigned to Matthew's case and collected data on the decreased functional use of his left lower extremity. Additional tests administered were the following:

1. Good-Lite Peripheral Vision Test
2. Porto Clinic Glare Tests (right-foot simple and complex reaction times, glare recovery, night accommodation and motor depth perception)
3. Titmus Vision Test (far acuity, color identification, depth perception, sign recognition and **heterophoria** (failure of the visual axes to remain parallel after stimuli have been eliminated[14]
4. Trailmaking—Parts A and B
5. Motor-Free Visual Perceptual Test
6. Minnesota Spatial Relations Test (A/B board only)
7. Wechsler Adult Intelligence Scale—Revised (subtests: Digit Span, Block Design, Picture Completion and Picture Arrangement)

The OTR scheduled Matthew for a functional behind-the-wheel evaluation with the COTA driving evaluator. All predriving assessment information was recorded on the Predriving Evaluation form and conveyed to the COTA. A portion of this form is presented in Figure 26-6.

Results of the in-car assessment indicated that Matthew could benefit from continued occupational therapy services for driver retraining to improve right-handed steering techniques using a spinner knob steering device. Equipment recommendations for a right side signal extension, spinner knob steering device (positioned at 4 o'clock), and automatic transmission were made for Matthew to consider when purchasing another vehicle. The most significant observation was that Matthew's left hand and arm would

Occupational Therapy Department
Driving Assessment and Educational Program
Johnston-Willis Hospital, Richmond, VA

Predriving Evaluation

Part I. Biographical Data Interview

Name: Mathew   Date: 4-10-xx   **Status:**
Address: 1401 JWH Ave   DOB: 5-17-xx   ☐ Inpatient REhab
         Richmond, Virginia 23235   Age: 24   ☐ Day Program
Phone:(W) 366-1645 (H) 379-9834   Sex: WM   ☐ Out Patient
SSN#: 226-74-4743   A/MR#:   700100   **Referral:**
Diagnosis: THI   BI#:   10022330   ☐ Physician Bonner

Marital St:	Single

☐ DRS _____
☐ Other _____

Past Medical History

				Hearing Aid: No

Dominance: right

Y N	Visual Probls.	2	Years w/dx	Glasses:	yes

Insurance:

Y N	Hearing Probls.	Y N	Fainting

☐ MediCareAid

Y N	Spasticity	Y N	Dizziness

Education: ☐ BC/FEP BC

Y N	Epilepsy	Y N	Convulsions

☐ Student   ☐ Other Work Comp

Y N	Diabetes	NO	Seizures

☐ High School Grad.   **Uses:**

Y N	Drugs/Alcohol	Y N	Contractures

☐ College-Certificate ☐ No Equipment

Y N	Heart Ailments	Y N	Behaviors

☐ Military Trained   ☐ St. Cane

Y N	Ambulates	Y N	Incontinent

☐ Vocational School
☐ Other

Driving Needs   ### Driving Record   ### Vehicle Descrip.   ### Medications*:

Driving Needs	Driving Record	Vehicle Descrip.	Medications*:
☐ To School	6 Years Driving	☐ No Vehicle	☐ None
☐ To work	3 Demerits	☐ Power Brake	☐ Antivert, Benadryl
☐ Job requires	? Safepts	☐ P Wind/Locks	☐ Bentyl, Cystospaz
☐ Independence	0 # MVAs	☐ Power Seat	☐ Parafon DSC, Robaxin
☐ Public	1 Violations	☐ Power Steer	☐ Percocet, Tylenol 3
transportation	Y N Dr Ed	☐ Bench Seat	☐ Robitussin AC
not accessible	Y N Copy Record	☐ Bucket Seat	☐ Donnagel PG
		☐ Manual	☐ Phenobarb, Tegreto
License Status		☐ Automatic	☐ Elabil, Desyrel
☐ Never Licensed		☐ Truck	☐ Mellaril, Thorazine
☐ Valid Lic/Perm		☐ Van	☐ Compazine, Phenergan
State VA # 226-74-4743		☐ 2-Door	☐ Valium, Xanax
		☐ 4-Door	☐ Dalmane, Halcion
Expires 4-30-xx		☐ VA Auto Ins	☐ Pilocar, Propine
☐ Invalid License		'87 Ford EXP	☐ Lioresol
☐ Restrictions * glasses			

Figure 26-6. *Pre-driving evaluation.*

Occupational Therapy Department
Driving Assessment and Educational Program
Johnston-Willis Hospital, Richmond, VA

<u>Pre-Driving Evaluation</u>

Part I.   Biographical Data Interview

Name: Mathew

Address: 1401 JWH Ave

              Richmond, Virginia 23235

Phone:(W) 366-1645   (H) 379-9834

SSN*: 226-74-4743

Diagnosis: THI

Date: 4-10-xx

DOB: 5-17-xx

Age: 24

Sex: WM

A/MR*: 700100

BI*:   10022330

<u>Status:</u>

☑ Inpatient REhab

☐ Day Program

☐ Out Patient

<u>Referral:</u>

☑ Physician <u>Bonner</u>

☐ DRS _____

☐ Other _____

Past Medical History

Ⓨ N	Visual Probls.	_2_	Years w/dx
Y Ⓝ	Hearing Probls.	Y Ⓝ	Fainting
Ⓨ N	Spasticity	Y Ⓝ	Dizziness
Y Ⓝ	Epilepsy	Y Ⓝ	Convulsions
Y Ⓝ	Diabetes	NO	Seizures
Y Ⓝ	Drugs/Alcohol	Y Ⓝ	Contractures
Y Ⓝ	Heart Ailments	Y Ⓝ	Behaviors
Ⓨ N	Ambulates	Y Ⓝ	Incontinent

_____

_____

Marital St: Single

Hearing Aid: No

Dominance: right

Glasses: yes

Education:

☐ Student

☑ High School Grad.

☐ College-Certificate

☐ Military Trained

☑ Vocational School

☐ Other

<u>Insurance:</u>

☐ MediCareAid

☐ BC/FEP BC

☑ Other <u>Work Comp</u>

<u>Uses:</u>

☐ No Equipment

☑ St. Cane

Driving Needs

☐ To School

☑ To work

☐ Job requires

☐ Independence

☐ Public
transportation
<u>not</u> accessible

License Status

☐ Never Licensed

☑ Valid Lic/Perm
    State <u>VA</u> * <u>226-74-4743</u>

              Expires <u>4-30-xx</u>

☐ Invalid License

☑ Restrictions *   glasses

Driving Record

_6_ Years Driving

_3_ Demerits

_?_ Safepts

_0_ * MVAs

_1_ Violations

Ⓨ N Dr Ed

Ⓨ N Copy Record

Vehicle Descrip.

☐ No Vehicle

☑ Power Brake

☐ P Wind/Locks

☐ Power Seat

☑ Power Steer

☐ Bench Seat

☑ Bucket Seat

☑ Manual

☐ Automatic

☐ Truck

☐ Van

☑ 2-Door

☐ 4-Door

☑ VA Auto Ins

'87 Ford EXP

Medications*:

☐ None

☐ Antivert, Benadryl

☐ Bentyl, Cystospaz

☐ Parafon DSC, Robaxin

☐ Percocet, Tylenol 3

☐ Robitussin AC

☐ Donnagel PG

☑ Phenobarb, Tegreto

☐ Elabil, Desyrel

☐ Mellaril, Thorazine

☐ Compazine, Phenergan

☐ Valium, Xanax

☐ Dalmane, Halcion

☐ Pilocar, Propine

☐ Lioresol

Figure 26-6. *Continued.*

Occupational Therapy Department
Driving Assessment and Educational Program
Johnston-Willis Hospital, Richmond, VA

Pre-Driving Evaluation

Part II.   Biographical Data Interview

Communication:

(Y) N   Verbal Intact _____
(Y) N   Nonverbal Intact _____
(Y) N   Language Intact _____
(Y) N   Speech Intact _____
(Y) N   Object Recognized _____
(Y) N   Follows Directions _____
(Y) N   Understands Phrases _____

General Mental Status:

0 x (Person) (Place) (Time) (Situation)
(Y) N   ST Memory Intact
(Y) N   LT Memory Intact

Coordination:

	LUE	RUE	
Gross Motor	intact	intact	Minnesota Rate of Manipulation
Fine Motor	intact	intact	9 hole peg test (total of 2 trials)

Sensation:

	LUE	RUE	LLE	RLE	Balance:
Light Touch	int	int	int	int	Sitting, static ___good___
Proprioception	abs	int	abs	int	Sitting, dynamic ___good___
Pain/Temp	int	int	int	int	Sit < - > Stand ind. using (R) UE push off
Stereognosis	int	int	int	int	

Home Situation:

Lives where ___Richmond, Apt.___
Lives with ___alone___

Y (N)   Garage
Y (N)   Curb Parking
(Y) N   Driveway
Y (N)   Bus Route Available _____
(Y) N   Transportation Service ___hospital van___
(Y) N   Family/Friend Driver ___several resources___

Y (N)   Door Opener
(Y) N   Curb Cut
Y (N)   Sloped   (Y) N   Paved

Transfers: (Y) N

Ambulates   (Y) N
WC < - > Car   (Ind) Dep

_____

_____

_____

_____

Figure 26-7. *Pre-driving evaluation, Part 2.*

<u>Cognitive, Visual/Perceptual/Motor:</u>

Part II. pg. 2

Visual Acuity	Daytime	Night time	Color perception	(3 /3)
Both Eyes	20 / 40 (20/40)	20 / 40 (>20/70)	Visual Depth Perc	(3 /3)
Right Eye	20 / 40 (20/40)		Sign Recognition	Pass Fail
Left Eye	20 / 40 (20/40)			

Lateral Phoria   6.5   Pass Fail (4-13)   Vertical Phoria   4   Pass Fail (3 - 5)

Field of Vision	Left Eye	Right Eye
nasal/temporal horizontal............	40 º 90 º (100º)	45 º 90 º (100º)
both eyes total degrees.................	135 º (135º)	

Night Accommodation ....   1.5   seconds (< 8 secs)

Glare Recovery   2   seconds (< 9 secs)

Motor Depth perception ....   1.5   " (≤ 3")

Reaction Times 33   seconds, simple (≤ .37 sec)

                     .54   seconds, complex (≤ .67 sec)

Visual Language Test ....   5 / 6   (≥ 4)

Mini – Mental Status   ....   20/20   (≥ 12)

Minnesota Rate of Manipulation

	1 Hand Placing	1 Hand Turning/Placing
left hand	unable	unable
right hand	WNLs	WNLs

Motor – Free Visual Perceptual Test   Minnesota Spatial Relations Test

1) <u>Response Behavior</u> WNLs/Und. Res.   1) B -> A boards

     Left   Sug/Ind   2) A -> B boards   99 % Rank Performance

     Right   Sug/Ind   99 % Rank Accuracy

2) <u>Raw Score</u>: WNLs; _____ pts below normal   OR

3) <u>Performance Behavior</u>:   3) D -> C boards

     Left ___ /21   Right ___ /15   4) C -> D boards   ___ % Rank Performance

4) <u>Processing Time</u> WNLs: ___ sec slower   ___ % Rank Accuracy

Trailmaking Tests

1) Part A __35__ sec. (< 60 sec.)

2) Part B __119__ sec. (≥ 120 sec.)

Captains Log

1) Attention skills Module

     8 subtests _____

2) Visual/Motor Skills Module

     5 subtests _____

3) Conceptual Skills Module

     5 subtests _____

Symbol Digit Modalities Test

_____ / _____ per 90 sec (Written-Oral)

   Y   N   Suggests cerebral dysfunction

WAIS

9	Digit Span Test: Forward (≥ 7)
6	Digit Span Test: Backward (≥ 5)
15	Digit Span Test: Total (≥ 18)
/90	Digit Symbol Test (≥ 39)
37	Block Design (≥ 25)
18/20	Picture COmpletion (≥ 13)
15	Picture Arrangement (≥ 10)

VPDT

_____	Figure Ground
_____	Visual Discrimination
_____	Dot Patterns
_____	Visual Memory
_____	Traffic Test
_____	

Figure 26-7. *Continued.*

move into a strong synergistic pattern with greater effort while steering. The COTA fabricated a wrist/seatbelt to secure his left extremity in a comfortable position and to avoid interference with steering.

Program Discontinuation

The COTA provided four sessions of driver retraining for Matthew. Once established goals had been achieved and after consultation with the OTR, he was discharged from the driving assessment and retraining program. It was recommended that his vehicle be modified as previously discussed and a follow-up visit scheduled to reassess equipment operation. At that time assistance would also be provided regarding his pursuit of the state Department of Motor Vehicles medical clearance and license renewal. The OTR prepared a discharge summary using the COTA's progress notes and the therapist's documentation of evaluations.

Summary

This chapter presents an overview of occupational therapy services for evaluation and treatment of the occupational performance skill of driving. The characteristics and credentials of occupational therapy practitioners are unique for providing this service; however, such programs require therapists and assistants to seek additional training to develop all necessary skills. The therapeutic intervention process of driving evaluation and retraining is complex and diverse. Guidance may be found in the evaluation process by using the occupational behavior frame of reference.

Independence in transportation affects all age groups. For example, the young child who participates in activities requiring driving-related skills will have a better chance to become a safe driver, the adolescent often seeks success in driving as a symbol of independence and having reached adulthood, the adult may depend on success in driving to pursue vocational and leisure goals, and the elderly may strive to maintain their driving ability to fulfill a sense of self-worth as well as maintaining independence.

In many cases, rehabilitation programs, personnel and reimbursement agencies have yet to include driving as a vital and necessary activity. Those who have acknowledged the need and instituted such programs are highly committed and thoroughly knowledgeable about the required regulations and credentials of personnel, as well as equipment needs, before establishing them. A supportive staff who endorses the driving program is necessary for success.

Related Learning Activities

1. Visit the Department of Motor Vehicles, the Department of Commerce or the Department of Education in your state and determine the training required to become a driving evaluator/instructor.

2. Conduct an informal interview with at least two individuals who are disabled drivers. Discuss their experiences in terms of driver retraining.

3. Visit a local company that modifies vehicles for drivers who are disabled. Look at vehicles being modified and note specific devices and methods used.

4. What are some of the major life-style changes you would need to make if you were unable to drive? How would these changes affect your independence?

References

1. Gowland C, Simoes N: *A Driver Training Program for Persons with Physical Disabilities*. 2nd Edition. Downey, California, Rancho Los Amigos Medical Center, 1984.
2. American Occupational Therapy Association: *Physical Disabilities Special Interest Section Newsletter* 10, No.4, December, 1987.
3. Reed KL: *Models of Practice in Occupational Therapy*. Baltimore, Williams & Wilkins, 1984.
4. Access Designs, Inc. Cycl-one (brochure). Portland, Oregon, Access Designs, undated.
5. Rowcycle (brochure). Fresno, California, Rowcycle, Inc., undated.
6. Taira ED (Ed): *Assessing the Driving Ability of the Elderly: A Preliminary Investigation*. New York, Haworth Press, 1989.
7. Less M: *Evaluating Driving Potential of Persons with Physical Disabilities*. Albertson, New York, Human Resource Center, 1978.
8. Cimolino N, Balkovec D: The contribution of a driving simulator in driving evaluation of stroke and disabled adolescent clients. *Can J Occup Ther* 55:3, 1988.
9. *Visual Perceptual Diagnostic Testing and Training Programs*. New York: Educational Electronics Techniques, Ltd., 1984.
10. Engum E, Cron L, Hulse C, et al: Cognitive behavioral driver's inventory. *Cognitive Rehabilitation* 6(5):34-45, 1988.
11. Schweitzer J, Gouvier W, Horton C: Psychometric predictors of driving ability among able-bodied and disabled individuals. Paper presented at RESNA Annual Conference, San Jose, California, 1987.
12. Sivak M, Kewman D, Henson D: Driving and perceptual/cognitive skills: Behavioral consequences of brain damage. *Arch Phys Med Rehabil* 62:476-483, 1981.
13. Van Zomeren A, Brouwer W, Rothengatter J, et al: Fitness to drive a car after recovery from severe head injury. *Arch Phys Med Rehabil* 69:90-96, 1988.
14. Miller BF, Keane CB: *Encyclopedia and Dictionary of Medicine, Nursing, and Allied Health*, 5th Edition. Philadelphia, WB Saunders, 1992.

Section V
MANAGEMENT

Documentation

Service Operations

Management of occupational therapy programs involves a great variety of tasks and skills. A primary area is timely and accurate documentation, which is a vital and essential component of communication among service providers. Basic principles are presented and a variety of formats and forms will acquaint the reader with the documentation requirements of various treatment settings.

A chapter on service operations defines and discusses the many facets of day-to-day management of an occupational therapy department. The reader will find useful information related to scheduling, record maintenance and analysis, preparation, maintenance and safety of the work setting, managing supplies and equipment, reimbursement procedures and accreditation. Aspects of program evaluation and quality assurance are also presented together with other related topics. Jones states that, "Although service management is primarily an administrative function, it is supported by all levels of personnel."

Documentation

Harriet Backhaus, MA, COTA

Introduction

According to Pagonis,[1] the current health care environment requires both timely and accurate documentation, which is viewed as the most vital and essential component of overall communication among providers of services. She goes on to state that "recent regulations and social pressures (have) greatly altered the quality and the quantity of necessary administrative and clinical recording and reporting in occupational therapy."[1]

This chapter discusses the purposes and principles of documentation as they specifically relate to the provision of services throughout the occupational therapy process. COTA documentation responsibilities are addressed and examples of various documentation formats and content are provided as they relate to particular areas of occupational therapy inter-vention. Information is also included on reimbursement, as well as other considerations.

Purposes

A primary purpose of all documentation is to provide both a serial and a legal record of the condition of the patient throughout the course of occupational therapy intervention. Records that detail all pertinent information from admission to discharge must be maintained.[1]

Another important purpose is to provide a source of information for patient care. Depending on the nature of the therapeutic intervention, a significant number of health care providers will read and contribute to the patient's medical record. Accurate documentation enhances communication among them.[1,2]

KEY CONCEPTS

Purposes and principles

Primary areas

Problem-oriented medical record

Individualized Education Plan

Individualized Family Service Plan

Medicare requirements

Computerized formats

Reimbursement implications

ESSENTIAL VOCABULARY

Documented records

Confidentiality

Initial note

Progress note

Discharge summary

Subjective

Objective

Assessment

Plan

Functional performance

Due to the realities of the information age of our society and the increasing demands for exacting, specific facts and data, we have had to increase our efforts to produce quality documentation. Other factors that influence this mandate include the marked increase in malpractice suits and challenges of reimbursement claims by third-party payers. Documentation records are often called into evidence by the courts in legal cases. As costs for health care services continue to soar, payers are scrutinizing documentation more closely than ever before. Another factor is the need to adequately protect occupational therapy practitioners from liability suits.

Of equal importance is the need for occupational therapy practitioners to continually review documentation as it relates to maintaining the provision of the highest quality services that result in effective treatment. All occupational therapy practitioners have both a professional and an ethical responsibility to provide services that meet the highest standards. Review of documentation is one means of assuring this process.

Documented records are legal documents that protect the rights of both the patient and the person providing treatment. They are also public documents that are read by a variety of individuals, including hospital administrators, insurance claim reviewers and a host of health care personnel. Impressions about the necessity, efficiency and effectivenss of occupational therapy services will often be formulated solely on review of the existing documentation. All occupational therapy practitioners should view their documentation as an important "window" that provides others with a view of the profession and the services provided.

Documentation records can also be used as part of quality assurance reviews for ensuring accountability in health care. Additional information on this topic is presented in Chapter 28.

Finally, documentation can be used to provide data for research studies, for educational purposes and to develop new intervention strategies and tools, as well as for overall institutional planning and program expansion or reduction.

Principles

Every COTA and OTR must adhere to rigorous standards and principles when writing any type of documentation. The following factors are important.

Level of responsibility: The OTR has the ultimate responsibility for all occupational therapy documentation, with the COTA contributing to the necessary documents and written reports. Depending on the setting, COTAs may have complete responsibility for the preparation of certain reports.[2] Specifically, the COTA contributes to the screening

and evaluation data, treatment plan, treatment implementation and progress data, any necessary revisions in treatment based on reassessment, and the discharge summary. Although the primary responsibility does indeed rest with the supervising OTR, the COTA is responsible for the accuracy and timeliness of the documentation he or she is providing.

Co-signature requirements: Requirements for co-signature of the COTA's documentation may be mandated by the facility's accrediting bodies. These groups include the Joint Commission on Accreditation of Healthcare Organizations (JCAHO), the Commission on the Accreditation of Rehabilitation Facilities (CARF), and the Comprehensive Outpatient Rehabilitation Facilities (CORF). Third-party payers, including Medicare and Medicaid, also have requirements. State laws, particulary those related to licensure, registration and certification, may also contain requirements regarding co-signature of notes. Each facility offering occupational therapy services must adhere to the guidelines established by these parties. Current information is available from the American Occupational Therapy Association (AOTA).

General principles and requirements: Ten elements of documentation published by the AOTA outline general principles and requirements for all documentation.[1,3] These are presented in Figure 27-1.

The **ten elements of documentation** as presented in the American Occupational Therapy Association's *Guidelines for Occupational Therapy Documentation*

1. Patient's full name and case number on each page of documentation.
2. Date stated as month, day, and year for each entry.
3. Identification of type of documentation and department name.
4. Signature with a minimum of first name, last name, and designation.
5. Signature of recorder directly at the end of the note without space left between the body of the note and the signature.
6. Countersignature by an OTR on documentation written by students and/or COTAs if required by law or facility.
7. Compliance with confidentiality standards.
8. Acceptable terminology as defined by the facility.
9. Facility approved abbreviations.
10. Errors corrected by drawing a single line through the error and the correction initialed (liquid correction fluid and/or erasures are not acceptable), or facility requirements followed.

Figure 27-1. *Ten elements of documentation. From "Functions of a Manager in Occupational Therapy" by Jacobs and Logigian, SLACK Inc., Thorofare, NJ, 1989.*

It is essential to clearly organize all documentation. Writing must follow the facility format and be "clear, concise, complete, accurate, current, objective and legible."[1] Language must be used correctly, including proper overall composition and accurate spelling and grammar. Professional jargon must be avoided. Uniform terminology adopted by the profession[4] should be utilized. To assure permanence and accurate photo copying, black ink should be used for all handwritten notes.

Confidentiality: **Confidentiality** (maintaining secrecy) must be maintained at all times. According to the American Medical Association (AMA), all information in the medical record that refers to reports on examinations, treatment, observation or conversation with a patient is confidential.[5,6] The patient has the right to view the medical record. The patient may also give permission for the record to be released for other purposes such as litigation, reimbursement or for other medical assessment.[5,6] Information such as the name and address of the patient, name of spouse or nearest relative, and the name of the patient's employer are not considered confidential in some settings.[5]

Document protection requirements: In large facilities, all documentation records are organized and stored by the medical records department. In smaller departments the department head is reponsible for ensuring that the records are preserved in a safe, secure and accessible manner. Most states have laws that regulate the length of time medical records must be stored.

Primary Areas

Service Management

A number of areas of documentation and reporting are the responsibility of occupational therapy practitioners. In addition to those related directly to patient service provision, which is detailed in following sections, the COTA will also be required to prepare other reports routinely or periodically, including the following:

1. Incident reports
2. Equipment and supplies ordered and received
3. Inventory control
4. Patient equipment loan records
5. General equipment maintenace records

Although each of these areas is important, they are not discussed in this chapter (see Chapter 28).

Service Provision

The COTA contributes to the occupational therapy process. Details of this responsibility are outlined in the document *Entry-Level Role Delineation for Registered Occupational Therapists (OTRs) and Certified Occupational Therapy Assistants (COTAs).*[7] Basic components

outlined in the section entitled Service Provision are reviewed as they relate to documentation.

Assessment. Occupational therapy intervention in the area of assessment has two components: screening and evaluation. During the screening process an entry-level COTA might document personal observations of a patient engaged in a structured activity of daily living task using a checklist format. This information would then be reported to the supervising OTR who would determine the need for intervention based on this checklist, together with other supporting data. After establishing the required level of competency, as determined by the OTR, the COTA may carry out the screening component and related documentation with supervision.

The evaluation component is a process of gathering a database and interpreting the findings for the development of a treatment plan. After demonstrating competence, the COTA, working under the supervision of an OTR, can administer standardized tests, score test protocols, complete and record data collection procedures such as record reviews, interviews, general observations and behavioral checklists. The COTA can also report factual data either orally, in writing or both.

Information from the assessment is incorporated into the **initial note.** An initial note written after an initial assessment includes the following information:[2]

1. Patient's name, hospital or case number if applicable, and the date (month, day, year, and time seen)
2. Referral source, reason for referral and when the referral was received
3. Information obtained during the first session
4. Plans for further occupational therapy intervention, including long-term and short-term goals determined by the patient and the therapist, methods to achieve those goals, frequency of treatment and anticipated outcome of treatment
5. Signature and title

More detailed information on the actual writing of initial notes is addressed in a later section.

Program Planning. Program planning involves preparation of the treatment plan. Because the OTR is responsible for the outcome of the occupational therapy intervention, he or she has the primary responsibility for establishing the treatment goals and formulating the plan in collaboration with the patient. The COTA contributes to goal development and can assist the OTR in developing the written treatment plan. Written goals should reflect the patient's needs. It is of critical importance to consider these needs in relation to establishing patient goals. By asking the patient what is relevant to him or her, the OTR and the COTA can make a more informed decision about the final written treatment plan. Goals need to reflect a patient action, a specific time frame and a qualifier of the action. The following is an example of a well-stated goal: *The patient will independently prepare an entree in a meal preparation group within one week.*

Treatment Implementation. Occupational therapy treatment is the implementation of the treatment goals and the subsequent intervention or treatment plan. The OTR is responsible for the outcome of the plan. The documentation of the occupational therapy treatment plan and the patient's response to it are written in the **progress note.** The COTA is highly involved in writing progress notes, as it is the assistant who provides a substantial number of treatment services.

Progress notes may be written once a week, once a month or as dictated by the facility or agency. Different formats may be used when writing progress notes, depending on the requirements of the setting. Two specific formats will be discussed in greater detail in a subsequent section. Some settings require a daily notation in the patient's medical record, which reflects the patient's response to treatment on that day. The COTA must be familiar with the time frame for documentation in the specific setting where he or she is employed.

The following information should be included when writing progress notes:[2,6]

1. A statement reflecting the patient's response to treatment
2. A summary of the patient's progress or lack of progress since the last note, stating in what activities the patient has been participating and the frequency of the participation. The type of therapeutic media used should also be noted such as dressing training with compensatory techniques or adaptations, participation in a cooking group or community mobility training
3. Any new information or important observations since the last note
4. A documented plan for the need for continuing occupational therapy treatment with any changes in the plan, including revision of goals, if needed, is stated (see section on reassessment).

The progress note is important to document the patient's functional performance in order to justify continuation of occupational therapy services. The means by which the patient is working toward achieving the goals should be stated as well.

Reassessment. Periodic reassessment is the process of gathering current data to decide whether to continue treatment, revise the treatment plan, or discontinue treatment. Tasks and documentation relevant to the screening and evaluation process apply to reassessment. The COTA can determine the need for reassessment and report any changes in performance that might indicate such need. Reassessment data may also indicate the need to make a written referral to another health care service provider.

Discontinuation of Intervention. When a person receiving occupational therapy services achieves the goals established by the occupational therapy process, or if the goals were unable to be met, the service is discontinued. The planning for discharge begins when the patient is first seen by occupational therapy practitioners.

Discontinuation of occupational therapy services is documented in the **discharge summary** or discharge note. The OTR is usually responsible for writing the discharge note, with the COTA assisting in determining the need for assessment of the discharge status. The discharge note is a summary of the course of the patient's treatment and includes the following components:

1. The number of sessions the patient attended
2. The report of the patient's progress, including the status of the goals
3. Changes in the patient's performance since the initial treatment
4. Any recommendations for further occupational therapy intervention or the need for other service

Specific Procedures for Reporting Services

Problem-oriented Medical Record

One commonly used procedure to structure documentation is the problem-oriented medical record (POMR).[6] The POMR consists of three sections: database, list of problems and the plan for resolving the problems.[2] Notes may be written in a narrative or paragraph form, as long as the problems are clearly identified and the plan and the goals are stated.

Many facilities use the POMR in the form of the subjective objective assessment plan or SOAP note.[6,8] Each section of this documentation format requires inclusion of specific information.

The **subjective** portion of an initial note written in the SOAP format refers to what the patient said, as well as what family members or significant others reported. This information can include the previous life-style or home situation, attitudes or feelings, complaints, and the patient's verbal response to treatment. At times, information from other disciplines may also be included. Subjective information is based on what has been reported and is not measurable.[6,7]

The **objective** portion of the SOAP note focuses on measurable and observable data obtained during the initial evaluation.[8,9] Objective data are derived from the results of tests and measurements such as the Purdue Pegboard Test and the Minnesota Rate of Manipulation Test. It is also obtained through measurements for range of motion and muscle strength, activities of daily living evaluations and sensory and cognitive assessments.

The **assessment** part of the note refers to the therapist's opinion as to how the limitations noted during the initial assessment will affect the patient's functional performance.[8] Any problems discovered as a result of the objective data collected are listed here. Examples include deficits in activities of daily living status, decreased strength or diminished problem-solving ability. Problems are listed and numbered in this part of the note. The problem list forms the basis for determining goals.

The last part of the SOAP note is the **plan**. This section describes the long-term goals (LTGs) and short-term goals (STGs) that have been set. The frequency and length of treatment are also stated.

An example of an initial note written in the SOAP format is shown in Figure 27-2.

Progress notes, which document the treatment given, may also be written in the SOAP note format. These notes are usually written weekly, unless the facility has other requirements. When writing a progress note in this format, the following content should be included:

1. *Subjective part*: What the patient reports about the treatment
2. *Objective part*: Patient's performance based on data found through specific evaluations, observations and the use of therapeutic activities

---

72-year-old patient with the diagnosis of status post right hip replacement with posterior approach secondary to degenerative joint disease, referred to O.T. by Dr. J Smith on 2-17-93 for O.T. consult for ADLs. Surgery date 2-15-93. Patient is toe-touch weight-bearing. Patient initiated on 2-18-93.

S. Patient complains of some hip pain. Patient states that she lives in a one-story house with the laundry facilities in the basement. She is a widow, but has a daughter who assists with shopping and heavy cleaning as needed. Patient states that she has had some difficulties with homemaking tasks before the surgery.

O. Chart reviewed. Past medical history unremarkable except for history of degenerative arthritis. UE ROM: WNL (upper extremity range of motion within normal limits).

Sensation, coordination: no deficits noted.

Functional transfers: moderate assistance of one from bed to chair.

ADL status: limitations in hip in LE ROM secondary to precautions for total hip replacement, and requires maximum physical assistance for lower extremity dressing. Patient reports she is independent in UE bathing and dressing, but tires easily and needs to rest frequently.

A. Patient is cooperative and motivated to become as independent as possible. Patient shows good understanding of the hip precautions necessary for ADLs and understands the need for adaptive equipment and training in regard to the precautions.

Problem List:
1. Decreased performance in ADLs
2. Decreased endurance for ADLs

Rehabilitation potential: good.

P. Patient to be seen once daily for ADL training and energy conservation techniques.

STGs (short-term goals):
1. Patient will bathe and dress lower extremities with adaptive equipment and minimum physical assistance in two days.
2. Patient will transfer to commode with minimum physical assistance in one week.
3. Patient will verbalize energy conservation techniques as instructed for ADL tasks in one week.

LTGs (long-term goals):
1. Patient will bathe and dress lower extremities independently using adaptive equipment by discharge.
2. Patient will transfer to commode using appropriate safety equipment by discharge.

Treatment plan: Instruct in use of adaptive equipment. Instruct in appropriate energy conservation techniques. Train in safe commode transfers.

Treatment initiated; Problem #1 addressed.
Patient was able to participate in treatment planning.

Jane Doe, OTR
2-18-93

Figure 27-2. *Occupational Therapy Initial Note (SOAP).*

3. *Assessment part*: The effectiveness of treatment and any changes needed; the status of the goals, and the justification for the need for continuing occupational therapy treatment
4. *Plan part*: Treatment modalities to be used during next treatment session, and the frequency and duration of treatment; the need for further evaluations, recommendations and any new goals

Examples of a progress note and a discharge summary note using the SOAP format are shown in Figures 27-3 and 27-4, respectively.

Different methods may be used to incorporate SOAP notes into the documentation process, and formats may vary slightly depending on the type of facility and the patient population being treated. Some SOAP formats are more formal than others. Practitioners must adhere to the specific documentation format used in the facilities where they are employed.[10] If the SOAP note format is not used, one may still want to use the principles of the format to organize note writing. Figure 27-5 is an example of a progress note using a modified SOAP format, and Figure 27-6 provides an example of a narrative progress note.

Individualized Education Plan

Centralized documentation is referred to as the Individualized Education Plan (IEP) in the public school system. These plans are required for all children receiving services under Public Law 94-142 of the Education for All Handicapped Children Act and cover ages 3 to 21 years.[10]

Individual education plans must be established in writing before special education and related services can be provided.[11] The occupational therapy portion of the IEP is a collaborative effort by a team usually comprised of a supervisory person, the child's parents, the child (if appropriate), and others involved in the child's care, as well as the OTR and the COTA. The COTA provides the supervising therapist with input based on the treatment conducted throughout the school year. The OTR is responsible for completing the necessary documentation after the end of the year evaluations.

Each school system has its own IEP outline; however, federal regulations specify that the following information be included:[11,12]

1. Present level of functioning
2. Goals and short-term objectives
3. Special education and related services to be provided
4. Dates for initiation and duration of services
5. Criteria for evaulating the achievement of the goals and objectives

Every discipline involved in providing services for the student contributes its plan of treatment, which then is incorporated into the Master IEP. Additional information and an example of documentation in an IEP format may be found in Chapter 6.

Individualized Family Service Plan

While somewhat similar to the IEP, the Individualized Family Service Plan (IFSP) was developed as a form of documentation as a direct result of the enactment of Public Law 99-457, Education of the Handicapped Amendments.

February 25, 1993

S: "I am using the adaptive equipment with the nurses."

O: Problem #1: Decreased performance in ADLs
Patient is able to put on and take off slacks and socks with long-handled dressing equipment with occasional minimum assistance. Patient transfers to the commode with raised seat and rails with minimal assistance to maintain weight-bearing status. Patient instructed in energy conservation techniques and was given printed materials.

A: Patient is limited by need for verbal cues at times to maintain toe-touch weight-bearing status. STGs achieved. LTGs reviewed and remain appropriate. Occupational therapy intervention continues to be needed to progress to independence in ADLs.

P: Continue to see patient once a day for ADL instruction.
New STG #4:
Patient will bathe and dress lower extremities with verbal cues and use of adaptive equipment in three days.
Continue to see per plan; patient able to participate in treatment planning.

Sally Smith, COTA
2-25-93

Figure 27-3. *Progress note (SOAP).*

Initial visit: 2-18-93

Discharge visit: 3-1-93

Patient with diagnosis of status post right hip replacement referred by Dr. J. Smith on 2-17-93 for ADL training.

S. Patient states she will have her daughter help her but she states she can dress herself.

O. Problem #1: Decreased performance in ADLs.

Patient is independent in lower extremity bathing and dressing using adaptive equipment (reacher, long-handled sponge, sock donner and dressing stick). Patient performs a sink bath. Patient transfers to the commode with raised seat and rails independently.

Problem #2: Decreased endurance for ADLs.

Patient instructed in energy conservation techniques.

Patient able to to verbalize techniques appropriately.

A. Patient was independent in use of adaptive equipment, showed good judgment and was able to follow posterior precautions.

Rehabilitation potential: good.

Status of goals:

STG #1: Patient will bathe and dress lower extremities using adaptive equipment and requiring minimum assistance in two days. Achieved.

STG #2: Patient will transfer to commode with minimum assistance in one week. Achieved.

STG #3: Patient will verbalize energy conservation techniques as instructed in one week. Achieved.

STG #2: Patient will bathe and dress lower extremities with verbal cues in three days. Achieved.

LTG #1: Patient will bathe and dress lower extremities using adaptive equipment independently by discharge. Achieved.

LTG #2: Patient will transfer to commode using appropriate safety equipment independently by discharge. Achieved.

P. Patient discontinued from O.T. secondary to discharge to home with daughter.

Recommendations: Continue to use recommended adaptive equipment for duration of precautions.

Follow-up: Home health O.T.

Jane Doe, OTR
3-1-93

Figure 27-4. *Occupational Therapy Discharge Summary (SOAP).*

This law mandates early intervention services for children from birth through two years of age.[13] Documentation contained in the IFSP must contain information about the "child's status, family, projected outcomes of intervention, and the methods, criteria, and time lines."[14] Additional information on this topic may be found in Chapter 4.

Use of Computerized Formats

Many occupational therapy departments use computerized formats that simplify documentation procedures and reduce the time necessary to write the required information. The computer generates a form that is customized to the particular type of documentation required. Using a word-processing program or a specific documentation software program, one types the specific information in the appropriate blank. Initial notes, IEPs, progress notes, and discharge summaries are frequently written in this way. Related reports also are often produced in this manner and may be sent to physicians, employers, schools and others. Computer-assisted evaluation programs are also being used in areas such as work hardening and hand rehabilitation where state-of-the-art technology records data. Smith[15] reports that some occupational therapy departments use the computer to compare admission and discharge data and to generate a graph illustrating the results of therapeutic intervention.

The Occupational Therapy Functional Assessment Compilation Tool (OT FACT), a computerized format designed by Roger Smith, is also available in a paper and pencil version, although the computer software provides the most

S: The Patient states that she is more interested in her appearance this week.

O: Orientation: the patient is oriented to person and place. She requires verbal cues for the day of the week.

ADLs: Patient is independent in selecting appropriate clothing and in taking her dress out of the closet. Minimum assistance is needed in putting her dress over her head.

A: The patient has been cooperative during the dressing program this week. She has improved from needing minimum assistance in choosing outfits and removing clothes from the closet to performing both tasks independently. Continued occupational therapy treatment is necessary to increase functional ADL performance.

P: Continue to see patient three times per week for orientation and ADL training.

Goal: Patient will require supervision with AM dressing only.

Sue Smith, COTA
3-1-93

Figure 27-5. *Progress note (modified SOAP).*

Carol Smith
3-18-93

Patient has been seen by occupational therapy for feeding skills. Patient has progressed from feeding only finger foods to using utensils appropriately with minimum verbal cues. Patient has improved in participation, attending four of the last five sessions. Patient needs continued occupational therapy to increase activities of daily living skills. Plan: continue to see patient once daily to increase level of independence in activities of daily living.

Sue Jones, COTA

Figure 27-6. *Narrative Progress Note.*

complete information.[16] *OT FACT* provides a comprehensive method for reporting functional status and clearly identifies functional deficit areas. For example, the use of adaptive equipment is not viewed as a deficit in activities of daily living, even though the patient may have definite limitation in range of motion. OT FACT identifies the reasons for difficulty in performing functional tasks, thereby making treatment planning more meaningful. In addition, a distinct separation is made between impairment and disability. The OTR assumes responsibility for the information required for this computerized assessment, with the COTA collaborating and assisting as needed. Additional information on OT FACT may be obtained by contacting AOTA.

Reimbursement Implications

Payment for occupational therapy services comes from several sources, including federal, state, private, and com-

mericial insurers as well as self-pay by the service recipients.[17] Documentation standards and guidelines vary greatly among these agencies. Insurance programs have more definite guidelines relative to services covered in specific settings. Grant programs providing funding for services generally follow state or local regulations, which conform to broad national goals.[17]

Whatever the source or sources of funding, it is imperative that occupational therapy personnel comply with the documentation requirements of each agency being billed for reimbursement for services. Failure to do so is likely to result in denied payment.

Medicare Requirements

Because it is impossible to outline the various documentation requirements for the many third-party payers, Medicare has been selected to provide an illustrative example. The reference *Medicare Billing for Part B Intermediary Outpatient Occupational Therapy Services* outlines requirements implemented in 1989.[18] Although designed specifically for outpatient Part B services, the guide is a useful tool in determining whether all essential parts of documenation have been covered before submitting a reimbursement claim.

Among other stipulations, the Medicare guide states that all documentation must reflect the patient's *functional loss* and the *level of assistance* requiring occupational therapy patient intervention. Documentation must include the following areas:[18]

1. Activities of daily living dependence
2. Functional limitations that require occupational therapy intervention, including attention span, strength, coordination, balance, and environmental barriers
3. Safety dependence, ie, physically or cognitively unsafe
4. Current functional status and progress or lack of progress

5. Expected potential for improvement
6. Any change in level of assistance needed for functional tasks, ie maximum, moderate, minimal or standby assistance
7. Change in performance by decreased refusals or increased consistency in performing functional tasks
8. Initiating a new skilled functional activity or compensating for a loss with a skilled compensatory technique, with or without equipment

Medicare guidelines also contain useful information to consider when a duplication of services is apparent. For example, both physical therapy and occupational therapy personnel may be involved in teaching a patient to transfer independently. In this case, careful documentation is necessary to assure that this situation is not viewed as a duplication of services. Records must clearly state that the occupational therapy treatment used transfer techniques in relation to functional performance of activities, such as tub and toilet transfers, whereas physical therapy intervention emphasized safety measures.

Related Considerations

Review of the material presented thus far reveals that regardless of the documentation format used, certain areas should be consistently addressed, using acceptable occupational therapy terminology and reflecting **functional performance**. For example, a COTA notices that a patient participating in a day treatment program exhibits the following behaviors:

1. Improved attendence
2. More participation in activities
3. Increased participation in group activities
4. Ability to complete projects

All of these facts should be documented. Documentation of these observations may enable the patient to continue in occupational therapy; they indicate that progress is indeed being made.

In another example, a COTA who is conducting a dressing assessment with a patient with a left cerebral vascular accident observes that he has progressed from only putting on a shirt independently to putting on slacks and socks without assistance or prompts. Instead of stating that the patient has improved in his activities of daily living related to dressing, the COTA should specifiy which areas have improved compared with the first documentation. Changes in performance that represent a regression also need to be noted. The supervising occupational therapist should also be informed of the changes.

In addition to the various resources already identified, several others are also useful. *Guidelines for Occupational Therapy Documentation*, published by AOTA is highly recommended. Figure 27-1 provides information from this source.[3] *Uniform Terminology for Occupational Therapy* is another important resource for assuring that language used in all types of documentation is uniform and therefore readily understood[4] (see Appendix C).

Summary

Documentation is a critical component of occupational therapy intervention. Forms and formats are specific to each employment setting and the populations served. All written documentation must be clear, concise, complete, accurate, current, objective and legible. Uniform terminology and correct spelling, grammar and punctuation must always be used. All records must be compiled and maintained according to the requirements of the facility and the reimbursement sources. They must be in compliance with legal statutes. Documentation for service provision follows the occupational therapy process, from admission to discharge, requiring that specific records be documented at various intervals. Examples include the initial note, progress notes and the discharge summary. The problem-oriented medical record and the subjective objective assessment plan note are among those formats commonly used. Computerized formats are being used to generate many of these. The COTA, working under the supervision of the OTR, will contribute to this process and frequently plays a major role in writing progress notes and preparing independent reports.

Editor's Note

It is important for the reader to review the information on the occupational therapy process, which is found in Chapter 1, before studying this chapter. A thorough understanding of this material is essential to integrate learning relative to documentation and its relationship to the specific tasks and responsibilities that must be carried out during therapeutic intervention. Although the material is briefly reviewed in this chapter, it should not be viewed as a substitute for additional reading. Examples of documentation related to specific diagnostic problems and resulting deficits may be found in the case study and models of practice sections in this text.

Acknowledgments

The author wishes to extend appreciation to Sally E. Ryan, COTA, ROH, editor, and Jean Kalschuer, MA, OTR, both of the College of St. Catherine, for their constructive critique and organizational and content recommendations.

Related Learning Activities

1. Locate samples of the various types of documentation discussed in this chapter. Review them carefully to determine how the format and content differ from the examples presented in this chapter.

2. Working in collaboration with an OTR, practice writing information to be included in an initial note, a progress note and a discharge note. Seek feedback on ways to improve your documentation.

3. Interview one of your fellow students regarding their interests. Write short-term and long-term goals to help this person achieve an objective.

4. Discuss the importance of patient confidentiality with peers and the COTA's responsibility in this area.

5. Describe ways that the standardized reporting of functional performance in occupational therapy documentation benefits the profession.

References

1. Pagonis JF: Documentation. In Jacobs K, Logigian M: *Functions of a Manager in Occupational Therapy*. Thorofare, New Jersey, Slack, Inc., 1989, pp. 112-133.

2. Early MB: *Mental Health Concepts and Techniques*. New York, Raven Press, 1987.

3. American Occupational Therapy Association: Guidelines for occupational therapy documentation. *Am J Occup Ther* 40:830-832, 1986.

4. American Occupational Therapy Association: Uniform terminology for occupational therapy—second edition. *Am J Occup Ther* 43:808-815, 1989.

5. Rowland H, Rowland B: *Hospital Administration Handbook*. Rockville, Maryland, Aspen Systems, 1984.

6. Jones RA: Service Mangement. In Ryan SE (Ed): *The Certified Occupational Therapy Assistant: Roles and Responsibilities*. Thorofare, NJ, Slack Inc., 1986, pp 358-368.

7. American Occupational Therapy Association: Entry-level role delineation for occupational therapists, registered, (OTRs) and certified occupational therapy assistants (COTAs). *Am J Occup Ther*, 44:1089-1090, 1990.

8. Cole DM: Documentation. In Hopkins H, Smith H (Eds): *Willard and Spackman's Occupational Therapy*, 7th Edition. Philadelphia, JB Lippincott, 1988.

9. Hirama H: *Occupational Therapy Assistant: A Primer*, Revised Edition. Baltimore, Chess Publications, 1990.

10. Scott SJ: *Payment for Occupational Therapy Services*. Rockville, Maryland, American Occupational Therapy Association, 1988.

11. King-Thomas L, Hacker BJ: *A Therapist's Guide to Pediatric Assessments*. Boston, Little, Brown and Company, 1987.

12. Clark PN, Allen AS (Eds): *Occupational Therapy for Children*. St. Louis, CV Mosby, 1985.

13. American Occupational Therapy Association: Guidelines for occupational therapy services in early intervention and preschool services. Position paper, 1989.

14. Benham PK: Unpublished material, 1991.

15. Smith RO: Technological approaches to performance enhancement. In Christianson C, Baum C (Eds): *Occupational Therapy: Overcoming Human Performance Deficits*. Thorofare, New Jersey, Slack Inc., 1990.

16. Christiansen C: Occupational performance assessment. In Christiansen C, Baum C (Eds): *Occupational Therapy: Overcoming Performance Deficits*. Thorofare, New Jersey, Slack, Inc., 1990.

17. Struthers MS, Schell BB: Public policey and its influence on performance. In Christiansen C, Baum C (Eds): *Occupational Therapy: Overcoming Human Performance Deficits*. Thorofare, New Jersey, Slack, Inc., 1990.

18. Health Care Financing Administration: *Medicare Guidelines for Occupational Therapy Services*. Washington, Department of Health and Human Services, 1989.

Chapter 28

Service Operations

Robin A. Jones, BS, COTA, ROH

Introduction

Service operations is defined as a process that involves planning, organizing and evaluating occupational therapy facilities and services. Primary responsibility for service operations and their management belongs with the department or program director; however, certain aspects of the management function require the support of all occupational therapy personnel. The level of responsibility occupational therapy staff members assume for service operations and management will be depending on the specific task involved and the level of training necessary to perform the task. The role of the certified occupational therapy assistant in service management will vary depending on the type of agency or facility, their policies and procedures, the amount of supervision available, the patient population being served and the nature of the tasks to be performed.

This chapter describes the following components of service operations and management:

1. Scheduling
2. Maintaining records and compiling and analyzing service data
3. Preparation, maintenance and safety of the work setting
4. Inventorying and ordering supplies and equipment
5. Reimbursement procedures
6. Accreditation
7. Program evaluation and quality assurance
8. Meetings

KEY CONCEPTS

Scheduling

Maintaining records and analyzing data

Preparation, maintenance and safety

Inventory, supplies and equipment

Reimbursement procedures

Accreditation

Program evaluation and quality assurance

Continuing education

Public information

Research

ESSENTIAL VOCABULARY

Service operations

Time management

Indirect patient care activities

Cost-effectiveness

Safety awareness

Risk management

Negligence

Malpractice

In-service education

Public relations

In addition, continuing education, in-service training, public relations and research will be addressed. Although these areas do not specifically pertain to service operations management, they are essential, related components for the continued growth and development of occupational therapy practitioners and the profession of occupational therapy.

Service delivery is changing rapidly with the growth of outpatient clinics and other alternative treatment settings. Although methods given as examples in this chapter will need to be modified to accommodate changes in occupational therapy practice, it is important to assure that all of the components are addressed.

Scheduling

Structuring the day to accommodate the demands made on one's time is an important aspect to consider. The OTR and the COTA should be able to establish priorities and utilize **time management** skills to plan effectively. Time needed to perform both direct and indirect patient care activities as well as to attend regularly scheduled meetings and conferences must be allotted. Schedules need to be clearly communicated and coordinated with all persons involved.

Under the category of direct patient care, occupational therapy practitioners must take into account the frequency with which a patient requires occupational therapy services and the level of care required, such as one-to-one or group, and the degree of supervision needed. In the majority of situations, this decision will initially be made by the supervising occupational therapist. Throughout the course of treatment, the patient's needs will be jointly reassessed and the therapist will adjust his or her schedule accordingly. The availability of practitioners will significantly influence the time spent in direct patient care and will also be a factor in determining how patient care responsibilities are divided among the OTR and COTA staff members. **Cost-effectiveness** (producing optimum results in relation to money spent) will influence whether the manager chooses a COTA or an OTR to perform certain direct patient care services.

Each facility or agency will have a different policy for scheduling patient services. The type of setting and the population served will influence the process. For example, in an acute care setting the therapist appreciates that the patient's medical status is the primary focus and that occupational therapy treatment will be scheduled in accordance with the patient's medical needs. For example, an individual with a spinal cord injury who is positioned on a Stryker frame is able to work on self-feeding only when in a prone position. This situation requires coordination between the nursing staff and occupational therapy staff to schedule that patient's "turning times" so that they correspond to the times that meals are served.

In a community setting, the schedule may vary daily according to the particular needs of the OTR's and the COTA's patient population. Because the community setting offers less structure than the traditional medical setting, occupational therapy practitioners must have the ability to function relatively independently. However, the occupational therapy staff often does not have control over the external factors that influence the population they serve. Schedules must be coordinated with the family and other disciplines involved with the patient's care and should accommodate the person's life-style as much as possible. Community-based programs in which COTAs may be involved include, but are not limited to, psychiatric day treatment centers, adult day care centers, vocational workshops, independent living centers and early intervention programs.

The availability of a patient or family financial reimbursement plan, which includes coverage of occupational therapy services, influences the frequency and duration of the occupational therapy services received. The issue of reimbursement and how it affects service delivery will be discussed in more depth later in this chapter. Because an OTR's or a COTA's caseload may include several patients who require varying amounts of time for services, it is important that time be managed accordingly. Both OTRs and COTAs must carefully examine each patient's individual needs when planning their time.

Occupational therapy practitioners must also allocate time for **indirect patient care activities** (scheduling, treatment set-up, etc.), administrative tasks and professional activities. Participation in departmental or patient-related meetings, supervision meetings and patient documentation time must be considered. As a COTA becomes more experienced in an area of specialization, additional tasks may be assigned such as participation in program development, research and teaching. Priorities must be established for these professional activities in terms of other responsibilities. In most instances, occupational therapy practitioners will find it difficult to incorporate additional responsibilities into their daily schedules and will need to decide what other tasks they are willing to do, if any, outside of their regular working hours. Management may also be able to assist individual staff members in identifying ways to handle their schedule more effectively, thus allowing more time for professional activities.

An often neglected but important area for personal health and well-being is the need to allot time for lunch and periodic breaks. This time is essential to a healthy mind and body and facilitates optimal performance. Availability of this time is positive in terms of socialization as well as for a quiet time to think and reflect. It leads to increased job satisfaction and enhances working relationships, which indirectly increases productivity. These breaks contribute to maintaining the balance between work and leisure activities. They also promote professional and personal growth and development, essential aspects of quality care. A sample daily schedule for a COTA working in a rehabilitation setting is shown in Figure 28-1. An "X" indicates that the previously listed activity extends into or fills the next time slot. This schedule does not reflect two 15- to 20-minute breaks, which are taken morning and afternoon.

Recording and Reporting

Maintaining accurate records of patient performance, attendance, billing, and equipment ordered and received is an essential component in managing an occupational therapy service program. In addition, service data are used by administration to evaluate program function in the process of internal quality assurance and efficiency studies as well as for research purposes.

Documentation

The most important aspect of record keeping is documentation of patient performance. Other health professionals use this documentation when dealing with the patient's overall care. In addition, records of the treatment provided are often used to justify occupational therapy

charges to third-party payers such as private insurance companies, Medicare and Medicaid. It is the responsibility of both the OTR and the COTA to enter information in the patient's medical record that accurately reflects the course of the treatment process. This information includes the initial evaluation, a written plan of care, including long-term and short-term goals, periodic progress notes and a discharge evaluation. Written instructions given to the patient and/or family members concerning appropriate care after discharge from occupational therapy services must also be included. Documentation of equipment that is issued must include the functional purpose of the equipment and any training that was provided to ensure proper use of the equipment. Another primary consideration is that the documentation shows continuity and that the discharge summary relates directly to the functional status and goals identified at the time of the initial evaluation. In depth information on documentation may be found in Chapter 27.

Preparation, Maintenance and Safety of the Work Setting

Determining the use of space required to provide occupational therapy services, as well as the equipment and supplies needed, is primarily the responsibility of the administrator of the department. The most effective system for developing and maintaining a given work setting cannot be successful without the full cooperation and participation of all personnel who work in the area.

Environmental Considerations

The COTA and the OTR are responsible for identifying and communicating with the appropriate personnel about all issues and needs relevant to the patient population they serve. These concerns may include, but are not limited to, issues relating to the treatment environment itself. For example, accessibility, lighting, noise levels, ventilation, maintenance and proper storage of equipment and supplies, as well as security measures must all be considered. Identification of the type of treatment areas needed must be determined. Some patients require a low-stimulus rather than a high-stimulus environment, whereas others may need an open rather than an isolated environment.

Space may be used for different purposes at different times of the day, a factor that will require coordination of schedules. Available space within a facility may be at a premium, and it is valuable to the administrator if staff members can assist in developing creative ways to make use of space or identify alternative work areas. The goal is to maximally use available space for cost-effectiveness, efficiency and safety.

Continual monitoring of the work setting for evidence of

Day of the week: TUESDAY

8:30 AM—AM Dressing program with Mr. Smith
(RM. 549)

9:00 AM—Feeding group on spinal cord unit

10:00 AM—ADL eval. with Mrs. Rose (RM. 762)

11:00 AM—Individual treatment session with Mr. Johnson; clinic

12:00 PM—Lunch

12:30 PM—PT Care conference
—Mrs. Rose and Mr. Smith

1:00 PM—PT Care conference/documentation time

1:30 PM—Individual treatment session with Mr. Smith

2:00 PM—"X"

2:30 PM—Stroke group
(community out-trip with th. rec.)

3:00 PM—"X"

3:30 PM—Staff inservice—infection control

4:00 PM—Documentation time; supervision meeting with Carol

Figure 28-1. *Daily schedule.*

worn out, broken or depleted supplies and equipment is the responsibility of all occupational therapy personnel. A specific staff member, either an OTR or a COTA, may be assigned the responsibility of coordinating the repair or replacement of equipment and supplies. Many departments use nonprofessional staff, if available, for this function.

Safety Factors

Safety awareness (knowledge of situations with potential for risk, injury or loss) in the work setting is essential. Policies and procedures regarding the maintenance of a safe working environment are mandated by the majority of accrediting bodies. Safety includes but is not limited to factors such as the following:

1. Adherence of all staff members to infection control procedures
2. Proper storage of toxic chemicals and flammable substances
3. Use of proper clothing during the operation of certain equipment such as power tools
4. Knowledge of departmental and facility fire and other emergency plans
5. Observance of precautions as they relate to specific diagnosis

Risk Management and Negligence

Risk management is the title given the branch of management that deals with issues of liability. Negligence and malpractice are the primary liability areas that occupational therapy personnel need to be aware of in the work setting.

Negligence is a safety concern that refers to the failure to perform a task that, under normal circumstances, would be properly attended to. It is often caused by heedlessness and carelessness.[1] Prevention is the key to maintaining a safe environment. All staff members should be aware of policies and practice them daily. Examples include monitoring patients in reception areas and rest rooms and enforcing smoking and emergency regulations.

Malpractice relates to misconduct and the lack of skill or care when performing professional duties. The COTA and OTR can protect themselves from being named in a malpractice suit by adhering to a high degree of patient care as dictated in the standards of practice for occupational therapy.[2] Both the OTR and COTA should carry professional liability insurance. Most facilities maintain coverage for their personnel, but it is the responsibility of the individual practitioner to determine whether coverage is available and adequate. Related information appears in Chapter 30.

Accident Prevention and Emergency Procedures

The proper storage of toxic chemicals and flammable substances is particularly important in the occupational therapy clinic due to the presence of such items frequently used for avocational pursuits, as well as the fabrication of orthotic devices and equipment. The use of proper protective clothing when using such substances and during the operation of power tools and equipment is essential. Face masks and gloves are recommended when working with toxic chemicals. Use of goggles to protect the face and eyes when operating power tools should be mandatory. Training and periodic review of the proper use of equipment and chemicals typically found in the department may be incorporated into the facility's orientation program for new staff members. It is also important that the facility provide thorough training for new employees in the specifics of both the departmental and the institutional procedures for fire and other emergencies.

A number of facilities require members of the staff to maintain current cardiopulmonary resuscitation (CPR) certificates and provide periodic refresher courses. Knowledge of precautions as they relate to a given diagnosis is also essential as a preventive measure. Training in how to monitor a pulse rate or take a blood pressure reading, manage a seizure, or assist an individual who is choking is important for all occupational therapy personnel.

Incident reports should be completed and filed whenever they occur and in accordance with the policies of the facility. In addition to choking, seizure management and CPR, other situations should also be documented. These include falls, cuts, burns, and ingestion or ocular involvement of foreign objects and substances.

Infection Control

Infection control procedures have specific implications for occupational therapy departments because of the storage and use of food in the clinic setting. Proper storage and preparation of food are essential to minimize the growth and spread of bacteria. Considerations include hand washing, hair nets, adequate cooking times and refridgeration. Adherence to infection control procedures is particularly important when working with a patient who is at risk for infecting others (eg, AIDS, herpes, hepatitis and urinary tract and respiratory infections) or whose immune system is weakened due to their physical condition (eg, AIDS). Specific information about patients with AIDS may be found in Chapter 15.

Managing Supplies and Equipment

Essential to the efficient operation of an occupational therapy program is an adequate supply of equipment and materials necessary to carry out treatment and operate the clinic efficiently. Responsibility for this particular function varies within a given facility and must often be coordinated by the management body; however, the COTA may participate in some phase of this process.

To maintain an adequate supply of equipment and materials, some form of inventory system should be instituted. The complexity of the system will vary and will depend on factors such as the following:

1. Size of the occupational therapy department
2. Quantity of supplies used during a given time period
3. Availability and adequacy of storage space
4. "Shelf life" of the materials
5. Accessibility to vendors
6. Delivery time for receiving ordered items
7. Price of the items including discounts given for quantity orders

Well-formulated inventory systems can greatly enhance the efficiency of reordering necessary supplies and equipment.

Large occupational therapy departments are often able to maintain a sizable inventory of supplies and equipment, whereas smaller departments may only be able to maintain an inventory of items for departmental use. As health care costs continue to escalate, administrators will be stressing the need to keep inventories as low as possible to decrease funds "tied up" and to maximize the use of storage space, possibly for other purposes. In addition, they will weigh any problems associated with the inability to provide equipment against the costs of processing purchasing orders. It is important that both the COTA and the OTR assist administration in identifying problems associated with maintaining an equipment supply and providing it for patient purchase, as they have direct contact with the consumer and can identify needs.

The departmental or institutional procedures for ordering equipment and supplies will influence the type of inventory system. Information obtained through the use of an inventory system will be used by the facility and departmental administration as well as by staff members. One example of the way in which administration uses the occupational therapy department's inventory records is to determine the facility's total assets. Inventory records are also used as a basis for budget planning by administrators and may be utilized by occupational therapy personnel when determining the availability of equipment for patient issue or use.

An inventory system that may be used for recording equipment that is loaned for temporary patient use is referred to as a check-out system. The occupational staff member who loaned the piece of equipment records on the appropriate form the patient's name, a description of the equipment, the date loaned, the anticipated date of return, and the name of the responsible therapist or assistant. When the equipment is no longer needed, the OTR or the COTA records the date that the equipment was returned on the original form and files it and also checks the overall condition of the item. For example, suction cups may be missing from an adapted grab bar and may need to be replaced before being issued to another patient. This procedure allows for an ongoing accounting and maintenance system of equipment in use as well as equipment available for use. A sample form is shown in Figure 28-2. More complex forms of inventory management may be utilized, and the role of occupational therapy practitioners will vary in maintaining these systems.

The specific procedures for ordering supplies and equipment will be determined be administration and the department head in most cases. Occupational therapy practitioners should keep abreast of new products on the market by reviewing professional journals, participating in continuing

---

XYZ REHABILITATION CENTER
EQUIPMENT LOAN RECORD

Patient name _____

Address _____

_____

Telephone number _____ Home _____ Work

Description of equipment _____

_____

Condition _____

Date loaned _____ Date of expected return _____

Date returned _____ Condition _____

Comments _____

Authorized by _____

Issued by _____

Received by _____

Figure 28-2. *Patient equipment loan form.*

education activities and attending exhibits held at state and national conferences. Information may also be obtained from the "Buyers Guide," published yearly in the *American Journal of Occupational Therapy*.

Reimbursement Procedures

Financial management of an occupational therapy department is the responsibility of the administrative staff. The department head establishes the budget and guidelines for expenditures, and the institutional management establishes the fees. Input into the development of the budget may be solicited from staff members to assist the director in determining money needed for capital expenditures such as major pieces of equipment and furniture, continuing education and program development.

Occupational therapy is a revenue-producing service in most settings, and it is the responsibility of individual therapists and assistants to submit accurate charges, either by units of time or for the specific cost of the occupational therapy service provided. Funding for occupational therapy services is obtained from both public and private sources, including state and federal governments, private insurance companies, charities, foundations, endowments and direct patient payment.

Medicare and Medicaid

The major sources of public funding come from Medicare and Medicaid. Medicare and Medicaid, established by Title XVII of the Social Security Act, are federally funded insurance programs that provide medical benefits primarily for the aged. Benefits may also be received by persons who have been disabled for more than 24 months and those with low incomes.[3] The standards for eligibility and services are established by the federal government. Previously, under this program, hospitals and other eligible health care facilities were reimbursed for their services under a cost-based reimbursement system whereby Medicare provided payment for services rendered based on what it cost the facility to provide a particular service.[4] Studies showed that the payments made for particular procedures or treatments were not consistent among service providers and no apparent difference in the quality of care accounted for the discrepancies.[4] This payment plan led to cost inflation in the health care field. There was no incentive for hospitals to operate more efficiently.

Tax Equity and Fiscal Responsibility Act

The Tax Equity and Fiscal Responsibility Act of 1982 (TEFRA) was a major move toward changing hospital reimbursement under Medicare. This legislation included steps that placed limits on a hospital's inpatient charges. Adjustments were made to reflect each hospital's case mix, a term used to describe the type of diagnosis treated. In addition, it placed limits on the yearly rate of increase in total costs per patient treated and provided for incentive payments to hospitals that were below the limits.[4] Historically, hospitals were reimbursed after a patient was discharged. Under the new system, reimbursement is determined prospectively.

Diagnostic-Related Groups and Medicare

Further study by the Department of Health and Human Services resulted in the initiation of a new reimbursement procedure, based on the diagnosis of the patients treated, known as diagnostic-related groups (DRGs). This system calls for a fixed price to be paid for each episode of illness, regardless of the number of days spent in the hospital or the number of procedures performed.[4] Patients are classified according to 468 disease categories and conditions, including medical, surgical, psychiatric and rehabilitation diagnoses. These categories were originally developed by researchers at Yale University and then used in the hospital reimbursement system of New Jersey, Maryland and other states before becoming part of the Medicare system.[3] DRGs are assigned to a Medicare patient on discharge from a hospital based upon the following factors:[4]

1. Principal diagnosis
2. Principal operating room procedure, if any
3. Other diagnoses and procedures
4. Age, sex and discharge status

Hospitals are paid a fixed rate for each Medicare patient, regardless of the actual cost of treatment. Provisions are available under the system to receive additional payment in cases where the hospital stay is unusually long and for patients who have accrued costs that exceed the DRG payment rate. These additional payments, however, must be reviewed by the Peer Review Organization who will determine whether the additional costs are medically necessary and reasonable.[5]

The impact of the Medicare DRGs on occupational therapy is not yet fully known. In light of the high cost of health care and restrictions imposed on reimbursement for services, it is important that occupational therapy treatment be provided in the most efficient and cost-effective manner possible. This goal will have a direct implication for staffing patterns, and more jobs will be available for the COTA. Increased emphasis is being placed on occupational therapy practitioners in terms of productivity levels and the feasibility of increasing treatment times, while at the same time decreasing the length of time it takes to achieve goals. All occupational therapy practitioners should be familiar with reimbursement procedures and their impact on the services they provide.

Accreditation

Accreditation is the process by which an institution or facility is evaluated for its compliance to predetermined qualifications or standards by an agency or organization.[2] Most facilities are subject to some type of regulations. These facilities include acute care and rehabilitation hospitals and long-term care institutions, as well as mental health agencies and facilities. This chapter addresses two major accrediting bodies: The Joint Commission on Accreditation of Healthcare Organizations (JCAHO) and the Commission on Accreditation of Rehabilitation Facilities (CARF).

JCAHO is a private, voluntary, nonprofit organization comprised of representatives of the American Hospital Association, the American Medical Association, the American College of Physicians and the American College of Surgeons.[2] Accreditation by JCAHO has been used as a guideline and a requirement for certain public programs and funding agencies such as Medicare. Through periodic on-site surveys, in which they review standards of care, methods of documentation, referrals and management operations, JCAHO gathers data that support its decision to grant either full accreditation or provisional accreditation.[2] Each department within a facility receives a request to present data that demonstrate their compliance with the standards set forth by the Joint Commission on Hospital Accreditation.

The Commission on Accreditation of Rehabilitation Facilities is similar to JCAHO except that it emphasizes the provision of rehabilitation services for the disabled population. Accreditation by CARF has become linked to funding agencies and public programs in much the same manner as JCAHO. Facilities may be accredited by more than one agency depending on the population they address and the services they provide. For example, hospitals may provide both medical care and rehabilitation services. Individual states may require a process similar to an accreditation process in order for a facility to receive a license to operate.

Program Evaluation and Quality Assurance

Program evaluation is an ongoing method of examining clinical outcomes that offers a factual, ready reference for both the staff and the consumer relative to what the program is accomplishing and how well it is being accomplished. First, the objective(s) of the program must be clearly established; then, a set of measurable criteria can be developed. If an area of the program demonstrates a decrease in its effectiveness, additional staff training or changes or additions to the current program may be needed. For example, if on completion of a specialized program patients are required to complete a program evaluation form that includes questions relating to areas of the program that did not meet their needs, program staff members will be able to examine the identified areas and take steps toward making improvements. CARF emphasizes program evaluation in their accreditation process. Methods may include an interview with selected occupational therapy program participants or significant others using a standard set of questions. An example of an individual program evaluation is shown in Figure 28-3.

The results of this form of program evaluation would be used to make ongoing changes in current programming. Four objectives can be met with program evaluation:[6]

1. Reviewing care provided to all patients
2. Measuring the outcomes achieved
3. Reporting of treatment results on a regular basis
4. Providing feedback to the department regarding the achievement of goals

In addition, program evaluation is an informational system that provides objective data that can be used in the decision-making process, research and program planning. All levels of the staff are involved in the process of program evaluation. They may participate indirectly by providing feedback to administration and by maintaining accurate records of patient performance for evaluation purposes. As new programs are developed, a method of evaluation is also helpful to justify treatment outcomes to third-party payers and continuation of the program.

Quality assurance, also referred to as total quality management (TQM), is another process that monitors patient care service delivery and its related components to assure that quality of care is maintained. Quality assurance programs are designed to use ongoing monitors to identify problems in the delivery of a service and to take steps toward remediating them. Focused studies may also be developed to demonstrate clinical outcomes. JCAHO requires that an effective quality assurance program be in place as a condition of accreditation.

The process of quality assurance involves five stages.[7] The initial stage is the process of identifying significant problems in patient care and establishing priorities. Stage two requires the application of some instrument for measuring the problem such as standards of care. The third stage in the process is to produce plans that are directed toward improving the problem. The fourth stage includes the actual implementation of a plan to improve a given problem. The final stage is the reassessment of the identified problem to determine whether the action has been effective. Documentation of these various steps must be kept and is reviewed during accreditation visits from JCAH. An example of a quality assurance issue and its relationship to documentation is shown in Figure 28-4.

Development of a quality assurance program is a manage-

Please check appropriate response and comment, if so desired.

1. Do you feel that you have increased your awareness of how to plan for and actually get around in the community?

 _____ Yes _____ No

 Comment:

2. Do you feel that the information presented in this group related to your situation and/or needs?

 _____ Yes _____ No (If no, why not?)

 Comment:

3. Was there a particular program that you found to be:

 A. Most useful? (Why?)

 B. Least useful? (Why?)

4. Is there any additional information that you would like to see presented?

5. Do you feel that you will carry over the skills you learned in this group when in the community?

 _____ Yes _____ No

 Comment:

6. Do you feel that this group aided in your adjustment to your disability?

 _____ Yes _____ No

 Comment:

7. Please list any ideas that you have that would improve this program.

8. Do you feel prepared to return to the community?

 _____ Yes _____ No

 Comment:

Thank you for taking time to complete this evaluation. The information will help us in improving the program for future participants.

Good luck!! And our best wishes!!

_____

*Developed by the Quadriplegic Reentry Group Committee, 1984.

Figure 28-3. *Program Evaluation: Quadriplegic community reentry group. Reprinted with permission of Rehabilitation Institute of Chicago, Chicago, Illinois.*

Question: How can I get better reimbursement for services for patients with psychiatric diagnoses, especially in long term care.

Answer: Documentation of the services you are providing is an essential element in the reimbursement for you services. One of the first criteria that we use in reviewing documentation of services is whether the specialized skills of occupational therapy personnel are needed. It is critical that this review criteria is met 100%. Our experience in reviewing long-term care documentation in the psychosocial area suggests that the treatment being documented does not consistently indicate specialized skill is necessary. Evidence on ongoing evaluation has been missing. It is also difficult to measure progress without a clear idea of the outcome that is expected from the treatment that is being given. Clear statements that reflect your occupational therapy skills and your expected outcome must be documented. Periodic evaluation must be evident. Progress towards your expected outcome must be within a reasonable period of time. It is unreasonable to expect a third party payer to reimburse six months of daily treatment

aimed at increasing the resident's ability to socialize with another resident for two minutes one out of five times. We have reviewed charts that had such goals. Obviously the "reasonable period of time" was used and treatment should have been discontinued. One last area of documentation needs to be clearly addressed and that is the area of functional performance. Goals must be related to function. How is this resident going to improve in activities of daily living because occupational therapy personnel are working with him/her? Is there a correlation between the dependency of individuals and their expected survival? Our documentation must address what gains the resident has made and how that has impacted his/her role in the living situation. It does not matter to a third party payer that the resident is working on a birdhouse to increase his/her attention span. What matters is that an increased attention span will allows this resident to be more independent in his/her daily routine, reducing dependence on others and the cost of care.

Cathy Brennan, MA, OTR, FAOTA
Quality Assurance Committee Co-Chair
Minnesota Occupational Therapy Association

Figure 28-4. *Quality assurance issue. Minnesota Occupational Therapy Association Newsletter 90 (15):1, 1991. Used with permission.*

ment function. Staff members participate indirectly through identifying problem areas and reporting them to administration, by assisting administration in developing and implementing a plan that addresses the problem, and through ongoing feedback regarding the success or failure of the plan.

Meetings

Employee meetings are defined in the document *Uniform Terminology for Reporting Occupational Therapy Services—Second Edition* as meetings of occupational therapy departmental staff members, both OTR and COTA, for the following purposes:[8]
1. Disseminating and receiving information
2. Conveying information about the administrative policies of the institution or conditions of employment
3. Discussing issues relevant to the management of the program
4. Discussing issues relating to the development of the department or institution and its relationship to total health care

Individual staff members are responsible for having knowledge and understanding about the policies and procedures of a given department or facility. This information can be disseminated most effectively through such employee meetings. Attendance at these meetings is usually mandatory and should

be considered a professional responsibility. Active participation in these meetings is strongly recommended.

Program-related conferences are interdepartmental meetings that are held to communicate issues relevant to the planning, development and management of specific programs.[8] COTAs report directly on issues relating to programs they are involved in or issues relevant to their role in the department.

Supervisory meetings between the OTR and COTA may be formal or informal. The type of supervision available (close or general) and the needs of the individual COTA will influence the frequency of such meetings. Additional information on supervision may be found in Chapters 2 and 3.

Continuing Education and In-service Training

Regardless of experience, participation in continuing education and in-service training is a necessary part of professional life and required by most accrediting agencies. **In-service education** refers to "in-house" seminars, regularly scheduled classes and special training sessions that are provided within or outside of the facility.[8] It is the general purpose of such programs to provide an opportunity for practitioners to enhance their knowledge, skills and attitudes and for new staff to acquire basic skills. Programs may be related to clinical techniques, interpersonal skills, administrative issues, issues relevant to practice, supportive functions such as infection control, CPR, and emergency procedures or interdisciplinary sharing of expertise and services available (eg, special programs, new equipment, demonstration of a treatment technique and clarification of roles).

In-service educational opportunities allow for dissemination of information regarding programming, equipment demonstrations, research results, utilization of staff, etc. and provide a good opportunity for staff to develop teaching skills. The COTA may be involved in the planning and implementation of such programming. The department should establish priorities for continuing education needs that address current trends in patient care. The frequency of departmental in-service programs will be determined by the individual facility and may be held jointly with other disciplines. Many larger institutions have designated staff positions for the planning and implementation of such programs whereas others delegate this responsibility to clinical staff.

Continuing education refers to on-going educational experiences beyond the basic educational level, which enrich or enhance the individual's knowledge, skills and attitudes toward work performance.[8] Continuing education programs are designed to provide occupational therapy personnel with an opportunity to maintain or upgrade their knowledge, skills and performance level. Mandatory participation in continuing education is not currently required by the American Occupational Therapy Certification Board for maintenance of certification in occupational therapy; however, a number of state regulatory boards do require continuing education as a requirement for their annual or biannual recredentialing process. Whether or not continuing education is required, it remains the responsibility of both the COTA and the OTR to maintain a level of knowledge that incorporates the current trends of the profession.

The availability of funding for participating in continuing education programs may be limited in some facilities. The individual occupational therapy practitioner must be prepared to assume at least a portion of the costs associated with these programs.

The poor availability of continuing education programs designed to meet the needs of the COTA has been a persistent problem for many years. Recent efforts have been made to increase program offerings for COTAs at the AOTA national conference, and state associations have been strongly encouraged to promote continuing education programs for the COTA.

Public Relations

A **public relations** program aimed at increasing the public awareness of occupational therapy through marketing of services and publicity can increase the visibility of the profession and its services at a time when competition in health care is high. Occupational therapy is not yet a household word and often is misunderstood. The individual COTA and OTR working in the field must promote their services to other healthcare professionals, third-party payers, legislators, consumers and the public. A public relations program can serve a number of purposes, including the following:[9]

1. Enhancing the role of the profession in the community
2. Bringing available services to the attention of potential patients
3. Increasing the visibility of occupational therapy within the practice setting
4. Attracting potential students
5. Demonstrating the value of services to society

Public awareness of occupational therapy has increased in recent years, in part due to the heightened awareness of all occupational therapy personnel in regard to the importance of educating the public about their services. Licensure has increased the visibility of occupational therapy on the state level, whereas the work of the Government and Legal Affairs Division of AOTA has resulted in national attention. The AOTA has developed a manual targeting occupational therapy in public relations activities, which is available to the membership. It provides ideas and suggestions for the development of public relations strategies and materials. In addition, AOTA has a number of brochures, posters, videotapes and films that the membership may use to promote occupational therapy.

Individual facilities may choose to develop their own plan for education and promotion. A variety of methods may be implemented, such as in-service training for other health professionals, developing a display that depicts occupational therapy procedures and services, sponsoring an open house in the occupational therapy department, developing audiovisual materials to be used for promotional purposes, providing tours of their clinics, and participating in local health fairs or career days.

Research

Research, as defined in the document, *Uniform Terminology for Reporting Occupational Therapy Services*, refers to the formalized investigation of activities for the purposes of improving the quality of occupational therapy patient care by means of recognized scientific methodologies and procedures.[8] Traditionally, therapists and assistants have not been research oriented. Concern for the lack of attention given to research was the subject of a portion of an editorial written by Charles Christiansen, in *The Occupational Therapy Journal of Research*. He states that ". . .research continues to be viewed commonly as an activity foreign to our clients (patients) and irrelevant to our practice."[10] Christiansen argues that we cannot remain competitive in a time of limited resources for health care dollars unless we have research to validate our claims of efficacy and value.[10] Research begins in the clinic. Practitioners need to substantiate what they do and determine what is true and what is false.[11]

The American Occupational Therapy Foundation (AOTF), a sister body to the American Occupational Therapy Association, has assumed much of the responsibility for guiding the research of the profession. Through the foundation, a number of grants and educational money have been made available for research activities. In addition, the Foundation maintains a resource library available to students, practitioners and researchers and publishes the *Occupational Therapy Journal of Research* (OTJR).

Research skills are usually taught at the advanced master's level of our profession. Professional level students generally are provided with basic principles and methods, whereas technical level students receive minimal information. The clinic is an important site of research activities and COTAs may assist in the development of the research question or questions through reporting observations and by identifying potential areas for research. In addition, they may also assist in the research process through compiling, posting and recording specific data.

Summary

All practitioners should have a clear understanding of the service management functions in the facility or institution where they are employed. Knowledge of their roles in the areas of scheduling, record maintenance, preparation and safe maintenance of the work area, inventorying and ordering supplies is of the utmost importance. Accreditation procedures, program evaluation and quality assurance activities all have components that directly involve the occupational therapy assistant. Although service management is primarily an administrative function, it is supported by all levels of personnel. Responsibilities and specific tasks will be assigned by administration or the supervising occupational therapist. The *Entry-level Role Delineation for Occupational Therapists, Registered (OTRs) and Certified Occupational Therapy Assistants (COTAs)* provides a framework for the administrator, supervisor and staff person to follow. As experience is gained, COTAs may increase their participation and assume greater responsibility for service management functions.

Equally important is that one recognize the value of meetings, continuing education, public relations and research activities, all of which relate to personal growth,

growth of the facility where one is employed, and to the profession in general.

Acknowledgments

The author wishes to express sincere thanks and gratitude to Shari Intagiata, MS, MPA, OTR/L for her encouragement and persistence throughout the many phases of writing this manuscript. The project could not have been completed without her guidance and support. Special appreciation is also extended to the author's many colleagues at the Rehabilitation Institute of Chicago for their support and understanding.

Related Learning Activities

1. Conduct an informal interview with three OTR/COTA teams—one working in a physical dysfunction setting in a hospital, one employed in a psychosocial dysfunction community-based center, and one working in a geriatric long-term care facility. Determine the service operations management tasks they perform regularly. Compare and contrast the results in light of the text material and discuss the findings with classmates.

2. Visit a hospital-based and a community-based occupational therapy department and determine what type of records and reports are required.

3. Design a brochure to be given to physicians that explains the types of services provided by an occupational therapy program.

4. Plan and construct a display for an open house designed to provide information about occupational therapy to the general public.

References

1. Rowland H, Rowland P: *Hospital Administration Handbook.* Rockville, Maryland, Aspen, 1984.
2. American Occupational Therapy Association: *Manual on Administration.* Rockville, Maryland, American Occupational Therapy Association, 1978.
3. Levine R: Community health care—the homebound patient. In Hopkins H, Smith H, (Eds): *Willard and Spackman's Occupational Therapy,* 6th Edition. Philadelphia, JB Lippincott, 1983.
4. Executive summary of the department of health and human services report to congress on hospital prospective payment for medicare. *Federal Report.* Rockville, Maryland, American Occupational Therapy Association, 1983.
5. Medicare prospective payment. *Occup Ther Newspaper,* 38:4, 1984.
6. Joe BE: Quality assurance consultants add program evaluation to repertoire. *Occup Ther Newspaper,* 38:5, 1984.
7. Ostrow PC: Quality assurance—improving occupational therapy. In Hopkins H, Smith H,(Eds): *Willard and Spackman's*

Occupational Therapy, 6th Edition. Philadelphia, JB Lippincott, 1983, p 862.

8. American Occupational Therapy Association: *Uniform Terminology for Reporting Occupational Therapy Services, 2nd Edition*. Rockville, Maryland, American Occupational Therapy Association, 1989.

9. Publicity and professionalism. *Occup Ther Newspaper* 37:7, 1983.

10. Christiansen C: Research: An economic imperative. *Occup Ther J Res* 37:195-198, 1983.

11. Yerxa EJ: The occupational therapist as a researcher. In Hopkins H, Smith H, Eds: *Willard and Spackman's Occupational Therapy*, 6th Edition, Philadelphia, JB Lippincott, 1983, p 870.

Section VI
CONTEMPORARY ISSUES AND TRENDS

The theme for the final section of this text is recapitulation and integration. In other words, the goals of the authors and the editor, in part, are to restate, review and summarize various issues related to the education and practice of occupational therapy practitioners. Several concepts are combined and unified as a professional whole. The major focus is fourfold.

Beginning with a review of the maturation process of the COTA in terms of intraprofessional relationships and socialization, the content builds to encompass principles of occupational therapy ethics as they relate to a variety of practice situations. The credentialing process within the profession is also described.

The concluding chapter redefines the impact of social forces in relation to the culture of occupational therapy. Values are reexamined in terms of historical, current and future impact. Gilfoyle states: "Through transformation we will direct our future. The time for promotion of the idea 'health through doing' is now. It is the era where occupational therapy can proclaim its uniqueness as the therapeutic use of occupations to facilitate abilities so that individuals can influence the state of their own health."

Intraprofessional Relationships and Socialization

A MATURATION PROCESS

Toné F. Blechert, MA, COTA, ROH
Marianne F. Christiansen, MA, OTR

Introduction

This chapter describes how a certified occupational therapy assistant (COTA) becomes socialized into the profession of occupational therapy. **Professional socialization** includes the acquisition of skills and knowledge to do the work of an occupation, the development and orientation of attitudes and behaviors that are needed for the specific role, and identities and commitments that motivate the person to pursue the occupation and feel accepted by the professional community.[1]

A student entering the field of occupational therapy has a partially developed value and belief system that has contributed to attitudes and behaviors that have compelled the person to enter a health care field. Through the use of a process model, steps in the development of socialization will be outlined as shown in Figure 29-1. These steps include:

1. Mastery of entry-level knowledge and skills
2. Practical application of technical knowledge and skills (ie, fieldwork experiences)
3. Entry-level work experience
4. Self-enhancement activities leading to new dimensions of knowledge, skill and sensitivity[2]

KEY CONCEPTS

Choosing a career

Mastery of entry-level knowledge and skills

Supervision

Entry-level work experience

Relationships

Motivation

Self-enhancement

Socialized self

ESSENTIAL VOCABULARY

Professional socialization

Adaptability

Flexibility

Ministration

Mastery

Maturation

Sustenance

Perceived conflict

Manifest behavior

Mentors

5. Commitment to lifelong learning and to the profession; the socialized self

Within this framework, topics are discussed that focus on the steps of choosing a career in occupational therapy and the progression of educational and practice experiences that lead to socialization within the profession. Interpersonal relationships, conflict management principles and professional motivation also will be discussed.

Choosing a Career in Occupational Therapy

Women and men who begin to consider a career in occupational therapy at the professional or technical level come from a diverse group representing a broad range of developmental needs, attitudes, values and behaviors. Studies have shown, however that one value held in common is the wish to contribute to the welfare of others.[3,4]

The careful planner goes through certain steps to make career choices. These steps are as follows:

1. *Discovery*: The individual examines past accomplishments and present activities and plans for the future. At this point usually some dissatisfaction motivates the person to explore alternatives.
2. *Focus*: The individual spends time and energy searching for information related to possible alternatives. Exploration of levels of occupational therapy education should occur at this point. This early orientation process begins the socialization process.
3. *Validation*: In this stage, the planning and choices become more integrated and the individual begins to share decisions with others to receive feedback and confirmation.
4. *Implementation*: In this stage the action toward the decision occurs. A time commitment is made and a school is selected, beginning a new phase of learning.[5]

Acquisition and Mastery of Entry-level Knowledge and Skills

Occupational therapy assistant education molds the student's orientation to his or her work. Several basic frames of reference are used in these curricula. Whichever frame of reference is favored, the curriculum must be tied to that framework which creates an organized body of knowledge. A variety of teaching methods are used to convey this material. With close attention to the *Essentials and Guidelines of an Accredited Educational Program for the Occupational Therapy Assistant*, developed by the American Occupational Therapy Association, a curriculum design may include focus on principles and technical concepts in a

variety of disability areas, fieldwork experiences to enhance that learning, opportunities to develop communication skills, and general education components. Involvement in this educational process may reinforce existing attitudes and values or allow them to change. Behaviors and even personalities may be altered. These changes occur as the student is exposed to the new concepts and experiences that the curriculum has to offer.

All students receive feedback during their education. The activities learned in the occupational therapy program provide unique opportunities for the student to receive feedback from nonhuman objects as well as instructors, clinical supervisors, patients and peers. This ongoing feedback is the beginning of the student's ability to make critical changes in thinking and actions. As a result, students begin to perceive themselves as interpersonally and technically competent. This sense of mastery enables them to progress to higher levels of socialization.

Practical Application

Mastery of occupational therapy concepts and the altered or reinforced beliefs and attitudes are the basis for the next step in the socialization process—practical application of knowledge and skills. In a professional or technical education program, fieldwork is used to provide this practical experience. During fieldwork, a student not only will apply already acquired information but also will be exposed to new knowledge and methods. The problem-solving skills gained during academic preparation are used as the student discovers possible alternatives in relating to patients and providing treatment. This process also requires adaptability and flexibility on the part of the student.

Adaptability refers to the skill enabling one to easily and quickly conform to new and strange circumstances. **Flexibility** is the willingness and openness that one must have to be able to adapt. A rigid person is less able to adapt to new situations that arise, including to new patient treatment techniques and approaches as well as relating to and interacting with new people, such as supervisors and co-workers.

Philosophies of treatment are changing in the health care field, and facilities and agencies will vary in their styles and methods of treatment. The continuum may range from a predominant focus on prevention and the issues of health and wellness to the traditional medical model still found in many hospitals. It is hoped that the student can face these varied situations with a flexible attitude. One should be able to use the problem-solving skills, creativity and the baseline of knowledge gained during classroom experiences to adapt to and meet new challenges.

Supervision

One necessary competence is acceptance of supervision. The relationships that are formed between students and

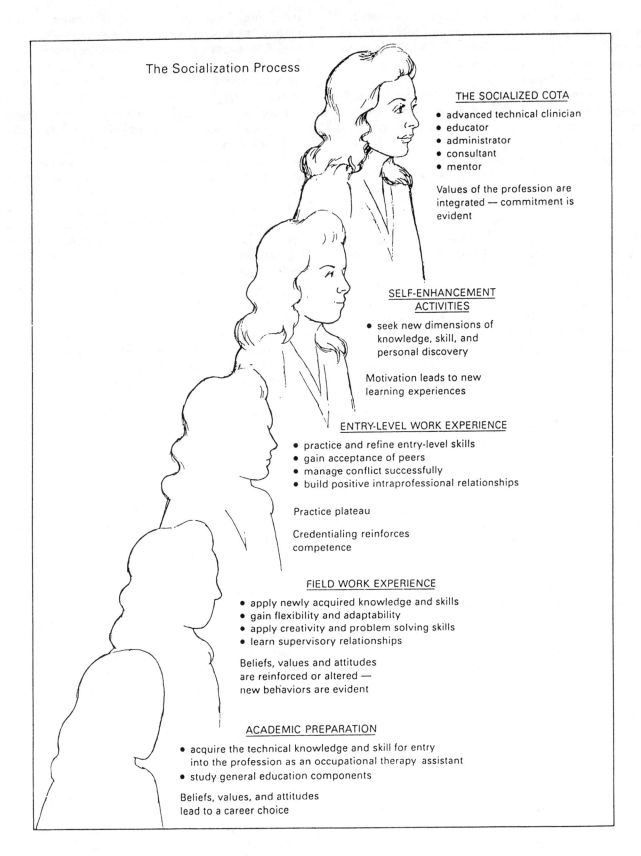

The Socialization Process

THE SOCIALIZED COTA
- advanced technical clinician
- educator
- administrator
- consultant
- mentor

Values of the profession are integrated — commitment is evident

SELF-ENHANCEMENT ACTIVITIES
- seek new dimensions of knowledge, skill, and personal discovery

Motivation leads to new learning experiences

ENTRY-LEVEL WORK EXPERIENCE
- practice and refine entry-level skills
- gain acceptance of peers
- manage conflict successfully
- build positive intraprofessional relationships

Practice plateau

Credentialing reinforces competence

FIELD WORK EXPERIENCE
- apply newly acquired knowledge and skills
- gain flexibility and adaptability
- apply creativity and problem solving skills
- learn supervisory relationships

Beliefs, values and attitudes are reinforced or altered — new behaviors are evident

ACADEMIC PREPARATION
- acquire the technical knowledge and skill for entry into the profession as an occupational therapy assistant
- study general education components

Beliefs, values, and attitudes lead to a career choice

Figure 29-1. *The socialization process.*

supervisors are crucial in the socialization process. It is primarily the supervisor who defines the relationship between supervisor and student during a fieldwork experience. The supervisor's behavior signals to the student the dimensions of their relationship.

The sooner that a student can understand the social system and goals of a particular fieldwork setting, the more likely the student is to have success. The idea of a psychological contract between an individual and a work place seems to have been originated in 1962 by Levinson, a clinical psychologist who became interested in mental health and work. As Levinson studied workers entering a new company, he observed a process of fulfilling mutual expectations and satisfying mutual needs in the relationship between a person and his or her work. Levinson described this process as *reciprocation*. Reciprocation is a process of carrying out a psychological contract between a person and company or any other institution where one works.[6]

According to Levinson's observations, an individual entering a work situation has certain expectations and needs, many of which are subconscious. Whether one is a student entering a fieldwork setting or a person beginning a new job, there is a hope that the work environment, the job itself and relationships with supervisors and co-workers will fulfill these needs and expectations.

A fieldwork setting's expectations may be very clear and in writing regarding objectives and assignments, but where behavior is concerned the expectations may be less clear. Whether the student is expected to be independent, warm, assertive or distant with other therapists or the supervisor is seldom communicated formally; however, these expectations do exist and the student's ability to adapt quickly to the social system is a strong predictor of success. So it is in any work situation as the individual worker wants the work setting to satisfy his or her needs and the work place wants the individual to satisfy its needs and help achieve its goals.

The fulfillment of this psychological contract depends on the level of reciprocity. If the individual student or worker and the work place are able to satisfy each others needs, the individual will tend to identify with the work place and consider his or her role appreciated and important.

The psychological contract identified by Levinson and introduced in Chapter 3 describes three needs that each person has when entering a work situation: **ministration, mastery** and **maturation**.[6]

Ministration needs for a student refer to needs for feeling close to others in the work setting and for support, guidance and protection.[6] Some students may need a significant amount of support in their work, whereas others may require very little. Students are not likely to tell a supervisor how much support is needed in order to function effectively; however, a supervisor will often sense these needs in their behavior. It is important for students to take responsibility

and communicate any feelings of discomfort or lack of support. If the supervisor is unable to provide the support needed by the student, he or she should be prepared to offer the student other sources of gratification. If students' needs for ministration are met, they are likely to perceive the work place as "caring."

The need for mastery is concerned with the desire to explore, understand and, to some extent, control oneself and an environment.[6] A fieldwork supervisor who is sensitive to the student's need for mastery will provide the student with an appropriate measure of control early in the fieldwork experience. This control may take the form of offering choices in assignments or patient groups, for instance. Supervisors usually appreciate a student's interest in achieving more independence; therefore, it is important to verbalize one's goals and needs. For the occupational assistant student, important competencies to be achieved must include more than those relevant to patient treatment. For example, the ability to deal adequately with professionals from other departments, as well as other occupational therapy personnel, should be an important goal.

If maturation needs are met a person unfolds; if they are not the person vegetates.[6] Fieldwork provides reality testing opportunities for a student as concepts learned in school are applied in a real situation. This reality testing takes the form of feedback from supervisors and patients as a result of one's efforts. Feedback provides a student with the sense of growth necessary for some maturation to take place.

These concepts of the psychological contract and the reciprocation process, as it is adapted to the interaction between fieldwork supervisors and students, are summarized in Figure 29-2. Both supervisor and student bring expectations to the relationship. If the reciprocation process works, the student's needs will be satisfied and he or she will be able to perform at the best level. Just as the supervisor satisfies the student's needs, so the student—even though he or she does not have control of the relationship—can potentially satisfy the supervisor's needs for ministration and mastery, but not for maturation. The supervisor also has some need for closeness, warmth and caring as well as for mastery of the environment. These concepts, as they relate to team building, are discussed in greater depth in Chapter 3. More information on supervision may be found in Chapter 2.

Entry-level Work Experience

After the required fieldwork experiences, the student has fully completed the formal educational process and is ready to enter the work arena. Although there may be anxiety associated with leaving familiar environments to enter a new work environment, there is also a feeling of excitement and

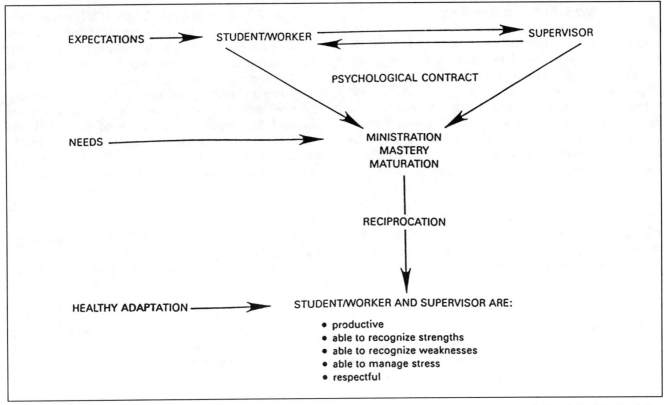

Figure 29-2. *Psychological contract and reciprocation process. Adapted from Levinson, H, Men, Management, and Mental Health. Cambridge, Massachusetts, Harvard University Press, 1962.*

of competence, which is then reinforced after successful completion of the certification examination.

As a COTA begins a first work experience, another phase in the maturing process begins. Many of the experiences, feelings and behaviors that were initially, and perhaps superficially, developed during fieldwork will be enhanced and encountered in more depth during the first work experience. The new COTA will be meeting new challenges, practicing and refining skills and continuing to gain acceptance from peers, patients and the public.

Acceptance

Feeling accepted is a crucial phase in the socialization process of the COTA. Without a feeling of respect and acceptance, particularly from the supervisor, it will be difficult for the COTA to perform adequately and feel confident and satisfied. If dissatisfaction occurs, motivation to achieve may decline, indicating that ministration needs are not being met. At this point the COTA may examine choices. If there is an investment in the profession and job because of other satisfactions, there will be energy to remedy the situation. If other satisfactions or investments are not present, the COTA may choose a different path such as a new job or different training.

There are many ways to remedy the situation and to gain acceptance if one chooses to try. First, it is important to enmesh oneself in the culture of the facility. Learning what is acceptable in terms of dress, language and general expectations and establishing oneself as a member of a multidisciplinary team will strengthen one's connection with a particular workplace. As a COTA begins to feel increased acceptance and respect, relationships will develop and the assistant will feel bonded to the setting. Four major aspects of work that encourage bonding are as follows:[7]

1. The general nature of the work, its challenge and the talents it requires
2. Freedom to perform the work, to use personal ideas, to feel vital in the efforts bringing about work accomplishment and to make decisions about work
3. Opportunities to grow and to develop through training and feedback on performance and to receive a reasonable variety of assignments
4. Recognition of work achievement in a forthright, sincere and timely manner

The needs for ministration, mastery and maturation also remain constant from the student role to the worker role. As the ministration and mastery needs are met, maturation will occur. The work experience allows even more time for this process than the fieldwork experience because both work investment and time commitment are greater.

Team Building Relationships

Review of the principles and concepts introduced in Chapter 3 points to the importance of developing and maintaining intraprofessional and interprofessional relationships within a teamwork and team building context. Establishing these ties often begins in the classroom. These ties then grow during the fieldwork experience and in the employment setting as people become increasingly more committed to the benefits and opportunities team work provides. Effective team building relationships with one's colleagues requires cooperation, flexibilty and creativity to form a closely knit, smoothly coordinated and synchronized group.[8] Relationships require maintenance and **sustenance** as well. Sustenance may be viewed as providing nourishment to a relationship. For example, taking extra time to talk with a fellow student or co-worker who is experiencing frustration or self-doubt often provides the needed sustenance to help the person during a difficult time.

Managing Conflict

Despite all of the positive aspects and efforts of teaming, it is inevitable that conflict sometimes will arise. Conflict does not have to be a negative factor and can, in fact, improve situations and stimulate personal growth if it is identified and handled appropriately. It should be noted, however, that effective problem solving aimed at confilct resolution cannot take place without some conflicts over ideas and opinions.

Preexisting conditions involving relationships and situations can lead to conflict. These conditions can include a conflict of interest between two people; physical, emotional or time factors that lead to communication barriers; economic or emotional dependence of one person on another; or previous unresolved conflicts.[9]

These preexisting conditions can lead to either perceived or actual conflict. **Perceived conflict** is that which is felt by a person that may or may not lead to actual conflict. The *actual conflict* is that which does happen. It usually involves an awareness of disagreement and may involve personal hostilities.

The **manifest behavior** is the reaction of the individuals that occurs in response to the conflict. It may be in the form of an argument, debate or any type of confrontation. It may also be less overt but is evident in nonverbal body language between two people.

The resolution or suppression phase is perhaps the most crucial. If the conflict and related feelings are suppressed, the aftermath will bring the cycle back to the beginning and more conflict will occur. It is important in this phase to find some way of resolving the conflict so that the outcome leads to improved relationships.

Several factors are important during this phase to enable resolution of conflict. The primary factor is that both people must be willing to try to resolve things. If only one person is willing, no amount of effort will improve the situation. This situation can be frustrating so it is hoped that with proper understanding and communication, both persons will be willing to attempt resolution.

As with the conflict process itself, there are many models for resolution. One such model is integrative decision making.[9] This method involves several steps. First, the involved parties must identify and adjust any particular physical or situational factors that might be causing difficulty. For instance, the conflict may relate to a lack of office space, which could be remedied by stating the problem to each other and or to a supervisor who may be able to make different arrangements. If this is not possible, a shift in scheduling may allow the two parties to share space more comfortably.

The next two steps important in this type of resolution are examination of each person's perceptions and attitudes. What is the other person feeling (overburdened, insecure, moody or inadequate)? What are one's own feelings (resentment, dependency, fear or aggression? The next step would be for the two people to sit down and actually describe their perceptions to each other. It is important to own your own feelings by using the personal pronoun and verb "I feel. . .." Often a misunderstanding is clarified and the two people can easily remedy the situation. If the conflict still cannot be resolved, at least a mutual understanding of each other's feelings and perceptions may have occurred, which will then allow the problem to be identified.

Many times, the actual problem is buried beneath negative feelings and therefore is never accurately stated. Once the problem has been defined, a search process for solutions can begin. During this process, both people offer as many solutions as possible. Solutions from others may also be included. This search phase can include brainstorming, discussion groups and surveys. Anything that can be looked at in an effort to resolve the problem should be considered. After this phase, a narrowing down process should begin until there is mutual agreement. During this evaluation and final stage, it is important to keep the original problem in mind and to be open about one's feelings so that they do not hamper reaching a satisfying solution.

Case Study

A new COTA is starting her first job in an activities department with a staff of two others and a supervisor. The supervisor and the two staff members have been employed at the facility for several years and have an established program, but an increase in caseload created the need for additional staffing. After a month of employment, the assistant begins to feel comfortable with the supervisor, but is having difficulty with the staff members regarding their choice of programming and their approach to patients. The

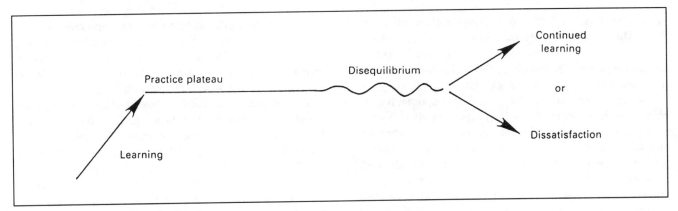

Figure 29-3. *Adaptations to entry-level work.*

COTA talks to the other staff members and expresses her concerns and new ideas but is met with resistance. Subsequently, the others become less friendly to her and continue with their routines, excluding her from any decision making.

At this point the preexisting conditions are present, and both perceived and actual conflict have become manifest in behaviors. The COTA has several choices. She can choose to ignore the situation and continue to feel uncomfortable and dissatisfied, quit the job, talk to the supervisor about it, or approach the staff members again in an effort to resolve the situation.

If the COTA decides to talk with the other staff, it would first be helpful to express her feelings rather than making suggestions. If the assistant can be open with her own feelings of frustration and perhaps rejection, others may be able to discuss their feelings. It is possible that they are feeling bored with the existing programming, yet threatened by a new staff member with new ideas. Once these feelings have been expressed, a problem can be more clearly defined. It may be a general programming problem that exists within the department.

If the emotions and feelings have been recognized, it will be easier and less threatening to resolve the problem together. The problem becomes less personalized and can be shared by all members of the department. Books and periodicals may be consulted or other programs contacted to identify new ideas for the old programs. With a pool of new ideas, the staff can decide together what programming would best meet the needs of the patients.

In summary, the relationship with co-workers and supervisors depends largely on openness of communication, mutual respect and understanding and cooperation rather than competition. If one senses conflict or dissatisfaction, it is important to identify the problem and proceed with necessary steps to resolve it; otherwise a weakened team structure may result.

Motivation

Entry-level work experience allows the COTA to practice and refine existing skills. A person will feel satisfied and comfortable for a period of time. Of course the mind is open to learn splinter skills that relate to a particular work setting, but for a while new learning is essentially stopped. The occupational therapy assistant is on a practice plateau enabling total integration of the technical knowledge and skills previously learned.

After some time has passed, and this differs for each individual, the COTA will desire to move off the plateau and begin a new learning experience. This feeling is not always understood on an intellectual level. Rather, there may just be a desire operating on the will that causes one to act. This desire or motivation occurs because of a feeling of *disequilibrium* or a sense of dissatisfaction associated with the need to know or grow.

Among the many factors that create this need to know are newly emerging goals, competition or curiosity, wish for success, quest for novelty or change and affiliation with a mentor. These motivators enable a person to move off the plateau and seek new learning experiences.

New learning takes several forms. Many people pursue increased specialization skills in occupational therapy. Others may seek knowledge in a totally different area to satisfy personal needs. Some may choose to pursue an education at the professional level to become an OTR. Whatever form the self-enhancement takes, it may serve as an example of healthy adaptation. If a person does not heed feelings of disequilibrium, a growing sense of dissatisfaction will occur. Relationships with peers and supervisors are likely to weaken and self-esteem will decrease. Figure 29-3 depicts this continuum.

Self-Enhancement

Continuing Education

Continuing education should be a lifelong and self-directed process. COTAs who value and pursue lifelong learning truly care for themselves. The COTA's role is "caretaker of others." The most competent caretakers are those who continually care for and renew their own lives. Continuing education may be seen as a means of renewal and an investment in oneself, in the profession of occupational therapy and in society in general.

One may continue to seek learning opportunities to enhance technical competence in occupational therapy or to gratify maturation needs through further study of other arts and sciences. The pursuit of learning in areas not directly related to one's profession helps lay a firm foundation for occupational excellence.[2] Study or experience in diverse interest areas broadens one's perspectives and offers new insights into one's personal and work life. Self-directed learning is a pleasurable activity and provides restful change and relaxation to help one achieve a healthy balance.

Continued education goals related to maintaining competence in the profession may be set by state associations, state regulatory boards or the individual. Such programs are offered through colleges, universities, technical schools and health agencies. Many learning programs award the continuing education unit (CEU). CEUs are based on specific standards that assure some measure of quality to the learner. Although CEUs are not currently required, in the future the American Occupational Therapy Association (AOTA) may choose to use them to measure participation in continuing education. It is possible that this form of measurement will be one option in a specialty certification process.[10]

The AOTA and affiliated state associations also offer continuing education programs and resources to the membership. Conferences, workshops, seminars, programmed learning packets and audiovisual materials may assist practitioners in maintaining competence. Publications such as the *American Journal of Occupational Therapy* and *Occupational Therapy Week* offer pertinent articles and information that also contribute to lifelong learning.

To become more fully socialized, however, one must expand on these concepts of continuing education. Most COTAs see the need for learning new theory and techniques that are directly applicable to a specific work role. More assistants must begin to recognize the learning potential related to volunteer activities such as participation on commissions, committees and task forces to serve the local, state and national occupational therapy associations.

The AOTA and the state affiliates draw their strength from each individual's contributions. These contributions are in the form of time, intellectual and emotional energy, and financial support. In turn, active involvement in the association activities is essential if a COTA is to realize his or her full potential. Extended and expanded exposure to the practice of occupational therapy is only one part of becoming socialized into the profession. One must also experience an extended exposure to and investment in association activities. This investment offers multidimensional continuing education opportunities. Participation in association

affairs aids the further development of communication and problem-solving skills. This work also contributes to one's understanding of the profession and its central mission. Increased understanding leads to inquiry, action and further learning, increased growth and new challenges.

Volunteerism also leads to the development of professional and personal relationships outside of the work place. These relationships expand one's support system, which is essential to the healthy practitioner. The wise COTA seeks social support as a means of preventing "burnout." Burnout is a popular term used to describe a state of mental fatigue that may be encountered during one's work life. Practitioners who suffer "burnout" experience an inability to generate energy for their job or think creatively. Burnout can be disabling and COTAs need to think in terms of prevention. Social support systems are an important part of one's renewal plan in order to maintain a high energy level and motivation for learning.

The Socialized Self

A socialized person is involved in lifelong learning as new personal goals continue to evolve. In addition, expectations of the profession and individuals within it increase significantly.[2] A COTA who has reached this level of maturation has a recognized area of expertise, which he or she is expanding and sharing through teaching, specializing in a clinical area, managing, speaking, publishing, creating audiovisual tools, developing computer programs, consulting and mentoring others.

The COTA as Advanced Clinician

A majority of COTAs maintain their roles as clinicians; however, after reaching this level of maturation and socialization, they can be designated as advanced clinicians with a specialized area of expertise.

During the initial educational process, the focus was on general occupational therapy education with exposure to a variety of disability areas and problems. Students received a framework of knowledge and learned therapeutic application of purposeful activity as it related to these areas. This approach prepared a student to seek employment in a number of different settings. When a COTA seeks entry-level employment, he or she begins in one area and may remain there. Some COTAs choose to work in a variety of practice areas during their first few years of experience before they begin to specialize.

Whichever route one takes, there usually is a desire to seek additional training in a particular area. Some of this training may occur on the job. Other training obtained through continuing education may offer a specialty certification from a particular agency. As experience increases, specialization permits a feeling of increased competence.[11] This feeling is an important source of self-gratification and mastery for the COTA and allows the patient to receive the best possible treatment.

Within one's area of expertise, it is important for each clinician to view that specialty as a part of the whole profession and not as a separate entity. Although terminology and techniques may vary, the philosophical base of occupational therapy remains central, and the connections to the profession and other clinicians must be maintained. For example, one COTA may be working in geriatrics while another specializes in psychiatry; however, the common base of activity should allow these COTAs to share problems, ideas and goals. In addition to specialized skills, this ability to be an integral part of the total profession is a strength of a COTA who is an advanced clinician.

The COTA as Administrator

Proficient COTAs may seek new dimensions of work experience in a management or administrative position. Examples of these kinds of positions held by COTAs include director of activities in long-term care settings, coordinator of volunteer services in community settings, and self-employed practitioners who manage others in offering supportive services to the elderly and others living at home.

Some individuals demonstrate a remarkable capacity to master management methods and principles through life and work experience. Others seek academic preparation to enhance their skills and knowledge. It has been said, however, that no program develops a manager; one develops oneself.[8] Educational programs, whether formal or informal, only assist a person in gaining awareness of strengths, limitations and growth possibilities and then encourage self-directed learning. The motivation to acquire knowledge and ability in management must be strong within the individual. More information on management may be found in Chapters 22 and 28.

The COTA as Educator

An increasing number of COTAs are becoming educators in both professional and technical level academic programs as well as in fieldwork.

In occupational therapy education the primary goal is to prepare people to function as practitioners.[12] Although many techniques can be used in this preparation, a helpful one is to involve the learner as much as possible. This technique can be compared to one of the basic tenets of the occupational therapy profession—the "doing of purposeful activity."

It is important to view education as a facilitation process in which the learner is assisted toward the goal of acquiring skills and knowledge that enable independent functioning.[13] The steps of developing rapport or establishing a comfort level, setting learning objectives and providing methods for the student to achieve these objectives are similar to the process used in any therapeutic interaction.

Some of the qualities that can assist an educator in facilitating the learning process include keeping current in the subject, making ideas understandable and pertinent, using creativity to stimulate the student's desire to learn, and being open with the students and realizing that they also have knowledge to offer.[14]

Writing, Speaking and Research

Whether a COTA chooses to become an educator, administrator or advanced clinician, writing, speaking and research permit further growth of the individual and the profession. Experienced COTAs are encouraged to share their knowledge in a formal way.

The purpose of writing and speaking is to communicate ideas and information, to share knowledge or create change. Writing and speaking are major forces in facilitating progress within the profession. COTAs contribute articles to professional journals and state and national newspapers. They are involved in the development of pamphlets, scripts and lessons for educational and public relations purposes. Speaking is a natural extension of writing. COTAs speak at national and state conferences, schools, seminars and workshops.

Research is currently one of the focal points of the science of occupational therapy. If members of the profession become active consumers of research, the demand will increase and the supply will expand.[15]

The role of consumer begins in the educational process with the studying and reading of information. It is hoped that the student will continue to read and study after graduation, but this does not always happen. One method of encouraging on-going education is to initiate a journal club among the staff where one is working. Journal clubs can assume a variety of formats, the basis being to read, share and discuss current articles that are being published. This approach promotes the concepts of research and development within the profession in addition to providing new dimensions of knowledge to the members involved.

The role of contributor to research is often perceived incorrectly as overwhelming. Contributing to research can begin by becoming a careful recorder of information. The complete recording of data such as patient ages, diagnoses, treatment techniques, length of treatment and responses to treatment can be a basis for developing research projects. The actual design and implementation of the project may require collaboration with an OTR or someone else with expertise; however, the compiling of data is the foundation of research.

Consuming or contributing to research is necessary to stimulate and validate the profession of occupational therapy as well as to allow all members of the profession to further their own growth. It is important for COTAs to seek out ways in which they can become actively involved in the research process.

The COTA as Consultant

The experienced and well-informed COTA may be asked to serve as a consultant in an area of expertise. The main goal of consulting is to provide a service or resolve a problem. Consulting can occur formally or informally. Informally, it may be the sharing and offering of information to a colleague. Formally, it can involve conferring regularly with other individuals or agencies to provide advice and guidance.

As advanced clinicians, administrators and educators, COTAs have served as consultants with directors of adult day care and senior citizen centers, designers of adaptive equipment, building planners and educators.

The COTA as Role Model and Mentor

Role models stimulate and inspire others through example and encouragement.[2] In this process, observing and copying are the primary methods of learning.

Role modeling differs from **mentoring**. Mentorship involves much more of a commitment and sharing between two people. The word mentor is used to mean a wise and faithful counselor or guide and originated from Greek mythology.[16] Mentoring can occur at different levels, depending on the needs of the person who is seeking additional personal and professional growth experiences. The mentor can focus on academics, work or professional activities. Acting as a mentor to others can be viewed as a form of ministration, which helps another person reach a higher level of maturity.

Being a mentor requires certain personal characteristics, including providing direction, being open and sensitive to another's needs, recognizing the potential strengths and limitations in others, being responsive and available, and desiring to have influence on the next generation.[16]

Some specific actions one can take to be a mentor may include inviting another COTA to work alongside oneself in any professional activity on a state or national level. While working with this person, one has the opportunity to introduce him or her to other members in the field. After working with this person, the next step would be to affirm strengths and identify areas for growth. Feedback and suggestions can be made to encourage growth. The mentor can then begin to recommend his or her colleague to others. For example, one might nominate the individual for committee membership or chairmanship in the state association. The ultimate goal would be for the colleague to be self-motivating and able to seek out new challenges independently to become enmeshed in the professional organizations. When involvement has become integrated and comfortable, it is hoped that the person will consider mentorship of another.[17]

Summary

Socialization is change or development toward increased maturity and responsibility. In general, the concept of socialization includes both the content that must be learned and the activities that one must participate in to create potential for integration of learning and continued growth. The content in occupational therapy includes the norms, values, beliefs and skills required for both the social integration of the person and the stability of the profession. Socialization can be said to be successful for both the individual and the profession if it provides for integration of the technician into the profession and mutual integration, understanding and acceptance of both levels of occupational thearapy personnel into the health care community[18]. For COTAs to be truly socialized, they must have extended exposure to the profession through education, practice and involvement in professional activities. Experience gained in these formal and informal settings enables COTAs to recognize themselves and be recognized by others as competent, contributing members of the profession of occupational therapy.

Editor's Note

Although the focus of this chapter is on the COTA, many of the points apply to the occupational therapist student and practitioner as well.

Related Learning Activities

1. Discuss factors that contribute to the socialization of an individual into a profession.

2. List ways feedback can be helpful? What types of feedback do you appreciate?

3. Discuss the importance of role models and mentors with your peers.

References

1. Simpson I: *From Student to Nurse: A Longitudinal Study of Socialization.* New York, Cambridge University Press, 1979, p. 6.
2. Houle C: *Continuing Learning in the Professions.* San Francisco, Jossey-Bass, 1980, pp. 47-48, 67-89, 114-115, 309-315.
3. Holstrom E: Promising prospects: Students choosing therapy as a career. *Am J Occup Ther* 10:608-614, 1975.
4. Madigan J: Characteristics of students in occupational therapy educational programs. *Am J Occup Ther* 1:41-46, 1985.
5. Buck J, Daniels M, Harren V (Eds): *Facilitating Students' Career Development.* San Francisco, Jossey-Bass, 1981, p 7.
6. Levinson H: *Men, Management, and Mental Health.* Cambridge, Massachusetts, Harvard University Press, 1962, pp. 39, 147-184.

7. Terry G: *Principles of Management*. Homewood, Illinois, Richard Irwin, 1977, pp. 227-228, 395.

8. Beggs D, Ed: *Team Teaching: Bold New Venture*. Indianapolis, United College Press, 1964, pp. 44-47, 131, 465.

9. Filley A: *Interpersonal Confict Resolution*. Glenview, Illinois, Scott Foresman, 1975, pp. 8, 92-93.

10. Robertson S, Martin E: Continuing education: A quality assurance approach. *Am J Occup Ther* 5:314-315, 1981.

11. Gillette N, Kielhofner G: The impact of specialization on the professionalization and survival of occupational therapy. *Am J Occup Ther* 1:20-28, 1979.

12. Shapiro D, Shanahan P: Methodology for teaching theory in OT basic professional education. *Am J Occup Ther* 4:217-224, 1976.

13. Bowen A: Carl Rogers' views of education. *Am J Occup Ther* 4:220-221, 1974.

14. Hansen E: Plain talk about good teaching. *Improving College and University Teaching* 1:23-24, 1978.

15. Gilfoyle E: Caring: a philosophy for practice. *Am J Occup Ther* 8:517-521, 1980.

16. Rogers J: Sponsorship: Developing leaders for occupational therapy. *Am J Occup Ther* 5:309-313, 1982.

17. Robertson S (Ed): *Find a Mentor or Be One*. Rockville, Maryland, American Occupational Therapy Association, 1992.

18. Gubrium J, Buckholdt D: *Toward Maturity*. San Francisco, Jossey-Bass 1977, pp. 126-144.

Principles of Occupational Therapy Ethics

Sister Genevieve Cummings, CSJ, MA, OTR, FAOTA

Introduction

Ethics has to do with the rightness or wrongness of an action. It relates to what it is that "ought" to be done. Moral principles, rules and standards are formulations of what "ought" to be done personally and professionally. Professional ethics is the rule or standard by which the rightness or wrongness of choices and behaviors are determined. Ethics is usually stated in terms of principles, rather than a list of rules. Basic attitudes and qualities define what is ethical.

Primary Values

All ethical principles are based on four values: **prudence, temperateness, courage** and **justice**. These four values form the foundation for ethical choices and behavior.

Prudence

Prudence refers to choosing the right means (ie, using foresight and care in what must be done). The opposite of prudence is negligence or recklessness. When occupational therapy practitioners act with prudence, they are knowledgeable about what they are doing and use good judgment in evaluation, treatment planning and implementation. They are able to predict the consequences of what they do. For instance, beginning treatment without evaluation or planning would be imprudent and unethical. Another example of imprudence, that is, not using foresight and care, is using treatment modalities without the appropriate education.

Temperateness

Temperateness, also referred to as temperance, means moderation. Another way to define temperateness is a regard for decency in behavior. The opposite, cruelty or insensibility, helps

KEY CONCEPTS

Primary values

Secondary values

Ethical theory

Professional ethics

Occupational therapy code of ethics

ESSENTIAL VOCABULARY

Prudence

Temperateness

Courage

Justice

Reverence

Fidelity

Teleologic

Deontologic

Beneficence

Fraudulent

to clarify what temperateness means. Any behavior that treats the patient inhumanely, that discriminates against the person or that ridicules the individual is intemperate behavior.

Courage

Courage is a value that shows itself in patience, tenacity and perseverance. Being willing to do what is known to be right, in spite of difficulties or problems, is an example of how the value of courage relates to ethical principles. Occupational therapy personnel have at times been discontinued in their work or even left positions because they took action in circumstances of unethical behavior on the part of others. It takes courage to stand up for what is right when that action will have adverse effects, even to the point of depriving the person of their employment. 'I don't want to get involved' is a common statement in our society.

Justice

Justice requires that each person be treated with integrity and honesty. This value is perhaps most obviously related to ethics. Any act that is dishonest is also unethical. Occupational therapy personnel owe their patients quality treatment that is carefully planned and implemented and accurately reimbursed. Giving persons their due is justice.

Secondary Values

Other values basic to ethical behavior include **reverence, fidelity,** awareness of responsibility, truthfulness and goodness. Although these values may seem abstract, they are the foundation of ethical principles. For instance, reverence requires respect for each person. Each one must be treated in a manner that recognizes the dignity of each human being. Fidelity or faithfulness can be applied in relationships both with patients and employers. It is expressed in contract keeping. Awareness of responsibility provides a framework for ethical behavior. No therapist or assistant should be able to say "I didn't know doing that would be unethical." We have an obligation to know. Not knowing is itself unethical. Truthfulness is at the heart of informed consent and of all relations with patients, families, colleagues and other professionals. Goodness has to do with rightness, aptness, fitness and excellence. Poor treatment, inappropriately carried out, cannot be ethical treatment.

Ethical Theory

Although there are many ethical theories, most ethicists define two basic theories—**teleologic** and **deontologic.**

Teleologic relates to the end; thus it focuses on the consequences of the act. It is also referred to as the consequential approach. If the end is good, then the means are ethical. The principle of **beneficence** comes from teleologic theory. It indicates that we must act so as to promote good consequences for others. The principle of utility, also flowing from teleologic theory, says that we must promote the greatest good for the greatest number of people.

Deontologic theory says that acts are right in themselves. This theory is also referred to as the formalist approach. The basic aspect of deontologic theory is duty. We have a duty to other persons that requires us to always consider the individual's rights over the rights of society as a whole.

It is important to have a framework for ethical decision making. Ethicists debate which of these basic theories is most correct, a debate that is beyond the scope of this chapter. Nevertheless, understanding the theoretical approaches to ethics and making an informed choice of what theoretical base to use are important for each person. Although many people combine these two approaches, such a combination is not always feasible. In some circumstances the common good and the good of the individual cannot be be accommodated.

Professional Ethics

One of the hallmarks of a profession is that it has a set of ethical principles to which it adheres and a mechanism to assure that its practitioners behave ethically. For many years, the American Occupational Therapy Association (AOTA) had a statement in its by-laws indicating that all occupational therapists and assistants were bound by a code of ethics; however, the Association did not have an established, clearly articulated code. In 1977, the Association adopted principles of occupational therapy ethics and established them as a "guide to appropriate conduct of its members." The Standards and Ethics Commission of the Association, under the leadership of Carolyn Baum, studied the ethical principles of many other professions in developing those appropriate for occupational therapy. In 1980, guidelines were completed to accompany each of the ethical principles. The document, *Principles of Occupational Therapy Ethics,* was revised in 1988 and published as the *Occupational Therapy Code of Ethics.* In this revision, the principles were reduced from 13 to 6.

The Standards and Ethics Commission of the AOTA has developed a system of enforcement that enables the Association to act when ethical principles are violated. The American Occupational Therapy Certification Board (AOTCB), through its Disciplinary Action Committee, is able to invoke reprimands, censure, suspension or revocation of certification when it determines that any occupational therapy practitioners have behaved unethically. In addition, if the person practices in a state with some type of statutory regulation such as licensure, the regulatory board in that state is notified of the AOTCB's action. In some situations, the regulatory board may take action first and inform the AOTCB of the sanctions imposed. Additional information on this subject may be found in Chapter 31.

Elements Essential to Ethics

Some of the elements essential to the ethical behavior for any professional and therefore for the occupational therapist and the assistant are as follows:

Universalism: Universalism means that the therapist and the assistant treat persons regardless of age, race, socioeconomic status, personality, likableness or any other considerations. It is unethical to be selective in who is treated for any reason other than professional judgment of ability of the person to benefit from treatment.

Disinterestedness: An occupational therapist or an assistant should not be motivated by profit or self-interest. Treatment has to be the best that can be provided under the circumstances. This element does not mean that occupational therapy practitioners should not be reimbursed appropriately for treatment.

Cooperation: A truly ethical person cooperates with colleagues and is supportive of them. Sharing knowledge about advancements in theory and practice is one sign of cooperation.

Occupational Therapy Code of Ethics

Each of the principles of occupational therapy ethics can be considered in detail, and examples are given of some of the ways that the particular principle can be carried out or violated. The ethical principles of the profession are stated in a way so that both the therapist's and the assistant's roles and obligations in the delivery of services are discussed. The AOTA document *Occupational Therapy Code of Ethics* contains six principles which are described in the following sections.

Principle 1: Beneficience/Autonomy

Confidentiality is a basic part of any professional health care relationship. The recipient of services has a right to expect and demand confidentiality. Judgment is needed to determine what information must be shared among the team members dealing with a particular person and what information must remain confidential. It is a breach of confidentiality to discuss a client or patient in any manner other than professionally. Recipients of services deserve the respect of all professionals working with them. There is a potential conflict of ethical

principles when the therapist or assistant learns information in a therapeutic relationship that affects the well-being of another person. In these rare instances, it may be necessary to break confidentiality to protect the other person.

Another aspect of this principle is related to fees and other administrative areas. Honesty is the hallmark of all relationships with employers and payers. These relationships must be carried out with integrity in all areas. In accepting employment, therapists and assistants accept the job description, policies and procedures of the facility and are obligated to follow them or to use appropriate means to change them. Such things as charging for services not rendered, engaging in "kickbacks" in purchasing materials, using favoritism in the choice of vendors or using supplies and equipment without approval all constitute unethical behavior.

Because not all services needed by the patient are reimbursable by third-party payers, there is a tendency to try to provide these services by charging them under another reimbursable service. The purpose of this practice often is to lead payers to believe that they are paying for a type of service that was not rendered. Looked at in this way, such a practice is dishonest, although the motive for doing this may be to benefit the patient. Unless there is a clear understanding that a related service is a part of occupational therapy and may be billed as such, it is unethical to bill in this manner.

Fees for service should reflect costs and be appropriate and justifiable. An appropriate profit may be built into a fee schedule.

The principle of beneficience/autonomy also applies to the area of research. All members of the profession have responsibility to advance the theory and practice of the profession. Reasearch is the primary way to achieve this goal. When conducting research, it is essential to protect the rights of the subjects.

A number of codes have been developed that deal with principles of ethical research. The American Occupational Therapy Foundation (AOTF) has adopted a statement of Ethical Considerations for Research in Occupational Therapy. Issues covered in that document include the following:

Privacy: All subjects in a research study must be given anonymity, and confidentiality must be maintained at all times.

Consent: Informed voluntary consent is absolutely essential. Persons must have the capacity to understand the possible effects of participation in the research and must be free to choose to participate. This issue presents particular problems in relation to research with children, prisoners, persons with head trauma or those with mental illness. Informed consent means that a complete explanation must be given to the persons being asked to participate, or to those who have the responsibility to make decisions for them. During a research project, a subject must be able to withdraw from the study. There can be no coercion to continue when the person chooses not to be involved further. If it becomes clear that the patient would benefit from a different treatment than that involved in a research project, the treatment of greatest benefit to the patient must be used.

Rewards and promises: The researcher must fulfill any promises made to subjects in regard to rewards. There should be a clear understanding before the start of the research study about rewards to be granted and the time they will be granted. If a subject withdraws from the study, rewards connected to the completed parts of the study must be given.

Protection: Persons participating in a study have the right to expect that no harm will come to them because of the study. The researcher has the responsibility to see that all persons are protected from physical or psychological harm.

Information: The researcher must disclose any relevant information to the subjects in an understandable manner. Persons need to know how the information will be used—whether it will be published or presented or if it will be used in additional studies.

Debriefing: Time must be allowed to discuss with the subjects their experiences in the study. Methods used should be adequately explained.

Approval: The investigator must adhere to the policies and procedures of the facility in which the research is taking place. All facilities that conduct research have committees to review the research design and the protection of the rights of human subjects. A facility may have additional rules to govern the use of persons in studies.

Permission: Any copyrighted or patented material may be used in research only with the written permission of the owner of the material.

Biomedical research: Beneficial results must be anticipated from the research. When using human subjects, the results must not be possible to achieve by other means, and the anticipated results must justify inconvenience or risk to the persons.

Responsibility for others: The person who is the principal investigator is responsible for the actions of all those assisting in the study. It is important to assure that all assisting in any way understand the ethical implications of the study and its methods.

Analysis and reporting of data: It is important to report negative as well as positive findings. Negative findings may prove useful in application of the research and in designing future studies.

Publishing: It is essential to report results accurately and to make known any reservation about the validity or reliability of the research study. If preliminary results are being reported, particular care must be taken. It is unethical to misrepresent the results of the study, to discard data that do not fit the intended results, or in any other way to falsify the results of research.

Principle 2: Competence

An occupational therapist has a high level of professional competence; an occupational therapy assistant has a high degree of technical competence. Each of these practitioners must continue to increase competence. It is obvious that health care is a constantly changing environment. To maintain skills at any one level is not sufficient; the therapist and assistant must improve skills to keep pace through further formal, academic education, self-study, participation in conferences, making use of a mentor or through an experiential study in an occupational therapy treatment facility.

Competence must be represented accurately to other professionals, to the patient, to the patient's family and to the public. Occupational therapy practitioners are asked to function in many different capacities as part of the health care team. Care must be taken not to allow others to presume capabilities that are not present.

All occupational therapy practitioners must be aware of their abilities and skills and the functions they may perform based on their education and background. They should not assume professional duties that are not within their area of competence. In a competitive health care climate, there may be a drive to make individual personnel indispensable by having them do "all things." The supervising occupational therapist must use professional judgment to determine what may ethically be done by those being supervised, as well as what exceeds the parameters of the profession.

Occupational therapy assistants must understand when the needs of the patient go beyond the assistant's ability to meet those needs. It may be necessary to refer the person to an occupational therapist who has the required skills, or to someone in another profession. The COTA should not hesitate to refer the patient to the person who will be best able to provide the services needed.

Principle 3: Compliance with Laws and Regulations

All acts that are legal are not necessarily ethical, but usually illegal acts are also unethical. A number of laws govern or relate to the delivery of health services. It is the duty of all occupational therapy personnel to be knowledgeable about those laws and to act in conformity with them.

Fraudulent (false) billing to government programs such as Medicare and Medicaid is both illegal and unethical. This practice can have a profoundly negative effect on health care professionals.

In recent years, health professionals have sometimes been accused of treating patients inhumanely, particularly patients with emotional or mental disabilities. When patients are particularly vulnerable and cannot protect themselves, this kind of behavior takes on exceptional seriousness. Ethical violations that have a direct effect on the patient are more serious than those that affect the profession or other occupational therapy personnel.

Another aspect of compliance with laws and regulations relates to records. Keeping records and writing and making reports are a part of professional duties. The therapist and the assistant must conform to legal requirements and to the policies of the institution or facility. An important part of treatment is to accurately record and report the process and result of treatment. Objective data should be used whenever appropriate. Subjective data may be valuable when based on sound professional judgment and on available objective data. It is important for the therapist to know what objective measurements are appropriate, to use them with skill, and to report and interpret the findings accurately. Generally, the occupational therapy assistant does not interpret such data, but should be skilled in the administration of structured assessment tools.

Falsifying records for reimbursement purposes is dishonest and unethical. Recording that a patient was treated when the person did not receive treatment is an example of falsifying records. Recording falsely that the occupational therapy assistant was supervised by a registered occupational therapist during treatment is, of course, dishonest.

Occupational therapy practitioners must be alert to the pressures of producing income. While recognizing the need for adequate income to the facility or private practice group, it is never ethical to achieve this income through the falsification of records. A therapist or assistant who is asked to do such recording must report this fact to the next person in the chain of authority. In some instances, it may be necessary for the occupational therapy personnel involved to leave their position(s) because persons in authority require unethical behavior.

Principle 4: Public Information

In the past, professions did not advertise; in fact, advertising was considered unethical. Today, however, advertising may be very appropriate. For example, in private practice, it would be very difficult to inform potential patients of the occupational therapy services available without advertising.

Truthful advertising is essential. Examples of dishonest advertising are promising a result from treatment that cannot be guaranteed, misleading the public about qualifications of personnel, and depreciating another therapist or service. An occupational therapy assistant usually will not advertise, but may be involved in a private practice or a health care facility that advertises.

Principle 5: Professional Relationships

This principle focuses on the issue of respect that must be shown toward colleagues in occupational therapy and in other professions. Each therapist and assistant represents the entire profession, and the quality of each one's service is a concern to all. The behavior of each reflects on all members of the profession.

The reputation of colleagues must be protected. Com-ments concerning the quality of treatment should be considered carefully. Often, such evaluations are subjective. When information, such as evaluations, indicates a problem in the quality of treatment being provided, the matter should be handled discretely. Poor quality of treatment should not be ignored or protected; but rather should be addressed according to official policy.

Occupational therapists and assistants must understand the role and educational background of other persons involved in treating the patient. Respect for their role and service is a necessary part of ethical behavior. Occupational therapy practitioners must be concerned with the quality of all services delivered to the patient; therefore, it is a concern of the therapist and the assistant if related health care personnel are not performing at a competent level.

When using work developed by others, it is essential that credit be given to the originators. Sometimes work developed by many therapists and built on by the profession is copyrighted by an individual. Because the work really belongs to the profession as a whole, this practice is not ethical. When a therapist or assistant makes a significant contribution to the work, that is, revises, updates or changes it, then the person has the right to be identified with the work. It is always necessary to give credit to those who contributed substantially to the work.

When occupational therapy practitioners work closely with other persons, some delegation of services to others may be desirable. Occupational therapists and assistants must not delegate when the skills needed are those of occupational therapy. Professional judgment must be used to determine which aspects of treatment can be taught and delegated to others and those that require the level of service of the therapist or assistant. When students are involved in providing treatment, the supervising therapist or assistant is responsible for determining the competency of the student to render the service.

One of the most difficult situations for occupational therapy practitioners is unethical behavior by others. If a COTA or OTR becomes aware of possible unethical behavior by others, he or she has an obligation to act. When possible, discussing and clarifying the situation with the person may be all that is necessary. It is possible for a health care professional to be unaware that the behavior is not considered ethical or may be questionable. When such discussion is not possible or does not result in change, the next step is to report the situation to the appropriate body, which may be a standards and ethics committee of a district or state professional association or a regulatory board. In a case concerning occupational therapy practitioners, both the Standards and Ethics Commission of AOTA and the Disciplinary Action Committee of the AOTCB may need to be informed. Both of these bodies have procedures for bringing a charge of unethical behavior against occupational therapy practitioners.

The procedures for both groups are detailed and relatively prolonged to ensure that the rights of all individuals are protected. Because the charge of unethical behavior is very serious, it is appropriate to allow adequate time for prudent decision making. Each of these bodies has an initial information investigation into the alleged violation. If it is judged that a possible breach of ethics has occurred, the person involved is informed and a preliminary investigation is undertaken. Formal investigation of the charges may follow. An appeal mechanism is an essential part of each procedure. The complete procedures may be obtained from the chair of the Standards and Ethics Commission and from the Executive Director of the AOTCB.

It is the responsibility of each therapist and assistant to know the principles of occupational therapy and to know the standards of the profession. The document, *Standards of Practice of Occupational Therapy* published by AOTA has been reprinted in this text (Appendix A). The AOTA develops, adopts and publishes these standards, which should be a guide for the performance of occupational therapists and assistants.

All occupational therapy personnel must be aware of changes in the field. One important way to obtain this information is by reading professional journals. Involvement in local, state and national associations helps therapists and assistants not only to know the changes but also to participate in the development of the profession.

Principle 6: Professional Conduct

This principle states that "occupational therapy personnel shall not engage in any form of conduct that constitutes a conflict of interest or that adversely reflects on the profession." Several of the principles of ethics previously discussed overlap with this principle. Any action that takes advantage of a patient's condition, any inhumane act, or anything that discriminates against a patient is an aspect of misconduct. Behavior that is not related to the direct responsibilities of the therapist or assistant, but which is illegal, reflects on the profession and is unethical. Stealing, driving while intoxicated and embezzlement of funds are examples of possible illegal actions not directly related to professional duties, but nevertheless unethical.

If it is brought to the attention of the AOTCB that a therapist or assistant is convicted of a felony, the board's disciplinary action committee will consider the case on an individual basis. If it is deemed that the crime is such that the person would not be able to practice in a safe, proficient or competent manner, disciplinary sanctions may be invoked. A student may not be eligible to take the national certification examination if convicted of a felony and the nature of the felony is such that it may affect the person's ability to practice safely, proficiently or competently.

Other Considerations

The broader issues of biomedical ethics must be of concern to all occupational therapy practitioners. They need to be concerned about all health care issues and how such issues affect society.

Health care professionals today face many bioethical issues. The defining of health, the allocation of scarce medical resources, the problems of informed consent for both treatment and psychosurgical procedures are among these issues. In addition, the prolongation of life or of dying, behavior control and the selection of persons to receive treatment are some of the many problems facing the health care worker. Occupational therapy practitioners must keep informed about these issues. New problems and concerns are discussed in the popular press almost daily.

Bioethical issues usually do not have a clear answer as to what is right or what is wrong. Some of the steps occupational therapy practitioners can take to understand these issues and respond to them are the following:

Clarify the question: Often it is necessary to look at an issue from many different viewpoints to clarify the basic question. The question that appears on the surface may not be the real one. To begin to deal with the issue, it is important to be as clear and succinct as possible when stating the question.

Identify values: When the answer to a bioethical issue is not apparent or agreed upon by all, it is usually because there are competing values about the issue, either among individuals or in society in general. There is no general agreement as to which values are relative and which are absolute. Identifying and clarifying values help determine the decisions.

Explore world views: A number of ethical theories determine how an issue will be approached and what will be an acceptable decision in relation to an issue. It is important to be clear about the implications of each theory. An individual's personal philosophy and religious beliefs will be important factors in one's world view and will greatly influence how ethical issues will be resolved.

Examine data: It is essential to make use of all available information. Analyzing the present situation by applying all the facts and knowledge will help to develop the possibilities and the alternatives in action so that a reasoned decision can be made.

Looking at bioethical issues from these viewpoints helps the professional to form a basis for decision making. Even if occupational therapy practitioners are not directly involved in making a decision, it is important to clarify the aspects related to any bioethical issue and to assist society in understanding the basis of decision making.

Conclusion

Ethical behavior is essential to the occupational therapist and the occupational therapy assistant. Such behavior is often a matter of attitude and not of rule following. All principles of occupational therapy ethics are stated positively. It is important to view them as guidelines of positive behavior. Whether or not a particular action is unethical depends on a number of circumstances. A person's knowledge, intention and motivation may all contribute to a decision about determining whether a particular behavior may in fact be unethical.

If occupational therapy practitioners always keep the good of the patient and the profession in the forefront of their considerations in making decisions about their behavior, those decisions, in all likelihood, will be ethical. Occupational therapy practitioners can then be proud of their behavior and of their profession.

Summary

All ethical principles are based on the four values of prudence, temperateness, courage and justice. Secondary values related to ethical behavior include reverence, fidelity, awareness of responsibility, truthfulness and goodness. One of the hallmarks of a profession is that it has a set of ethical principles that it adheres to as a means to assure that its practitioners behave ethically. Elements essential to professional ethics are universalism, disinterest and cooperation. The AOTA has adopted an *Occupational Therapy Code of Ethics*, which outlines six principles that all occupational therapy practitioners must uphold. These principles relate to beneficience/autonomy, competence, compliance with laws and regulations, public information, professional relationships and professional conduct.

Ethical behavior is essential for all occupational therapy practitioners. Practitioners must act according to the good of the patient and the profession as to assure ethical decisions and behavior.

Related Learning Activities

1. Make six cards with a principle of occupational therapy ethics on each. Divide the class into two teams and conduct the "ethics game" according to the following rules:

   a. One student turns over a card.
   b. A member of team one gives an activity or behavior that is indicated by the principle on the card.
   c. A member from team two gives an activity or a behavior that violates that principle.
   d. Score one point for each correct answer and continue until all the cards have been turned over.
   e. The team with the most points at the end wins.

2. Consider the following two scenarios and address the specific items stated at the conclusion as they relate to both:

   a. Mrs. J, an extremely confused 89-year-old woman, seems to be getting minimum results from her occupational therapy treatment and is quite belligerent toward all staff at the nursing home where she is a resident. It is suggested that her occupational therapy be discontinued.
   b. Three new patients have been referred to occupational therapy today, but because of limits of staff time, only two patients can be added to the work load of the department.

Discuss what your decision/action would be in these two examples, considering these additional points:
   - Determine what additional information you would want to know.
   - Decide what values are involved.
   - Specify the prevailing world views that have an impact on the situations.
   - Determine the religious beliefs that are relevant.
   - Decide what, if any, ethical principles are involved.

3. Review your local newspaper for reports of biomedical issues. Select an article and discuss it with peers, considering the four areas Cummings stresses as important in reaching decisions about such matters.

The Credentialing Process in Occupational Therapy

Madelaine Gray, MA, MPA, OTR, FAOTA

Introduction

In today's world, occupational therapists and occupational therapy assistants need to be aware of how the profession of occupational therapy relates to the various aspects of the entire health care delivery system. One major component of this system is the regulation of employment qualifications and scope of practice for thousands of health care workers. The credentialing of health care personnel has an impact on the quality and cost of services, the accessibility of delivery systems and the supply of personnel. This chapter presents both an historical chronology and a description of the nature and purpose of contemporary credentialing practices in the profession of occupational therapy in the United States.

Definition of Terms

It is important to understand the basic terminology used to discuss the credentialing process in occupational therapy. The following terms are commonly used:

Credentialing: The term **credentialing** refers to a process that gives title or approval to a person or a program. Credentialing can take three forms:

1. **Accreditation** of educational programs
2. **Certification** and/or **registration** of individuals by a state or private agency
3. State regulation, ie **licensure**, statutory certification and registration of individuals by a government agency.

Accreditation: An agency or organization institutes a process to evaluate and recognize

---

ESSENTIAL VOCABULARY

Credentialing

Accreditation

Certification

Registration

Licensure

Essentials

Specialty certification

Standards

Special accommodations

Psychometric

KEY CONCEPTS

Historical background

Eligibility requirements

Relationship to state credentialing

Recertification and relicensure

Role of AOTCB

Role of state regulatory boards

Disciplinary action

an institution or program of study in terms of its ability to meet certain predetermined criteria or standards.[1]

Certification: This term is used to denote a form of public recognition that can be provided by a state agency under state law (statutory certification) or awarded by a private, nongovernmental agency and is voluntary. To become certified, an individual must meet predetermined qualifications. Eligibility requirements generally involve education, experience and examination or a combination thereof. Certification is a form of "title protection" because only those individuals who are certified may use certain titles or credentials.

Registration: This is the listing of the names of individuals on an official roster that is maintained by a governmental or nongovernmental agency. In some instances, the agency may establish qualifications for registration and minimum practice standards; however, other agencies may permit anyone to register.

Licensure: This is the process by which a government agency grants permission to a person to engage in a given occupation upon finding that the applicant has attained the minimum degree of competence necessary to ensure that the public health, safety and welfare will be reasonably well protected. Licensure is a more encompassing regulation of a profession than certification because it establishes the scope of practice and prohibits unlicensed persons from performing specific functions cited in the statute.[2]

American Occupational Therapy Certification Board (AOTCB): The AOTCB is a private, nongovernmental agency that has the sole responsibility for the establishment and administration of the national, voluntary certification program that offers the credentials of Occupational Therapist, Registered (OTR) and Certified Occupational Therapy Assistant (COTA) to those individuals who have met specific educational, fieldwork and examination requirements.

American Occupational Therapy Association (AOTA): The AOTA is the national, voluntary membership association representing OTRs, COTAs and occupational therapy students who are members of the association. The AOTA provides a variety of services to meet member needs, such as continuing education programs and publications, public education and legislative and lobbying activities to promote the understanding and use of occupational therapy services.

Historical Background

The profession of occupational therapy was one of the first health care professions to develop a credentialing system during the 1930s and 1940s. This early credentialing program took the form of accreditation of occupational therapy educational programs and the registration of individuals who had met specific education, experience and examination requirements to become an Occupational Therapist, Registered (OTR).[3,4]

After establishing the minimum standards for training occupational therapists, the AOTA began registering occupational therapists in 1931. The first Directory of Qualified Occupational Therapists was published by the AOTA in 1932 with the names of 318 registered therapists.[5] The AOTA Register contained a Main Register for persons who qualified by having approved professional training and subsequent successful work experience of at least one year. During the early years of registration, the AOTA also used a Secondary Register to register individuals as "Occupational Assistant, Registered." These persons were "practical workers," qualified on the basis of work experience, but who did not possess the educational background required for admission to the Main Register.[6] Beginning in 1937, only graduates of accredited occupational therapy programs were admitted to the Register, thus ending the Secondary Register and closing admission by work experience only.[7]

Certificaton requirements later were expanded to include passage of a written examination, then called the Registration Examination. After exploring the use of an essay examination for registration in 1939, the AOTA decided in 1946 to administer an objective, multiple-choice question examination because it was the most valid, reliable, and efficient type of assessment instrument available. The first multiple-choice Registration Examination was given in 1947 and included 300 questions in 35 content areas. The candidate's examination score accounted for 80% of the total requirement and the remaining 20% was the field work performance score.[4]

Initially, beginning in the late 1930s, the certification and registration program of the AOTA was only for occupational therapists; however, in the late 1950s, educational programs for occupational therapy assistants were developed and certification as a Certified Occupational Therapy Assistant (COTA) was granted to those individuals who completed an approved occupational therapy assistant education program. Certification was also granted to those who had worked a minimum of two years in one disability area and who were recommended by three qualified individuals, one of whom was an OTR under whom the applicant was working. The AOTA adopted this "grandfather" plan in 1957 and terminated the plan in 1963.[8,9] The certification examination was implemented first in the field of psychiatry and a few years later in general practice. The certification examination for COTAs was first administered in 1977, after the AOTA completed a role delineation study that identified the expected, entry-level competencies of OTRs and COTAs.

In 1971, the AOTA adopted a policy that allowed qualified COTAs the opportunity to apply for a new program called the Career Mobility Program. This program was designed to allow COTAs to become OTRs without having to satisfy the academic degree requirements for the OTR level. A COTA with at least four years of qualified work experience could submit a self-study plan and once this plan was approved, the COTA could enter into the therapist-level, six-month field work requirement under the supervision of an OTR. Once the fieldwork requirement was passed, the COTA was approved to take the certification examination for OTRs.[10]

The first COTA met all the Career Mobility Program requirements and passed the OTR examination in 1973. During the 17 years in which the program was in operation, a total of 163 COTAs became OTRs through the Career Mobility Program. The AOTA terminated the program in 1982, although it allowed COTAs who were already in the program to finish the program by 1988. Since the end of the Career Mobility Program, the AOTA has encouraged the development of educational programs to meet the needs of COTAs who want to become OTRs.

Creation of the AOTCB

In 1986, the AOTA decided that it would be in the best interest of the public to separate the certification program from the membership-focused association and create a separate entity to administer the certification program under the auspices of the AOTA. In allowing this change, the AOTA recognized that there was an inherent conflict of interest for a membership-driven organization to be in charge of and have control over a certification program that should serve the purpose of protecting the public.

Therefore in July 1986, the AOTA membership approved an AOTA by-laws change that allowed for the creation of a separate autonomous body to handle the certification program. After receiving membership approval, the AOTA created the American Occupational Therapy Certification Board (AOTCB) to develop and administer all aspects of the occupational therapy certification program. Although the certification program was administratively and financially independent from the AOTA, the program was still conducted under the auspices of the AOTA.

The AOTA appointed two OTRs, two COTAs and four public members to serve on the AOTCB's initial and interim Board of Directors. The Board of Directors also included an AOTA Executive Board liaison to facilitate communication between the AOTA and the AOTCB. An AOTCB office was located in the AOTA building and office staff were hired, including an Executive Director.

In 1988, the AOTA and the AOTCB decided to separate by having the AOTCB become an independent corporation. Consequently, on November 22, 1988, the AOTCB, Inc. was formed, thus allowing the certification program

to function completely independently from the AOTA.[11] The AOTA and the AOTCB developed a service agreement whereby the AOTCB contracted with the AOTA for the provision of certain services, eg, the use of the AOTA computer system to maintain the database for all certification records.

Thus, a workable, cooperative relationship was established by two independent organizations so that each could focus on their respective missions of membership services and promotion of the profession (AOTA) and protection of the public (AOTCB). After being developed and administered by the AOTA for over 50 years, the certification program is now the sole responsibility of the AOTCB.

Current Requirements for AOTCB Certification

The AOTA initially established the eligibility requirements that individuals must meet to be certified as either an OTR or COTA. The AOTCB adopted these same requirements when the certification board was formed in 1986. The AOTCB requirements for certification are listed in Figure 31-1.

The AOTCB issues certificates verifying certification to all individuals who have met the certification requirements. Certificates are reissued every five years except to those OTRs and COTAs whose certification has been suspended or revoked.

Relationship of AOTCB Certification to State Regulation

In the mid-1970s, the occupational therapy credentialing system started to expand to include state regulation, in the form of licensure, or in some states, statutory certification, and/or registration, or trademark laws.[12]

Although there are a few exceptions, the AOTCB certification requirements are used by most of the occupational therapy state regulatory boards. Thus, if an individual is credentialed by the AOTCB as either an OTR or a COTA, in most cases the person will also be able to meet the state requirements. The few exceptions, made by a small number of state boards, are related to nonacceptance of OTRs who have achieved this designation through the AOTA Career Mobility Program and to some foreign trained occupational therapists who have a diploma in occupational therapy, rather than a bachelor's degree.

For the most part, once an individual has met the AOTCB requirements, the OTR or COTA does not have to meet any new or additional requirements of the state regulatory board. A few state boards require an OTR or

I. Current requirements for graduates from schools in the United States:
   A. Occupational Therapist, Registered (OTR)
      To become an OTR, an individual must:
      1. Be a graduate of an accredited occupational therapist educational program and have successfully completed all therapist level fieldwork required by the educational program (but not less than six months)
      2. Have successfully completed the Certification Examination for Occupational Therapist, Registered
   B. Certified Occupational Therapy Assistant (COTA)
      To become a COTA, an individual must:
      1. Be a graduate of an accredited/approved occupational therapy assistant educational program and have successfully completed all assistant level fieldwork required by the educational program (but not less than twelve weeks)
      2. Have successfully completed the Certification Examination for Occupational Therapy Assistant
II. Requirements for Graduates from Foreign Schools to Become OTRs:
   Graduates from foreign schools are required to pass the Certification Examination for Occupational Therapist, Registered. The eligibility requirements for taking the certification examination are as follows:
   A. Graduates of Approved Occupational Therapy Programs
      Successful completion of all academic and clinical/ fieldwork requirements of a program approved by a member association of the World Federation of Occupational Therapists (WFOT)
   B. Occupational Therapists Educated in Countries That Are Not Members of the World Federation of Occupational Therapists
      Eligibility for writing the examination shall be determined for each individual by the AOTCB after evaluation of each individual's education as compared to the educational standards for the United States and WFOT-approved schools.

Figure 31-1. *Requirements for Certification from the AOTCB.*

COTA who has not been employed in occupational therapy for a number of years to retake the certification examination in order to receive a credential from the state board.

Recertification and Relicensure

Because lifetime certification is not necessarily an adequate way to protect the public, the health professions and numerous regulatory agencies have been involved in extensive discussions and research studies focusing on the best way to periodically recredential health care personnel.

During the 1970s, the AOTA, through the Continuing Certification Program, investigated and proposed several types of requirements for periodic recertification.[13] Mandatory continuing education as well as reexamination were proposed to the AOTA Representative Assembly; however,

each proposal was rejected by the AOTA membership. Since then, some state regulatory boards have established a mandatory continuing education requirement for relicensure.

Recredentialing continues to be of concern to the AOTCB, state regulatory boards, employers, third-party payers, OTRs and COTAs and the public. The problem concerns how to develop a recredentialing program that identifies those who have kept up to date with current knowledge and skill required for the practice of occupational therapy. Because evidence of participation in continuing education is not necessarily evidence of an OTR's or COTA's current knowledge and skills, there is a concern over the use of mandatory continuing education requirements for recredentialing. On the other hand, there is also concern that requiring periodic passage of a written examination may not be fair for those OTRs and COTAs who have become specialized in a specific area of occupational therapy practice. The debate over these concerns continues and it is hoped that a solution will some day be found to the complex problem of recredentialing.

Role of The American Occupational Therapy Association

Beginning in the 1930s, the AOTA established a relationship with the American Medical Association for the accreditation of occupational therapy training programs. Now the AOTA is responsible for the accreditation of professional level occupational therapy educational programs in collaboration with the Committee on Allied Health Education and Accreditation (CAHEA) of the American Medical Association. In the 1950s, standards for occupational assistant (technical level) educational programs were established, and the AOTA became the sole agency that approved occupational therapy assistant educational programs. In 1991, CAHEA also began to accredit the occupational therapy assistant programs in collaboration with AOTA. The AOTA has been exploring the feasibility of seeking independent status as an accrediting agency. The AOTA Representative Assembly is expected to act on this decision in 1993. In the meantime, the AMA decided that it would discontinue CAHEA. Plans are underway to replace CAHEA with an independent agency to handle accrediting responsibilities.

Educational standards, also referred to as the **Essentials**, for the academic and fieldwork programs are used to review and determine whether the educational programs have met these standards and are therefore eligible for accreditation.

This credentialing service is provided by CAHEA and the AOTA Department of Accreditation along with the AOTA

Accreditation Committee, a group of volunteer OTRs and COTAs, and with the public members and CAHEA representatives.

The AOTA is also responsible for the development and distribution of the fieldwork evaluation forms that are used by the fieldwork supervisors to evaluate the performance of OTR and COTA students during their required fieldwork. Once the student has completed all of the academic fieldwork requirements, the program director notifies the AOTCB that the student is eligible to take the AOTCB certification examination.

Another credentialing program that the AOTA is developing is a voluntary **specialty certification** program. The specialty certification program is designed to recognize and credential occupational therapists who have specialized in an area of practice. The AOTA has selected pediatrics as the first area to offer specialty certification. A written examination was administered to qualified candidates in 1992. At this time no plans have been introduced to offer specialty certification to COTAs.

Role of The AOTCB

The purposes of the AOTCB are as follows:
1. To encourage high standards of performance by occupational therapy personnel in order to promote the health, safety and welfare of the public.
2. To establish, maintain and administer standards, policies and programs for the professional certification and registration of occupational therapy practitioners.
3. To sponsor and/or conduct research and/or educational activities related to the above.

The AOTCB is responsible for developing and revising the certification policies and procedures as needed. The AOTCB determines the requirements for an individual's certification as either an OTR or a COTA. The AOTCB requirements for certification specify graduation from an accredited or approved occupational therapy education program, and the AOTCB has accepted the accreditation and approval **standards** (requirements for measurement of compliance)and process of CAHEA and the AOTA.

Another responsibility of the AOTCB is to develop certification examinations that are administered twice a year by a testing agency, under contract with the AOTCB. OTR candidates and COTA candidates take different examinations. At the present time, the examinations consist of 200 multiple-choice questions, and candidates are given four hours to complete the test. The examinations are developed from job analysis data that indicate the expected responsibilities and competencies for entry-level (beginning) OTRs and COTAs. The test questions are application oriented and are directly related to the practice of occupational therapy. Sample questions, as well as other related information, may be found in the AOTCB Candidate Handbook.

Candidates with disabling conditions—including visual, orthopedic or hearing impairment; health impairment; learning disability; or a multiple disability condition—may request **special accommodations** or arrangements for taking the examination. Such requests must be made in writing and include documentation of the history and diagnosis of the impairment by a *qualified health professional*, (not the program director) and a description of the specific special accommodations requested. All requests must be reviewed and approved by the testing agency.

The examinations are developed by the AOTCB Certification Examination Development Committee (CEDC), a group of content experts (COTAs and OTRs) drawn from a wide variety of work environments and geographic areas. In addition, the AOTCB Academy of Content Experts has been established and trained to provide questions for consideration by the CEDC members. The test questions for the OTR and COTA examinations are finalized by the CEDC, with **psychometric** (measurement of mental traits, abilities and processes) advice and guidance provided by the testing agency. Sensitivity tests are carried out to assure that the test questions are free of gender, racial and cultural bias. COTA and OTR test items are kept in separate item banks and are used only on their respective examinations.[14]

Every administration of the certification examination uses a unique combination of items drawn from the item bank. The OTR and COTA examinations each have a separate content outline that indicates the percentage of items to be included in each major area of the examinations. This process ensures that the same emphasis on the various content areas is consistent with each administration. The content outlines are found in the *AOTCB Candidate Handbook*, which is sent to an OTR or COTA candidate when the program director notifies the AOTCB that a student is eligible to take the certification examination.

The AOTCB, with guidance from the testing agency, performs a cut-score study and determines the minimum passing score for the examinations upon approval of the AOTCB Board of Directors. The testing agency scores the examinations and sends the candidates a notice of the passing or failing score. Those candidates who pass the examinations are sent an AOTCB certificate that verifies their certification as an OTR or a COTA. Thus an individual is certified immediately after passing the examination. No additional application process or fee is required; nor is there any renewal requirement or renewal fee.

The AOTCB is responsible for the maintenance of the records of all examination candidates and persons who are certified as an OTR or a COTA. These records are maintained on a computer and are used to verify certification as requested by employers and state regulatory boards. Examination scores are only released after written authorization is received from the examinees.

Presently, about 5,000 candidates take the AOTCB certification examinations each year. Approximately 3,500 take the OTR examination and about 1,500 take the COTA examination. The pass rate for US graduates who are first-time examinees for the OTR examination is generally in the 92% to 94% range; the pass rate for first time examinees for the COTA examination is typically around 88% to 90%. As of January 1993, approximately 71,447 persons have been certified: approximately 54,043 OTRs and 17,404 COTAs.

The AOTCB grants candidates an unlimited number of opportunities to take the examination; however, some state regulatory boards impose a limit on the number of times a candidate may take the examination for state regulatory board purposes.

The certification examinations are given twice a year, on the fourth Saturday in January and the fourth Saturday in July. The examination is administered by the testing agency at test centers located in major cities throughout the United States and overseas. Candidates may select, from the list of test centers, the test center most conveniently located.

When a candidate applies to take the certification examination, he or she may indicate on the examination application form if a score report is to be sent to a state regulatory board. The testing agency charges a small fee for each report sent to each state regulatory board.

After the examination results are given to the candidate and the AOTCB, the testing agency sends educational program directors a summary of the results for their school. These results do not contain scores by name, but use an identification number to protect the confidentiality of the candidate. The program directors may use this information for program evaluation and other research purposes.

The Role of State Regulatory Boards

As of April 1993, there were 48 states plus the District of Columbia and Puerto Rico that had some form of state regulation for occupational therapists and/or occupational therapy assistants. The two other states are in the process of seeking state regulation. State regulation can be in several different forms, such as licensure, statutory certification, and/or registration. As mentioned previously, most states will credential an individual who has met the AOTCB certification requirements for OTRs and COTAs.

If an OTR or a COTA wishes to use the title and/or practice occupational therapy in a jurisdiction that has licensure, statutory certification or registration, the OTR or COTA must contact the regulatory board and meet the requirements of the board before working in the state/ jurisdiction. Some regulatory boards provide a temporary

permit or a temporary license to students waiting to take the certification examination. To use the title or practice without first meeting the requirements of the regulatory board is illegal, and the OTR or COTA may be subject to a fine and/or disciplinary action by the board.

If a state does not have any regulation for occupational therapists or assistants, it is up to the employer to decide if AOTCB certification as an OTR or a COTA is required. Most, but not all, employers require certification.

Information about state regulation may be obtained from the state regulatory board. Contact information may be obtained from the state occupational therapy association, the AOTA or the AOTCB.

Disciplinary Action Programs

State regulatory boards, the AOTA and the AOTCB have disciplinary action policies and procedures to handle complaints against OTRs, COTAs and occupational therapy students. Each of the groups may take disciplinary action independent of the other groups. For example, a state regulatory board may take disciplinary action against an OTR or a COTA licensee in the state, but the AOTCB and the AOTA may decide not to take disciplinary action or vice versa.

The state boards, the AOTA and the AOTCB have established the grounds for disciplinary action and the type of sanctions that can be applied to persons who have been found guilty of a violation. Some state boards may revoke the state credential (eg license), may impose a fine, may suspend a license or may censure or reprimand an individual. Likewise, the AOTCB, through the AOTCB Disciplinary Action Committee may revoke or suspend certification or it may reprimand or censure an individual. The AOTA, acting through its Standards and Ethics Commission, may revoke membership and may censure or reprimand a member who is an OTR, COTA or student.

The AOTCB is a clearinghouse for the exchange of disciplinary action information among the state boards, the AOTA and the AOTCB. The AOTCB publishes a periodic report called the Disciplinary Action Information Exchange Network (DAIEN) that contains a master list of the names of persons who have been reported to have had disciplinary action taken against them by a state regulatory board, the AOTA and/or the AOTCB. The DAIEN facilitates the exchange of information so that employers, the public and regulatory bodies can be informed of action that has been taken against an OTR, a COTA or an occupational therapy student.

Information about the grounds, sanctions and disciplinary action procedures used by each state board, the AOTA and the AOTCB is available by contacting the respective organizations. In general, disciplinary action cases usually consist of a complaint by another OTR or COTA, by an employer or by a patient or client. The complaint is investigated, and a determination is made whether the complaint is true and is related to the grounds for disciplinary action. The defendant is given an opportunity to present his or her view of the situation and may be offered the opportunity to participate in an administrative hearing to present further information and to answer questions. The case may be dismissed if there are no grounds for disciplinary action or if there is not enough evidence for sanctions, or sanctions may be made against the individual. Each case is handled individually.

To date, most types of cases have been complaints about fradulent billing for occupational therapy services, some form of patient harm or injury, misrepresentation or falsification of credentials, sexual misconduct or impairment due to alcohol or substance abuse.

Summary

The credentialing of occupational therapists and occupational therapy assistants is an important component of the health care delivery system. Various organizations, such as the AOTA, the AOTCB and state regulatory boards, participate in the ongoing administration of the credentialing process. Credentialing in occupational therapy not only involves the award of initial certification as an OTR or a COTA and the state regulatory board credentials, but it also involves the continuing monitoring of occupational therapy practice and ethical behavior through the disciplinary action programs conducted by the AOTA, the AOTCB, and the state regulatory boards. A summary of significant milestones in the credentialing process in occupational therapy is presented in Figure 31-2.

1923	Minimum standards of training for occupational therapists established.
1932	First directory of qualified occupational therapists published, containing the names of 318 OTRs. A Main Register and a Secondary Register, for persons qualified through work experience, are used.
1937	Registration requirements are changed. Only graduates of accredited schools are admitted to the Registry.
1939	An essay examination is used for Registration.
1947	First, multiple-choice Registration Examination is administered.
1957	Plans approved for development of occupational therapy assistant training programs and certification as COTAs.
1961	First Directory of COTAs published. There are 553 COTAs and six approved training programs. Some COTAs qualify under a grandfather plan on the basis of work experience.
1963	Grandfather program for COTAs is discontinued. Certification requires graduation from an approved training program.
1968	Puerto Rico passes first liscensure law for occupational therapists.
1971	AOTA approves Career Mobility Program for qualified COTAs to become OTRs.
1971	AOTA Delegate Assembly passes resolution #300, the Continuing Certification Program. AOTA embarks on study of possible recertification policies and procedures.
1973	First COTA passes the certification examination for OTRs under the auspices of the Career Mobility Program.
1973	AOTA completes the Role Delineation Study for entry-level OTRs and COTAs.
1975	New York and Florida are the first states to pass licensure laws for OTRs and COTAs.
1977	First Certification Examination for COTAs administered. Certification as a COTA requires passage of the certification examination.
1982	Career Mobility Program is terminated.
1986	AOTA membership approves by-laws change to create the American Occupational Therapy Certification Board (AOTCB) as a separate and autonomous entity under the auspices of the AOTA.
1988	AOTA membership approves by-laws change to allow for the creation of the AOTCB as a separate corporation, no longer affiliated with the AOTA. AOTCB becomes incorporated in November, 1988.
1990	AOTCB publishes first issue of the Disciplinary Action Information Exchange Network.
1991	AOTCB Job Analysis Study completed. Results to be used to update certification examinations to reflect current entry-level practice of OTRs and COTAs.
1993	A record breaking number, over 5,000, candidates expected to take the certification examinations. Effective with the January examinations, the certification examinations changed to reflect changes in entry-level practice identified through the Job Analysis Study.
1993	A total of 50 jurisdictions have some form of regulation governing occupational therapists and occupational therapy assistants.

Figure 31-2. *Milestones in the Occupational Therapy Credentialing Process.*

Related Learning Activities

1. Discuss the purposes of credentialing and the primary functions of the AOTCB.

2. Describe the differences between certification and licensure.

3. Contact the state regulatory board in your state or a neighboring state. Determine the procedures to become credentialed.

References

1. US Department of Health, Education and Welfare: *Licensure and Related Health Personnel Credentialing*. Washington, DC, Department of Health, Education and Welfare, 1971.

2. American Hospital Association: *Report on Voluntary Certification of Health Care Personnel*. Chicago, Illinois, American Hospital Association, 1990.

3. Brandt H: How shall occupational therapists be registered: The written examination. *Am J Occup Ther* 1:18-21, 1947.

4. Brandt H: The AOTA registration examination: Past, present, and future. *Am J Occup Ther* 10:281-287, 1956.

5. American Occupational Therapy Association: *National Directory of Qualified Occupational Therapists*. New York, AOTA, 1932.

6. American Occupational Therapy Association: *Directory of Qualified Occupational Therapists*. New York, AOTA, 1934.

7. American Occupational Therapy Association: *Directory of Registered Occupational Therapists*. New York, AOTA, 1940.

8. American Occupational Therapy Association: *Directory of Certified Occupational Therapy Assistants*. New York AOTA, 1961.

9. Hirama H: The COTA: a chronological review. In Ryan S (Ed): *The Certified Occupational Therapy Assistant: Roles and Responsibilities*. Thorofare, New Jersey, Slack Inc, 1986.

10. Adams N: Ladder to professional certification: The career mobility program. *Am J Occup Ther* 35:328-331, 1981.

11. Baum C, Gray M: Certification: Serving the public interest. *Am J Occup Ther* 42:77-79, 1988.

12. Davy J, Peters M: State licensure for occupational therapists. *Am J Occup Ther* 36:429-432, 1982.

13. Gray M: Recertification and relicensure in the allied health professions. *J Allied Health* 13:22-30, 1984.

14. American Occupational Therapy Certification Board: *AOTCB and State Regulation: A Partnership to Protect the Public*. Rockville, MD: AOTCB, 1991.

Chapter 32

The Future of Occupational Therapy

AN ENVIRONMENT OF OPPORTUNITY

Elnora M. Gilfoyle, DSc, OTR, FAOTA

Introduction

During the 1990s and the beginning of the 21st century, several forces will provide an environment of opportunity for occupational therapy. As a profession, we must realize that the environment is created both by historical and contemporary social, political and economic forces. We are not dependent on those forces; rather, we can be a part of the forces. Occupational therapy can have an influence on its environment, as well as being affected by its forces. Because environment profession is a **transactional process** (act of carrying on business, negotiations and other activities), occupa-

tional therapy practitioners must work together to create opportunities that facilitate growth and development of the profession and address the needs of society. By so doing, our profession will expand its services and society will benefit.

Identifying social, economic and political forces gives us direction for informed planning. An awareness of these forces, plus attention to today's technologic forces, is the first step in providing occupational therapy practitioners with abilities to create opportunities for themselves. This chapter presents an overview of environmental trends and implications from the profession's history.

KEY CONCEPTS

Maturation of America	Power of values
Mosaic society	Legacy of value system
Redefinition of individual and society roles	OT value system
Information-based economy	Dimensions of practice
Globalization	Trends in educational preparation
Personal and environmental health	

ESSENTIAL VOCABULARY

Transactional process

Change drivers

Globalization

Trends

Mosaic

Cultural shift

Transformation

Values

Integration

Adaptation

Naisbitt forecasts that the 1990s will be the most important decade for our society, as it is a period of innovation in technology, unprecedented opportunities in our economy, political reform and rebirth of cultural interests.[1] Of particular importance are the predictions of this futurist for the 1990s to be a decade of women in leadership, a period of triumph for individuals, an age of biology, free-market socialism, global economic boom, privatization of the welfare state, global life-styles and cultural nationalism. The United Way of America's Environmental Scan Committee identified nine leading forces, which they term **change drivers** (concepts or elements that lead future societal modifications) that can be considered as key developments in American society.[2] The nine change drivers include the maturation of America, our developing mosaic society, the redefinition of individual and societal roles, the exploding information-based economy, **globalization** (worldwide activities), economic restructuring, attention to personal and environmental health, redefinition of family and home and the rebirth of social issues. A listing of predictions and trends is presented here to orient the reader to some of the contemporary forces and predictions that will influence occupational therapy. (Information on these trends was compiled, in part, as a report to the Intercommission Council, Future's Task Force of the American Occupational Therapy Association.)

The Maturation of America

Demographics of America's population is maturing as the "baby boom" generation grows older. Our older population will be more active and affluent than in previous generations. Our society is being transformed from an era focused on youth to one that is more realistic, responsible, conservative and tolerant of diversity.[2]

Major social, economic, political and technologic **trends** (general course or tendency) affecting society are enumerated in Figures 32-1 through 32-4. Review of these marked changes indicates that they will certainly have many implications for occupational therapy personnel, some which are listed here.

- Clientele will change; dramatic increase in needs of those over age 75.
- Increased employment by corporations to conduct services and educational programs for employees concerning problems related to caring for the elderly.
- Increasing demands for occupational therapy personnel to work in long-term care facilities and with home-based care.
- Occupational therapy personnel become entrepreneurs responding to eldercare markets.
- Increase in opportunities for therapists and assistants to provide job assessment and job training to elderly populations.
- Expansion of roles of occupational therapy personnel, ie, OTR—manager, educator, researcher, consultant, supervisor and evaluator; COTA—active practitioner; aides become an important component of practice.
- Increase in the number of therapists and assistants in private practice serving the elderly.
- Occupational therapy positioned and marketing itself as the expert for eldercare.
- Occupational therapy personnel become political activists for needs of the aging population.
- Profession demonstrating the cost-effectiveness of its services to the elderly.

To be prepared for service delivery in this rapidly changing environment, the profession will need to make changes that assure the delivery of needed services. These changes include the following:

- Preparing students with knowledge, skills and attitudes necessary to provide services to the elderly (Biopsychosocial development theories with elderly, human performance with elderly, effects of the aging process on human performance).
- Political and economic implications affecting elderly and the impact of the maturation of America upon political, economic and social aspects.
- Knowledge and skills needed for clinicians to participate in efficacy studies to validate intervention studies as service delivery models.
- Knowledge related to reimbursement and uninsured health care processes.
- Greater understanding of the various roles for occupational therapy personnel, including OTR, COTA and aide.
- Ethical issues affecting elderly.

Mosaic Society

A growing population of elderly individuals adds an element of diversity to our society. In addition, increasing ethnic diversity, more single-person households, increasing number of persons with disabilities and growth of the US population due to increasing immigration transforms our society from a "mass" toward a **mosaic**, a society with distinctive identities.[2] Examples of social and economic trends seen in our mosaic society are summarized in Figures 32-5 and 32-6.

In the political arena, it is likely that special interest groups will increase[2] and minorities will have greater political influence.[1,2,5,9] Decentralization of government will continue[2] and, due to shifts in populations, representatives will change in number, particularly in the Northeast, South

- Slowing of population growth.[2]
- Population older, with median age rising.[2]
- Decline in proportion of children in total population.[2]
- Decline in number of young adults.[2]
- Increase in numbers of persons age 35-54.[2]
- Senior population (65-74) stable through year 2000.[2]
- Dramatic increase in population over age 75.[2]
- Higher education recruits older Americans as students.[2]
- By 2020, the number of people age 50 or older increases 74%: the number under age 50 grows a mere 1%.[3]
- One in four Americans age 50 by 2020.[3]
- Exact size of older market will depend on trends in mortality rate and on the following factors: application of new medical techniques, presence of environmental pollutants, improvements in exercise and nutrition, rate of violent crimes, new diseases, rate of cigarette smoking, drug and alcohol abuse, extent to which people take responsibility for their own health and changes in society's conception of value of life.[3]
- By 2000, number of people age 50 and older could grow by as much as 21% or as little as 16%; because of age of "baby boomers," number of people in their 50s expected to grow between 38% and 42%.[3]
- By year 2000, number of people in 60s will rebound.[3]
- Year 2000 begins boom in retirement-related industries.[3]
- Between 1990 and 2020, number of men in their 60s will increase by 75% to 17 million; number of women in their 60s will increase 68% to 19 million; most optimistically, number of men in their 60s will double between 1990 and 2020.[3]
- When first "baby boomer" turns 65, in 2011, men could live as many as 18 more years, on the average; women an additional 23 years.[3]
- Today, women age 65 outnumber men by 50%—86 men for every 100 women in their 60s; by 2010 there will be 92 men for every 100 women; for men and women in their 70s, the ratio could improve from 71 to 85 men for every 100 women.[3]
- Wives will outlive husbands through 2020, but longer life expectancies for both sexes will keep spouses together longer.[4]
- By 2050, more than one American in five (23%) will be 65 (12% today).[3]
- For every American in a nursing home, two others with similar needs live in the community.[4]
- Home-based elderly may be eligible for local services, but often depend on network of family and friends for transportation, shopping, personal care, meal preparation, financial management and home repair.[4]
- Nearly 7 million Americans provide unpaid personal care to elderly friends and family members.[4]
- 75% of caregivers are women, and over 50% hold full-time or part-time jobs; 40% also have responsibility for children (referred to as the "sandwiched" Americans).[4]
- More than 95% of 40-year-olds have at least one surviving parent; in the 50-year-old group, proportion is 80%.[4]
- Approximately 28% of workers age 30 and older are providing some form of care for an older person. Responsibilities take from 6 to 10 hours a week, and 8% of the workers spending 35 hours a week with eldercare responsibilities averaging 5 to 6 years.[4]
- Travelers Companies Foundation has documented greater than average absenteeism among employees with responsibility for an elderly person.[4]
- Caregivers need information on where to go for help.[4]
- Travelers Companies sponsor "caregiving fairs" where service providers and referral agencies gather to respond to caregiver's questions.[4]
- Predict increase in involvement for corporations; eg company-paid counselor running support groups for employee caregivers; offering flexible work schedules.[4]
- As population ages, need for caregivers increases and more older persons rely on relatives who work; result is that eldercare is an employee issue.[4]
- Increase in entrepreneurs responding to eldercare market.[4]
- Increased goal is helping elderly stay in their homes as long as possible.[4]
- Increased numbers of elderly will need long-term care facilities.[4]
- Three of four caregivers to elderly or other relatives are women; this will affect professions that are predominately female.[4]
- Graying of population will affect education, health care, job market, retirement age rules, nursing homes, consumerism, work force and health care.[1]

Figure 32-1. *Social Trends—Maturation of America.*

- Era of America's youth-driven economy will diminish.[3]
- Better educated labor force necessary to increase economic production.[3]
- Corporate "elite" and highly educated "gold collar" worker will emerge.[2]
- Median income of families will grow.[2]
- Savings rate will increase.[2]
- Labor force will grow older with workers having more experience.[2,3]
- Flexible work schedules and retirement options will be offered in an effort to reverse trend toward early retirement.[2]
- More middle-aged workers will start new careers.[2]
- The declining young population and increasing elderly population means that by 2050 there will be approximately one worker for each social security beneficiary; presently, the ratio is about 3:1, and by the year 2000 the ratio will be 2:1.[3,5]
- By 1995, there will be fewer young people to enter the workforce, and these scarce young workers will have to be highly productive to keep our economy growing and to maintain our standard of living.[6]
- Between 1980 and 2000, the 18-year-olds to 24-year-olds in the United States population will decline by 19%, while the overall population will increase by 18%.[6]

Figure 32-2. *Economic Trends—Maturation of America.*

- More pragmatic activism, reflecting aging of society.[2]
- Increase in public policy to address issues facing the elderly.[5]
- More government dollars allocated to programs for the elderly.[3]
- Fewer dollars spent on issues for youth, such as education.[5]

Figure 32-3. *Political Trends—Maturation of America.*

- Research will increase to discover ways to ease the affects of aging.[2]
- Computer technology to assist with communication from home base.[3]
- Technology to be readily available for increasing dependent living environments.[4]

Figure 32-4. *Technologic Trends—Maturation of America.*

- Greater proportional growth of minorities.[2]
- Greatest increase in US population will be with immigration.[1,2,5]
- Immigration will affect classrooms as ethnic/racial diversity increases.[1,2]
- Alternative methods for teacher certification to alleviate teacher shortage.[2]
- Alternative educational options increase—year-round schools, flexible schedules, evening-weekend programs, home-based courses, etc.[1,2]
- In year 2000, 85% of new entrants to the nation's workforce will be members of minority groups and women.[6]
- Number of people with disabilities who can get out into the workplace will increase.[7]
- America is changing, particularly in the composition of its young—blacks and Hispanics are now 25% of schoolchildren; by the year 2000, they will be 47%.[8]
- By 2010, one in every three 18-year-olds will be black or Hispanic, compared to one in five in 1985.[6,9]
- Changing demographics will affect the composition of the future workforce. Of new workers entering the labor force by the year 2000, only 15% will be white men; the rest will be either white women, members of minority groups or immigrants.[6,9]
- Of the 4 million scientists and engineers in the United States, only 2% identify themselves as disabled.[9]
- Projected shortfalls of future BS degree holders are related to the declining number of young people in our population.[6,9]
- American Indians enrolled in the 278 recognized tribes in the lower 48 states and 300 Aleut and Eskimo villages in Alaska number 1.4 million, or 6% of the US population.[9]
- Asian Americans make up only 2% of the US population; blacks are 12% of the American population; Hispanic population is the fastest-growing minority group, comprising 9% of the population.[6,9]
- An estimated 36 million people of working age in the United States have some disability (numbers uncertain because many people with disability do not identify themselves on surveys).[6,7,9]
- Women are now 51% of the population and 45% of the nation's workforce.[3,6,9]
- Poverty continues to grip a large number of children, including a disproportionate share of minority children.[6,9]
- Nation faces a serious shortage of scientists and engineers in the coming decades.[9]
- Asian and Hispanic immigration is highest to the region where the greatest concentration of Hispanic and Asian Americans reside.[5,6,9]
- Women, minorities and immigrants will make up 80% of all new entrants into the job market in the next decade; increased importance of flexible work schedules, leaves of absence, flextime, and working at home.[2,6,9]

Figure 32-5. *Social Trends—Mosaic Society.*

and Southwest.[5]

Technologic trends indicate that advances in technology will enable more persons to obtain products, services, publications and information that are targeted to their particular ethnic characteristics, economic status and personal preferences.[2]

The many implications for occupational therapy include the following factors:

- OT products, services, publications and information targeted to individuals by considering each person's ethnic/racial characteristics, economic status and personal preferences. OT information resources must target specific populations and be readily available.
- OT practitioners involvement with state politics and special interest groups.
- OT practitioners involvement with ethnic minority populations will have an influence on the political decisions related to occupational therapy services.
- Increase of OT personnel with ethnic minority backgrounds and persons with disability.
- Occupational therapy personnel must become bilingual.
- OTRs and COTAs working closely with the implementation of programming enacted from the Americans with Disabilities Act (ADA).

In response to the needs of an increasingly mosaic society, occupational therapy practitioners will need to develop knowledge and skills to assure that these needs are indeed met. Among the changes necessary are these:

- The education curriculum in OT must have a multicultural perspective and sensitivity, as well as be multilingual.
- OT education programs must focus on recruitment and retention of persons from ethnic minority backgrounds.
- OTRs and COTAs must promote themselves as the leading resource in how to access technology by persons with disability.

Redefinition of Individual and Societal Roles

The 21st century will see a blurring of boundaries that traditionally defined our roles as individuals, families and organizations. Included in the redefinition is the increased opportunities for women in leadership positions.[2] Societal, economic and political trends related to this redefinition of the individual and roles are shown in Figures 32-7 through 32-9, respectively.

Technologic trends indicate that computer technology will be available for very small firms to allow them to compete successfully.[2] Concern about privacy will increase as more data are collected electronically.[2] The increased availability of computers, modems and other equipment will help people maximize technology for lifelong learning opportunities.[1,5]

Implications for occupational therapy related to the redefinition of the individual and society roles include some of the following:

- Increase in number of OTs in management and consulting positions.

- Market "niches" will increase, reflecting increasing diversity.[2]
- Business to operate through networks rather than consolidated under one roof.[2]
- Organizations to be either "very large" or "very small."[1,3,5]
- Increase in two-income households; single parent households decreasing.[2,5]
- Growth of urban, minority underclass to continue.[2,5]
- Labor force to be increasingly multicultural and multilingual.[2]
- Women's representation in top management positions will increase.[1,2,6]
- Child care benefits and flexible hours in workplace will be necessary to accommodate workers.[1,2]

Figure 32-6. *Economic Trends—Mosaic Society.*

- Women in top management positions will increase.[1]
- Child-care benefits and flexible hours will be necessary to accommodate the increase in women in the workplace.[1]
- Businesses will operate through networks rather than being consolidated under one roof.[1]
- There will be an increase in two-income households, with single-parent households decreasing.[1]
- There will be increased sensitivity to the importance of "the human resource."[1]
- Wellness activities will become increasingly important.[2]
- Rise in practice of holistic medicine.[2]
- Increased growth in self-help movement.[1,2]
- Growth of entrepreneurial activity, self-employment, and multiple careers.[1,2]
- Individuals more willing to act on their own rather than depend on large institutions.[1,2]
- Business more directly involved in social issues such as education, health and human services.[1,2,5]
- Federal deficit will continue to constrain federal action on social problems, thus more involvement from private sector.[1,2]

Figure 32-7. *Social Trends—Role Redefinition.*

- Business and industry will be more directly involved in social issues, such as education, health and human services.[1,2,5]
- Employees to have increased autonomy and be in closer contact with customer.[2]
- Highly educated "gold collar" worker will emerge.[2]
- Union membership will decline.[2]
- Traditional roles of government and business blur as private sector spending on social issues increases.[2]

Figure 32-8. *Economic Trends—Role Redefinition.*

- There will be an increase in the number of women serving in local, state and national government positions.
- Although federal deficit will remain, society will put pressure on government to increase funding for some human service programs.[1,2]
- Pressure to deregulate industries such as telecommunications will emerge.[2]
- State government influence on social issues to increase, with decline in federal government's influence.[1,2]
- Private sector will perform services formerly carried out by government via contracts.[10]
- Increase in referenda on a wide variety of issues.[2]

Figure 32-9. *Political Trends—Role Redefinition.*

- Increased proportion of services by OTRs and COTAs outside the health arena.
- Increasing numbers of OT personnel in political activities.
- Increased OT participation/partnership with business to deliver health and human services.
- OT practitioners will be computer literate.
- OT practitioners will maximize technology for lifelong learning opportunities.
- OTRs and COTAs compete successfully as a "small business," using computer technology to manage.
- Wellness/self-help movement provides positive impact on OT; public requests OT services directed toward prevention, enhancement of independence, self-care and education.
- Prevention a major goal for OT service.
- OT practitioners service provision via contracts with the private sector.
- Accountability for OT services required.

Knowledge and skills needed by occupational therapy practitioners to prepare them to respond to these changes include the following areas:

- Management and leadership roles
- Increased content related to communication, emphasizing conflict resolution, negotiation, networking and marketing

- Accounting, financing and economics
- Public policy
- Business ethics
- Concepts of "wellness" activities
- Principles of establishment of a small business
- Marketing
- Reimbursement, ethics and managed health care
- Cost-effectiveness and efficacy studies

Information-Based Economy

Explosion of information creates an information-based society. Advancements in communication technology provide necessary tools for information management. Our upcoming information-based economy will be a different structure and system than our current industrial economy. Both types are related and will influence us throughout the upcoming decade.[2] The many technologic trends that influence our information based economy are presented in Figure 32-10.

The implications for occupational therapy practitioners are many and include the following examples:

- Providing programs for persons who have health effects from working at computer terminals.

- Business will operate through networks rather than consolidate under one roof.
- Increased use of information technology as a teaching and learning aid.
- Telephone to increasingly become the gateway to sophisticated communications.
- Mobile communications environment to increase and be readily available.
- Desktop and electronic publishing to become more important.
- Factory automation to experience growth.
- In urban areas, every individual will have computers in the home or workplace by the year 2000.
- Devices (home computers, Fax machines, video cassette recorders) in homes will increase.
- Automation to increase pressure on executives to become "hands-on" managers.
- Cable television to offer more and draw an increasing audience share.
- Information overload to become an increasing issue.
- Technologic "haves" and "have-nots" to develop.
- Health issues and effects of working at computer terminals will be a major focus for individuals and industry.
- Advances in technology will improve ability to diagnose illness.
- Biology-based industries to grow in economic importance.

Figure 32-10. *Technologic Trends—Information Based Economy[2].*

- Collaborating with bioengineers for development of devices.
- Increase in the demand for personnel to work in industry in "back to work" programs and prevention related to effects of technology.
- Participating in continuing education programs using information technology as teaching and learning aids, programs for self-study at home via videocassette recorders, and networking via computers.
- Home-based OT employment increase.

To assure adequate preparation for these new roles, greater knowledge and skills will be needed by therapists and assistants. Educational curricula in OT must include information on technology, computer literacy, networking and programming.

Globalization

Many factors are contributing to the transformation from our US-based society to a global economy. Foreign ownership of US companies and an increasing presence of American firms in foreign countries will affect our economy. Increased travel, immigration, the growth of internation associations, and the proliferation of advanced technology for media all contribute to the growth of multiculturalism and respect for diversity.[2] Social trends seen in this area are summarized in Figure 32-11.

The implications for occupational therapy focus on the following factors:

- Increased internal competition
- Increase in practitioners in organizations such as Peace Corps
- Increase in foreign OTs working in the United States
- International programs of AOTA and its state associations
- Global market trend information and market research provided to membership of AOTA
- Increased understanding by AOTA members of relationship between the international scene and their "own back yard"
- Non-US members included in AOTA and state associations
- AOTA expertise made available to foreign clients
- Databases that incorporate massive amounts of research from other countries created by AOTA
- AOTA services capacities built through technology rather than through dependency on people

Occupational therapy practitioners need a broad base of knowledge to address a global society. Educational programs must include a multicultural perspective and content related to the economics of globalization. Occupational therapy education should include opportunities for internships in foreign countries.

Personal and Environmental Health

Key areas of public concern will include health promotion, prevention of illness and disability, quality of life

---

- Growth of the US population increasingly dependent on immigration.[1,2,10]
- Increasing foreign ownership of industry.[1,2]
- Relative economic power of United States declining as other nations develop.[2]
- Americans directing volunteer time and dollars to global issues, as well as national causes.[2]
- Foreign-owned firms to play a growing role in philanthropy.[1,2]
- Globalization is a fundamental part of association's strategic plan.[10]
- Associations must serve their members by providing global market trend information and market research members' needs.[10]
- Associations need to be in a key position to assist members in understanding the relationship between the international scene and their "own back yard."[10]
- Professional associations should consider closer relationships with US embassies overseas.[10]
- Professions and their associations must consider ways in which they can influence non-US members.[10]
- Associations/professions need to be considering how their expertise can be translated into products for foreign clients.[10]
- Associations should explore creation of databases that incorporate massive amounts of research from tort litigation.[10]
- Global trends toward decentralization mean that developing countries will increasingly rely on nongovernmental solutions to social problems.[10]
- US associations could be prime consultants in the creation of new associations.[10]
- To compete for members, many associations will have to offer teleconferencing and electronic mail, and plan for the next wave of information need, such as video newspapers and interactive, on-line databases accessible by members.[10]
- Associations will build service capacity through technology rather than people.[10]

Figure 32-11. *Social Trends—Globalization.*

issues and the state of the environment. The transformation of the "biomedical era" to an era of "wellness" is an opportunity for occupational therapy. The many social trends reflected in this arena may be found in Figure 32-12. Economic trends related to personal and environmental health are shown in Figure 32-13.

Political trends indicate that Congress may pass national health insurance for the 37 million Americans without health insurance, and Medicare hospital reimbursement will be modified to incorporate a severity index on all inpatients on diagnostic-related groups (DRGs).[11] Hospitals and health systems must cut costs by at least 3% to 5% annually, and management layoffs are predicted which will reduce senior and middle managers by 5%.[11]. In addition, hospitals will eliminate unprofitable or uncompetitive services.[11]

Trends indicate a rapid turnover rate in new technologies.[2] Concern will grow about health effects of working at computer terminals, and health providers will see increasing numbers of individuals seeking health care services for these problems. On the other hand computer technology will be a boon for workers with existing disabilities, with bedside computing and technologic substitutions becoming common.[7,11] Advanced technology will also provide tools for increased research in health promotion.

Change drivers and trends reported in the literature provide an environment of opportunity for occupational therapy; however, the culture of occupational therapy must be modified to adapt to today's rapidly changing society. In the process of modification, social forces become the primary impetus for a change or shift in the profession's culture. A **cultural shift** is a response to social forces and is viewed as dynamic change or **transformation**. Transformation is a new seeing, insight, vision; it is a period of shift in ideas or new ways of thinking about old concepts. The original concepts and ideas that made the profession in the beginning is the historical force behind the success of its transformation and future.

Occupational therapy services have evolved into a variety of specializations and the need for two levels of personnel. A diverse profession can continue to meet the demands of the environment and expand its services as long as there is continuity in the profession's philosophy. The beliefs and values that make up the philosophy of occupational therapy provide continuity to the profession's practices, whereas contemporary demands for services promote diversity among practice. History and tradition interact to form the strength of our philosophical base that provides the security to react to social forces and create opportunities for ourselves.

Our profession's legacy has provided basic concepts, beliefs and values that form the reality of occupational therapy. The professions's reality is in its culture, and culture's real existence lies in the hearts and minds of its people. Webster defines culture as "the integrated pattern of human behavior that includes thought, speech, action and artifact. . .culture depends on man's capacity for learning and transmitting knowledge to succeeding generations." Therefore, the growth and development of our profession his not only in the tools of scientific management, but in the people that make the profession work. The culture of occupational therapy becomes a synthesis of objective and subjective contributions that makes us a profession.[12]

- Key area of public concern includes quality of life issues, particularly the health of person and state of environment.[1,2]
- AIDS epidemic to become increasingly critical.[2,11]
- Concern relative to substance abuse continues.[2,11]
- Continued concern for issues regarding long-term care will grow.[2,11]
- Issues related to biomedical ethics will increase.[11]
- Environmental issues will gain prominence.[2]
- Rising violence by youth.[2]
- Increasing concern regarding safety and security.[2]
- Family violence to be critical problem.[2]
- People skills will be an essential executive asset.[11]
- Strategic vision will play a key role in the success of tomorrow's hospitals and health systems.[11]
- Health care executives must be more intuitive than logical; long-term and less short-term in perspective; innovative and less traditional; conceptual and less pragmatic; risk-taking and less conservative; customer oriented and less marketing oriented.[11]
- By year 2000, 50% of all patients will receive medical care from managed health-care systems, compared to only 10% in 1985.[11]
- Majority of Americans favor a health care system like Canada's, in which government uses taxes to pay most of the costs of health care and sets all hospital and physician fees.[11]
- Malpractice crisis is continuing to grow.[2]
- Community-oriented primary care (COPC) new "buzz word" in health care.[11]
- Trend emerging to hire foreign trained therapists.[2,11]

Figure 32-12. *Social Trends—Personal and Environmental Health.*

- Currently 7.5 million disabled persons aged 16 to 64—about 40% have completed 4 years of high school and another 30% have gone on to college.[6]
- One in five adults with a work disability has an income that falls below the poverty level.[2]
- Among people age 16 to 64 with a work disability, only 36% of men and 28% of women are in the labor force.[7]
- Men without disabilities who work full-time earn an average of $30,000; men with disabilities average $24,000. Women without disabilities earn $19,000 compared with $16,000 for women with disabilities.[7]
- Shortage of entry-level workers created by declining birth rates in late 1960s and 1970s is forcing businesses to hire workers with disabilities.[7]
- People with disabilities are the largest, best educated, least tapped employment resource in America.[7]
- Advertisers who target the disabled population directly can expect rewards.[7]
- Marketers looking for ways to increase their consumer base will find that people with special needs have a special appreciation for good service.[7]
- US health industry can expect rising costs, financial losses, staff cuts, hospital closures and no significant Medicare reimbursement increases in the next decade.[11]
- Hospital length of stay will rise by a half-day and occupancy will gain 1% to 2% due to longer stays and rising admissions.[11]
- Rural hospitals will strengthen their financial viability by transporting more complex, long-stay inpatients to regional medical centers.[11]
- Hospital closures will rise to more than 100 per year for the next 3 years.[11]
- Turnover of health-care executives will continue at rates above 20% per year.[11]
- Wage inflation will spiral upward with hospital and health-care workers.[11]
- Despite higher wages, labor shortages among hospital and health-care workers will get worse due to AIDS, lack of career advancement, and private sector opportunities.[11]
- To save labor costs, hospitals will spend from 2.5% to 5% of budget for new information systems and technologic substitutions that save labor hours.[11]
- Hospitals will invest millions in "continuum of care campuses" with multilevel facilities and services.[11]
- Employers will cut inpatient stays down to less than 10 days for alcohol and drug abuse and psychiatric care.[11]
- Hospital conversion of 10% to 20% of empty beds to extended care and "swing beds."[11]
- Health maintenance organizations (HMOs) will use more nursing homes without prior hospitalization.[11]
- Hospitals and health systems will adopt the value system for the "consumer's choice-buyer's market."[11]
- Pay for performance will gain popularity.[11]

Figure 32-13. *Economic Trends—Personal and Environmental Health.*

Central to the culture of occupational therapy is "the science and art of the occupational process which facilitates meaning and order to the lives of persons with disabilities."[12] The therapeutic use of occupation to promote fullness of life is the basic value, which is the heart of our culture. During transformation, our value system will remain and our basic concepts and beliefs will expand into a science of occupation and an art of purposefulness.

Through our transformation process, the roles and functions of occupational therapy personnel will change. Occupational Therapists, Registered (OTRs) will assume professional health care roles, with the majority of services being provided through consultation, monitoring and supervision. Increasing numbers of OTRs will be involved in research, theory development, education and administration. Certified Occupational Therapy Assistants (COTAs) will continue to provide direct patient care and work closely with OTRs in carrying out services. As we direct our profession into contemporary society, COTA/OTR collaborative efforts will increase, with more opportunities for COTAs to carry out independent practices. The escalating costs of health care, as well as society's shift from the biomedical model,[13] to a more comprehensive health model will provide opportunities and dictate a need to change the current roles and functions of occupational therapy practitioners. Change in roles and functions necessitates a change in educational preparation and professional regulations. Change can be a positive force; however, the profession's value system must be central to directing its change.

The Power of Values

Occupational therapy's value system is based on basic concepts and beliefs, and forms the heart of our profession's culture. **Values** become the essence of our philosophy, as values state what it is that we believe and do. Therefore, our values communicate what is unique about occupational therapy.[14]

The rapidly changing society of the 1990s and consequences of "future shock" demand accurate and logical choices. The most reliable guide for making logical choices is an awareness of our values. Bryan Hall states that clarification of values is not a skill that stands apart from those of science, but rather value clarification integrates the facts of science by bringing present knowledge into a more holistic focus.[15] Values are essential not only to occupational therapy, but also to each therapist and assistant, as values are the integrating force that bring all elements of the profession into focus. Through the profession's clarification of its value system, the power and uniqueness of occupational therapy can be understood.[15]

Values involve an internal choosing by the profession, not an external giving or demand by society.[15] A profession must view itself as a subject freely controlling its own destiny, not as an object at the beck and call of others.[15] Hall proposed that controlling one's own destiny and becoming dependent on others are alternative ways of conceptualizing oneself and are designated by the terms **integration** and **adaptation**.[15]

Integration results from the capacity to adapt oneself to reality plus the critical capacity to make choices and transform that reality. To the extent that man loses his ability to make choices and is subjected to the choices of others, man is no longer integrated, rather, he has adapted; he has adjusted. . .Passive obedience, conformity, external approval, and reliance on the directions of others characterizes the adaptive person, while independence, creativity, self-confidence and self-directiveness are typical of the integrated person.[15]

Occupational therapy must not succumb to being an adaptive profession; rather, our future must be directed to the recognition of our value system so that we can clarify the power of our profession, direct choices and transform the reality of occupational therapy toward a vital profession that can sustain a continual interactive process with society.

The transactional process of our profession and environment will result in a shift in the reality of occupational therapy, including its concepts, beliefs and values. A newly emerging value system will be defined in response to social forces and research findings, providing opportunities for expansion. Although a new value system is presently emerging, future and present are based on the past. Therefore, an understanding of our historical roots is necessary for us to prepare for the future.

Legacy of Our Value System

Our roots have been traced to Galen, 172 AD, in the statement, "Employment is nature's best physician and is essential to human happiness."[16] The early Egyptians and Greeks used music, games and physical and mental activities to improve one's state of health. During the 18th and 19th centuries, reports of the use of occupations for restoration of mental health appeared in the literature and the term "moral treatment" was initiated. In 1873, a Frenchman named Pinel wrote a book on moral treatment in which he discussed benefits of occupation for the mentally ill.[17] The idea of occupation or work for the mentally ill spread rapidly in Europe and to the United States.

Moral treatment continued to be popular in caring for the mentally ill until the time of the Civil War. After the war, the concept of moral treatment declined; however, in the early 1900s, Dr. Herbert Hall and nurse Susan E. Tracy rediscovered the idea of moral treatment and began to write about it.[18] Further writings proclaimed the value of occupation, and in 1909, Haviland stated: "The therapeutic value of occupation for the insane is axiomatic and is based on sound psychological laws."[12] Haviland's statement was one of the first to relate the therapeutic value of occupation with rudiments of theory.

In 1914, George Barton, speaking at a conference in Massachusetts, coined the term, *occupational therapy*. Mr. Barton had been a patient at Clifton Springs Sanatorium, where he helped his own recovery by engaging in manual work, primarily carpentry and gardening. He was so successful in influencing his own recovery that he became an advocate for the value of "doing" as a means to influence one's own health. Barton's term *occupational therapy* was so descriptive of the value of occupation and the idea of "doing" that the term caught on, replacing earlier terms such as moral treatment and ergotherapy.[19]

Just as the legacy of our values can be traced to the early 1900s, the legacy of essential characteristics of occupational therapy personnel can be traced to Hall's book, *Occupational Therapy—A New Profession*.[20] According to Hall, occupational therapy is a well-paid and attractive new profession for educated young women! He also wrote that occupational therapy is a full-time job and demands health, energy, an attractive personality, an interest and facility in handicrafts, a desire to serve crippled humanity and very special education! Mr. Hall declared: "The girl who undertakes training should be at least 20 years old. The age limit the other way is elastic—but few women over 35 should attempt the work."[20] Social transformation, particularly the feminist movement, has had a profound impact on the essential characteristics of occupational therapy personnel.

The National Society for the Promotion of Occupational Therapy was formed in 1917. Objectives of the Association were developed and statements of principles, which adopted occupational therapy as a method of treatment by means of purposeful occupation, were endorsed. Thus during the early 1900s, the values of occupation and of the patient's "doing" emerged, characteristics of occupational therapy practitioners were described, and an Association was formed to promote the ideas of occupational therapy.

Because of social forces, the early ideas of "occupation"

and "doing" were modified by the demands of both World War I and World War II. Wounded soldiers needed rehabilitation, and early ideas of the use of games, handicrafts and work evolved into values of exercise, constructive activities and activities of daily living. Concepts of work simplification and training in the use of adaptive equipment and prosthetic and orthotic devices became the therapeutic media for occupational therapy, and the original values of occupation were modified. Medical technology expanded and specialization led to the emergence of allied health fields. Occupational therapy identified itself with medicine and the profession's media and practices began to adopt biomedical ideals.

By the 1950s and 1960s, occupational therapy programs for persons with physical disabilities were based on sensorimotor rehabilitation techniques borrowed from physical therapy. The concept of the therapeutic use of self in the treatment of psychiatric disorders was borrowed from psychology and the therapeutic use of occupations was deemphasized. By 1950, the profession's services and its educational preparation began to identify two areas of specialization: physical disabilities and psychosocial disabilities.

With further advances in medical technology, life-saving techniques emerged, with more infants surviving birth trauma and congenital disorders. Knowledge about early development began to appear in the literature and therapy based on developmental concepts began to be reported. The recognition of a pediatric specialty for occupational therapy practice emerged.

By the 1960s and 1970s, the idea of "purposeful activity" was introduced and the term "occupation" dropped. The value of activity based on a neurobehavioral or occupational behavioral orientation or on the biopsychosocial model became popular, and the need for theory became a professional issue.[21] Professionals began to cry for a unifying theory, and the concept of adaptation as the unifying or single theory for occupational therapy began to appear in our literature.[22,23] Kielhofner modified the early concepts of occupational behavior and proposed "human occupation" as the unifying force of the profession[24]; occupational therapy practitioners once again began to include "occupation" as a descriptive term.

During the past decade, the change in the age of the population has had an impact on health care services, and occupational therapy has begun to expand its services in the area of gerontology. Current values and practices of occupational therapy, as well as its educational preparation, are based on a false dichotomy of two diagnostic groups (physical and psychosocial) and the dichotomy of two age groups (pediatrics and gerontology). Diversity based on two disabilities and two age groups does not provide the profession with a clear sense of its values or directions.

Another major development in our legacy was an official philosophy statement adopted by the Association in 1979. The statement was developed to describe our belief system and declare our uniqueness.[25] Although the statement is an attempt to provide continuity to our culture, our philosophy does not appear to provide us with a certainty about our day-to-day practices; it does not give us convincing responses about the therapeutic value of occupation and does not provide a sense of direction for our services. Consequently, recent literature in occupational therapy communicates an internal debate about the efficacy and credibility of activity as therapeutic media.[26]

During the 1980s, the profession of occupational therapy developed uncertainty about its values, therapeutic media and methods and dimensions of practice. This uncertainty, together with the social forces of the decade, provided an opportunity to research beliefs and philosophy. Historical concepts about activity were transformed into new perspectives of "occupation" and "occupational." The profession's value system, based on the concept of "occupation" as "action" with events of the environment, and the dimension of "occupational." as the "process of action" in which the patient becomes the action agent or "doer," became the unifying forces that provided continuity to the philosophies and theories of occupational therapy.[12] Occupational therapy entered the 1990s with a renewed spirit and pride about its professional uniqueness and value to society.

Occupational Therapy Value System

The following theoretical statements are presented to summarize the profession's concepts and beliefs. The statements provide a framework for understanding our value system.

1. Human beings have the capacity to influence their own state of health.
2. Human beings can achieve a state of healthfulness through the processes of adaptation and integration.
3. Adaptation and integration occur through dynamic transactions of an individual with his or her biopsychosocial environment.
4. Transactions with one's biopsychosocial environment take place through human occupations.
5. Human occupations include self-care, play/leisure activities, work/school work and rest.
6. Active processes of biopsychosocial transactions can influence a person's state of health as he or she functions as an open system.

Inherent in the preceding statements is the value system that forms the culture of occupational therapy. Our value system includes the core values of:

1. Human occupations as therapeutic media
2. Active participation with biopsychosocial events as

the occupational process to promote development, change or modification

3. Adaptation and integration as processes by which a person can influence his or her own state of health
4. Therapists and assistants as action facilitators, with the patient being the action agent
5. Each patient as a unique individual

Thus, concepts of "doing," "action," "occupation," and value of the patient as unique and the 'doer' or action agent are the integrating forces that bring the science and art of purposeful occupation into focus as the heart of our culture.[12]

Through science, explanations and rational knowledge about the values of the profession will be identified and measured. Clarifying a value system provides direction for the profession's research efforts, whereas research measures the efficacy of concepts and values. Although science is primary to defining the uniqueness of occupational therapy, the art of therapy is also a powerful force that exemplifies our uniqueness. The art of therapy provides us with an awareness or intuitive knowledge. Therapeutic art is a relationship in which the patient receives from the therapist, but it is the patient who has the capacity to influence his or her fulfillment of life. The value of occupational therapy therapeutic relationships is not in external giving by the therapist or assistant but in the internal receiving by the patient. "It is through internal receiving that occupational experiences become purposeful."[12] Through our scientific findings we will be able to predict and explain the uses of occupations as therapeutic media, but the purposefulness of the occupational process will remain a value that cannot be explained through scientific measurements. As such, the purposefulness of occupation remains our unique therapeutic art.

In summary, our legacy provides the basic concepts and beliefs that form the reality of occupational therapy. Throughout history, society's forces have had an impact on the growth and development of our ideas. Our basic values in occupation were modified and the media of therapy expanded. The biomedical model and theories of development influenced our practices. Our past provides a heritage in which change was gradual, whereas our present is characterized by rapid change and the demand to act quickly. "In this era, professions are presented with a need and the pressure to respond to that need without the necessary time to reflect on the knowledge and skills required to respond effectively."[27] Effective response depends on the profession's abilities to make choices, and the profession's values are essential for accurate and logical choice-making. A value system based on the concepts of "occupation" and "occupational" will be the integrating force that brings the science and art of occupational therapy into cultural focus. A strong culture provides the profession with abilities to react to the present, integrate the past, and prepare for the future.

Dimensions of Practice: Diversity Within Community

A unifying value system provides occupational therapy with needed continuity so that logical diversity within its practices can emerge. Practice diversity must be complementary to philosophy; then diversity can add strength and power to the profession. Our early roots found occupational therapy practitioners working in hospital settings and the medical model dictating practice diversity. Operating from the medical model, practice was defined as the "art of healing through guided prescription."[27] Dimensions of practice were hospital-based and occupational therapists were identified as members of treatment-oriented medical teams.[27]

Diversity of practice was founded on diagnosis or disabilities. As medical technology expanded to life-saving techniques and developmental theories influenced medicine, practice dimensions added diversity based on age, but a focus on disability remained paramount. From the 1920s until the 1970s, practice dimensions were based on the medical model, with diversity among practitioners having no identification with philosophic continuity, but rather with diagnosis and age.

Because our diversity was based on disabilities, our profession diminished its values with our "unique perspective and focus on asset, abilities, competencies and satisfying performance in all areas of human existence."[26] In the 1970s and 1980s, however, social forces began to provide the opportunity for our profession to reidentify itself with human performance. Society began to lose its allegiance to medicine, and occupational therapy began to respond with a change in its focus from treatment orientation to one of health promotion. The cost of medical care is a major factor influencing the decline in society's allegiance to the biomedical model.[13] These social forces provide an opportunity for occupational therapy to "call up" earlier concepts and values and adapt those to society's needs. Through integration of our past values with present practices, occupational therapy is evolving into a comprehensive health profession. Consequently, our roles in health promotion and the prevention of disability are expanding.[27]

In 1978 Yerxa stated: "As occupational therapists, we are at home with the mundane stuff of everyday living, but society does not yet value the commonplace, everyday activities of play, leisure and self-maintenance."[28] Yerxa proposed that "society does need us but it has not yet found that out."[28] In her address, Yerxa challenged the profession to

reaffirm to ourselves and society the significance of the mundane stuff of daily living. If we can hold on, articulate, and perpetuate the valuing of everyday activity, we can give society the opportunity to catch up with us. For what we value is what existence is about, finding meaning in all that we do.[28]

In the present decade, society is beginning to catch up with occupational therapy, and the opportunity for our profession to influence its own dimensions of practice is now. Diversity within our practice will no longer be based on disability but on the continuity of our value systems; thus, dimensions of occupational therapy services will have logical diversity.

Two economic and political forces have had major ramifications on our dimensions of practice: legislation in the late 1970s that delineated occupational therapy as an education-related service rather than a medical service, governmental decisions in 1983 that created the prospective payment system resulting in economic influences on where health services are provided.

The term *related service* has influenced changing dimensions of our practices. Education-related services cannot be limited to direct treatment approaches. Although most handicapping conditions serviced by occupational therapy personnel in the school systems can be described as medical in their origin, the effect and amelioration of the conditions is not through medical treatment, but through education.[12] Through opportunities to provide services in school environments, occupational therapists and assistants have expanded their practice.

One example of the expansion of occupational therapy services created by social and political forces is the current reestablishment of our concepts and values related to work, vocational rehabilitation, and a person's rights for a productive and purposeful life.[29] Opportunities to identify our services with vocational readiness programs resulted from social forces placed on the public educational system. Consumers advocated for education and community agencies to work together to provide programs that focus on students' transition from school systems to community systems.

In the 1980s, the United States Department of Education identified "transition" as a funding priority. Occupational therapy responded with the development of successful transition programs. Our values of work as human occupation had a major impact on the concepts of transition and subsequent programs for supported employment. Both COTAs and OTRs will continue to be important personnel in transition programs.

The future of education-related occupational therapy practices will see an increase in the need for consultation and supervision, participation in research, and development of cost-effective services, as well as management of resources. Thus, OTRs will increase their roles with indirect services, with direct therapist-student relationships carried out primarily by COTAs.

Prospective payment has changed concepts of acute medical care within medical environments. An awareness of the importance of personal responsibility or self-care has emerged, and home health and other community programs are being developed in response to economic forces. With government stressing the need for cost containment, occupational therapy practitioners are struggling with reimbursement issues for certain services.[3] In response to reimbursement issues, the Association authorized funding for efficacy studies to demonstrate the cost-effectiveness of occupational therapy. Cost-containment issues have opened up new opportunities for occupational therapy personnel to provide services through home health and other community agencies. Identifying ourselves with cost-effective services that can be offered outside the domain of the hospital setting has complemented the profession's efforts to reestablish our values in the promotion of human performance.

Another example created by social and economic forces to return the disabled to productive life is the newly developed programs in work evaluation, work hardening, and work capacity. Social forces prevalent today provide advantages for our profession to proclaim human occupation as therapeutic media and the occupational process as a cost-effective method to promote healthfulness. In this decade, OTRs must become actively involved in research and management of cost-effective services. Thus, an increasing number of COTAs will be employed in schools, home health and community agencies, with expansion of their roles in direct services.

Trends in Educational Preparation

As service delivery patterns expand and diversity of practice is determined by the system where services are provided, the roles and functions of occupational therapy practitioners must be altered to meet the evolving focus on health promotion and prevention of disabilities. In response to transformation, the Association must reexamine the delineation of roles and functions of the OTR and COTA. No longer must the delineation be solely determined by current practices; the impact of future trends on OTR and COTA practices must be considered. Through delineation of predicted roles of the entry-level therapist and assistant, knowledge, skills and attitudes needed by each of the personnel groups must be identified. Only then can appropriate educational preparation of the OTR and COTA be implemented.

The demands for OTRs to assume roles in consultation and supervision, to conduct research, develop theories, and manage cost-effective programs will require knowledge and skills associated with graduate level programs. The demands for COTAs to function more independently will require knowledge and skills about occupational therapy theory and practice as well as liberal arts or basic general education courses. Liberal arts and sciences provide basic knowledge necessary for problem-solving skills. General studies are necessary for individuals to analyze critically and to make interconnections required for appropriate clinical judgments and professional competence. The level of general knowledge plus the skills, attitudes and information specific to the practice of occupational therapy requires a minimum of four years of higher education. For COTAs to function more independently in the areas of evaluation, planning and treatment, an increased number of years in higher education will be necessary. Independent practices require problem-solving abilities and skills to analyze and synthesize complex information. Thus, additional educational preparation will be necessary.

Summary

The future of occupational therapy will be influenced by our current environment of opportunity. Social, political, economic and technologic forces are all affecting occupational therapy health care services. Demands for cost-effective programs and concepts of health promotion, advanced technology, and our changing demographics, together with society's recognition of the importance of one's own responsibilities toward maintaining health, will promote an expansion of our service.

Our profession is in a period of transformation, with the emergence of a value system based on occupation and the process of occupational providing sensible continuity for practice. Dimensions of practice will include diversity of our services as offered through community, education and medical systems. Philosophy and practice will evolve from treatment orientation to health promotion, where our services can focus on the patient's assets and abilities.

Occupational therapy practitioners will modify their roles and functions to meet the demands for services. As roles change, so must the educational preparation for both the OTR and COTA.

Through transformation, we will direct our own future. The time for promotion of the idea of "health through doing" is now. Today occupational therapy can proclaim its uniqueness as the therapeutic use of occupations to facilitate abilities.

Related Learning Activities

1. Plan a "think-tank" discussion with a group of peers. Envision what a typical occupational therapy clinic might look like ten years and 20 years from now. Who are the primary recipients of services? What methods and modalities are used? What changes will be necessary in the delivery of services?

2. Obtain a copy of the AOTA Directions for the Future Report from your state representative. What are some of the implications for COTA education and practice in the future? Compare these with Gilfoyle's predictions.

3. Research the environment in your locale, and make a list of the changes that you have observed in relation to the trends cited in this chapter. Discuss how these changes are affecting you, your family and significant others.

References

1. Naisbitt J, Aburdene P: *Megatrends 2000*. New York, William Morrow & Co., 1990.
2. Lynch AE: *What Lies Ahead: Countdown to the 21st Century*. Alexandria, Virginia, United Way Environmental Scan Committee, United Way Strategic Institute, 1990.
3. Exter T: How big will the older market be? *American Demographics*, June 1990, pp. 33-36.
4. Buglass K: The business of eldercare. *American Demographics*, June 1990, pp. 33-36.
5. Hodgkinson H: Colorado: The state and its educational system. Lecture presented at Colorado State University, March, 1990.
6. The dynamic west: A region of transition. Report of the Western Region, Council of State Governments, San Francisco, California, 1990.
7. Waldrop J: From handicap to advantage. *American Demographics* April 1990, pp. 33-35, 54.
8. Willard T: *Why Study the Future*. Washington, DC, American Speech and Hearing Association, 1988.
9. Changing America: The new face of science and engineering. *Interim Report of the Task Force on Women, Minorities, and the Handicapped in Science and Technology*. Washington, DC, Author, 1988.
10. Kurent H: Voices of action. *Association Management*, June 1990, pp. 109-112.
11. Coile R, Grossman R: Tomorrow's macrotrends. *Healthc Forum J*, November/December 1988, pp. 51-53.
12. Gilfoyle E: Transformation of a profession. *Am J Occup Ther* 38:578-582, 1984.
13. Capra F: *The Turning Point: Science, Society, and the Rising Culture*. Toronto, Canada, Bantam Books, 1983, pp. 158-159.
14. Deal TE, Kennedy AA: *Corporate Cultures: The Rites and Rituals of Corporate Life*. Reading, Massachusetts, Addison-Wesley, 1982, pp. 21-25.
15. Hall BP: *The Development of Consciousness: A Confluent Theory of Values*. New York, Paulist Press, 1976, pp. 8, 11, 20-21, 26.
16. Willard H, Spackman C: *Occupational Therapy*. Philadelphia, JB Lippincott, 1947, p. 1.
17. Kidner TB: *Occupational Therapy, The Science of Prescribed Work for Invalids*. Stuttgart, Germany, W Kohlhanne, 1930.
18. Licht S: The founding and founders of the American Occupational Therapy Association. *Am J Occup Ther* 23:269-277, 1967.
19. Barton GE: *Teaching the Sick: A Manual of Occupational Therapy and Re-education*. Philadelphia: WB Saunders, 1914, p. 4.

20. Hall H: *Occupational Therapy—A New Profession*. Concord, New Hampshire, Rumfort Press, 1923, p. 15.

21. Hopkins H, Smith H (Eds): *Willard and Spackman's Occupational Therapy*, 6th Edition. Philadelphia, JB Lippincott, 1983, p. 3.

22. King LJ: Toward a science of adaptive responses. *Am J Occup Ther* 32:429-430, 1978.

23. Gilfoyle E, Grady A, Moore J: *Children Adapt*, 2nd Edition. Thorofare, New Jersey, Slack, Inc., 1990.

24. Kielhofner G (Ed): *Health Through Occupation: The Theory and Practice of Occupational Therapy*. Philadelphia, FA Davis, 1983.

25. The Philosophical Base of Occupational Therapy. American Occupational Therapy Association, Resolution #531, April, 1979.

26. West W: A reaffirmed philosophy and practice of occupational therapy for the 1980s. *Am J Occup Ther* 38:15-23, 1984.

27. Jaffe E: Transition in health care—Critical planning for the 1990s. *Am J Occup Ther* 39:432-434, 1985.

28. Yerxa E: The philosophical base of occupational therapy. In *Occupational Therapy: 2001 AD*. Rockville, Maryland, American Occupational Therapy Association, 1978.

29. Davy J: Status report on reimbursement for occupational therapy. *Am J Occup Ther* 38:295-297, 1984.

Appendices

Appendix A
STANDARDS OF PRACTICE
FOR OCCUPATIONAL THERAPY

Preface

These standards are intended as recommended guidelines to assist occupational therapy practitioners in the provision of occupational therapy services. These standards serve as a minimum standard for occupational therapy practice and are applicable to all individual populations and the programs in which these individuals are served.

These standards apply to those registered occupational therapists and certified occupational therapy assistants who are in compliance with regulation where it exists. The term *occupational therapy practitioner* refers to the registered occupational therapist and to the certified occupational therapy assistant, both of whom are in compliance with regulation where it exists. The minimum educational requirements for the registered occupational therapist are described in the current *Essentials and Guidelines of an Accredited Educational Program for the Occupational Therapist* (American Occupational Therapy Association [AOTA], 1991a). The minimum educational requirements for the certified occupational therapy assistant are described in the current *Essentials and Guidelines of an Accredited Educational Program for the Occupational Therapy Assistant* (AOTA, 1991b).

Standard I: Professional Standing

1. An occupational therapy practitioner shall maintain a current license, registration, or certification as required by law.
2. An occupational therapy practitioner shall practice and manage occupational therapy programs in accordance with applicable federal and state laws and regulations.

3. An occupational therapy practitioner shall be familiar with and abide by AOTA's (1988) *Occupational Therapy Code of Ethics*.
4. An occupational therapy practitioner shall maintain and update professional knowledge, skills, and abilities through appropriate continuing education or in-service training or higher education. The nature and minimum amount of continuing education must be consistent with state law and regulation.
5. A certified occupational therapy assistant must receive supervision from a registered occupational therapist as defined by the current *Supervision Guidelines for Certified Occupational Therapy Assistants (AOTA, 1990) and by official AOTA documents. The nature and amount of supervision must be provided in accordance with state law and regulation.*
6. An occupational therapy practitioner shall provide direct and indirect services in accordance with AOTA's standards and policies. The nature and scope of occupational therapy services provided must be in accordance with state law and regulation.
7. An occupational therapy practitioner shall maintain current knowledge of the legislative, political, social, and cultural issues that affect the profession.

Standard II: Referral

1. A registered occupational therapist shall accept referrals in accordance with AOTA's *Statement of Occupational Therapy Referral* (AOTA, 1989) and in compliance with appropriate laws.
2. A registered occupational therapist may accept referrals for assessment or assessment with intervention in occupational performance areas or occupational per-

formance components when individuals have or appear to have dysfunctions or potential for dysfunctions.

3. A registered occupational therapist, responding to requests for service, may accept cases within the parameters of the law.

4. A registered occupational therapist shall assume responsibility for determining the appropriateness of the scope, frequency, and duration of services within the parameters of the law.

5. A registered occupational therapist shall refer individuals to other appropriate resources when the therapist determines that the knowledge and expertise of other professionals is indicated.

6. An occupational therapy practitioner shall educate current and potential referral sources about the process of initiating occupational therapy referrals.

Standard III: Screening

1. A registered occupational therapist, in accordance with state and federal guidelines, shall conduct screening to determine whether intervention or further assessment is necessary and to identify dysfunctions in occupational performance areas.

2. A registered occupational therapist shall screen independently or as a member of an interdisciplinary team. A certified occupational therapy assistant may contribute to the screening process under the supervision of a registered occupational therapist.

3. A registered occupational therapist shall select screening methods that are appropriate to the individual's age and developmental level; gender; education; cultural background; and socioeconomic, medical and functional status. Screening methods may include, but are not limited to, interviews, structured observations, informal testing, and record reviews.

4. A registered occupational therapist shall communicate screening results and recommendations to appropriate individuals.

Standard IV: Assessment

1. A registered occupational therapist shall assess an individual's occupational performance components and occupational performance areas. A registered occupational therapist conducts assessments individually or as part of a team of professionals, as appropriate to the practice settings and the purposes of the assessments. A certified occupational therapy

assistant may contribute to the assessment process under the supervision of a registered occupational therapist.

2. An occupational therapy practitioner shall educate the individual, or the individual's family or legal guardian, as appropriate, about the purposes and procedures of the occupational therapy assessment.

3. A registered occupational therapist shall select assessments to determine the individual's functional abilities and problems as related to occupational performance areas; occupational performance components; physical, social, and cultural environments; performance safety; and prevention of dysfunction.

4. Occupational therapy assessment methods shall be appropriate to the individual's age and developmental level; gender, education, socioeconomic, cultural and ethnic background; medical status; and functional abilities. The assessment methods may include some combination of skilled observation, interview, record review, or the use of standardized or criterion-referenced tests. A certified occupational therapy assistant may contribute to the assessment process under the supervision of a registered occupational therapist.

5. An occupational therapy practitioner shall follow accepted protocols when standardized tests are used. Standardized tests are tests whose scores are based on accompanying normative data that may reflect age ranges, gender, ethnic groups, geographic regions, and socioeconomic status. If standardized tests are not available or appropriate, the results shall be expressed in descriptive reports, and standardized scales shall not be used.

6. A registered occupational therapist shall analyze and summarize all collected evaluation data to indicate the individual's current functional status.

7. A registered occupational therapist shall document assessment results in the individual's records, noting the specific evaluation methods and tools used.

8. A registered occupational therapist shall complete and document results of occupational therapy assessments within the time frames established by practice settings, government agencies, accreditation programs, and third-party payers.

9. An occupational therapy practitioner shall communicate assessment results, within the boundaries of client confidentiality, to the appropriate persons.

10. A registered occupational therapist shall refer the individual to the appropriate services or request additional consultations if the results of the assessments indicate areas that require intervention by other professionals.

Standard V: Intervention Plan

1. A registered occupational therapist shall develop and document an intervention plan based on analysis of the occupational therapy assessment data and the individual's expected outcome after the intervention. A certified occupational therapy assistant may contribute to the intervention plan under the supervision of a registered occupational therapist.
2. The occupational therapy intervention plan shall be stated in goals that are clear, measurable, behavioral, functional, and appropriate to the individual's needs, personal goals, and expected outcome after intervention.
3. The occupational therapy intervention plan shall reflect the philosophical base of occupational therapy (AOTA, 1979) and be consistent with its established principles and concepts of theory and practice. The intervention planning processes shall include:
   a. Formulating a list of strengths and weaknesses.
   b. Estimating rehabilitation potential
   c. Identifying measurable short-term and long-term goals.
   d. Collaborating with the individual, family members, other caregivers, professionals, and community resources.
   e. Selecting the media, methods, environment, and personnel needed to accomplish the intervention goals.
   f. Determining the frequency and duration of occupational therapy services.
   g. Identifying a plan for reevaluation.
   h. Discharge planning.
4. A registered occupational therapist shall prepare and document the intervention plan within the time frames and according to the standards established by the employing practice settings, government agencies, accreditation programs, and third-party payers. The certified occupational therapy assistant may contribute to the formation of the intervention plan under the supervision of the registered occupational therapist.

supervision of a registered occupational therapist.
2. An occupational therapy practitioner shall implement the intervention plan through the use of specified purposeful activities or therapeutic methods to enhance occupational performance and achieve stated goals.
3. An occupational therapy practitioner shall be knowledgeable about relevant research in the practitioner's areas of practice. A registered occupational therapist shall interpret research findings as appropriate for application to the intervention process.
4. An occupational therapy practitioner shall educate the individual, the individual's family or legal guardian, noncertified occupational therapy personnel, and non-occupational therapy staff, as appropriate, in activities that support the established intervention plan. An occupational therapy practitioner shall communicate the risk and benefit of the intervention.
5. An occupational therapy practitioner shall maintain current information on community resources relevant to the practice area of the practitioner.
6. A registered occupational therapist shall periodically reassess and document the individual's levels of functioning and changes in levels of functioning in the occupational performance areas and occupational performance components. A certified occupational therapy assistant may contribute to the reassessment process under the supervision of a registered occupational therapist.
7. A registered occupational therapist shall formulate and implement program modifications consistent with changes in the individual's response to the intervention. A certified occupational therapy assistant may contribute to program modifications under the supervision of a registered occupational therapist.
8. An occupational therapy practitioner shall document the occupational therapy services provided, including the frequency and duration of the services within the time frames and according to the standards established by the employing facility, government agencies, accreditation programs, and third-party payers.

Standard VI: Intervention

1. An occupational therapy practitioner shall implement a program according to the developed intervention plan. The plan shall be appropriate to the individual's age and developmental level, gender, education, cultural and ethnic background, health status, functional ability, interests and personal goals, and service provision setting. The certified occupational therapy assistant shall implement the intervention under the

Standard VII: Discontinuation

1. A registered occupational therapist shall discontinue service when the individual has achieved predetermined goals or has achieved maximum benefit from occupational therapy services.
2. A registered occupational therapist, with input from a certified occupational therapy assistant where applicable, shall prepare and implement a discharge plan that is consistent with with occupational ther-

apy goals, individual goals, interdisciplinary team goals, family goals, and expected outcomes. The discharge plan shall address appropriate community resources for referral for psychosocial, cultural, and socioeconomic barriers and limitations that may need modification.

3. A registered occupational therapist shall document the changes between the intial and current states of functional ability and deficit in occupational performance areas and occupational performance components. A certified occupational therapy assistant may contribute to the process under the supervision of a registered occupational therapist.

4. An occupational therapy practitioner shall allow sufficient time for the coordination and effective implementation of the discharge plan.

5. A registered occupational therapist shall document recommendations for follow-up or reevaluation when applicable.

Standard VIII: Continuous Quality Improvement

1. An occupational therapy practitioner shall monitor and document the continuous quality improvement of practice, which may include outcomes of services, using predetermined practice criteria reflecting professional consensus, recent developments in research, and specific employing facility standards.

2. An occupational therapy practitioner shall monitor all aspects of individual occupational therapy services for effectiveness and timeliness. If actual care does not meet the prescribed standard, it must be justified by peer review or other appropriate means within the practice setting. Occupational therapy services shall be discontinued when no longer necessary.

3. A registered occupational therapist shall systematically assess the review process of patient care to determine the success or appropriateness of interventions. Certified occupational therapy assistants may contribute to this process in collaboration with the registered occupational therapist.

Standard IX: Management

1. A registered occupational therapist shall provide the management necessary for efficient organization and provision of occupational therapy services.

2. A certified occupational therapy assistant, under the supervision of a registered occupational therapist,

may perform the following management functions:

a. Education of members of other related professions and physicians about occupational therapy.

b. Participation in (1) orientation, supervision, training, and evaluation of the performance of volunteers and other noncertified occupational therapy personnel, and (2) developing plans to remediate areas of skill deficit in the performance of job duties by volunteers and other noncertified occupational therapy personnel.

c. Design and periodic review of all aspects of the occupational therapy program to determine its effectiveness, efficiency, and future directions.

d. Systematic review of the quality of service provided, using criteria established by professional consensus and current research, as well as established standards for state regulation; accreditation; American Occupational Therapy Certification Board (AOTCB) certification; and related laws, policies, guidelines and regulations.

e. Incorporation of a fair and equitable system of admission, discharge, and charges for occupational therapy services.

f. Participation in crossdisciplinary activities to ensure that the total needs of the individual are met.

g. Provision of support (i.e., space, time, money as feasible) for clinical research or collaborative research when such projects have the approval of the appropriate governing bodies (e.g., institutional review board) and the results of which are deemed potentially beneficial to individuals of occupational therapy services now or in the future.

References

American Occupational Therapy Association. (1979). The philosophical base of occupational therapy. *American Journal of Occupational Therapy, 33,* 785.

American Occupational Therapy Association. (1988). Occupational therapy code of ethics. *American Journal of Occupational Therapy, 42,* 795-796.

American Occupational Therapy Association. (1989). Statement of occupational therapy referral. In *Reference manual of the official documents of the American Occupational Therapy Association, Inc.* (AOTA) (p. VIII.1). Rockville, MD: Author (Original work published 1969, revised 1980).

American Occupational Therapy Association. (1990). Supervision guidelines for certified occupational therapy assistants. *American Journal of Occupational Therapy, 44,* 1089- 1090.

American Occupational Therapy Association. (1991a). *Essentials and guidelines of an accredited educational program for the occupational therapist.* Rockville, MD: Author.

American Occupational Therapy Association. (1991b). *Essentials and guidelines of an accredited educational program for the occupational therapy assistant.* Rockville, MD: Author.

Reprinted from AJOT, 46, pp. 1082-1085, American Occupational Therapy Association, Inc, 1992. Reprinted with permission.

Standards of Practice reprinted from American Journal of Occupational Therapy, 46 pp. 1082-1085, American Occupational Therapy Association, 1992. Reprinted with permission.

Appendix B
RESOURCE GUIDE

Visually Impaired

American Foundation for the Blind
Aids and Appliances Catalog
15 West 16th Street
New York, NY 10011

Be O.K. Self-Help Aids
Fred Sammons, Inc.
P.O. Box 32
Brookfield, IL 60513

Hammocker-Schlemmer
147 East 57th Street
New York, NY 10022

Large Print Publications

Dialogue
Dialogue Publications, Inc.
3100 South Park Avenue
Berwyn, IL 60402
(Quarterly; a variety of articles, poems, and stories)

Guideposts
Guideposts Associates, Inc.
Carmel, New York 10512
(Monthly; interfaith subjects)

Ideals
Ideal Publishing Corporation
P.O. Box 2100
Milwaukee, WI 53201
(Bimonthly; photographs, poems, stories usually on seasonal topics)

Musical Mainstream
National Library Service for the Blind and Physically
   Handicapped
Music Section
Library of Congress
Washington, DC 20542
(Bimonthly; original and reprinted articles; additions to the
National Library Service Collection)

Reading Materials in Large Type
National Library Service for the Blind and Physically
   Handicapped
Library of Congress
Washington, DC
(Reference circular)
New York Times/Large Type Weekly

New York Times Company
Large Print Edition
P.O. Box 2570
Boulder, CO 80302
(Weekly; current events, news)

Readers Digest
Readers Digest Large Type Edition
P.O. Box 241
Mt. Morris, IL 61054
(Monthly; condensed stories and variety of articles)

Sunshine Magazine
Sunshine Magazine Large Print Edition
P.O. Box 40
Litchfield, IL 62056
(Monthly; family focus)

World Traveler
Alexander Graham Bell Associates
4317 Volta Olace NW
Washington, DC 20007
(Monthly; science and social studies)

Oscar B. Stiskin
Ulverscraft Large Print Books
P.O. Box 3055
Stamford, CT 06905

Hearing Impaired

SHHH (Self-Help for Hard of Hearing People, Inc.)
1800 Wisconsin Avenue
Bethesda, MD 20814

National Information Center on Deafness
Gallaudet College
900 Florida Avenue, NE
Washington, DC 20002

General Safety

Home Safety Checklist
U.S. Consumer Products Safety Commission
Washington, DC 20207
1-800-638-2772

Various Sensory Deficits

BIT Corporation
(Boston Information & Technology)
52 Roland Street
Boston, MA 02129

Gadgets, Gizmos, Thingamabobs
P.O. Box 891
McLean, VA 22101
(Specify presenter guide or resource directory)

Maddock Inc.
Pequannock, NJ 07440-1993

Homecare Product Reference
USA and Canada

Official Directory of Homecare Suppliers
Medical Device Register, Inc.
Stamford, CT 06905

Appendix C
UNIFORM TERMINOLOGY FOR OCCUPATIONAL THERAPY—SECOND EDITION

Uniform Terminology for Occupational Therapy—Second Edition delineates and defines **Occupational Performance Areas** and **Occupational Performance Components** that are addressed in occupational therapy direct service. These definitions are provided to facilitate the uniform use of terminology and definitions throughout the profession. The original document, *Occupational Therapy Product Output Reporting System and Uniform Terminology for Reporting Occupational Therapy Services*, which was published in 1979, helped create a base of consistent terminology that was used in many of the official documents of The American Occupational Therapy Association, Inc. (AOTA), in occupational therapy education curricula, and in a variety of occupational therapy practice settings. In order to remain current with practice, the first document was revised over a period of several years with extensive feedback from the profession. The revisions were completed in 1988. It is recognized and recommended that a document of this nature be updated periodically so that occupational therapy is defined in accordance with current theory and practice.

Guidelines for Use

Uniform Terminology—Second Edition may be used in a variety of ways. It defines occupational therapy practice, which includes **Occupational Performance Areas** and **Occupational Performance Components**. In addition, it will be useful to occupational therapists for (a) documentation, (b) charge systems, (c) education, (d) program development, (e) marketing, and (f) research. Examples of how **Occupational Performance Areas** and **Occupational Performance Components** translate into practice are provided below. It is not the intent of this document to define specific occupational therapy programs nor specific occupational

therapy interventions. Some examples of the differences between **Occupational Performance Areas** and **Occupational Performance Components** and programs and interventions are:

1. An individual who is injured on the job may be able to return to work, which is an **Occupational Performance Area**. In order to achieve the outcome of returning to work, the individual may need to address specific **Performance Components** such as strength, endurance, and time management. The occupational therapist, in cooperation with the vocational team, utilizes planned interventions to achieve the desired outcome. These interventions may include activities such as an exercise program, body mechanics instruction and job modification, and may be provided in a work-hardening program.

2. An individual with severe physical limitations may need and desire the opportunity to live within a community-integrated setting, which represents the **Occupational Performance Areas** of activities of daily living and work. In order to achieve the outcome of community living, the individual may need to address specific **Performance Components**, such as normalizing muscle tone, gross motor coordination, postural control, and self-management. The occupational therapist, in cooperation with the team, utilizes planned interventions to achieve the desired outcome. Interventions may include neuromuscular facilitation, object manipulation, instruction in use of adaptive equipment, use of environmental control systems, and functional positioning for eating. These interventions may be provided in a community-based independent living program.

3. A child with learning disabilities may need to perform educational activities within a public school setting. Since learning is a student's work, this educational activity would be considered the **Occupational Per-**

formance Area for this individual. In order to achieve the educational outcome of efficient and effective completion of written classroom work, the child may need to address specific **Occupational Performance Components**, including sensory processing, perceptual skills, postural control, and motor skills. The occupational therapist, in cooperation with the team, utilizes planned interventions to achieve the desired outcome. Interventions may include activities such as adapting the student's seating to improve postural control and stability and practice motor control and coordination. This program could be provided by school district personnel or through contract services.

4. An infant with cerebral palsy may need to participate in developmental activities to engage in the **Occupational Performance Areas** of activities of daily living and play. The developmental outcomes may be achieved by addressing specific **Performance Components** such as sensory awareness and neuromuscular control. The occupational therapist, in cooperation with the team, utilizes planned interventions to achieve the desired outcomes. Interventions may include activities such as seating and positioning for play, neuromuscular facilitation techniques to enable eating, and parent training. These interventions may be provided in a home-based occupational therapy program.

5. An adult with schizophrenia may need and desire to live independently in the community, which represents the **Occupational Performance Areas** of activities of daily living, work activities, and play or leisure activities. The specific **Occupational Performance Areas** may be medication routine, functional mobility, home management, vocational exploration, play or leisure performance, and social skills. In order to achieve the outcome of living alone, the individual may need to address specific **Performance Components** such as topographical orientation, memory, categorization, problem solving, interests, social conduct, and time management. The occupational therapist, in cooperation with the team, utilizes planned interventions to achieve the desired outcome. Interventions may include activities such as training in the use of public transportation, instruction in budgeting skills, selection of and participation in social activities, and instruction in social conduct. These interventions may be provided in a community-based mental health program.

6. An individual who abuses substances may need to reestablish family roles and responsibilities, which represents the **Occupational Performance Areas** of activities of daily living and work. In order to achieve the outcome of family participation, the individual may need to address the **Performance Components** of roles, values, social conduct, self-expression, cop-

ing skills, and self-control. The occupational therapist, in cooperation with the team, utilizes planned intervention to achieve the desired outcomes. Interventions may include role and value clarification exercises, role-playing, instruction in stress management techniques, and parenting skills. These interventions may be provided in an inpatient acute care unit.

Because of the extensive use of the original document (*Uniform Terminology for Reporting Occupational Therapy Services*, 1979) in official documents, this revision is a second edition and does not completely replace the 1979 version. This follows the practice that other professions, such as medicine, pursue with their documents. Examples are the *Physician's Current Procedural Terminology First-Fourth Editions (CPT1-4)* and the *Diagnostic and statistical Manual First-Third Editions (DSM-I—III-R)*. Therefore, this document is presented as *Uniform Terminology for Occupational Therapy—Second Edition.*

Background

Task Force Charge

In 1983, the Representative Assembly of the American Occupational Therapy Association charged the Commission on Practice to form a task force to revise the *Occupational Therapy Product Output Reporting System and Uniform Terminology for Reporting Occupational Therapy Services*. The document had been approved by the Representative Assembly in 1979 and needed to be updated to reflect current practice.

Background Information

The *Occupational Therapy Product Output Reporting System and Uniform Terminology for Reporting Occupational Therapy Services* (hereafter to be referred to as *Product Output Reporting System* or *Uniform Terminology*) document was originally developed in response to the Medicare-Medicaid Anti-Fraud and Abuse Amendments of 1977 (Public Law 95-142), which required the Secretary of the Department of Health and Human Services to establish regulations for uniform reporting systems for all departments in hospitals. The AOTA developed the documents to create a uniform reporting system for occupational therapy departments. Although the Department of Health and Human Services never adopted the system because of antitrust concerns relating to price fixing, occupational therapists have used the documents extensively in the profession.

Three states, Maryland, California, and Washington, have used the *Product Output Reporting System* as a basis for statewide reporting systems. AOTA's official documents have relied on the definitions to create uniformity. Many occupational therapy schools and departments have used the definitions to guide education and documentation. Although the initial need was for reimbursement reporting systems, the profession has used the documents primarily to facilitate uniformity in definitions.

Task Force Formation

In 1983, Linda Kohlman McCourty, a member of the AOTA Commission on Practice, was appointed by the commission's chair, John Farace, to chair the Uniform Terminology Task Force. Initially, a notice was placed in the *Occupational Therapy Newspaper* for people to submit feedback for the revisions. Many responses were received. Before the task force was appointed in 1984, Maryland, California, and Washington adopted reimbursement systems based on the *Product Output Reporting System*. Therefore, to increase the quantity and quality of input for the revisions, it was decided to postpone the formation of the task force until these states had had an opportunity to use the systems.

In 1985, a second notice was placed in the *Occupational Therapy News* requesting feedback, and a task force was appointed. The following people were selected to serve on the task force:

Linda Kohlman McGourty, MOT OTR, Washington (Chair)

Roger Smith, MOT, OTR, Wisconsin

Jane Marvin, OTC, California

Nancy Mahon Smith, MBA, OTR, Maryland and Arkansas

Mary Foto, OTR, California

These people were selected based on the following criteria:
1. Geographical representation
2. Professional expertise
3. Participation in other current AOTA projects
4. Knowledge of reimbursement systems
5. Interest in serving on the task force

Development of the Uniform Terminology— Second Edition

The task force met in 1986 and 1987 to develop drafts of the revisions. A draft from the task force was submitted to the Commission on Practice in May of 1987. Listed below are several decisions that were made in the revision process by the task force and the Commission on Practice.

1. To not replace the original document (*Uniform Terminology for Reporting Occupational Therapy Services,* 1979) because of the number of official documents based on it and the need to retain a *Product Output Reporting System* as an official document of the AOTA.
2. To limit the revised document to defining **Occupational Performance Areas** and **Occupational Performance Components** for occupational therapy intervention (i.e., indirect services were deleted and the *Product Output Reporting System* was not re-

vised) to make the project manageable.
3. To coordinate the revision process with other current AOTA projects such as the Professional and Technical Role Analysis (PATRA) and the Occupational Therapy Comprehensive Functional Assessment of the American Occupational Therapy Foundation (AOTF).
4. To develop a document that reflects current areas of practice and facilitates uniformity of definitions in the profession.
5. To recommend that the AOTA develop a companion document to define techniques, modalities, and activities used in occupational therapy intervention and a document to define specific programs that are offered by occupational therapy departments. The Commission on Practice subsequently developed educational materials to assist in the application of uniform terminology to practice.

Several drafts of the revised *Uniform Terminology—Second Edition* document were reviewed by appropriate AOTA commissions and committees and by a selected review network based on geographical representation, professional expertise, and demonstrated leadership in the field. Excellent responses were received, and the feedback was incorporated into the final document by the Commission on Practice.

Outline

OCCUPATIONAL THERAPY ASSESSMENT
Occupational Therapy Intervention

I. Occupational Therapy Performance Areas
   A. Activities of Daily Living
      1. Grooming
      2. Oral Hygiene
      3. Bathing
      4. Toilet Hygiene
      5. Dressing
      6. Feeding and Eating
      7. Medication Routine
      8. Socialization
      9. Functional Communication
     10. Functional Mobility
     11. Sexual Expression
   B. Work Activities
      1. Home Management
         a. Clothing Care
         b. Cleaning
         c. Meal Preparation and Cleanup
         d. Shopping
         e. Money Management
         f. Household Maintenance
         g. Safety Procedures

    2. Care of Others
    3. Educational Activities
    4. Vocational Activities
       a. Vocational Exploration
       b. Job Acquisition
       c. Work or Job Performance
       d. Retirement Planning
  C. Play or Leisure Activities
    1. Play or Leisure Exploration
    2. Play or Leisure Performance
II. Performance Components
  A. Sensory Motor Component
    1. Sensory Integration
       a. Sensory Awareness
       b. Sensory Processing
         (1) Tactile
         (2) Proprioceptive
         (3) Vestibular
         (4) Visual
         (5) Auditory
         (6) Gustatory
         (7) Olfactory
       c. Perceptual Skills
         (1) Sterognosis
         (2) Kinesthesia
         (3) Body Scheme
         (4) Right-Left Discrimination
         (5) Form Constancy
         (6) Position in Space
         (7) Visual Closure
         (8) Figure-Ground
         (9) Depth Perception
         (10) Topographical Orientation
    2. Neuromuscular
       a. Reflex
       b. Range of Motion
       c. Muscular Tone
       d. Strength
       e. Endurance
       f. Postural Control
       g. Soft Tissue Integrity
    3. Motor
       a. Activity Tolerance
       b. Gross Motor Coordination
       c. Crossing the Midline
       d. Laterality
       e. Bilateral Integration
       f. Praxis
       g. Fine Motor Coordination/Dexterity
       h. Visual-Motor Integration
       i. Oral-Motor Control
  B. Cognitive Integration and Cognitive Components
    1. Level of Arousal
    2. Orientation

    3. Recognition
    4. Attention Span
    5. Memory
       a. Short-Term
       b. Long-Term
       c. Remote
       d. Recent
    6. Sequencing
    7. Categorization
    8. Concept Formation
    9. Intellectual Operations in Space
    10. Problem Solving
    11. Generalization of Learning
    12. Integration of Learning
    13. Synthesis of Learning
  C. Psychosocial Skills and Psychological Components
    1. Psychological
       a. Roles
       b. Values
       c. Interests
       d. Initiation of Activity
       e. Termination of Activity
       f. Self-Concept
    2. Social
       a. Social Conduct
       b. Conversation
       c. Self-Expression
    3. Self-Management
       a. Coping Skills
       b. Time Management
       c. Self-Control

Occupational Therapy Assessment

Assessment is the planned process of obtaining, interpreting, and documenting the functional status of the individual. The purpose of the assessment is to identify the individual's abilities and limitations, including deficits, delays, or maladaptive behavior that can be addressed in occupational therapy intervention. Data can be gathered through a review of records, observation, interview, and the administration of test procedures. Such procedures include, but are not limited to, the use of standardized tests, questionnaires, performance checklists, activities, and tasks designed to evaluate specific performance abilities.

Occupational Therapy Intervention

Occupational therapy addresses function and uses specific

procedures and activities to (a) develop, maintain, improve, and/or restore the performance of necessary functions; (b) compensate for dysfunction; (c) minimize or prevent debilitation; and/or (d) promote health and wellness. Categories of function are defined as **Occupational Performance Areas** and **Performance Components. Occupational Performance Areas** include activities of daily living, work activities, and play/leisure activities. Performance Components refer to the functional abilities required for occupational performance, including sensory motor, cognitive, and psychological components. Deficits or delays in these **Occupational Performance Areas** may be addressed by occupational therapy intervention.

I. **Occupational Performance Areas**
  A. Activities of Daily Living
    1. *Grooming*—Obtain and use supplies to shave; apply and remove cosmetics; wash, comb, style, and brush hair; care for nails; care for skin; and apply deodorant.
    2. *Oral Hygiene*—Obtain and use supplies; clean mouth and teeth; remove, clean and reinsert dentures.
    3. *Bathing*—Obtain and use supplies; soap, rinse, and dry all body parts; maintain bathing position; transfer to and from bathing position.
    4. *Toilet Hygiene*—Obtain and use supplies; clean self; transfer to and from, and maintain toileting position on bedpan, toilet, or commode.
    5. *Dressing*—Select appropriate clothing; obtain clothing from storage area; dress and undress in a sequential fashion; and fasten and adjust clothing and shoes. Don and doff assistive or adaptive equipment, prostheses, or orthoses.
    6. *Feeding and Eating*—Set up food; use appropriate utensils and tableware; bring food or drink to mouth; suck, masticate, cough, and swallow.
    7. *Medication Routine*—Obtain medication; open and close containers; and take prescribed quantities as scheduled.
    8. *Socialization*—Interact in appropriate contextual and cultural ways.
    9. *Functional Communication*—Use equipment or systems to enhance or provide communication, such as writing equipment, telephones, typewriters, communication boards, call lights, emergency systems, braille writers, augmentative communication systems, and computers.
    10. *Functional Mobility*—Move from one position or place to another, such as in bed mobility, wheelchair mobility, transfers (bed, car, tub, toilet, chair), and functional ambulation, with or without adaptive aids, driving, and use of public transportation.
    11. *Sexual Expression*—Recognize, communicate, and perform desired sexual activities.
  B. Work Activities
    1. *Home Management*
      a. *Clothing Care*—Obtain and use supplies, launder, iron, store, and mend.
      b. *Cleaning*—Obtain and use supplies, pick up, vacuum, sweep, dust, scrub, mop, make bed, and remove trash.
      c. *Meal Preparation and Cleanup*—Plan nutritious meals and prepare food; open and close containers, cabinets, and drawers; use kitchen utensils and appliances; and clean up and store food.
      d. *Shopping*—Select and purchase items and perform money transactions.
      e. *Money Management*—Budget, pay bills, and use bank systems.
      f. *Household Maintenance*—Maintain home, yard, garden appliances, and household items, and/or obtain appropriate assistance.
      g. *Safety Procedures*—Know and perform prevention and emergency procedures to maintain a safe environment and prevent injuries.
    2. *Care of Others*—Provide for children, spouse, parents or others, such as the physical care, nurturance, communication, and use of age-appropriate activities.
    3. *Educational Activities*—Participate in a school environment and school-sponsored activities (such as field trips, work-study, and extracurricular activities).
    4. *Vocational Activities*
      a. *Vocational Exploration*—Determine aptitudes, interests, skills, and appropriate vocational pursuits.
      b. *Job Acquisition*—Identify and select work opportunities and complete application and interview processes.
      c. *Work or Job Performance*—Perform job tasks in a timely and effective manner, incorporating necessary work behaviors such as grooming, interpersonal skills, punctuality, and adherence to safety procedures.
      d. *Retirement Planning*—Determine aptitudes, interests, skills, and identify appropriate avocational pursuits.
  C. Play or Leisure Activities
    1. *Play or Leisure Exploration*—Identify interests, skills, opportunities, and appropriate play or leisure activities.
    2. *Play or Leisure Performance*—Participate in play or leisure activities, using physical and psychosocial skills.

a. Maintain a balance of play or leisure activities with work and activities of daily living.

b. Obtain, utilize, and maintain equipment and supplies.

II. **Performance Components**

  A. Sensory Motor Component

    1. *Sensory Integration*

      a. *Sensory Awareness*—Receive and differentiate sensory stimuli.

      b. *Sensory Processing*—Interpret sensory stimuli.

        (1) *Tactile*—Interpret light touch, pressure, temperature, pain, vibration, and two-point stimuli through skin contact/receptors.

        (2) *Proprioceptive*—Interpret stimuli originating in muscles, joints, and other internal tissues to give information about the position of one body part in relationship to another.

        (3) *Vestibular*—Interpret stimuli from the inner ear receptors regarding head position and movement.

        (4) *Visual*—Interpret stimuli through the eyes, including peripheral vision and acuity, awareness of color, depth, and figure-ground.

        (5) *Auditory*—Interpret sounds, localize sounds, and discriminate background sounds.

        (6) *Gustatory*—Interpret tastes.

        (7) *Olfactory*—Interpret odors.

      c. *Perceptual Skills*

        (1) *Sterognosis*—Identify objects through the sense of touch.

        (2) *Kinesthesia*—Identify the excursion and direction of joint movement.

        (3) *Body Scheme*—Acquire an internal awareness of the body and the relationship of body parts to each other.

        (4) *Right-Left Discrimination*—Differentiate one side of the body from the other.

        (5) *Form Constancy*—Recognize forms and objects as the same in various environments, positions, and sizes.

        (6) *Position in Space*—Determine the spatial relationship of figure and objects to self or other forms and objects.

        (7) *Visual Closure*—Identify forms or objects from incomplete presentations.

        (8) *Figure-Ground*—Differentiate between foreground and background forms and objects.

        (9) *Depth Perception*—Determine the relative distance between objects, figures, or landmarks and the observer.

        (10) *Topographical Orientation*—Determine the location of objects and settings and the route to the location.

    2. *Neuromuscular*

      a. *Reflex*—Present an involuntary muscle response elicited by sensory input.

      b. *Range of Motion*—Move body parts through an arc.

      c. *Muscular Tone*—Demonstrate a degree of tension or resistance in a muscle.

      d. *Strength*—Demonstrate a degree of muscle power when a movement is resisted as with weight or gravity.

      e. *Endurance*—Sustain cardiac, pulmonary, and musculoskeletal exertion over time.

      f. *Postural Control*—Position and maintain head, neck, trunk, and limb alignment with appropriate weight shifting, midline orientation, and righting reactions for function.

      g. *Soft Tissue Integrity*—Maintain anatomical and physiological condition of interstitial tissue and skin.

    3. *Motor*

      a. *Activity Tolerance*—Sustain a purposeful activity over time.

      b. *Gross Motor Coordination*—Use large muscle groups for controlled movements.

      c. *Crossing the Midline*—Move limbs and eyes across the sagittal plane of the body.

      d. *Laterality*—Use a preferred unilateral body part for activities requiring a high level of skill.

      e. *Bilateral Integration*—Interact with both body sides in a coordinated manner during activity.

      f. *Praxis*—Conceive and plan a new motor act in response to an environmental demand.

      g. *Fine Motor Coordination/Dexterity*—Use small muscle groups for controlled movements, particularly in object manipulation.

      h. *Visual-Motor Integration*—Coordinate the interaction of visual information with body movement during activity.

      i. *Oral-Motor Control*—Coordinate oropharyngeal musculature for controlled movements.

  B. Cognitive Integration and Cognitive Components

    1. *Level of Arousal*—Demonstrate alertness and responsiveness to environmental stimuli

    2. *Orientation*—Identify person, place, time, and situation.

3. *Recognition*—Identify familiar faces, objects, and other previously presented materials.
4. *Attention Span*—Focus on a task over time.
5. *Memory*
   a. *Short-Term*—Recall information for brief periods of time.
   b. *Long-Term*—Recall information for long periods of time.
   c. *Remote*—Recall events from distant past.
   d. *Recent*—Recall events from immediate past.
6. *Sequencing*—Place information, concepts, and actions in order.
7. *Categorization*—Identify similarities of and differences between environmental information.
8. *Concept Formation*—Organize a variety of information to form thoughts and ideas.
9. *Intellectual Operations in Space*—Mentally manipulate spatial relationships.
10. *Problem Solving*—Recognize a problem, define a problem, identify alternative plans, select a plan, organize steps in a plan, implement a plan, and evaluate the outcome.
11. *Generalization of Learning*—Apply previously learned concepts and behaviors to similar situations.
12. *Integration of Learning*—Incorporate previously acquired concepts and behavior into a variety of new situations.
13. *Synthesis of Learning*—Restructure previously learned concepts and behaviors into new patterns.

C. Psychosocial Skills and Psychological Components
   1. *Psychological*
      a. *Roles*—Identify functions one assumes or acquires in society (eg, worker, student, parent, church member).
      b. *Values*—Identify ideas or beliefs that are intrinsically important.
      c. *Interests*—Identify mental or physical activities that create pleasure and maintain attention.
      d. *Initiation of Activity*—Engage in a physical or mental activity.
      e. *Termination of Activity*—Stop an activity at an appropriate time.

   f. *Self-Concept*—Develop value of physical and emotional self.
   2. *Social*
      a. *Social Conduct*—Interact using manners, personal space, eye contact, gestures, active listening, and self-expression appropriate to one's environment.
      b. *Conversation*—Use verbal and non-verbal communication to interact in a variety of settings.
      c. *Self-Expression*—Use a variety of styles and skills to express thoughts, feelings, and needs.
   3. *Self-Management*
      a. *Coping Skills*—Identify and manage stress and related reactors.
      b. *Time Management*—Plan and participate in a balance of self-care, work, leisure, and rest activities to promote satisfaction and health.
      c. *Self-Control*—Modulate and modify one's own behavior in response to environmental needs, demands, and constraints.

References

American Medical Association. (1966–1988). *Physicians' current procedural terminology first-fourth editions (CPT 1–4)*. Chicago: Author.

American Occupational Therapy Association. (1979). *Occupational therapy output reporting system and uniform terminology for reporting occupational therapy services*. Rockville, MD: Author.

American Psychiatric Association. (1952–1987). *Diagnostic and statistical manual of mental disorders first-third editions (DSM-I–III-R)*. Washington, DC: Author.

Medicare–Medicaid Anti-Fraud and Abuse Amendments (Public Law 95–142). (1977), 42 U.S.C. §1305.

Prepared by the Uniform Terminology Task Force (Linda Kohlman McGourty, MOT OTR, Chair, and Mary Foto, OTR, Jane Marvin, MA, OTC, CIRS, Nancy Mahon Smith, MBA, OTR, and Roger O. Smith, MOT, OTR, task force members) and members of the Commission on Practice, with contributions from Susan Kronsnoble, OTR, for the Commission on Practice (L. Randy Strickland, EdD, OTR, FAOTA, Chair).

Approved by the Representative Assembly April 1989.

Appendix D
OCCUPATIONAL THERAPY CODE OF ETHICS

The American Occupational Therapy Association and its component members are committed to furthering people's abilities to function fully within their total environments. To this end the occupational therapist renders service to clients in all stages of health and illness, to institutions, to other professionals and colleagues, to students, and to the general public.

In furthering this commitment, the American Occupational Therapy Association has established the Occupational Therapy Code of Ethics. This code is intended to be used as a guide to promoting and maintaining the highest standards of ethical behavior.

This Code of Ethics shall apply to all occupational therapy personnel. The term *occupational therapy personnel* shall include individuals who are registered occupational therapists, certified occupational therapy assistants, and occupational therapy students. The roles of practitioner, educator, manager, researcher, and consultant are assumed.

Principle 1 (Beneficence/Autonomy)
Occupational therapy personnel shall demonstrate a concern for the welfare and dignity of the recipient of their services.

   A. The individual is responsible for providing services without regard to race, creed, national origin, sex, age, handicap, disease entity, social status, financial status, or religious affiliation.
   B. The individual shall inform those people served of the nature and potential outcomes of treatment and shall respect the right of potential recipients of service to refuse treatment.
   C. The individual shall inform subjects involved in education or research activities of the potential outcome of those activities.
   D. The individual shall include those people served in the treatment planning process.
   E. The individual shall maintain goal-directed and objective relationships with all people served.

   F. The individual shall protect the confidential nature of information gained from educational, practice, and investigational activities unless sharing such information could be deemed necessary to protect the well-being of a third party.
   G. The individual shall take all reasonable precautions to avoid harm to the recipient of services or detriment to the recipient's property.
   H. The individual shall establish fees, based on cost analysis, that are commensurate with services rendered.

Principle 2 (Competence)
Occupational therapy personnel shall actively maintain high standards of professional competence.

   A. The individual shall hold the appropriate credential for providing service.
   B. The individual shall recognize the need for competence and shall participate in continuing professional development.
   C. The individual shall function within the parameters of his or her competence and the standards of the profession.
   D. The individual shall refer clients to other service providers or consult with other service providers when additional knowledge and expertise is required.

Principle 3 (Compliance With Laws and Regulations)
Occupational therapy personnel shall comply with laws and Association policies guiding the profession of occupational therapy.

   A. The individual shall be acquainted with applicable local, state, federal, and institutional rules and Association policies and shall function accordingly.

B. The individual shall inform employers, employees, and colleagues about those laws and policies that apply to the profession of occupational therapy.

C. The individual shall require those whom they supervise to adhere to the Code of Ethics.

D. The individual shall accurately record and report information.

Principle 4 (Public Information)

Occupational therapy personnel shall provide accurate information concerning occupational therapy services.

A. The individual shall accurately represent his or her competence and training.

B. The individual shall not use or participate in the use of any form of communication that contains a false, fraudulent, deceptive, or unfair statement or claim.

Principle 5 (Professional Relationships)

Occupational therapy personnel shall function with discretion and integrity in relations with colleagues and other professionals, and shall be concerned with the quality of their services.

A. The individual shall report illegal, incompetent, and/or unethical practice to the appropriate authority.

B. The individual shall not disclose privileged information when participating in reviews of peers, programs, or systems.

C. The individual who employs or supervises colleagues shall provide appropriate supervision, as defined in AOTA guidelines or state laws, regulations, and institutional policies.

D. The individual shall recognize the contributions of colleagues when disseminating professional information.

Principle 6 (Professional Conduct)

Occupational therapy personnel shall not engage in any form of conduct that constitutes a conflict of interest or that adversely reflects on the profession.

Reprinted from American Journal of Occupational Therapy, 42(12), 795-796, The American Occupational Therapy Association, Inc., 1988. Reprinted with permission.

Bibliography

Chapter 1. Therapeutic Intervention Process

Brooks B: COTA issues: Yesterday, today, and tomorrow. *Am J Occup Ther* 36:568, 1982.

Lamport NK, Coffey MS, Hersch GI: *Activity Analysis Handbook.* Thorofare, New Jersey, SLACK Inc., 1993.

Schell BAB: Guide to classification of occupational therapy personnel. *Am J Occup Ther* 39:803-810, 1985.

Shriver D, Foto M: Standards of practice for occupational therapy. *Am J Occup Ther* 37:802-804, 1983.

Uniform occupational therapy evaluation checklist. *Am J Occup Ther* 35:817-818, 1981.

Commission on Practice: Standards of practice for occupational therapy. *Am J Occup Ther* 46:1082-1085, 1992.

Chapter 2. COTA Supervision

Clakeley GL: Designing job enrichment projects. In Johnson JA (Ed): *Certified Occupational Therapy Assistants—Opportunities and Challenges.* New York, Haworth Press, 1988.

Christie BA, Joyce PC, Moeller PL. Fieldwork experience. Part 2: The supervisor's dilemma. *Am J Occup Ther* 39:675-681, 1985.

Hawkins TR: Supervising the occupational therapy assistant student. *Administration and Management Special Interest Section Newsletter.* 7:1, 1991.

Puccetti DD: Supervisio nof the COTA: Developing a knowledge base. *Occup Ther Health Care* 5(2/3):23-25, 1988.

Chapter 4. The Child with Visual Deficits

American Occupational Therapy Association: *Family Centered Care: An Intervention Resource Manual.* Rockville, Maryland, American Occupational Therapy Association, 1989.

Dunn W: *Pediatric Occupational Therapy.* Thorofare, New Jersey, SLACK Inc., 1991

Dunn W (Guest Ed): Special issues on early intervention. *Am J Occup Ther* 43:717-776, 1989.

Semmler CJ, Hunter JG: *Early Occupational Therapy Intervention: Neonates to Three Years.* Gaithersburg, Maryland, Aspen, 1990.

Warren DH: *Blindness and Early Childhood Development.* New York, American Foundation for the Blind, 1977.

Chapter 5. The Child with Mental Retardation

Currie C: Evaluating function of mentally retarded children through the use of toys and play activities. *Am J Occup Ther* 23:1, 1969.

Dunn ML: *Pre-Dressing Skills.* Tucson, Arizona, Communication Skill Builders, 1983.

Dunn W: *Pediatric Occupational Therapy.* Thorofare, New Jersey, SLACK Inc., 1991.

Lederman EF: *Occupational Therapy in Mental Retardation.* Springfield, Illinois, Charles C. Thomas, 1984.

Popovich D: *A Prescriptive Behavioral Checklist for the Severely and Profoundly Retarded.* Volume II. Austin, Texas, Pro-Ed, Inc., 1981.

Pratt PN, Allen AS: *Occupational Therapy for Children.* St. Louis, Mosby-Year Book, 1989.

Chapter 6. The Child with Cerebral Palsy

American Occupational Therapy Association: *Guidelines for Occupational Therapy in School System.* Rockville, Maryland, American Occupational Therapy Association, 1987.

Batshaw M, Perret Y: *Children with Hadicaps: A Medical Primer.* Baltimore, Maryland, Paul H. Brookes, 1981.

Cerebral Palsy. Rockville, Maryland, Practice Division, American Occupational Therapy Association, 1983.

Colby IL: *Pediatric Assessment of Self-Care Activities.* St. Louis, CV Mosby, 1978.

Dunn W: *Pediatric Occupational Therapy.* Thorofare, New Jersey, SLACK Inc., 1991.

Erhardt R: *Developmental Hand Dysfunction.* Laurel, Maryland, Ramsco, 1982.

Feeding and Dressing Techniques for the Cerebral Palsied. Chicago, National Society for Crippled Children and Adults.

Finnie N: *Handling the Young Cerebral Palsied Child at Home,* Edition 2. New York, EP Dutton, 1975.

Friedman B: A program for parents of children with sensory integrative dysfunction. *Am J Occup Ther* 36:586-589, 1982.

Gilfoyle EM: *Training: Occupational Therapy Educational Management in Schools.* OSERS Grant #G007801499. Rockville, Maryland, American Occupational Therapy Association, 1980.

Hanft BE (Ed): *Family-Centered Care: An Early Intervention Resource Manual.* Rockville, Maryland, American Occupational Therapy Association, 1989.

Healy H, Stainback SB: *The Severely Motorically Impaired Student.* Springfield, Illinois, Charles C. Thomas, 1980.

Howison M: Occupational therapy with children—cerebral palsy. In Hopkins H, Smith H (Eds): *Willard and Spackman's Occupational Therapy,* 6th Edition. Philadelphia, JB Lippincott, 1983.

Levitt S: *Treatment of Cerebral Palsy and Motor Delay.* Philadelphia, JB Lippincott, 1977.

Powell HS (Ed): *PILOT: Project for Independent Living in Occupational Therapy.* Rockville, Maryland, American Occupational Therapy Association, 1986.

Royeen CB (Guest Ed): Special issue on occupational therapy in the schools. *Am J Occup Ther* 42:695-762, 1988.

Smith J: *Play Environments for Movement Experience.* Springfield, Illinois, Charles C. Thomas, 1980.

Stainback SB, Healy HA: *Teaching Eating Skills, A Handbook for Teachers.* Springfield, Illinois, Charles C. Thomas, 1982.

Wendt E, Black T, Wilson C, Walski T (for Commission on Education): *Final Report: Ad Hoc Committee to Study Pediatric Education and Fieldwork at the Technical Level.* Rockville, Maryland, American Occuaptional Therapy Association, 1990.

Chapter 9. The Adolescent with Chemical Dependency

Diepenbrock EC: *Understanding Adolescents.* Silver Springs, Maryland, Unpublished paper, 1980.

Henderson DC, Anderson SC: Adolescents and chemical dependency. *Social Work in Health Care* 14(1):87-105, 1989.

Llorens LA: *Application of a Developmental Theory for Health and Rehabilitation.* Rockville, Maryland, American Occupational Therapy Association, 1976.

MacDonald DI: Diagnosis and treatment of adolescent substance abuse. *Curr Probl Pediatrics* 19:395-444, 1989.

Moyers P: *Substance Abuse: A Multi-Dimensional Assessment and Treatment Approach.* Thorofare, New Jersey, SLACK Inc., 1992.

Chapter 10. The Adolescent with Burns

Artz C, Moncrief J, Pruitt B: *Burns, A Team Approach.* Philadelphia, WB Saunders, 1979.

DiGregorio VR: *Rehabilitation of the Burn Patient.* New York, Churchill Livingstone, 1984.

Eagan M: Cultured skin grafts: Preserving lives, challenging therapists. *OT Week* 6:12-15, 1992.

Fisher SV, Helm PA (Eds): *Comprehensive Rehabilitation of Burns.* Baltimore, Williams & Wilkins, 1984.

Kaplan SH: Patient education techniques used at burn center. *Am J Occup Ther* 39:655-658, 1985.

Malick MH, Carr JA: *Manual on Management of the Burn Patient.* Pittsburgh, Harmarville Rehabilitation Center, 1982.

McGourty LK, Givens A, Fader PB: Roles and functions of occupational therapy in burn care delivery. *Am J Occup Ther* 39:791-794, 1985.

Salisbury RE, Newman NM, Dingeldein GP: *Manual of Burn Therapeutics.* Boston, Little, Brown, 1983.

Chapter 11. The Young Adult with a Spinal Injury

Wilson DJ, McKenzie MW, Barber LM, et al: *Spinal Cord Injury: A Treatment Guide for Occupational Therapists,* Revised Edition. Thorofare, New Jersey, SLACK Inc., 1984.

Hill JP (Ed): *Spinal Cord Injury: A Guide to Functional Outcomes in Occupational Therapy.* Rockville, Maryland, Aspen, 1986.

Tapper BE (Ed): Living with spinal cord injury. *OT Week* 6:16-21, 1992.

Chapter 12. The Young Adult with Schizophrenia

Allen CK: *Occupational Therapy for Psychiatric Diseases: Measurement and Management of Cognitive Disabilities.* Boston, Little, Brown, 1985.

American Psychiatric Association: *Diagnostic and Statistical Manual of Mental Disorders,* 3rd Edition—Revised. Washington, DC, American Psychiatric Association, 1987.

Evans A: Roles and functions of occupational therapy in mental health. *Am J Occup Ther* 39:799-802, 1985.

Malone J: *Schizophrenia: Handbook for Clinical Care.* Thorofare, New Jersey, SLACK Inc., 1992.

Mosey AC: *Activities Therapy.* New York: Raven Press, 1973.

Tiffany EG: Psychiatry and mental health. In Hopkins H, Smith H (Eds): *Willard and Spackman's Occupational Therapy,* 6th Edition. Philadelphia, JB Lippincott, 1983.

Chapter 13. The Young Adult with Rheumatoid Arthritis

American Occupational Therapy Association: Entry-level role delineation for registered occupational therapists (OTRs) and certified occupational therapy assistants (COTAs). *Am J Occup Ther* 44:1091-1102, 1990.

Entry-level OTR and COTA role delineation. *Occup Ther Newspaper* 35:8-18, 1981.

Feinberg J, Brandt KD: Allied health team management of rheumatoid arthritis patients. *Am J Occup Ther* 38:613-620, 1984.

Fries JF: *Arthritis: A Comprehensive Guide.* Reading, Massachusetts, Addison-Wesley, 1979.

Lorig K, Fries JF: *The Arthritis Helpbook.* Reading, Massachusetts, Addison-Wesley, 1986.

Melvin JL: *Rheumatic Disease in the Adult and Child: Occupational Therapy and Rehabilitation.* Philadelphia, FA Davis, 1989.

Swezey R: *Arthritis Rational Therapy and Rehabilitation.* Philadelphia, WB Saunders, 1979.

American Occupational Therapy Association: *The Role of the Occupational Therapist in Home Health Care.* Rockville, Maryland, American Occupational Therapy Association, 1981.

Chapter 15. The Adult with AIDS

Benza JF, Zumwalde RD: *Preventing AIDS: A Practical Guide for Everyone.* Cincinnati, Jalsco, 1986.

Denton R: AIDS: Guidelines for occupational therapy intervention. *Am J Occup Ther* 41:427-432, 1987.

Frutchey C, Christen P, Rittinger D: *AIDS 101 Manual.* San Francisco, San Francisco AIDS Foundation, 1988.

Galantino ML: *Clinical Assessment and Treatment of HIV: Rehabilitation of a Chronic Illness.* Thorofare, New Jersey, SLACK Inc., 1992.

Hopp JW, Rogers EA: *AIDS and the Allied Health Professions.* Philadelphia: FA Davis, 1989.

Marcil W, Tigges K: *The Person with AIDS.* Thorofare, New Jersey, SLACK Inc., 1992.

Schindler VJ: Psychological occupational therapy intervention with AIDS patients. *Am J Occup Ther* 42:507-512, 1988.

Chapter 16. The Adult with a Cerebral Vascular Accident

Carr JH, Shepherd RB: *A Motor Relearning Program for Stroke.* Rockville, Maryland, Aspen, 1987.

Christiansen C, Baum C (Eds): *Occupational Therapy, Overcoming Human Performance Deficits.* Thorofare, New Jersey, SLACK Inc., 1991.

Eggers O: *Occupational Therapy in the Treatment of Adult Hemiplegia.* Rockville, Maryland, Aspen, 1984.

Kottke FJ, Stillwell GK, Lehmann JF: *Krusen's Handbook of Physical Medicine and Rehabilitation,* 3rd Edition. Philadelphia, WB Saunders, 1982.

Zoltan B, Siev E, Freishtat B: *Perceptual and Cognitive Dysfunction in the Adult Stroke Patient: A Manual for Evaluation and Treatment,* 2nd Edition. Thorofare, New Jersey, SLACK Inc., 1986.

Chapter 17. The Elderly with Parkinson's Disease

Dahlin-Webb S: Brief or new: A weighted wrist cuff. *Am J Occup Ther* 40:363-364, 1986.

Dorros S: *Parkinson's: A Patient's View.* Cabin John, Maryland, Seven Locks Press, 1981.

Duuvoisin R: *Parkinson's Disease: A Guide for Patient and Family.* New York: Raven Press, 1980.

Gelbart A, Hamilton W: Parkinson's disease. *Fam Physician* 23:182-189, 1981.

Gauthier L, Dalziel S, Gauthier S: The benefits of group occupational therapy for patients with Parkinson's disease. *Am J Occup Ther* 41:360-365, 1987.

Hunt L: Care report: Continuity of care maximizes autonomy of the elderly. *Am J Occup Ther* 42:391-393, 1988.

Levy LL (AOTA Commission on Practice): Occupational therapy in adult day-care. *Am J Occup Ther* 40:814-816, 1986.

Lewis S: *Elder Care in Occupational Therapy.* Thorofare, New Jersey, SLACK Inc., 1989.

MacDonald KC, Epstein CF, Vastano S: Roles and functions of occupational therapy in adult day care. *Am J Occup Ther* 40:817-821, 1986.

Malone T (Ed): *Physical and Occupational Therapy: Drug Implications for Practice.* Philadelphia, JB Lippincott, 1988.

Marquit S: *Psychological Factors in the Management of Parkinson's Disease.* Miami, Florida, National Parkinson Foundation, 1981.

Trombly CA: *Occupational Therapy for Physical Dysfunction,* 3rd Edition. Baltimore, Williams & Wilkins, 1989.

Chapter 18. The Elderly with Alzheimer's Disease

Lewis S: *Elder Care in Occupational Therapy.* Thorofare, New Jersey, SLACK Inc., 1989.

Chapter 20. The Elderly with Hearing and Visual Impairments

Greenblatt SL: *Meeting the Needs of People with Vision Loss: A Multidisciplinary Perspective.* New York, Resources for Rehabilitation, Inc, 1991.

LaBuda DR (Ed): *The Gadget Book,* The American Society on Aging. Glenview, Illinois, Scott, Foresman, 1985.

Lewis S: *Elder Care in Occupational Therapy.* Thorofare, New Jersey, SLACK Inc., 1989.

Zoltan B, Siev E, Freishtat: *The Adult Stroke Patient.* Thorofare, New Jersey, SLACK Inc., 1986.

Chapter 21. Work Hardening

Isernhagen SJ: *Work Injury: Management and Prevention.* Frederick, Maryland, Aspen, 1988.

Ogden-Niemeyer L, Jacobs K: *Work Hardening: State of the Art.* Thorofare, New Jersey, SLACK Inc., 1990.

Rager R (Ed): Work hardening—21st Century. *OT Week* 5, 1991.

Reed KL: The role of the COTA in work and productive occupation programs. In Ryan SE (Ed): *The Occupational Therapy Assistant: Roles and Responsibilities.* Thorofare, NJ, Slack, Inc., 1986.

Spencer JC: The physical environment and performance. In Christiansen C, Baum C (Eds): *Occupational Therapy: Overcoming Human Performance Deficits.* Thorofare, New Jersey, Slack, Inc., 1991.

United States Department of Labor: *Dictionary of Occupational Titles,* 4th Edition. Menomonie, Wisconsin, Materials Development Center, University of Wisconsin-Stout, 1991.

Chapter 22. The Role of the COTA as an Activities Director

Crepeau EL: *Activity Programming for the Elderly.* Boston, Little, Brown, 1986.

Drake M: *Crafts in Therapy and Rehabilitation.* Thorofare, New Jersey, SLACK Inc., 1992.

Foster PM: *Activities and the Well Elderly.* New York, Haworth Press, 1983.

Foster PM: *Activities in Action.* New York, Haworth Press, 1991.

Greenberg P: *Visual Arts and Older People: Developing Quality Programs.* Springfield, Illinois, Charles C. Thomas, 1987.

Kiernat JM: *Occupational Therapy and the Older Adult: A Clinical Manual.* Gaithersburg, Maryland, Aspen, 1991.

Krawcyk A: The certified occupational therapy assistant as an activity director. *Occup Ther Health Care* 5:111-118, 1988.

Leitner MJ, Leitner SF: *Leisure in Later Life: A Sourcebook for the Provision of Recreational Services for the Elderly.* New York, Haworth Press, 1986.

Levete G: *The Creative Tree: Active Participation in the Arts for People Who are Disadvantaged.* London, Michael Russell, 1987.

Lewis SC: *Providing for the Older Adult.* Thorofare, New Jersey, SLACK Inc., 1983.

Mann M, Edwards D, Baum CM: OASIS: A new concept for promoting the quality of life for older adults. *Am J Occup Ther* 40:784-785, 1986.

Chapter 23. Traumatic Brain Injury

Barrer AE, Ruben DH: *Understanding the Etilogy of Brain Injury.* Framingham, Massachusetts, National Head Injury Foundation, undated.

Corthell DW, Tobman ML (Eds): *Rehabilitation of TBI— Twelfth Institute on Rehabilitation Issues.* Menomonie, Wisconsin, Materials Development Center, 1985.

Lezak M: *Neuropsychological Assessment,* 2nd Edition. New York, Oxford University Press, 1983.

Chapter 24. Stress Management

Christiansen C: Performance deficits as sources of stress. In Christiansen C, Baum C (Eds): *Occupational Therapy: Overcoming Human Performance Deficits.* Thorofare, New Jersey, SLACK Inc., 1991.

Hansen M, Ritter G, Gutmann M, et al: *Understanding Stress.* Rockville, Maryland, American Occupational Therapy Association, 1990.

Lazarus RS, Folkman S: *Stress, Appraisal and Coping.* New York, Springer, 1984.

Chapter 25. Hospice Care

Flanigan K: The art of the possible—occupational therapy in terminal care. *Br J Occup Ther* 45:274-276, 1982.

Picard H, Magno J: The role of occupational therapy in hospice care. *Am J Occup Ther* 36:592-598, 1982.

Tigges K, Holland A: The hospice movement: A time for professional action and commitment. *Br J Occup Ther* 44:373-376, 1981.

Tigges K, Marcil W: *Terminal and Life-threatening Illness: An Occupational Behavior Approach.* Thorofare, New Jersey, SLACK Inc., 1988.

Chapter 26. Driver Assessment and Education for the Disabled

Hutcherson D: Self monitoring of driving for the elderly: Evidence for the use of a driving diary. *Phys Occup Ther Geriatrics* 7:1-2, 1989.

Trombly CA (Ed): *Occupational Therapy for Physical Dysfunction,* 3rd Edition. Baltimore, Maryland, Williams & Wilkins, 1989.

Chapter 27. Documentation

Allen C, Foto M, Moon-Sperling T, et al: An approach to Medicare outpatient documentation. *Am J Occup Ther* 43:793-800, 1989.

Bair J, Gray M (Eds): *The Occupational Therapy Manager.* Rockville, Maryland, American Occupational Therapy Association, 1985.

Denton PL: *Psychiatric O.T.: A Workbook of Practical Skills.* Boston, Little, Brown, 1987.

Dunn W (Ed): *Pediatric Occupational Therapy: Facilitating Effective Service Provision.* Thorofare, New Jersey, SLACK Inc., 1991.

Kettenbach G: *Writing S.O.A.P. Notes.* Philadelphia, FA Davis, 1990.

McClain L: Reporting meaningful movement measures. *Occup Ther Pract* 1:73-83, 1990.

Smith RO: Administration and Scoring Manual. *OT Fact (Occupational Therapy Functional Assessment Compilation Tool).* Rockville, Maryland, American Occupational Therapy Association, 1990.

Weed LL: *Medical Records, Medical Examination and Patient Care.* Chicago, The Press of Case Western Reserve, 1970.

Chapter 28. Service Operations

Bair J, Grey M (Eds): *The Occupational Therapy Manager,* Revised Edition, Rockville, Maryland, American Occupational Therapy Association, 1992.

Baum C, Luebben A: *Prospective Payment System.* Thorofare, New Jersey, SLACK Inc., 1986.

Brollier C (Guest Ed): Special issue on management. *Am J Occup Ther* 41:279-332, 1987.

Christiansen C: Nationally speaking—research: Looking back and ahead after four decades of progress. *Am J Occup Ther* 45:391-393, 1991.

Early MB: *Mental Health Concepts and Techniques for the Occupational Therapy Assistant.* New York, Raven Press, 1987.

English CB: The art of leading meetings. *Am J Occup Ther* 41:321-326, 1987.

American Occupational Therapy Association: Guide for supervision of occupational therapy personnel. In *Reference Manual of the Official Documents of the American Occupational Therapy Association.* Rockville, Maryland, American Occupational Therapy Association, Chapter 5, 1983.

Howard BS: How high do we jump? The effect of reimbursement on occupational therapy. *Am J Occup Ther* 45:875-881, 1991.

HCFA moves to implement Medicare payment system. *Occup Ther Newspaper* 37:3, 1983.

Jacobs K: Marketing occupational therapy. *Am J Occup Ther* 41:315-320, 1987.

Jacobs K, Logigian M: *Functions of a Manager in Occupational Therapy.* Thorofare, New Jersey, SLACK Inc., 1989.

Joe BE: Study examines quality in Medicare. *OT Week* 4(48):9, 1990.

Talty PM: Time management in clinical practice. *Occup Ther Health Care* 2:95-104, 1985-1986.

Chapter 29. Intraprofessional Relationships and Socialization

Davis C: *Patient Practitioner Interaction.* Thorofare, New Jersey, SLACK Inc., 1989.

Hawkins TR: Supervising the occupational therapy assistant student. *Administration and Management Special Interest Section Newsletter* 7(1):1-2, 1991.

Chapter 30. Principles of Occupational Therapy Ethics

Ashley BM, O'Rourke KD: *Health Care Ethics.* St. Louis, Catholic Hospital Association, 1978.

American Occupational Therapy Certification Board: Procedures for disciplinary action. *Program Director's Reference Manual.* Rockville, Maryland, American Occupational Therapy Certification Board, 1989.

Beauchamp T, Walter L: *Contemporary Issues in Bioethics.* Belmont, California, Wadsworth, 1978.

Cassidy JC: Access to health care: A clinician's opinion about an ethical issue. *Am J Occup Ther* 42:295-299, 1988.

Davis C: *Patient Practitioner Interaction.* Thorofare, New Jersey, SLACK Inc., 1989.

Fagothy A: *Right and Reason.* St. Louis, CV Mosby, 1967.

Goodwin L: Ethical theory in the practical context. *SCAN* (St. Catherine's Alumnae News) 61:6-8, 1885.

Kyler-Hutchison P: Ethical reasoning and informed consent in occupational therapy. *Am J Occup Ther* 42:283-287, 1988.

Munson R: *Intervention and Reflection: Basic Issues in Medical Ethics.* Belmont, California, Wadsworth, 1979.

Occupational therapy code of ethics. *Am J Occup Ther* 42:795-796, 1988.

Research Advisory Council, American Occupational Therapy Foundation: Ethical considerations for research in occupational therapy. *Am J Occup Ther* 42:129-130, 1988.

Vollmer HM, Mills DL: *Professionalism.* Englewood Cliffs, New Jersey, Prentice-Hall, 1966.

Glossary

This glossary is provided to assist the reader in learning new words and acronyms and their meanings. The index of the textbook should be used to locate specific terms so they may be reviewed within context. In addition to the individual chapter definitions of terms, the following sources were used: *Uniform Terminology for Occupational Therapy*, 2nd Edition, 1989, (AOTA); *The Random House College Dictionary*, Revised Edition, 1990; *Roget's International Thesaurus*, 4th Edition, 1977; and the *Encyclopedia and Dictionary of Medicine, Nursing, and Allied Health*, 5th Edition, 1992.

AA— Alcoholics Anonymous.

AARP— American Association of Retired Persons.

Accreditation— A process by which an agency or organization evaluates and recognizes an institution or program of study as meeting certain predetermined criteria or standards.

Acetabulum— Hip socket that receives the head of the femur.

Activities consultant— Qualified individual employed by the facility to provide guidance to the activity director concerning all aspects of the activities program.

Activities director— Individual employed by a facility who has direct responsibility for carrying out an activities program.

Activities of daily living— Area of occupational performance that refers to grooming, oral hygiene, dressing, feeding and eating, medication routine, socialization, functional communication, functional mobility and sexual expression activities.

Activities program— On-going plan for providing meaningful activities determined in relation to individual needs and interests of those involved.

Activity analysis— Process to determine the therapeutic potential of activities by examining their elements related to factors such as age-appropriateness, inherent properties, potential for adaptation, relationship to interests of the patient, etc.

Activity categories— Types of activities such as physical, social, creative, productive, etc.

Activity components— Elements; constituent parts.

Activity configuration— A form that details the activities one engages in at specific times of the day.

Actual conflict— Conflict that does occur; involves an awareness of hostilities (see perceived conflict).

Acuity— Acuteness or clearness.

Adaptability— Skill enabling one to conform easily and quickly to new and strange circumstances.

Adaptation— Satisfactory adjustment to the environment over time.

Adaptive behavior (preschool)— Child's ability to use language, play with others and do things independently (AAMD).

Adaptive devices— Equipment used to assist with performance of tasks such as button hooks, zipper pulls, tub seats, etc.

ADC— AIDS dementia complex.

ADL— Activities of daily living.

Adolescence— Stage in human development characterized by significant changes in physical development; time of social awkwardness and desire to achieve independence and establish an identity.

Advanced-level practice— OTR or COTA who has three or more years of practice experience and has achieved the intermediate level.

Aerobic— Requiring air or free oxygen for life.

AFO— Ankle-foot orthosis.

Aggression— Angry and destructive behaviors aimed at dominance.

Agitation— Irregular action, unrest or disquiet.

AIDS— Acquired immunodeficiency syndrome.

AJOT— *American Journal of Occupational Therapy*.

Akinesia— An absence or poverty of motion.

Alanon— A support group for family members and significant others involved with alcoholics.

Alcohol dependence— Disease characterized by addiction to alcohol.

Algorithms— Sets of rules with a finite number of steps.

AMA— American Medical Association.

Anemic— Condition of reduced red cells and level of hemoglobin in the blood.

Antabuse— Drug used to treat alcoholism.

Anterolateral— In front and to one side.

Anticholinergic drugs— Medication that blocks transmission of nerve impulses through the parasympathetic nerves; used to prevent side effects caused by some antipsychotic drugs such as Parkinsonian symptoms.

Antideformity position (hand)— Maximum flexion of the metacarpophalangeal joints and full interphalangeal joint extension.

AOTA— American Occupational Therapy Association.

AOTCB— American Occupational Therapy Certification Board.

AOTF— American Occupational Therapy Foundation.

Aphasia— Impairment in using and understanding written and spoken language.

Apnea— Temporary cessation of breathing.

ARC— AIDS-related complex.

AROM— Active range of motion.

Arrhythmia— Abnormal heartbeat.

Arthroplasty— Surgical replacement, formation or reformation of a joint.

Assessment— Critical analysis and valuation or judgment of the quality or status of a particular situation or condition; a subsection of the problem-oriented medical record.

Ataxia/Ataxic— Failure of muscle coordination or irregularity of muscle action.

Atonic— Absence of muscle tone.

Attention span— Ability to focus on a task or tasks over a period of time.

Auditory— Receive, process and interpret sounds through the ears; includes the ability to localize and discriminate noises in the background.

Autogenic— Self-produced.

Autonomic dysreflexia— Dangerously high increase in blood pressure, usually due to distension or infection of the bladder.

AZT— Ziduvodine/Retrovir; a drug used to treat HIV.

Baseline evaluation— Basic assessment of functional abilities (OT).

Behavioral control— System of warnings and "time outs" for unacceptable behavior.

Beneficence— Actions are taken to promote good consequences for others.

Bereavement— Deprivation due to death.

BID— Twice a day.

Body mechanics— Specific methods for lifting, reaching, etc.

Boutonnière deformity— Condition of the finger or fingers resulting in proximal interphalangeal flexion and distal interphalangeal hyperextension.

Bradycardia— Slowness of heartbeat.

Bradykinesia— Abnormal slowness of motion.

Burnout— State of mental fatigue that results in an inability to generate energy from one's job or to think creatively.

CAHEA— Committtee on Allied Health Education and Accreditation; formed under the auspices of the Council on Medical Education of the American Medical Association.

Career enhancement— Opportunities for challenge, growth and advancement in relation to one's job.

CARF— Commission on Accreditation of Rehabilitation Facilities.

Causal map— Illustration of relationships between elements such as cause and effect.

CDC— Centers for Disease Control.

CEDC— Certification Examination Development Committee; a standing committee of the American Occupational Therapy Certification Board.

Cerebral palsy— Pertains to a number of nonprogressive movement and posture disorders resulting from damage to a child's immature brain; mental retardation, seizures, visual and auditory deficits, speech and language disabilities and behavior problems may also be present.

Certification— Process, which may be statutory or voluntary, that recognizes an individual as having met predetermined criteria.

CEU— Continuing education unit.

Change drivers— Concepts or elements that lead future societal modifications.

Choreoathetoid— A classification of cerebral palsy.

Close supervision— Direct, onsite, daily guidance and direction.

Cognition— Mental process involving perception, memory and reasoning, which leads to understanding and knowing.

Cognitive domains— Levels of performance abilities delineated in a hierarchy related to knowing and understanding.

COJ— *Classification of Jobs* manual.

Collaboration— Working with others in a shared, cooperative endeavor to achieve mutual goals.

Collagen disease— Condition that pertains to connective tissue and bones.

Coma— A state of prolonged unconsciousness.

Communication worksheet— Tool used with patients to help identify various communication factors, eg easiest, most difficult, barriers.

Conduct disorder— Persistent pattern of behavior in which the basic rights of others and the major age-appropriate social roles or expectations of others are violated.

Confidentiality— Maintaining secrecy regarding information such as medical records.

Conformers— Silastic elastomer inserts, custom molded to provide total contact with scar tissue.

Context— Refers to the social, physical and psychological milieu of the situation.

Contraindication— Condition that deems a particular type of treatment undesirable or improper.

Contralateral— Affecting the opposite side.

Cooperation— Working together to achieve common goals.

Coordination board— A device to practice motor skills such as manipulating snaps, buttons, zippers, etc.

COPC— Community oriented primary care.

CORF— Comprehensive Outpatient Rehabilitation Facilities.

Cost-effective— Producing the best results in relation to dollars spent.

Coup and counter-coup— Points where the brain impacts the hard skull as a result of an injury.

Courage— Willingness to stand up for what is right in spite of difficulties or problems.

CP— Cerebral palsy.

CPR— Cardiopulmonary resuscitation.

Creativity— Expression of originality of thought; unique ideas and methods.

Credentialing— Process that gives title or approval to a person or program such as certification, registration or accreditation.

Crepitations— Dry, crackling sounds or sensations associated with joints.

Cross addiction— Addiction to a variety of chemical substances.

CT scan— Computed tomography.

Cuing— Hints or suggestions that facilitate the appropriate response.

Cultural shift— Movement in response to societal forces that results in a dynamic change.

Curanderos— Folk healers of the Spanish culture.

CVA— Cerebral vascular accident.

Cytomegalovirus— A herpes type virus producing enlarged cells similar to infectious mononeucleosis.

DAIEN— Disciplinary Action Information Exchange Network sponsored by the American Occupational Therapy Certification Board.

Daily living skills— Those things done each day that sustain and enhance life such as dressing, grooming and eating.

Data collection— Process of gathering information.

DDI— Dideoxynsine (a drug used with HIV patients).

Debridement— Removal of foreign matter and contaminated and devitalized tissue.

Decerebrate (posture)— Hips and shoulders extend, adduct and rotate internally; elbows and knees extend; hyperpronation of the forearm is seen; wrist and fingers flex; feet are inverted in plantar flexion.

Decubiti— Ulcers that form over bony prominences.

Decubitus ulcers— See decubiti.

Deficit— Inadequate behavior or task performance.

Delirium tremens— Condition caused by acute alcohol withdrawal; may lead to convulsions.

Delusions— False beliefs based on incorrect interpretation of reality.

Dementia— Severe impairment or loss of intellectual capacity and personality integration.

Demyelinating— Destruction or removal of the myelin sheath of a nerve.

Deontologic— A theory of ethics that supports the position that acts are right in themselves; basic concept is duty to other persons in terms of considering the rights of the individual over the rights of society as a whole; also referred to as the formalistic approach.

Depression— A disorder of mood in which there is a loss of interest or pleasure in almost all activities; associated symptoms include disturbances in appetite and sleep, decreased energy and agitation, as well as others.

Developmental delay— Slowed physical, cognitive language and speech and psychosocial development and the attainment of age-appropriate self-help skills.

Developmental expectations— Age-appropriate goals.

Diagnosis— Description of the cause or nature of a condition or problem.

DIP— Distal interphalangeal.

Diplegia— Involvement of two extremities.

Discharge summary— Documented report of discontinuation of services.

Disequilibrium— A sense of dissatisfaction; being out of balance.

Disorientation— Inability to make accurate judgments about people, places and things.

Diuresis— Increased excretion of urine.

DME— Durable medical equipment.

DMV— Department of Motor Vehicles.

Documented records— Written legal records; protect the rights of the patient and the person providing treatment.

Dopamine— A neurotransmitter in the central nervous system produced in the substantia nigra of the brain stem.

DOT— Dictionary of Occupational Titles.

DRGs— Diagnostic-related groups.

Driver licensing regulations— Rules affecting the operation of motor vehicles such as operator restrictions, reexamination requirements, medical review board procedures, etc.

DSM III-R— *Diagnostic and Statistical Manual of Mental Disorders,* Third Edition, Revised .

DWI— Driving while intoxicated.

Dyadic— One-to-one interaction.

Dynamometer— A device used to measure the force of muscular contraction.

Dysadaptive— Refers to behavior that allows one to function marginally but may result in difficulty in coping effectively.

Dysarthria— Imperfect speech articulation.

Dyspraxia— Inability to motor plan.

Dysrhythmia— Disturbance of heart rhythm.

Dysthymic disorder— Mental depression; also any intellectual abnormality.

Edema— Abnormal accumulation of fluid in the intercellular spaces of the body.

Educable mentally retarded— Individual with approximate IQ of 55 to 70.

EEG— Electroencephalogram.

ELISA— Enzyme-linked immunoabsorbant assay; test used to detect HIV antibodies in the blood.

Embolism— Occlusion of a blood vessel.

EMR— Educable mentally retarded.

Endurance— Ability to sustain exertion over time; involves musculoskeletal, cardiac and pulmonary systems.

Energy conservation— Methods used to reduce energy expended such as sitting instead of standing to work, sliding objects rather than lifting, etc.

Entry-level practice— COTA or OTR who has had less than one year of practice experience.

EPI— Evaluation of Personal Independence.

Equipment modification— Alteration of item or its controls to promote more effective use.

Essentials— Educational standards of the AOTA.

Esthetic— Having sensation.

Evaluation— Component of the occupational therapy process to determine the patient's current level of functional performance and to identify performance deficits.

Exacerbation— Increase in the severity of a disease or condition.

Exercises— Performance of physical exertion designed to increase and/or maintain strength and endurance, improve health or correct physical deformity.

Expressive aphasia— Inability to find the right word or words to describe things.

Exudate— Fluid that has escaped from blood vessels and may be found in blisters of second-degree burns.

Feedback— Information that individuals receive about their behavior.

Feeding and eating— Skills of chewing, sucking, swallowing and the use of utensils.

Festination— Involuntary tendency to take short accelerated steps when walking.

Fibrillation— Involuntary muscle contraction.

Fidelity— Faithfulness.

Figure-ground discrimination— Ability to differentiate between background and foreground objects and forms.

Findings— Results; determination.

Fine motor coordination/dexterity— Ability to perform controlled movements, particularly in the manipulation of objects, through the use of small muscle groups.

First-degree burn— Involves only epidermis and heals in 3 to 5 days; skin is bright red, painful and sensitive.

Flexibility— The willingness and openness that one must have to adapt to change.

Follow-up— Part of the OT process involving gathering of information to determine the effectiveness of treatment, general adjustment outcomes and the degree to which the individual is able to resume roles.

Form constancy— Recognition of objects and forms as the same in different sizes, positions or environments.

Fraudulent— False.

FROMAJE— A test covering the seven areas of function, reasoning, orientation, memory, arithmetic, judgment and emotional state.

Functional communication— Ability to use communication devices and systems such as telephone, computer, call lights, etc.

Functional mobility— Ability to move from one position to another (eg in bed or wheelchair) or transfer to tub, shower, toilet, etc.; driving and use of other forms of transportation.

Functional performance— Motor and behavioral components required to carry out tasks.

Functional status— Level of ability to perform tasks and carry out roles.

GAS— Goal Attainment Scale.

General supervision— Frequent "face-to-face" meetings at the work place and regular interim communication via telephone, written reports, conferences, etc.

Genetic— Hereditary.

Geriatrician— Physician who specializes in working with older people.

Gestures— Body movements used to express ideas, opinions or emotions.

Glare— Harsh or very bright light.

Glioblastoma— A malignant tumor of the brain.

Globalization— Worldwide activities.

Goniometer— Device used to measure angles.

Graded activities— Activities that feature increasing levels of resistance, slow to rapid performance or simple to complex requirements.

Graded resistive exercises— Tasks that require increasing degrees of resistance such as sawing soft wood followed by sawing hard wood.

Gross motor coordination— Controlled movements are made using large muscle groups.

Gustatory— Receive, process and interpret tastes.

Habituation— Roles and habits that influence and guide occupational behavior.

Hallucinations— Sensory impressions that have no basis in external stimulation.

Hemiparesis— Slight or incomplete paralysis of one side of the body.

Hemiplegia— Paralysis of one side of the body.

Herpes simplex virus— An inflammatory skin disease that results in the formation of small vesicles (sacs containing liquid).

Heterophoria— Failure of the visual axes to remain parallel after stimuli have been eliminated.

Heterotopic ossification— Condition caused by deposits of osseous material at the knee, hip, elbow or shoulder leading to bony contractures and decreased range of motion.

Hip arthroplasty— Surgical formation or reformation of the hip joint.

HIV— Human immunodeficiency virus.

HMOs— Health maintenance organizations.

Holism— Refers to the complete life-style of the individual and provides a context for intervention; physical, psychological and social aspects are considered simultaneously (Girdano and Everly).

Home-based programming— Home visits and provision of some services in the living environment.

Hospice— Model of health care for people with advanced metastatic disease when there is no hope of cure and life expectancy is six months or less.

Hypertension— Persistently high blood pressure.

Hypertonicity— Abnormally increased tone or strength.

Hypertrophic— Increased volume of tissue such as in scar formation.

Hyperventilation— Excessively rapid and deep breathing.

Hypotension— Lowered blood pressure.

Hypotonic— See hypotonicity.

ICF— Intermediary care facility.

ICU— Intensive care unit.

IEP— Individualized education plan.

IFSP— Individualized Family Service Plan.

Incest— Sexual relationships between family members or very close relatives.

Incontinence— Lack of bowel and/or bladder control.

Indirect patient care activities— Tasks not involving actual treatment such as treatment set-up, scheduling, etc.

Individual vulnerability— Susceptibility of an individual to react to stressors based on personality characteristics and personal experience.

Individualized educational plan— Documentation of the services to be received and the goals of a child's program in a school setting.

Individualized family service plan— Documentation of the services to be received and the goals of a child's program, with strong emphasis on the collaboration of the family and the professional services.

Infarct/Infarction— Occlusion of the arterial supply or venous drainage as in the case of a thrombus or embolism.

Initiative— Ability for original conception and independent action.

Initial note— Form of documentation written after an initial assessment.

In-service education— Facility-based training sessions, seminars and classes.

Integration— Combining into an integral whole.

Interests— Activities that the individual finds pleasurable; those that maintain one's attention.

Intermediate-level practice— COTA or OTR who has one or more years of practice experience and is competent to carry out entry-level tasks.

Interphalangeal— Area between two contiguous phalanges.

IP— Interphalangeal.

Isometric— Muscle action occurring against resistance in a strong and motionless, pressing, contracting and flexing pattern

ITP— Individualized therapy plan.

IV— Intravenous.

IVDU— Intravenous drug user.

JCAHO— Joint Commission on Accreditation of Healthcare Organizations.

Job capacity evaluation— An assessment of the match between the individual's capabilities and the critical demands of a specific job.

Job description— A list of tasks one is expected to perform.

Job simulation— Replication of actual work tasks.

Job site visit— Observation of work in progress at the place of employment.

Joint preservation— Principles used to maintain joint function such as avoiding deforming postures and forces, maintaining range of motion and muscle strength, energy conservation, etc.

Justice— Treatment of everyone with integrity and honesty.

Kaposi's sarcoma— A malignant tumor that primarily involves the skin, although visceral lesions may also be present.

Kinesthesia— Ability to identify the sensation of movement, including its path and direction.

KS— Kaposi's sarcoma.

Laterality— Use of a preferred body part, such as the right or left hand, for activities requiring a high skill level.

Lazarus Project— Model of long-term care focusing on public policy and the politics of empowerment and based on a community model of democratic governance responsive to all member needs.

LD— Learning disability.

Leisure— Nonwork or free time spent in adult play activities that have an influence on the quality of life.

Lesion— Pathological or traumatic interruption in tissue or loss of function.

Liability— Legal responsibility.

License restrictions (driving)— Limitations imposed such as operating a vehicle during the daytime hours or only when wearing prescription glasses.

Licensure— A process by which an agency of the government grants permission to persons to engage in a given occupation once the minimum level of competency is attained to ensure protection of the public.

Life change— A different course in life such as marriage, new job, relocation, etc.

Locus— Place.

Long-term objective— Expected outcome of treatment.

Lordosis— Forward curvature of the lumbar spine.

Loss— Failure to keep or have such as the death of a loved one, being laid off a job, experiencing a broken engagement, etc.

LTGs— Long-term goals.

Lymphadenopathy— Condition characterized by enlarged lymph glands.

M-team— Multidisciplinary team.

Maladaptive— Behavior that is the result of one not having learned the skills and tasks required for role performance.

Malpractice— Any professional misconduct, unreasonable lack of skill or fidelity in performance of professional duties; immoral or illegal behavior.

Manifest behavior— Reaction of individuals that occurs in response to conflict.

Manual guidance— Providing physical assistance such as placing one's hands over another's to help guide the required movement.

Masceration— Softening of tissue.

Mastery— The desire to explore, understand, and to some extent, control oneself and an environment.

Maturation— Complete in natural growth or development; an "unfolding"; the opposite of vegetation.

MDS— Minimal data set.

Medication routine— Ability to obtain medication, operate containers and take medication at the required times.

Meningomyelocele— Condition in which the spinal cord fails to close and connect properly.

Mental retardation/mentally retarded— An overall slowness in development; significant subaverage general intellectual functioning and deficits in adaptive behavior.

Mental Status Questionnaire— A ten-item rating scale used to assess orientation and recent and remote memory.

Mentors— Wise and trusted counselors; those who provide guidance.

Metacarpophalangeal— Part of the hand between the wrist and the phalanges of the fingers.

Methyl methacrylate— Self-curing acrylic resin adherent used in surgical procedures such as hip arthroplasty.

Metida— Spanish folk term for "busy body" or nosy person.

Milieu— Social and physical environment; one's surroundings.

Ministration— The need to feel close to others and for support, guidance and protection.

MMT— Manual muscle test.

Mobility— Ability to physically move from one position or place to another.

Mobility toys— Vehicles used by children during play such as scooters, tricycles, skateboards and the like.

Monogamous— Marriage or exclusive commitment to one person.

Morale— Condition of a person or a group relative to cheerfulness, confidence and a positive attitude.

Moro reflex— Flexion of the thighs and knees; fanning and clenching of fingers, with arms thrust outward, then brought together as if embracing something.

Mosaic (society)— One with distinctive identities within.

MP— Metacarpophalangeal.

MRI— Magnetic resonance imaging.

MSQ— Mental status questionnaire.

Multidisciplinary team— A group comprised of several professionals.

Multisensory input— Treatment technique designed to elicit responses to various stimuli such as light, sounds, smells, etc.

Muscle tone— Degree of tension or resistance present in a muscle or muscle group.

Mycobacterium avium-intracellulare— An infectious disease involving lungs, skin and lymph nodes as well as other sites.

NA— Narcotics Anonymous.

NAAP— National Association of Activity Professionals.

Narcotics— Drugs that lessen or eliminate pain and cause sedation.

NDT— Neurodevelopmental treatment.

Negligence— Failure to perform a task that would have been carried out under normal circumstances; often caused by heedlessness and carelessness.

NIMH— National Institute of Mental Health.

NIOHS— National Institute of Occupational Health and Safety.

Noscomial— Diseases originating in hospitals.

Nystagmus— Involuntary, rapid, rhythmic movement of the eyeball.

Object manipulation— Skill in handling large and small objects such as keys, doorknobs and a calculator.

OBRA— Omnibus Budget Reconciliation Act of 1987.

Occupational behavior— Theoretical framework proposed by Reilly to guide therapeutic intervention; focuses on the individual's achievement, roles, play and work; influenced by abilities, interests, skills and habits.

Occupational capacity evaluation— Assessment of the match between the individual's capabilities and the critical demands of an occupational group.

Occupational performance (areas)— Participation in activities of daily living, work activities and play or leisure activities.

Occupational therapy aide— Individual who receives on-the-job training to perform routine tasks.

Olfactory— Receive, process and interpret odors.

Omnibus Budget Reconciliation Act— Law enacted in

1990 that included specific amendments for nursing home reform.

Opportunistic disease— One commonly found in the environment but governed by the immune response. Impairment of this response allows proliferation of infection within the body.

Oppositional behavior— Physical and verbal aggression.

Oral-motor control— Ability to exhibit controlled movements of the mouth, tongue and related structures.

Organization— Tendency of a person to develop a coherent system; to systematize.

Orientation— Degree to which one is able to correctly identify person, place, time and situation.

Orthosis— Device, such as a splint, used to prevent deformity and/or improve function.

Orthostatic hypotension— Rapid fall in blood pressure when assuming an upright position.

OTJR— *Occupational Therapy Journal of Research.*

Paralysis— Loss or impairment of motor function.

Paranoia— Mental disorder characterized by systematized delusions and projection of personal conflicts based on supposed hostility of others.

Paraplegic— Paralysis of the legs and in some instances the lower part of the body.

Parental priorities— Functional problems that are of concern to parents.

Patterns of response— Configurations or arrangements of answers or actions.

PCR— Polymerized chain reaction.

Peer interactions— Verbal and nonverbal interchanges with individuals of a similar age.

Pentamidine— Drug used to treat *Pneumocystis carinii* pneumonia.

Perceived conflict— That which is felt by a person that may or may not lead to actual conflict.

Perception— Information obtained as a result of interpretation of sensory information.

Performance— Actions produced through skill acquisition.

Performance areas— Activities of daily living, work and play or leisure.

Performance components— Elements of an activity such as sensory motor, cognitive and psychosocial.

Persistent generalized lymphadenopathy— Enlarged lymph glands; condition persists six months or longer.

Personal causation— Refers to the sense that one can effect change in the environment.

PGL— Persistent generalized lymphadenopathy.

Physiatrist— A physician who specializes in physical medicine.

PIP— Proximal interphalangeal.

Plan— Component of the problem-oriented medical record describing goals and frequency and length of treatment.

Plaque— Any patch or flat surface; often pertaining to the brain and nervous system (refers to demyelinating of nerve fibers in multiple sclerosis).

Play— An intrinsic activity that involves enjoyment and leads to fun; spontaneous, voluntary and engaged in by choice.

Play group— Therapy program where children engage in activities such as playing games according to rules, taking turns, being "good sports," etc.

Pneumocystis carinii pneumonia— A respiratory condition characterized by the development of ridgelike cysts and inflammation of the lungs.

PNF— Proprioceptive neuromuscular facilitation.

POMR— Problem-oriented medical record.

Position in space— The ability to determine the spacial relationship of objects and figures to self or to other objects and forms.

Posterolateral— In the rear and to one side.

Post-traumatic— Following injury produced by violence or other outside agent.

Postural balance— Maintaining equilibrium in different positions; see postural control.

Postural control— Ability to assume and maintain a position; proper alignment of body parts, orientation to midline, necessary shifting of weight and righting reactions are important elements for accomplishment.

Praxis— Ability to do motor planning and to perform purposeful movement in response to demands from the environment.

Prevention— Taking measures to keep something from happening.

PRN— Whenever necessary.

Problem solving— Process of studying a situation that presents uncertainty, doubt or difficulty and arriving at a solution through definition, identification of alternative plans, selection of a likely plan, organizing the necessary steps in the plan, implementing it and evaluating the results.

Professional socialization— Acquisition of skills and knowledge to do the work of an occupation; development and orientation of attitudes and behaviors needed for a specific role; identities and commitments that motivate one to pursue the occupation and feel accepted by its members.

Prognosis— Forecast of the probable course and outcome of a disease or condition.

Progress note— Documentation of the treatment plan and the patient's response.

PROM— Passive range of motion.

Prophylactic— An agent that tends to ward off disease.

Proprioception— Provides the individual with awareness of position, balance and equilibrium changes based on stimuli from muscles, joints and other tissues; gives information about the position of one body part in relation to that of another.

Prosthesis— Replacement part; artificial substitute.

Protective extension— Extension of the upper extremities in space during specific movement patterns that require anticipating precaution.

Protocol— Specific plan of action.

Prudence— Choosing the right means; using care and foresight.

Psychometric— Measurement of mental traits, abilities and processes.

Psychomotor— Refers to activity that combines both physical and psychic or cerebral elements.

Psychomotor retardation— Delays in motor responses to psychic or cerebral activity.

Public relations— Increased awareness via wide dessemination of information through methods such as newspaper articles, radio and television spots, etc.

PWA— Person with AIDS.

Quad pegs— Projections from the metal push rim on the wheels of a wheelchair.

Quadriplegia— Paralysis of all four limbs.

Quality of life— Concept that includes a combination of factors such as excellence of character, accomplishment, personal/social status and sense of personal well-being.

RA— Rheumatoid arthritis.

Range of motion— Movement of body parts through an arc.

RAPs— Resident assessment protocols.

Receptive aphasia— Difficulty in understanding explanations.

Reciprocity— Mutual giving and receiving or exchange.

Reevaluation— Process used to determine necessary program modifications or discontinuation and discharge planning.

Reflex— An involuntary muscle response due to stimulation.

Regimen— Regulated plan.

Registration— A process that requires an individual to file his or her name and address with a designated agency and is placed on an official roster.

Rehabilitation question— Objective of referral to a work hardening program.

Reimbursement— Repayment of costs.

Reinforcers— Preferences in food and activities that may be used to encourage and promote optimum performance.

Remission— Reduction or abatement of disease symptoms.

Resident care plan— A method used in extended care facilities to assess needs and problems systematically.

Resting tremor— Controlled shaking of the hand that occurs when a person is at rest and disappears when there is voluntary movement.

Retrolental fibroplasia— Bilateral condition causing blindness in infants; frequently caused by elevated oxygen levels.

Reverence— Respect for each person; recognizing the dignity of the human person.

Rheumatoid arthritis— A chronic systemic disease that produces inflammatory changes, which occur throughout the connective tissue and bones, resulting in progressive limitations and deformities.

Rheumatologist— Physician specializing in rheumatic diseases.

Right-left discrimination— Ability to discriminate one side of the body from the other.

Risk management— Involves dealing with issues of liability such as negligence and malpractice.

RLF— Retrolental fibroplasia.

Role dysfunction— Inability to carry out responsibilities.

Roles— Functions of the individual in society that may be assumed or acquired (homemaker, student, caregiver, etc.).

ROM— Range of motion.

Romberg's sign— Inability to maintain balance with one's eyes closed while holding arms out and feet placed together.

RPT— Registered physical therapist.

RUE— Right upper extremity.

Rule of Nines— Method used to determine the percentage of body surface area affected by burns.

Safety awareness— Knowledge of situations with potential for risk, injury or loss.

Schizophrenia— A group of mental disorders characterized by mental deterioration resulting in delusions, hallucinations, inappropriate affect and impairment in social and occupational roles.

SCI— Spinal cord injury.

Sclerosis— Hardening of tissue.

Screening— Process used to determine the need for intervention services.

Seclusion— Confinement or isolation.

Second-degree burn— Involves epidermis and part of dermis; skin is moist, red, and very painful with blisters; healing time approximately three weeks.

SED— Seriously emotionally disturbed.

Segmentation— Movement characterized by differentiating the head from the trunk.

Self-catheterization— Independent management of bladder drainage system.

Self-esteem— Respect for or a favorable impression of oneself.

Sensory integration— Ability to organize and process sensory input for use.

Sensory processing— Interpretation of sensory stimuli from sources such as visual, tactile, auditory and others; information is received, a motor response is made and sensory feedback is provided.

Sepsis— Presence of pathogenic microorganisms or their toxins in the blood or other tissues.

Sequelae— Abnormal conditions brought about by another event.

Service competence— Relates to performance and implies that two people can perform the same or equivalent procedures and obtain the same results.

Service operations— Process involving planing, organizing, managing and evaluating facilities and services.

Severely mentally retarded— Individuals who need help with most of their daily needs; some may never develop speech and may have severe handicaps such as those seen in cerebral palsy.

Sexually abused— One who has experienced forced sexual contact.

Shiva— Jewish ritual involving the gathering of family and friends after a death.

Short-term objectives— Contribute to the achievement of long-term goals; stated in achievable, measurable outcomes met within a short enough timespan to serve as record of improvement.

SNF— Skilled nursing care facility.

SOAP note— Subjective, objective, assessment and plan method of documentation.

Social conditions— Circumstances in society such as population, level of poverty, economic resources, etc.

Socialization— Ability to interact with others approriately with consideration to cultural and contextual factors.

Spasticity— Resistance to stretching by a muscle due to abnormally increased tension with heightened deep tendon reflexes.

Special accommodations— Individualized arrangements to accommodate a particular situation.

Specialty certification— Credential awarded to recognize occupational therapists who have specialized in an area of practice.

SSCE— Scoreable Self-Care Evaluation.

Standards— Requirements for measurement of compliance.

Sterognosis— Ability to use the sense of touch to identify objects.

STGs— Short-term goals.

Strength— Muscle power and degree of movement is demonstrated in the presence of gravity or resistive weight.

Subjective— Component of the problem-oriented medical record containing information that is not measurable such as what the patient said or what family members reported.

Subluxation— Partial dislocation of a joint.

Substance abuse— Continued use of alcohol, narcotics or marijuana for at least one month or more, despite recurring social, occupational or physical problems caused or exacerbated by substance use; does not meet criteria for substance dependence.

Substance dependence— Syndrome in which the person has impaired control over use of alcohol, narcotics or marijuana and continues use despite adverse consequences, which may be both behavioral and physiologic symptoms, including tolerance and withdrawal.

Substance-related disability— Impairment in social or occupational functioning due to a problem with use of chemical substances at least one month in duration.

Substantia nigra— Layer of gray substance separating the tegmentum of the midbrain from the the crus cerebri; located in the upper brain stem; area where dopamine is normally produced.

SUDS— Single use diagnostic system; test used to detect HIV antibodies.

Suicide— Taking one's own life.

Sustenance— Providing nourishment to a relationship.

Synergy— Correlated or cooperative action pattern.

Tachycardia— Abnormally rapid heartbeat.

Tactile— Use of skin contact and related receptors to receive, process and interpret touch, pressure, temperature, pain, vibration and two-point stimulation.

Takata's Play History— An assessment used to assist in measuring a child's play and family interactions in the home.

Tardive dyskinesia— A late-appearing impairment of voluntary motion.

Task analysis— See activity analysis.

Task skills group— Working with others on an assigned cooperative project to accomplish specific goals.

TBI— Traumatic brain injury.

TBSA— Total body surface area.

Teamwork— Smoothly coordinated and synchronized action achieved by a closely knit group.

TEFRA— Tax Equity and Fiscal Responsibility Act of 1982.

Teleologic— Refers to ethical theory and supports the position that if the end is good then the means are ethical; also known as the consequential approach.

Temperateness— Moderation; decency in behavior.

Tenodesis— Position of wrist extension and finger flexion.

THA— Total hip arthroplasty.

Thenar eminence— Fleshy part of the hand at the base of the thumb.

Third-degree burn— Both epidermis and dermis are destroyed; skin is dry and leather-like; may be black, yellow-brown or translucent; healing time varies.

Time management— Structuring the day to accommodate the demands made on one's time.

TMR— Trainable mentally retarded.

Topographic orientation— Ability to determine the route to a specified location; to identify the location of particular objects and settings.

Torque— Action or condition that produces rotation.

Toxoplasmosis— An infection similar to mononucleosis that may involve cerebral edema.

Trainable mentally retarded— Individual who is moderately mentally retarded and whose IQ is approximately 40 to 55.

Transactional process— Act of carrying on business, negotiations and other activities.

Transformation— Dynamic change.

Traumatic brain injury— Wound to the brain from an external source.

Tremors— Trembling movements.

Trends— General courses or tendencies.

Triage— Procedure used to determine priority of medical needs and proper place of medical treatment.

Trochanter— A process on the femur.

TQM— Total quality management.

UE— Upper extremity.

Unilateral neglect— To disregard or ignore one side of the body.

Values— Beliefs, feelings or ideas that are important, highly regarded and have value to the individual.

Venous stasis— A condition where blood flow in the vein is stopped or significantly reduced.

Vestibular— Receiving, processing and interpreting stimuli received by the inner ear relative to head position and movement.

Visual— Receive, process and interpret stimuli received by the eyes, such as acuity, color, figure ground and depth.

Vital signs— Pulse, respiration and temperature of the body.

VMI— Visual-motor integration.

Vocational exploration— Process of determining appropriate vocational pursuits through study of one's aptitudes, skills and interests.

Volition— A subsystem in the Model of Human Occupation that oversees the entire human system; symbolizes the need for exploration and mastery.

Volunteer— An unpaid worker who assists with various routine tasks.

WFOT— World Federation of Occupational Therapists.

WLNs— Within normal limits.

Work— Skill in socially productive activities, which include gainful employment, homemaking, child care-parenting and work preparation activities.

Work capacity evaluation— Assessment of the match between an individual's capabilities and the demands of the competitive environment.

Work conditioning— A biomechanical rehabilitation process that builds physical conditioning to a level similar to one's job demands.

Work hardening— A multidisciplinary therapeutic intervention program designed to return the injured worker to the competitive work force.

Work simplification— Reducing the number of steps required to complete tasks such as preparing one-course meals.

Workshop task group— Several choices of projects are offered for patient to work on independently; choices are geared toward success but allow for creativity and problem solving (Florey).

WPM— Words per minute.

Index